Second Edition

NEUROLOGICAL
SURGERY   *Volume 2*

A Comprehensive Reference
Guide to the
Diagnosis and Management of
Neurosurgical Problems

Edited by

JULIAN R. YOUMANS, M.D., Ph.D.

Professor, Department of Neurological Surgery,
School of Medicine, University of California
Davis, California

1982 **W. B. SAUNDERS COMPANY**
Philadelphia • London • Toronto • Mexico City • Sydney • Tokyo

W. B. Saunders Company: West Washington Square
Philadelphia, PA 19105

1 St. Anne's Road
Eastbourne, East Sussex BN 21 3UN, England

1 Goldthorne Avenue
Toronto, Ontario M8Z 5T9, Canada

Cedro 512
Mexico 4, D.F. Mexico

9 Waltham Street
Artarmon, N.S.W. 2064, Australia

Ichibancho, Central Bldg., 22-I
Chiyoda-ku, Tokyo 102, Japan

Library of Congress Cataloging in Publication Data

Youmans, Julian Ray, 1928–
  Neurological surgery.

  1. Nervous system—Surgery. I. Title.
[DNLM: 1. Neurosurgery. WL368 N4945]
RD593.Y68   1980   617'.48
ISBN 0-7216-9663-5 (v. 2)   80-21368

Volume 1 ISBN 0-7216-9662-7
Volume 2 ISBN 0-7216-9663-5
Volume 3 ISBN 0-7216-9664-3
Volume 4 ISBN 0-7216-9665-1
Volume 5 ISBN 0-7216-9666-X
Volume 6 ISBN 0-7216-9667-8
Six Volume Set ISBN 0-7216-9658-9

Neurological Surgery—Volume Two

Last digit is the print number: 9   8   7   6   5   4   3   2   1

Contributors

MAURICE S. ALBIN, M.D.

Ultrasound in Neurosurgery

Professor of Anesthesiology and Neurological Surgery, Department of Anesthesiology, University of Texas Health Science Center at San Antonio. Attending Anesthesiologist, Bexar County Hospital and Audie Murphy Veterans Administration Hospital, San Antonio, Texas.

JOHN F. ALKSNE, M.D.

Cerebral Death

Professor of Neurological Surgery, Chairman of the Division of Neurological Surgery, University of California at San Diego, School of Medicine. Attending Neurological Surgeon, University of California at San Diego Medical Center; Chairman of the Department of Neurological Surgery, Kaiser Medical Center, San Diego, California. Chairman of the Department of Neurological Surgery, Veterans Administration Medical Center, La Jolla, California.

LESLIE BERNSTEIN, M.D., D.D.S., M.B. B.Ch., D.L.O., F.A.C.S.

Neurotology

Professor of Otorhinolaryngology, Chairman of Department of Otorhinolaryngology, University of California, School of Medicine at Davis, Davis, California. Chief of Otorhinolaryngology, University of California Davis Medical Center at Sacramento, Sacramento, California.

ROGER CONLEY BONE, M.D.

Pulmonary Care and Complications

Associate Professor of Medicine, University of Arkansas School of Medicine. Chief of Pulmonary Medicine, University of Arkansas Medical Center; Consultant, Veterans Administration Hospital, Little Rock, Arkansas.

CHARLES E. BRACKETT, M.D., F.A.C.S.

Pulmonary Care and Complications, Arachnoid Cysts, Subarachnoid Hemorrhage, Post-Traumatic Arachnoid Cysts, Cordotomy

Professor of Neurological Surgery, Chairman of Department of Neurological Surgery, University of Kansas Medical Center, College of Health Sciences and Hospital. Chief of Neurological Surgery Service, University of Kansas Medical Center; Attending Staff, Kansas City Veterans Administration Hospital, Kansas City, Missouri.

SHELLEY N. CHOU, M.D., Ph.D., F.A.C.S.

Urological Problems; Scoliosis, Kyphosis, and Lordosis; Tumors of Skull

Professor of Neurological Surgery, Head of Department of Neurological Surgery, University of Minnesota Medical School. Chief of Neurological Surgery Service, University of Minnesota Hospitals; Consultant, Minneapolis Veterans Administration Hospital, Minneapolis, Minnesota.

GERALD A. GRONERT, M.D.

Neuroanesthesia

Professor of Anesthesiology, Mayo Medical School. Consultant, Anesthesiology, Mayo Clinic; Attending Staff, St. Marys Hospital, Rochester, Minnesota.

LAWRENCE C. HARTLAGE, Ph.D., F.A.P.A., F.A.A.M.D., F.A.O.A.

Psychological Testing

Professor of Neurology and Pediatrics, Medical College of Georgia, Neuropsychologist, Talmadge Memorial Hospital; Consultant, University Hospital and Veterans Administration Hospitals, Augusta, Georgia, and Eisenhower Army Medical Center, Fort Gordon, Georgia.

PATRICIA L. HARTLAGE, M.D.

Psychological Testing

Associate Professor of Neurology and Pediatrics, Medical College of Georgia. Attending Staff, Talmadge Memorial Hospital; Consulting Staff, University Hospital and Gracewood State School and Hospital, Augusta, Georgia.

SADEK K. HILAL, M.D., Ph.D

Interventional Neuroradiology, Tumors of Orbit

Professor of Radiology, Columbia University College of Physicians and Surgeons. Attending Radiologist, Presbyterian Hospital; Director of Neuroradiology, Neuroradiological Institute of New York, New York, New York.

ROBERT EDGAR HODGES, M.D.

Nutrition and Parenteral Therapy

Professor of Internal Medicine, University of Nebraska College of Medicine. Chief of Clinical Nutrition Section, University of Nebraska Medical Center, Omaha, Nebraska.

THOMAS McNEESE KELLER, M.D.

Cerebral Death

Attending Neurological Surgeon, Santa Rosa Memorial Hospital, Community Hospital, and Warrack Hospital, Santa Rosa, California.

DAVID J. KIENER, M.D.

Neurotology

Assistant Professor of Otolaryngology, University of California, School of Medicine at Davis, Davis, California. Attending Staff, University of California Davis Medical Center at Sacramento, Sacramento, California.

THOMAS WILLIAM LANGFITT, M.D., F.A.C.S.

Increased Intracranial Pressure

Charles Harrison Frazier Professor of Neurosurgery, Director of Division of Neurological Surgery, University of Pennsylvania School of Medicine. Vice President for Health Affairs, University of Pennsylvania, Philadelphia, Pennsylvania.

JOSEPH C. MAROON, M.D., F.A.C.S.

Ultrasound in Neurosurgery

Professor of Neurological Surgery, University of Pittsburgh School of Medicine. Attending Neurological Surgeon, Presbyterian–University Hospital, Pittsburgh, Pennsylvania.

J. A. McCRARY, III, M.D.

Neurophthalmology

Associate Professor of Ophthalmology and Neurological Surgery, Baylor College of Medicine. Attending Staff, Methodist Hospital and St. Luke's Episcopal Hospital; Consultant, Houston Veterans Administration Hospital and Ben Taub Hospital, Houston, Texas.

CAROL A. McMURTRY, M.A.

Neurotology

Clinical Instructor of Audiology, Department of Otorhinolaryngology, University of California, School of Medicine at Davis, Davis, California. Senior Audiologist, University of California Davis Medical Center at Sacramento, Sacramento, California.

W. JOST MICHELSEN, M.D., F.A.C.S.

Interventional Neuroradiology

Associate Professor of Neurological Surgery, Columbia University College of Physicians and Surgeons. Associate Attending Neurological Surgeon, Columbia–Presbyterian Hospital, New.York, New York.

JOHN D. MICHENFELDER, M.D.

Neuroanesthesia

Professor of Anesthesiology, Mayo Medical School. Consultant Neuroanesthesiologist, Mayo Clinic; Attending Neuroanesthesiologist, St. Marys Hospital and Rochester Methodist Hospital, Rochester, Minnesota.

CARL-HENRIK NORDSTRÖM, M.D., Ph.D.

Cerebral Metabolism

Teaching Staff, Department of Neurological Surgery, University Hospital, Lund, Sweden.

GUY L. ODOM, M.D., F.A.C.S.

General Operative Technique

James B. Duke Professor of Neurological Surgery, Duke University School of Medicine. Attending Neurological Surgeon, Duke University Hospital, Durham, North Carolina.

RAYMOND V. RANDALL, M.D., F.A.C.P.

Neuroendocrinology, Empty Sella Syndrome

Professor of Medicine, Mayo Medical School. Senior Consultant, Mayo Clinic; Consultant Physician, St. Marys Hospital and Rochester Methodist Hospital, Rochester, Minnesota.

KAI REHDER, M.D.

Neuroanesthesia

Professor of Anesthesiology and Physiology, Department of Anesthesiology and Department of Physiology and Biophysics, Mayo Medical School. Anesthesiologist, Department of Anesthesiology, Mayo Clinic; Attending Anesthesiologist, St. Marys Hospital and Rochester Methodist Hospital, Rochester, Minnesota.

MICHAEL H. REID, Ph.D., M.D.

Ultrasound in Neurosurgery

Associate Professor of Radiology, University of California, School of Medicine at Davis, Davis, California. Chief, Section of Computerized Tomography; Chief, Section of Mammography; Staff Radiologist, University of California Davis Medical Center at Sacramento, Sacramento, California.

ALBERT L. RHOTON, JR., M.D., R.D., F.A.C.S.

Micro-Operative Technique, Intracavernous Carotid Aneurysms and Fistulae

Keene Family Professor of Neurological Surgery, University of Florida College of Medicine. Chairman of Department of Neurological Surgery, University of Florida Teaching Hospitals and Clinics; Consultant, Veterans Administration Hospital, Gainesville, Florida.

GAYLAN L. ROCKSWOLD, M.D., Ph.D.

Urological Problems

Associate Professor of Neurological Surgery, University of Minnesota Medical School. Chief of Neurological Surgery, Hennepin County Medical Center, Minneapolis, Minnesota.

BO U. SIESJÖ, M.D., Ph.D.

Cerebral Metabolism

Professor, Medical Research Council Cerebral Metabolism Group, Research Department of University Hospital, University of Lund, Lund, Sweden.

W. EUGENE STERN, M.D., F.A.C.S.

Preoperative Evaluation, Prevention and Treatment of Complications; Bacterial Infections

Professor of Surgery/Neurological Surgery, University of California, School of Medicine at Los Angeles, Los Angeles, California. Chief of Neurological Surgery, University of California Los Angeles Center for Health Sciences; Neurological Surgeon Consultant, Wadsworth Veterans Administration Hospital, Harbor General Hospital, St. John's Hospital, Los Angeles, California, and Santa Monica Hospital, Santa Monica, California.

ROBERT H. WILKINS, M.D., F.A.C.S.

General Operative Technique

Professor of Neurosurgery, Duke University Medical Center. Chief of Division of Neurological Surgery, Duke University Medical Center, Durham, North Carolina.

EARL F. WOLFMAN, JR., M.D., F.A.C.S.

Nutrition and Parenteral Therapy

Professor of Surgery, University of California, School of Medicine at Davis, Davis, California. Attending Surgeon, University of California Davis Medical Center at Sacramento, Sacramento, California; Consultant in Surgery, David Grant Medical Center, United States Air Force, Travis, California; Martinez Veterans Administration Hospital, Martinez, California.

JULIAN R. YOUMANS, M.D., Ph.D., F.A.C.S.

Diagnostic Biopsy, Cerebral Death, Cerebral Blood Flow, Trauma to Carotid Arteries, Glial and Neuronal Tumors, Lymphomas, Sarcomas and Vascular Tumors, Tumors of Disordered Embryogenesis, Peripheral and Sympathetic Nerve Tumors, Parasitic and Fungal Infections.

Professor of Neurological Surgery, University of California, School of Medicine at Davis, Davis, California. Attending Neurological Surgeon, University of California Davis Medical Center at Sacramento, Sacramento, California; Consultant in Neurological Surgery, United States Air Force Medical Center, Travis Air Force Base, California; Veterans Administration Hospital, Martinez, California.

Contents

III

SPECIAL TESTS
AND EVALUATION

NEUROPHTHALMOLOGY

The eye and the structures associated with it are supplied by one half of the cranial nerves. Any careful evaluation of a neurosurgical patient should, therefore, include investigation for the ocular signs of neural damage. Although the ophthalmologist is best prepared to evaluate the eyes, a good examination can be made by anyone willing to spend a few additional minutes. The items needed for the examination are shown in Figure 17–1. With practice in the use of these instruments and in the interpretation of the findings, there are few major diagnostic eye signs that the neurosurgeon could overlook.

No matter how carefully the examination is performed, it is worth little if a detailed history is not included. Although physicians are trained as medical students to take good quality histories, the press of a busy practice may tend to interfere with detailed history-taking. It bears repeating that difficult diagnostic problems are more often solved by additional history than by further laboratory tests. The astute clinician distinguishes himself from the average clinician by taking a better than average history.

HISTORY

The neurosurgical patient is often incapable of giving a concise detailed account of the events that led to his present state of affairs. He may be dysphasic from a dominant hemisphere lesion or obtunded following seizures or a rise in intracranial pressure. One may have to rely on members of the family, friends, or total strangers for some historical clues to the nature of the patient's disorder. This is particularly true in children. One must rely on the parents for information about the patient's growth, development, behavior, and habits. Specific questions should be asked concerning difficulties during the pregnancy, labor, or delivery. The history of skin rash and low-grade fever during the first trimester of the pregnancy may explain retardation, nystagmus, and peculiar retinal pigmentation in an infant as being due to maternal rubella.

Old photographs are an important part of any history. They are especially helpful in those patients who have recently noticed the drooping of one upper eyelid, a small difference in pupil size, or the sudden onset of diplopia. A good look at several old photographs under bright light with a magnifier may save the patient needless hospitalization for evaluation of a congenital ptosis, or anisocoria (unequal pupil size), or an old strabismus. A modest head tilt in an old photograph may be all that is needed to explain the onset of vertical diplopia.

It is not sufficient merely to obtain the history of diplopia. It is equally important to know if it was of sudden onset (vascular) or slow (increased intracranial pressure), transient (myasthenia gravis), or progressive (neoplastic). If it is horizontal and worse at distance, a sixth nerve paresis or internuclear ophthalmoplegia is suggested. If the diplopia is vertical, it is usually worse when looking into the distance with disorders of the vertical rectus muscles and worse at near with disorders of the oblique muscles. It is also helpful to know if the diplopia increases when the patient looks to the right or left, up or down.

The symptomatic correlate of acquired nystagmus is oscillopsia, or the apparent to-and-fro movement of the environment. The patient with vertical oscillopsia may

J. A. McCRARY III

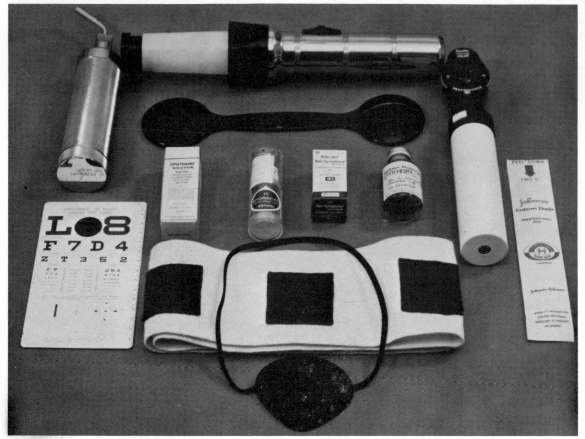

Figure 17–1 Examination materials. *Left to right, top row:* hand light, projector light, Maddox rod-occluder, and direct ophthalmoscope. *Middle row:* ophthalmic solutions. *Bottom row:* near card, opticokinetic tape, occluder patch, and cotton-tipped applicators.

describe it as though the vertical hold of a television picture were out of adjustment. Oscillopsia does not occur in congenital nystagmus.

Transient loss of vision may occur in one or both eyes. Transient obscurations of vision are unilateral or bilateral and generally last 5 to 15 seconds. They are associated with chronic papilledema and are described as brief "gray-outs" or "brown-outs" or occasionally as complete loss of vision in both eyes. There may be hundreds of such episodes per day, but *they always last seconds, not minutes.* Transient ischemic attacks (TIA's) may be unilateral (carotid artery disease) or bilateral (basilar artery disease) and consist of sudden loss of vision, often preceded and followed by a "curtain" or "shade" moving across the visual field. If the carotid circulation is involved, the attacks occur in one visual field (eye), and the "shade" may approach either horizontally

or vertically, almost always the latter. If the basilar arterial circulation is involved, the attack occurs in both visual fields. Often the lower half is involved more than the upper half, and in both types the attacks last 5 to 15 minutes. Occasional episodes may last up to 20 minutes. If an attack lasts over 20 minutes, there is usually some permanent impairment of visual field function. The major exception is the hemianopia associated with migraine.

Migraine is the most common cause for transient homonymous hemianopia; an attack may affect the visual field for more than 20 minutes without permanent damage. These hemianopias may occur without headache, nausea, emesis, scintillating scotomas, or any of the other usual stigmata of migraine (migraine equivalent). Migraine may affect the vascular supply of a single eye, rather than of the hemisphere, in which case a unilateral visual field disturb-

TABLE 17–1   DISEASES OF THE CENTRAL NERVOUS SYSTEM WITH PHOTOPHOBIA AS A RELATED COMPLAINT

Migraine
Subarachnoid hemorrhage
Aura preceding seizure or in the postictal state
Mass lesion
Arachnoiditis (viral, bacterial, chemical)
Postconcussion state
Encephalitis
Acromegaly
Trigeminal neuralgia

ance is found. Migraine is worsened by the use of oral contraceptives in young women. In menopausal women, estrogens can reactivate migraine. Many of the patients who develop vascular complications while using contraceptive medications have a previous history of migraine.

Photophobia is not uncommon in the history of neurosurgical patients. The causes for discomfort or headache brought on by exposure to light of even moderate intensity are many. Photophobia is most often related to primary ocular disease, such as glaucoma or uveitis, but it may be found in diseases of the central nervous system (Table 17–1).

Less than 5 per cent of all headache is due to disorders of the eye primarily. Certainly errors of refraction, ocular muscle imbalance, and glaucoma can cause discomfort about the eyes (asthenopia) or headache. Headache so related is usually noted later in the day, with increased use of the eyes, and is often frontal. The simple question regarding the relationship of headache to increased use of the eyes may help in deciding whether there may be an ocular cause for the headache.

Three common causes for frequent changes in glasses prescription are: glaucoma, cataract, and diabetes mellitus. Any patient who complains of variation in visual acuity from day to day or hour to hour should have a formal three-hour glucose tolerance test. Intraocular pressure should be measured.

The past history and family history must also be carefully reviewed. The patient presenting a history of blepharospasm may also have a history of previous encephalitis several years before. One would thus be attuned to a possible diagnosis of postencephalitic Parkinson's disease with blepharospasm as one of its features. A careful review of the patient's medications should always be included. It is wise not to ask what drugs the patient is taking, but instead to ask what medications are used. Some patients equate drugs with narcotics, to the exclusion of all other medications. The family history should include specific details concerning the ages of the patient's parents, and the cause of their death, if they are deceased. Also, it is helpful to know how many siblings were produced, how many are living, their medical histories (if pertinent), how many are deceased, and the exact causes of death. Other details of the medical and ocular history in close relatives may be important.

VISUAL ACUITY DETERMINATION

Accurate determination of the visual acuity is the foundation upon which the entire eye examination rests. Only the best vision for each eye should be recorded. Ideally, the eye that is not being tested should be completely occluded. Some type of patch is required for children. A black occluder with an elastic band works well and is inexpensive. When testing vision in a patient with glasses, a cleansing tissue may be placed between the lens and the closed eyelid. The best test of visual acuity consists in measurement at distance and near, if a distance (20-foot) Snellen chart is available. This should include the vision with and without glasses. The addition of a pinhole before the tested eye with poor vision will generally increase its visual acuity if the cause for decreased vision is refractive. It will reduce the acuity if the decrease in vision is due to opacities of the media (cornea, lens, vitreous) or a central scotoma. The patient should be encouraged to demonstrate the best possible acuity. Many times better visual acuity can be recorded if the examiner allows sufficient time for the patient to find the best head position and encourages an occasional guess.

If facilities do not allow the distance vision to be tested, the near card (reduced Snellen) should be used. The ideal near card should have letters, numbers, and sentences. A dysphasic patient may be capable of identifying numbers but not letters, letters but not numbers, or both letters and numbers when shown in an isolated manner, but be unable to read them accurately as used in sentences. The patient should be asked to move the card into the best reading position. An alert observer can detect a visual field defect by watching the position of the near card. A card held slightly off center often means that a central scotoma is present. The card held in the nasal field of each eye suggests chiasmal disease with a bitemporal hemianopia. Similarly, other positions may be the clues to a homonymous hemianopia or an altitudinal visual field loss. In patients over the age of 50, the acuity at near will be reduced simply because of the effects of presbyopia. The patient will tend to hold the card at an excessively long reading distance. The near vision should be tested with the patient's glasses in place. Presbyopia is the most common cause of visual complaints concerning near visual tasks in patients over the age of 40. Repeat testing of vision should be done in light similar to that used for the initial test. A near card held far from one eye and near to the other may imply: (1) anisometropia (unequal refractive error between the two eyes), (2) accommodative weakness in one eye—the card would be held further away than usual—suggesting impairment of cranial nerve III, or (3) increased depth of accommodation—common with Horner's syndrome—in which the card would be held closer than usual.

It may not be possible to test vision with the near card in some patients, especially if they are dysphasic, and one may have to rely on finger counting techniques in order to assess vision. The extended fingers are about the equivalent of the letters or numbers on the Snellen distance chart that should be visible to the normal eye at 200 feet. In the ophthalmologist's office, the patient who can just see these letters at 20 feet is given a vision of 20/200. A patient who must walk to within 5 feet of the letters before recognizing them is given a vision of 5/200. Using his fingers alone, the examiner can obtain a good estimate of the patient's vision by having him count the number of fingers presented at increasing distances from the bedside until the patient no longer responds correctly. In the dysphasic patient, one may have to communicate with sign language until he understands that he should hold up the same number of fingers as the examiner for a correct response. This can be time-consuming but really worth the effort; however, even this may be impossible, and the examiner may have to be content with a very gross estimate of visual acuity made by evaluating the patient's response to moving targets, such as a pen or hand light, his response to opticokinetic targets, or finally the pupillary response to light.

A special problem is encountered in testing the vision in children. The average visual acuity of children with increasing age is as follows:

Birth	10/400 (or 5/200)
1 year	20/200
2 years	20/40
3 years	20/30
4 years	20/25
5 years	20/20

It is possible to determine whether or not vision is present *even in the newborn infant* with the use of opticokinetic targets and pupillary responses to light. One should be able to elicit some ocular movement by using an opticokinetic tape. The child must be fully awake and not crying. The opticokinetic tape will produce responses in patients who have 5/200 or better visual acuity. A normal child will be able to fix and follow a hand light or another rather large target by the age of 3 months. Formal testing of visual acuity is not usually possible before the age of 3 years. The child must be learning some verbal skills. Sometime between the ages of 3 and 4 years, most children are capable of learning to play the "E game." They are asked to point one finger in the direction of the "legs" on the E. This can be taught at home by the parents, using a letter E cut from a piece of cardboard. When the parents have not been successful in teaching a child of 5 or 6 years to play the game, three possible causes of their failure are mental retardation, a parietal lobe lesion, and poor vision. After the age of 9 years, most children will be able to respond accurately to the adult vision test. In very young children, it is often best to test them with both eyes open initially, and later to test each eye individually.

EXTERNAL EXAMINATION

General inspection is important in the external examination. The subtle flattening of the nasolabial fold on one side of the face may be the clue to a central facial paralysis. Acne rosacea of the facial skin may point to chronic alcoholism as the cause for tremor and ataxia. It may also explain a sudden loss of vision from nutritional amblyopia. Careful attention to the color, quality, and texture of the skin is of great importance.

The eyelids should next be considered. The width of the lid fissures (maximum diameter between the edges of the upper and lower lids) should be measured or estimated. The average width of the lid fissure is 11 mm in the adult. A range of 8 to 12 mm is certainly within the limits of normal. The upper lid margin usually lies at or just about 1 mm below the upper limbus (junction of the cornea and sclera). In small children, especially under the age of 2 years, the upper lid usually rests at the upper limbus. The lower lid margin is usually at the limbus in children and adults. Knowing these simple landmarks, one can estimate very accurately whether the fissures are abnormally wide or narrow.

The fissures may be abnormally wide owing to extreme concentration, fear, sympathomimetic drugs, thyroid eye disease, or the pathological lid retraction seen with lesions of the posterior commisure (Collier's sign). Thyroid eye disease with its lid retraction and lid lag is usually easy to diagnose. Collier's sign is one of the very important external ocular findings in mesencephalic disease. Whereas the lid retraction of thyroid disease is often bilateral but asymmetrical, the lid retraction in Collier's sign is generally quite symmetrical unless there is a superimposed Horner's syndrome or

involvement of the nucleus of the third cranial nerve that is causing ptosis. Another common cause of unilateral widening of the lid fissure is a peripheral palsy of nerve VII. Supranuclear damage to the facial nerve complex causes paralysis of the lower side of the face, sparing the upper face, contralateral to the lesion. The lids are little involved except for some slight weakness of closure. The eyelids are little affected compared to the peripheral seventh nerve palsy because of the bilateral representation of the upper face in the supranuclear pathways. A handy clinical guide to the level of a lesion in the stem is: (1) a lesion above the nucleus of nerve VII causes a contralateral paralysis of the *central* face, arm, and leg; (2) the lesion at the level of the nucleus of nerve VII causes an *ipsilateral peripheral* facial palsy and *contralateral* hemiparesis; and (3) with one below the nucleus a contralateral hemiparesis occurs that spares the face. The lid fissure is widened not only by the weakness of closure of the upper lid and unopposed force of the levator, but also from the slight sagging downward of the lower lid (lagophthalmos). Because exposure of the cornea to drying and foreign bodies invites corneal ulcer formation, the eye should be kept moist with artificial tear solutions (Liquifilm, Isoptotears) or ointments (Lacri-lube). If it is not desirable to use these measures, the eyelids may be closed with tape or a minor surgical procedure, the lateral tarsorrhaphy (Fig. 17–2). Either of these protects the cornea. The tarsorrhaphy can be released at any time.

Narrowing of the lid fissure (ptosis) may

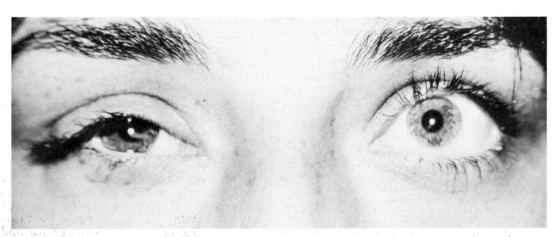

Figure 17–2 Right lateral tarsorrhaphy for exposure keratitis from facial palsy in postoperative angle tumor case.

occur in the following circumstances: (1) fatigue, (2) loss of sympathetic innervation of the smooth muscle of the upper lid (Müller's muscle), (3) lesions of the third cranial nerve (levator), (4) neuromyopathic diseases such as myasthenia gravis, (5) direct myopathic disease (chronic progressive external ophthalmoplegia), and (6) pseudoptosis due to inflammatory or infiltrative lesions of the upper lid that increase its weight and produce an apparent ptosis. Congenital ptosis may be separated from acquired ptosis by the history, old photographs, and its stability (acquired forms are often variable).

The most profound ptosis occurs with lesions of the oculomotor nerve. More common, but less impressive, is the ptosis seen with lesions of the sympathetic system. The amount of ptosis is often small (0.5 mm). It is variable, depending on the degree of alertness of the patient, the level of the lesion, and the length of time it has been present. The signs of oculosympathetic paralysis are listed in Table 17–2. Other less frequent eyelid signs of neurological disease are myokymia, myoclonic lid movements, lid nystagmus, lid fatigue in myasthenia gravis, fasciculations, blepharospasm, and apraxia of lid opening.

Exophthalmos is best discussed by classification according to the age of the patient, the presence or absence of pulsation of the globe, and the presence or absence of a bruit. The most common cause of pulsating exophthalmos without a bruit in childhood is neruofibromatosis with a defect in the orbital roof. In adults, the most common cause for pulsating exophthalmos without a bruit is a defect in the orbital roof (traumatic) and the most common cause with a bruit is the carotid-cavernous fistula. The most common cause of nonpulsatile exophthalmos in children under the age of 2 years is metastatic adrenal neuroblastoma;

TABLE 17–2 CLINICAL SIGNS OF OCULOSYMPATHETIC PARESIS

Ptosis—may be minimal
Miosis—may be minimal
Enophthalmos—more relative than real
Anhydrosis—variable, depends on level
Increased depth of accommodation
Transient increase facial skin temperature
Ocular hypotony
Heterochromia iridis—if damage occurs before age 2 years.

over the age of 2 the common causes are orbital hemangioma, lymphoma, dermoid, and glioma of the optic nerve.

Optic nerve glioma should be suspected when the eye is displaced down and outward, the optic nerve is undergoing progressive atrophy, and the optic foramen is enlarged on x-ray. A CT scan is usually diagnostic in such cases, although a pneumoencephalogram may be needed to assess chiasmal extension. These tumors occur most often in the first decade of life. They grow slowly and cause enlargement of the optic foramen by pressure from the expanding nerve substance and the proliferation of the overlying meningeal coverings. Gliomas should be suspected in children with evidence of neurofibromatosis who develop proptosis. Approximately 20 per cent of these gliomas are associated with café-au-lait spots or other signs of neruofibromatosis.

Rhabdomyosarcoma is the most common primary malignant tumor of the orbit in children. It is also the third most common tumor in children. Only leukemia and neuroblastoma precede it in frequency. This tumor presents as a rapidly enlarging mass in the orbit, often palpable through the lid, and usually located in the upper nasal quadrant of the orbit. It may cause papilledema or optic atrophy. Previously, radical surgical excision was the only treatment, but irradiation and chemotherapy have shown increased promise in the management of this highly malignant neoplasm.

In adults, exophthalmos is usually due to thyroid eye disease (Fig. 17–3). With proptosis the eye may be markedly injected or may appear completely normal in every respect. It is common to have bilateral protrusion of the globes, but this may be quite asymmetrical. The patient may be hyperthyroid, euthyroid, or hypothyroid by laboratory studies. Proptosis associated with a history of previous treatment with thyroid preparations, swelling of the upper eyelids, difficulty with vertical gaze, vertical diplopia, congestion of the conjunctiva, and retraction of the upper lids is thyroid eye disease, regardless of the laboratory results. *Thyroid eye disease is a clinical diagnosis.* It often advances more rapidly after treatment with radioactive iodine or subtotal thyroidectomy. The major complications are drying of the eye from exposure and corneal ulcer formation. A helpful aid to

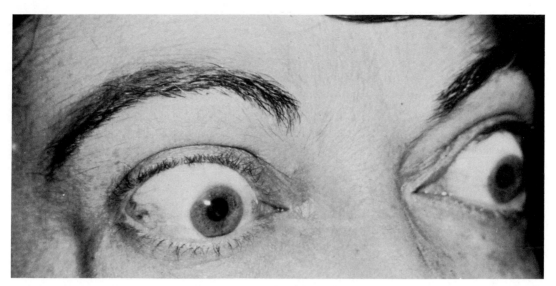

Figure 17-3   Thyroid eye disease.

diagnosis is the Werner thyroid suppression test. This is performed by determining the baseline radioactive iodine (RAI) uptake, following which the patient takes T_3 (Cytomel, 25-μg tablets) three times per day for 7 to 10 days, and the RAI uptake is retested. In the normal person, the uptake is depressed, but in the thyrotoxic patient it is not. This test will be positive in approximately 50 per cent of persons with thyroid eye disease.

Other causes of nonpulsating exophthalmos in adults are lymphoma, hemangioma, pseudotumor of the orbit, metastatic tumor from the breast or lung, lacrimal gland tumor, and meningioma arising either de novo in the orbit or as an orbital extension of a sphenoid wing meningioma. Lymphoma, hemangioma, pseudotumor, and meningioma are the most frequent causes of proptosis in adults with the exception of thyroid eye disease.

The presence of exophthalmos is best determined with the Krahn exophthalmometer. Serial measurements are the best method for following the progress of a patient under treatment for exophthalmos. Over 2 mm difference in the measurements between the two eyes is suggestive of proptosis; over 3 mm is pathological. It should be noted that the range of normal ocular protrusion is 12 to 21 mm with a mean of 16 mm.

Every medical student knows that the three common causes for a "red" eye are glaucoma, infection, and uveitis. The neurosurgeon should know that a red eye may be the clue to unilateral carotid insufficiency, Sturge-Weber syndrome, ataxia-telangectasia, Wyburn-Mason syndrome, sickle cell anemia, beginning carotid-cavernous fistula, or polycythemia vera. The presence of isolated or diffusely injected sclera (scleritis) is common in severe collagen disease, as is the conjunctival injection and furrow ulcer formation at the limbus in the diffuse arteritis of collagen disease. This may be of value diagnostically in certain patients with a history of seizures, syncopal episodes, transient ischemic attacks, or multisystem complaints and nervous system signs.

THE PUPIL

The pupil has three major functions: to control the volume of light entering the eye, to increase the depth of focus (as it contracts), and to decrease spherical and chromatic aberration. The normal pupillary diameter varies between 2 and 6 mm with an average diameter of 3.5 mm. The pupils tend to be small and resistant to dilation in infants and the elderly, large and easy to dilate in the teens and early adult life. In 17 per cent of normal persons there is a slight but perceptible anisocoria (unequal pupil size), and in 4 per cent the difference is pronounced (over 1 mm).

Anatomy of the Pupillary Pathways

Afferent Pathway

This begins in the retina at the rod and cone layer, and fibers concerned with the pupillary function proceed to the optic nerve. The fibers are scattered in a random distribution throughout the substance of the optic nerve. Whether the afferent pupillomotor fibers are the small or large fibers seen on careful histological analysis of the optic nerve is still open to debate.

After crossing in the chiasm, in equal proportions, the afferent fibers then enter the optic tract, the brachium of the superior colliculus (but not the colliculus proper), and the pretectum. From the pretectum, an equal number of fibers pass to the right and left sides of the commissure (partial decussation). They then proceed around the aqueduct in the periaqueductal gray matter until they enter the Edinger-Westphal nucleus. At this point another synapse occurs. *This is the beginning of the efferent limb of the pupillary reflex arc.*

Efferent Pathway

After synapsis, the parasympathetic fibers pass ventrally with the fibers of cranial nerve III through the substance of the midbrain. The pupillary fibers occupy the superior aspect of the nerve as it passes through the middle cranial fossa. They are in close relation to the tentorial margin and the hippocampal gyrus. The nerve then passes through the cavernous sinus and then to the superior orbital fissure. It divides into an upper and lower division. The upper division supplies innervation to the levator of the upper lid and the superior rectus muscle. The lower division supplies the medial rectus, inferior rectus, and inferior oblique muscles and the intrinsic muscles of the eye. Those fibers in the lower division that subserve the pupil and accommodation leave the inferior division at the lateral border of the inferior rectus. They then turn upward to enter the ciliary ganglion via the motor root. At this juncture, another synapse occurs, and finally the postganglionic fibers pass from the ciliary ganglion to the globe by the short ciliary nerves. They enter the posterior aspect of the globe and pass into the suprachoroidal space. They then proceed to the musculature of the pupil and the ciliary body. These pupillary fibers are parasympathetic and are the most important factor determining the size of the pupil. They affect the sphincter of the pupil and secrete acetylcholine at the myoneural junction.

Sympathetic Influence on the Pupil

The fibers of the sympathetic pupillary pathway arise in the hypothalamus and pass downward in the substance of the midbrain tegmentum. Gradually, they assume a more lateral position. In the pons, they lie in the reticular substance, and in the cervical cord, in the superficial layers of the cord just under the dentate ligaments. From C7 to T2, three cord segments, the first neuron sympathetic fibers synapse with the second neuron fibers at the ciliospinal center of Budge. The second neuron fibers pass out of the cord through the white rami to form the cervical sympathetic chain.

The pupillary fibers pass through the inferior and middle cervical sympathetic ganglia without synapsing. These fibers synapse only at the superior cervical ganglion. The fibers leaving this synaptic junction (third neuron) are the final pathway for sympathetic influence on the pupil. They pass upward wrapped about the sheath of the internal carotid artery, enter the cavernous sinus, then join with the first division of the fifth nerve to enter the orbit through the superior orbital fissure. The sympathetic fibers are then concentrated in the nasociliary division of nerve V. They enter the globe in the two long ciliary nerves and pass forward through the suprachoroidal space to form a plexus at the ciliary body. Finally, fibers from the ciliary plexus proceed to the dilator muscle of the iris. Norepinephrine is secreted at the myoneural junction.

Other intracranial fibers of sympathetic origin form the cavernous sympathetic plexus. Before it is formed, however, some of the fibers loop posteriorly over the petrous portion of the temporal bone and then course anteriorly. These enter the orbit with the two divisions of the oculomotor nerve to supply the Müller's muscle of the upper and lower lids. Those fibers of the sympathetic plexus that follow the course of the external carotid artery supply the innervation for facial sweating.

Reactions and Reflexes in Normal Pupils

Direct Light Reflex

In the normal person, the direct reaction of the pupil to light is at least as good as, and usually better than, the reaction to a *near* stimulus. If the direct light reflex of the pupil is poorer than the contraction to near, the term "light-near dissociation of the pupil" is used. When testing the direct light reflex, the patient's gaze must be fixed on a distant object and a bright light must be used. The most common cause for a misdiagnosis of light-near dissociation is a weak light source. The Welch-Allyn battery powered handle with the Finhoff transilluminator is the best light source for this purpose. The direct light reflex is graded from 1+ to 4+. If the response is less than 1+, it is recorded as *nil* or 0.

Consensual Reflex

In the normal person, when a strong light is placed before one eye, the pupil of the opposite eye responds by contracting as promptly and as forcefully as the pupil of the stimulated eye.

Near Pupillary Reflex

When the normal person makes an effort to focus the eye on an object near the face, the pupils promptly become miotic. By using the patient's finger as the object, this reflex can be tested even in a person who is totally blind. This may be of importance in separating blindness of ocular origin from that of cerebral origin. In a patient with bilateral acute compression of the anterior visual pathways, e.g., hemorrhage into a pituitary neoplasm, the visual loss may be quite severe with profound loss of the light response. The near response will still be present if the patient is cooperative and no oculomotor nerve dysfunction has occurred. Cortical blindness, on the other hand, is typified by normal pupillary light responses.

Pathological Pupillary Reactions and Reflexes

Oculosympathetic Paresis (Horner's Syndrome

This is the most common cause of pupillary inequality in neurosurgical practice. Careful observation will reveal that most patients who undergo direct carotid angiography develop a transient pupillary miosis. Bilateral decrease of sympathetic innervation to the pupil is difficult to prove without the aid of pupillography. Denervation of the sympathetic pathways may produce the signs listed in Table 17–2. The number of signs produced depends on the age of the patient and the level and magnitude of involvement of the pathways. Discovery of a Horner's syndrome when and where expected is very helpful in localizing neurological lesions.

Much has been made of the value of chemical testing to determine the level of involvement (first, second, third neuron) of sympathetic damage. Recent evidence obtained in patients with lesions of the first, second, and third neurons demonstrated the value of hydroxyamphetamine (Paredrine) in accurately localizing the level of the lesion.[10] The chemical test of most value is the cocaine test. It will be positive in lesions at all levels.

The cocaine test should be performed in the following manner. Since it is not reliable if the corneas have been manipulated, the cocaine should be the first drops instilled, and the testing of the corneal reflexes should be reserved for later. One drop of cocaine 10 per cent solution should be instilled in the lower cul-de-sac *in each eye*—this test depends on the comparison of the dilation of the normal versus the sympathectomized pupil. In 10 minutes, if the pupils have not begun to dilate, two more drops should be instilled. The response to cocaine is evaluated 30 to 45 minutes after the last instillation. A positive test is one in which the sympathectomized pupil remains at least 2 mm smaller than the normal one at the end of 30 minutes. The belief that a "central Horner's syndrome," a first neuron lesion, cannot have a positive

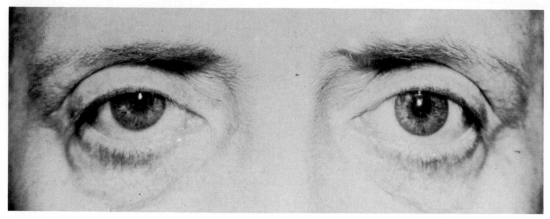

Figure 17–4   Right Horner's syndrome before cocaine instillation. Note the minimal miosis and ptosis, which could be easily overlooked.

cocaine test has been disproved. Positive cocaine tests do occur if the criteria for a positive test will allow for some dilation of the sympathetically denervated pupil (Figs. 17–4 and 17–5).

A few of the causes of oculosympathetic paresis that should be included in differential diagnosis are: (1) first neuron lesions—vascular accidents of the brain stem, syringomyelia, syringobulbia, tumors of the brain stem or cervical cord, meningitis, and meningomyelitis; (2) second neuron lesions—cervical rib, cervical trauma, infection or metastatic tumor to cervical nodes, and Pancoast's tumor; and (3) third neuron lesions—carotid aneurysm, carotid angiography, carotid inflammatory disease as with cranial arteritis or periarteritis nodosa, tumor at the base of the skull, otitis media (severe), cholesteatoma, Raeder's paratrigeminal syndrome, and skull fracture.

Tonic Pupil (Adie's Syndrome)

This pupillary abnormality results from the postganglionic denervation of the parasympathetic supply to the pupil (Fig. 17–6). Although it may follow a viral infection such as varicella or mumps, most often no cause is established. There are two common causes for the sudden onset of a dilated pupil, responding poorly to light, in an otherwise healthy young person: accidental instillation of atropine or some other cycloplegic medication into the eye (common in medical students, nurses, or young mothers who have children under treatment with cycloplegics) and Adie's tonic pupil. The clinical features of the tonic pupil are summarized in Table 17–3. It is incorrect to apply the term "Adie's pupil" to a pupil that responds poorly to light and near stimulus in a person with diabetes mellitus,

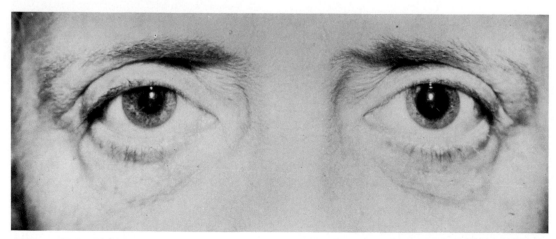

Figure 17–5   Right Horner's syndrome after cocaine instillation. Note the obvious value of the cocaine test in detecting a subtle sympathetic underaction.

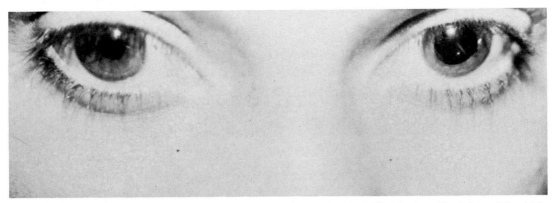

Figure 17–6 Left Adie's tonic pupil. Photograph taken in standard room illumination. The left pupil is widely dilated and responds poorly to light and near stimuli.

TABLE 17–3 CLINICAL FEATURES OF ADIE'S TONIC PUPIL

Unilateral in 80 per cent of patients
Affected pupil usually larger (dilated)
Direct light reflex almost abolished
Pupil dilates slowly in dark
Pupil contracts slowly on prolonged light exposure
During accommodation miosis occurs, may exceed that of
  normal pupil
Pupil dilates slowly when accommodation discontinued
Reacts normally to mydriatics
More common in females (20–30 age group)
Bilateral tonic pupils occur
Patient should be neurologically intact except for absence
  of knee and ankle jerks
Prompt miosis occurs with instillation of 2.5 per cent meth-
  acholine (Mecholyl)—this does not occur in normal eye
  If Mecholyl is not available, 0.0625 per cent pilocarpine
solution is useful as an alternative test

lues, alcoholic polyneuritis, or pineal tumors. Tonic pupils will show abnormal sensitivity to weak cholinergic solutions that would not constrict a normal pupil. The classic chemical test for the tonic pupil has been 2.5 per cent methacholine (Mecholyl). Because difficulty in obtaining this medication practically precludes its use, a 0.0625 per cent pilocarpine solution substitutes quite well. This can be prepared by any pharmacist by diluting 0.5 per cent pilocarpine to the proper concentration. It should be prepared in such a way as to maintain sterility. Two drops should be instilled in each eye, and a positive test is judged by the observation of marked constriction of the affected pupil, for which the normal pupil serves as a control.

Argyll Robertson Pupil

This pupillary abnormality is the most conclusive ocular sign of neurosyphilis. Approximately 13 per cent of patients with

tabes dorsalis and 8 per cent of those with general paresis have Argyll Robertson pupils. Over 70 per cent of patients with neurosyphilis will have some abnormality of pupillary function during the course of the disease. The Argyll Robertson pupil has very strict criteria, which include the following: (1) some vision must be present; (2) miosis, which may be unilateral; (3) dilates poorly to atropine, cocaine, and similar agents; (4) *does not react to light regardless of its intensity;* but (5) does react to accommodation. Irregular shape, though common, is not a requirement for diagnosis.

The Argyll Robertson–like pupil is more often seen in patients with neurosyphilis and is a pupil that does respond to light but not as well as to the near stimulus (light-near dissociation). These pupils may be large or small, may be round or irregular in shape, and respond normally to mydriatics and cycloplegics. The differential diagnosis of the Argyll Robertson–like pupil is as follows: (1) lues—especially juvenile paresis; (2) diabetes mellitus (diabetic pseudotabes); (3) pituitary tumors (tabes pituitaria); (4) lesions of the periaqueductal gray matter (midbrain); (5) primary amyloidosis; (6) myotonic dystrophy; and (7) misdirection in regeneration of nerve III (called the pseudo–Argyll Robertson pupil here because its size often varies with different directions of gaze). A positive test with 2.5 per cent methacholine (Mecholyl) can be found in the conditions listed in Table 17–4.

Miotic Pupils

The three most common causes for pupillary miosis are miotics, morphine, and pon-

TABLE 17–4 POSITIVE MECHOLYL TEST IN PUPILLARY DISORDERS

Argyll Robertson pupil
Myotonic dystrophy
Primary amyloidosis
Riley-Day syndrome (familial dysautonomia)

tine miosis. The latter is found usually in patients who have large pontine hemorrhages, and the pronounced miosis is a grave prognostic sign. It may result from destruction of the sympathetic and disruption of the inhibitory pathways to the Edinger-Westphal nucleus arising in the lower stem and the spinal cord.

Traumatic Mydriasis or Miosis

Direct ocular trauma may lead to either a dilated or miotic pupil. Dilation is usually the result of paralysis of the sphincter because of local damage to the nerve endings supplying it. It may also result from one or more tears of the sphincter muscle, in which case the pupil is often irregular in outline. Miosis after direct ocular injury is most often due to the associated intraocular inflammation.

Closed head trauma with increased intracranial pressure frequently produces a dilated pupil that responds poorly to light and near stimulus, the so-called Hutchinson's pupil. Most often this results from cerebral edema; subdural or intracerebral hematoma forces the uncus of the hippocampus downward, thus pressing on the superior aspect of the adjacent third nerve. The nerve is trapped between the uncus and the ten-

torium. At other times there may be horizontal shifting of the intracranial contents so that the mesencephalic pyramidal tract will press the third nerve against the tentorial edge. With a more or less unilateral increase in intracranial pressure, as with a rapidly expanding mass, one expects to see a contralateral hemiparesis and ipsilateral Hutchinson's pupil. In some patients, because of the horizontal shifting due to pressure, the patient may develop a hemiparesis ipsilateral to the lesion with a contralateral dilated and fixed pupil (Kernohan's notch).[6] Compression of the posterior cerebral artery may occur, causing a homonymous hemianopia. With sufficiently increased intracranial pressure, all parameters of third nerve function can be affected either unilaterally or bilaterally. Bilateral dilation of the pupils with increased intracranial pressure is a grave prognostic sign.

The Amaurotic Pupil

The five pupillary signs of the blind eye are: (1) no *direct* pupillary response with light on blind eye, (2) no *consensual* response with light on blind eye, (3) intact *direct* pupillary response with light on normal eye, (4) intact consensual response in blind eye with light on normal eye, and (5) near pupillary response normal in both eyes.

The Marcus Gunn pupillary phenomenon (swinging flashlight sign) indicates a defect in the afferent arc of the pupillary light reflex. It is invaluable as an aid to confirmation of visual loss resulting from a lesion anterior to the chiasm and is found in optic nerve disease even when the reduction in

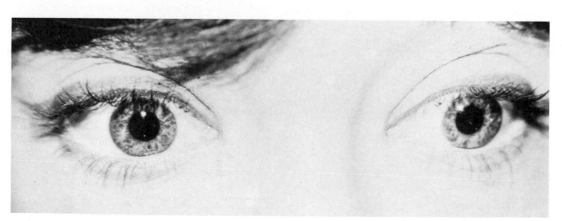

Figure 17–7   Patient with conduction defect of the left optic nerve in standard room illumination before testing for Marcus Gunn pupil.

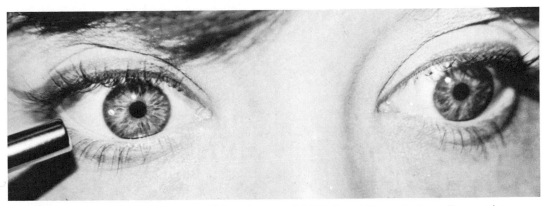

Figure 17–8 Conduction defect of left optic nerve. Light before right eye, both pupils constrict.

visual acuity is minimal (Figs. 17–7, 17–8, and 17–9). It is also present when visual loss is the result of retinal dysfunction, but the retina must be severely damaged. With the patient fixing at distance, a strong light is placed before the intact eye. A crisp contraction of the pupil is noted bilaterally, assuming no other lesions are affecting pupillary diameter. When the light is then moved quickly to the affected eye, the pupils will dilate slightly. This dilation continues for a short period while light is pouring into the eye. The pupils may then begin to contract. The light is then quickly moved to the sound eye and the pupils contract promptly. Unless vision is severely reduced, the direct pupil response may appear normal in the poorer eye. The swinging flashlight test is a very sensitive guide to minimal damage of the optic nerve.

The Pupils in Epilepsy

During the aura, the pupils are often miotic. As convulsions begin, they are usually dilated and often fixed to light. This is helpful in differentiating true from hysterical seizures. It is unusual for the pupils to become fixed to light in petit mal seizures.

DISORDERS OF OCULAR MOTILITY

Definition of Terms

Versions—both eyes turned to the right, left, up, or down; this is also a "conjugate deviation" of the eyes because they are moving in the same direction.

Ductions—movements of one eye.

Vergence—movement of both eyes in different directions. Convergence is the movement of each eye toward the midline. Divergence is the reverse of convergence. These are also called dysjugate or nonconjugate movements.

Eso—inward deviation of the eye (toward the midline).

Exo—outward deviation of the eye.

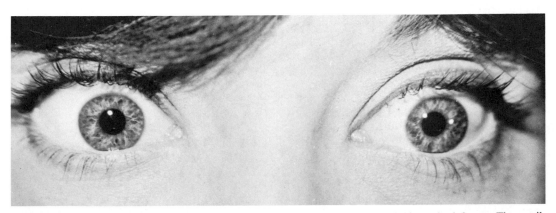

Figure 17–9 Conduction defect of left optic nerve with light now moved quickly to the left eye. The pupils dilate under the light for a short time before constriction occurs.

Hyper—upward deviation of the eye.

Phoria—a latent tendency for the eye to deviate. It is manifest when binocular fixation is disrupted by any means. When the disrupting "cover" is removed, the eye turns to pick up fixation again. With or without the cover, the opposite fixing eye never moves. In the cover-uncover test to determine the presence or absence of a phoria, one eye is allowed to fix on an object at all times while an occluder is placed before the other eye. When the cover is removed, if a phoria is present, the eye that was covered moves to pick up fixation. The eye that was used for fixation does not move during the test if a phoria is present. Normally a small esophoria is present when fixing on distant objects, and a small exophoria when fixing at near. If the eye does not move when the cover is removed, there is no phoria.

Tropia—a manifest deviation of the eye. This may be alternating (either eye can fix accurately and hold fixation), and the fixing eye may have good visual acuity. It may be monocular with only one eye used constantly for fixation while the deviating eye has poor visual acuity (amblyopia). In either case, when the cover-uncover test is performed and the cover is placed before the eye preferred for fixation, the uncovered eye makes a fixation movement; removal of the cover results in movement of *both* eyes as the preferred eye once again assumes fixation. This is the method of separating phorias from tropias.

Comitancy—a tropia with the same amount of deviation in all fields of gaze. A noncomitant deviation is characteristically found in recent palsies of nerves III, IV, and VI. They are easily recognized by the presence of "secondary deviation." When the alternate cover test is performed, the ocular deviation is greater when the eye with the paretic muscle fixes (secondary deviation) than when the nonparetic eye fixes (primary deviation).

Suppression amblyopia—the loss of usable vision in an eye that has not maintained a visual direction compatible with the other eye. This is due to central inhibition of the visual field of the deviating eye. It occurs as the result of inability to superimpose disparate retinal images simultaneously. This is found with constant ocular deviation occurring before the age of 6 years. After that age, the patient rarely develops amblyopia; instead, the usual result is the onset of diplopia. An ocular deviation in a child should prompt a careful ophthalmological examination. An unsuspected intraocular tumor may produce such a deviation.

Most of the ocular deviations occurring shortly after birth, or noted at birth, are the result of anatomical defects in the orbit. Those arising between the ages of 2 and 4 years are usually the result of an accommodation-convergence derangement. Most children with acquired unilateral visual loss will develop an esotropia, whereas most adults will develop an exotropia. Childhood esotropias may decrease in amount as the patient ages, although the vision in the deviating eye is poor. This is the reason some physicians make the error of telling the parents of children with strabismus that "they will grow out of it." The child may look cosmetically better as the esodeviation decreases, but the chance for treatment is usually lost. Severe bilateral loss of vision in childhood or adult life will infrequently produce strabismus.

Head Tilt, Face Turn, and Chin Position

It is vital to note the presence of any of these signs of motility dysfunction. Face turn in the horizontal plane is most pronounced in defects involving the horizontal rectus muscles. The face turns *toward* the paretic muscle. Minimal face turn may be present in patients with weakness of the vertically acting muscles. A face turn as the result of horizontal muscle dysfunction would be suggested by horizontal diplopia coupled with little tendency for head tilt or elevation or depression of the chin. The reverse would suggest a defect in vertical muscle action. The patient thus adapts himself to horizontal deviations with the face turn, to vertical deviations by elevating or depressing the chin, and to torsional defects by tilting the head. The position of head, face, and chin should be written down to be analyzed later. It is always worthwhile to compare old photographs with the present head position.

Action of the Ocular Muscles

The horizontal recti (1—the lateral recti) abduct the eye and are more effective in upward gaze, and (2—the medial recti) adduct the eye and are more effective in downward gaze.

The superior recti are primarily elevators but also adduct and intort.

The inferior recti are primarily elevators but also adduct and intort.

The inferior recti are primarily depressors but also adduct and extort.

The superior obliques are primarily depressors but also abduct and intort.

The inferior obliques are primarily elevators but also abduct and extort.

One can better understand the actions of the vertically acting muscles by a study of the anatomy. The vertical rectus muscles insert on the globe at an angle of 23 degrees from the anteroposterior plane of the globe and anterior and lateral to the sagittal plane of the globe. Their unique position produces essentially pure vertical movement of the eye when it is ABducted to an angle of 23 degrees. When the eye is in the ADducted position, the action of the vertical recti is more torsional. Conversely, the obliques insert at an angle of 51 degrees and thus are most effective in vertical movement of the eye when the globe is in the ADducted position. The vertical function of the obliques is almost pure when the eye is adducted to 51 degrees. When the eye is in the divergence position, the obliques become more efficient in torsion. This effect is greatest when the eye is abducted to 39 degrees.

When these facts are kept in mind, it is obvious that with complete paralysis of nerve III the only sign of an intact nerve IV would be some torsional movement of the eye. The eye is in the ABducted position when nerve III is paralyzed. This is the most favorable position for the torsional effect of the superior oblique. This also explains why the vertical recti are most important in control of the vertical position of the eye at distance, whereas the obliques are most important at near.

Tests for Weakness of an Ocular Muscle

The subjective red-glass test (cover-uncover) and the objective cover test (alternate cover) are adequate to identify any motility problem. The motility examination is best carried out with the patient wearing his glasses. It is good practice to obtain both the subjective and objective measurement of the patient's ocular deviation.

Subjective Red-Glass Test

By convention, the patient usually has the red glass placed before the right eye (Fig. 17–10). He is then asked to look at a light at distance with both eyes open. If no ocular deviation exists, he will see the red and white images superimposed as a single pink image. If the patient has an exophoric or exotropic deviation, he will see the red image to his left and the white image to his right (crossed diplopia). It may be helpful to assign a color to each hand and then have

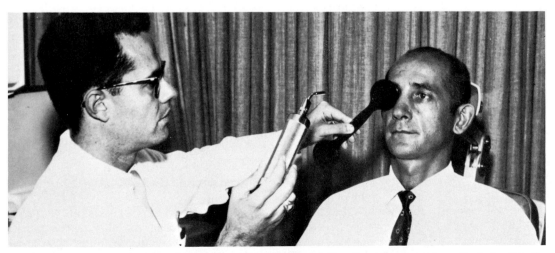

Figure 17–10 The subjective red-glass test. The red glass is before the right eye as the patient observes the hand light.

the patient show with his hands the relationship of the two images in space. For example, if the right hand is "red" and the left hand is "white," a patient with an exodeviation will cross his hands when asked to show the relationship of the lights to each other in space. (A useful mnemonic: There is an *x* in exo and an *x* is also a cross-crossed diplopia.) If the patient has an esodeviation, the red image is to the right and the white image to the left (uncrossed or homonymous diplopia). A hyperdeviation will be manifest as a vertical displacement of the images. This may occur alone or in combination with a horizontal deviation. If the right eye is deflected upward, the image is displaced downward or "the red light is lower than the white light."

The test light is then moved to about 33 cm from the patient with the red glass before the right eye. The light is moved into the cardinal fields of gaze and the patient is asked to comment on the relative separation of the red and white images. Again his hands may indicate the amount of separation. After the field of greatest separation is located, a cover test will make final determination of the paretic muscle. The amount of deviation can be measured by inserting prisms of the proper amount and direction before the eyes until the images are superimposed.

The Cover Test

This may be done with the eyes fixing at any distance, but for most neurosurgical examinations it is best done with the patient fixing at near (33 cm). The patient is asked to follow the movements of a hand light into the cardinal fields. The light is then held steady, and the patient's eyes are alternately covered by any convenient object (i.e., a hand or cardboard). The alternate cover test will disclose any tendency for the eyes to deviate when fixation with both eyes is disrupted. The cover-uncover test will determine if the deviation is a phoria or a tropia. It then remains to decide in which of the cardinal fields the deviation is maximal. One must also note whether the deviation is greater with the right or left eye fixing. It is usually abnormal to find hyperdeviations at near. Once the decision is made as to the cardinal field with the greatest deviation, and the amount of deviation with

TABLE 17–5 IDENTIFICATION OF A PARETIC EXTRAOCULAR MUSCLE

POSITION OF GAZE	MUSCLES INVOLVED	GREATEST DEVIATION
Right gaze	Right lateral rectus	Right eye fixing
	Left medial rectus	Left eye fixing
Up-right	Right superior rectus	Right eye fixing
	Left inferior oblique	Left eye fixing
Down-right	Right inferior rectus	Right eye fixing
	Left superior oblique	Left eye fixing
Left gaze	Left lateral rectus	Left eye fixing
	Right medial rectus	Right eye fixing
Up-left	Left superior rectus	Left eye fixing
	Right inferior oblique	Right eye fixing
Down-left	Left inferior rectus	Left eye fixing
	Right superior oblique	Right eye fixing

the right and left eye fixing is settled, the paretic muscle is identified (Table 17–5).

Confirmation of a superior oblique palsy can be made with the Bielschowsky head tilt test. Because the superior oblique muscle has a significant torsional effect even in straight ahead gaze, weakness of a superior oblique will allow the eye to extort. To compensate for this, the patient learns to tilt his head *away from the side with the paretic muscle*. Thus, one has a left head tilt with a right fourth nerve palsy. To prove the right fourth nerve is underacting, the patient is asked to tilt his head to the right. When this is done, the right eye shows further hyperdeviation. When the red glass is used, the patient notes improvement of diplopia when the head is tilted to the left. If an inferior oblique is involved, the patient tilts the head to the same side as the paretic muscle to avoid diplopia. The chin is elevated if an elevator is involved (superior rectus or inferior oblique) and depressed if a depressor is at fault. Using the outlined approach, a reasonable conclusion can be made as to which muscle is underacting.

Supranuclear Gaze Palsies

Supranuclear gaze palsies are differentiated from nuclear and infranuclear palsies primarily by loss of voluntary movement with retention of following ocular movement. Also, supranuclear gaze palsies are conjugate gaze problems. The patient often has great difficulty in moving the eyes on command, but can move them much better when following a moving target. The Bell's phenomenon is typically intact in supranuclear lesions.

Ocular Motor Apraxia

In this disturbance of ocular motility, the patient has full random movement capacity of the eyes. If he attempts to move the eyes purposefully toward a specific object, he experiences more difficulty than if random movements are used. The condition may be either congenital or acquired.

In congenital ocular motor apraxia there is loss of willed movements of the eyes with full movement in random gaze. Horizontal movement is selectively involved. Vertical movements are usually full on willed gaze. There is also a characteristic compensatory movement of the head to change the direction of gaze. The patient moves the head toward the object of regard, and this quick turn of the head produces a contraversive movement of the eyes away from the object. The head must then be turned past the object sufficiently far so that the eyes will eventually be brought about to fix on it. Once fixation is established, the head is then rotated until it is straight with the eyes. This movement of the head and eyes is not seen in any other abnormal state of gaze. Cogan suggested that this form of conjugate gaze disturbance implied no associated significant neurological defect. Yet this entity has been seen with significant intracranial defects such as porencephaly, hamartoma of the third ventricle, and agenesis of the corpus callosum. A child with this gaze disorder deserves evaluation. A CT scan may be in order before one can assure the parents that no neurological defect exists.

In acquired ocular motor apraxia the patient can turn neither eyes nor head voluntarily. Random movements may be somewhat restricted. There may be preferential loss of vertical rather than horizontal movements, as in the sylvian aqueduct syndrome. Lesions of the hemisphere commonly produce this type of motility disorder affecting horizontal gaze. Tumors, intracranial hemorrhage, and direct damage to the surface of the brain (contusion, laceration) are com-

TABLE 17–6 OCULAR SIGNS IN DISEASES AFFECTING SUPRANUCLEAR GAZE MECHANISMS

Sylvian aqueduct syndrome
  Retraction nystagmus
  Vertical nystagmus
  Difficult voluntary vertical gaze (especially upgaze)
  Vertical gaze better following or doll's head than on command. Bell's phenomenon intact
  Adduction movements with attempted vertical gaze
  Defective convergence
  Retraction movements of eyes with downgoing optico-kinetic targets
  Pupillary anomalies
  Collier's sign (pathological lid retraction)
Parkinsonism
  P = paresis of vertical gaze, pupillary changes
  A = accommodative paresis (drug and/or disease related)
  R = reflex blepharospasm, retraction upper lids (Collier's sign)
  K = keratitis from drying, cogwheeling ocular movements
  I = infrequent blinking
  N = nystagmus, vertical
  S = seborrheic dermatitis of lids and face
  O = oculogyric crises, opticokinetic dissociation, vertical
  N = no bifocals, no hemianopias
  I = impossible tonometry
  S = styes, Wilson's sign (inability to change direction of gaze without a blink)
  M = Myerson's sign (inability to suppress blinking when examiner taps on lateral orbital margin)
Progressive supranuclear palsy
  Early onset of downgaze weakness
  Horizontal gaze often affected but less than vertical gaze
  Following movements and doll's head ocular movements much better than ocular movements on command
  Dystonic neck rigidity
  Decreased mentation
  Dysarthria
  Occasional cerebellar and pyramidal tract signs
Pseudobulbar palsy
  Inappropriate affect
  Thickened speech
  Moderate dementia
  Exaggeration of jaw jerk
  Appearance of snout, suck, and palmarmental reflexes
  Eye movements slow, possible cogwheeling
  Conjugate gaze restricted in all fields, especially on command
  Corneomandibular reflex often present (lateral movement of jaw away from cornea stroked with cotton wisp)
  Usually due to bilateral destruction of corticobulbar pathways by vascular disease in the elderly or severe head trauma or demyelinizing disease in young adults

mon causes. The findings in other supranuclear gaze palsies are listed in Table 17–6.

Internuclear Ophthalmoplegia

The medial longitudinal fasciculus extends from the thalamus superiorly to the anterior horn cells of the spinal cord inferiorly. It functions in part by connecting the homolateral oculomotor nerve nucleus to the contralateral vestibular nuclei. A lesion in this fasciculus between the pons and mesencephalon produces a characteristic ocular motility disorder, the internuclear ophthalmoplegia. Recent neuropathological studies have proved that the lesion responsible for this gaze disorder is in the fasciculus ipsilateral to the paretic medial rectus. The clinical signs of internuclear ophthalmoplegia are defective adduction of the ipsilateral eye and dissociated nystagmus, with the nystagmus more pronounced in the abducting eye. Convergence may be intact or absent depending on the level of involvement of the brain stem. In anterior internuclear ophthalmoplegia, convergence is lost. This is found with lesions at the level of the upper stem, at or near the oculomotor nuclei. In posterior internuclear ophthalmoplegia, convergence is intact. This implies a lesion below the level of the oculomotor nuclei. Most internuclear palsies are of the posterior type.

Other clinical signs of subtle internuclear ophthalmoplegias are dysmetria and dissociation of horizontal opticokinetic responses. With minimal damage to the fasciculus, an internuclear ophthalmoplegia may be difficult to recognize. It can sometimes be made more apparent, however, by using horizontal opticokinetic targets and looking for dissociation of the responses between the two eyes. The same phenomenon may be seen if the patient is tested for ocular dysmetria by having him shift fixation of the eyes on command from the examiner's finger to his nose. A dysmetric overshoot of the abducting eye is often found.[9]

Unilateral internuclear palsies are of vascular etiology in 75 per cent of patients, and bilateral ones are related to disseminated sclerosis in over 90 per cent of patients. Bilateral internuclear palsies have been described in brain stem vascular accidents, brain stem encephalitis, Wernicke's encephalopathy, and syringobulbia, and a pseudointernuclear palsy has been reported with the ocular signs of myasthenia gravis.[4] Bilateral internuclear palsy is the most common sign in disseminated sclerosis, and retrobulbar neuritis is the most common ocular sensory manifestation. They usually occur separately.

Skew Deviation

The four major ocular signs of cerebellar disease are: nystagmus, ocular dysmetria, flutter-like oscillations, and skew deviation. The latter is also called the Hertwig-Magendie vertical divergence ocular position. Skew deviations may be classified as comitant, noncomitant, or laterally comitant.

Comitant Skew Deviation

When a patient experiences the onset of vertical diplopia that is comitant in all fields of gaze, there are only two possibilities. Either the patient has a previously unrecognized vertical muscle underaction with sudden loss of fusional amplitude, or a comitant skew deviation is present. The presence of a head tilt or face turn suggests the former. Patients with long-standing vertical muscle underactions also have the capacity to fuse large amounts of vertical prism power. Normal is 2 prism diopters; some of these patients can fuse as much as 10 prism diopters.

Noncomitant Skew Deviation

This mimics an isolated overaction or underaction of a vertical rectus or oblique muscle of recent onset. The vertical disparity is definitely greater in one field of gaze and greater with either the right or left eye fixing. Orbital disease must be ruled out prior to making the diagnosis of a noncomitant skew deviation.

Laterally Comitant Skew Deviation

This is the least difficult type of skew deviation to diagnose, as it presents with the sudden onset of vertical diplopia and a comitant hypertropia only in gaze right or left. A patient with this type of skew deviation will show little or no vertical separation in one field of gaze and a comitant deviation in the opposite field. It will measure the same with either eye fixing.

Many patients with skew deviations can be satisfactorily managed with vertical prism correction in their glasses. This may require frequent changes of glasses, and the patient must be so advised. Operation is rarely indicated and should not usually be done until more than six months have elapsed and at least three successive sets of measurements of the vertical imbalance are in agreement. Occasional patients are found with evidence of dysfunction at the midbrain level who also have vertical diplopia. The differential diagnosis is between a nuclear third nerve palsy and a midbrain skew deviation.

Isolated Cranial Nerve Palsies

Abducens Palsy

The most common cause for paresis of the sixth nerve is brain tumor. This is not usually the result of direct involvement of the nerve by tumor, but the result of increased intracranial pressure and stretching of the nerve over the crest of the temporal bone. It has a long intracranial course and innervates only the lateral rectus muscle. Underaction produces esotropia. It is especially vulnerable in basilar skull fracture. It is also commonly affected in patients with Wernicke's encephalopathy, but responds quickly to thiamine.[2]

Other less common causes of underaction of nerve VI are: demyelinating disease; otitis media; purulent meningitis; tumor, sarcoid, or amyloid at the orbital apex; painful ophthalmoplegia; diabetes mellitus (Fig. 17–11); herpes zoster; and cerebellopontine angle tumor or intrapontine neoplasm.

Spasm of the near reflex is commonly confused with unilateral or bilateral abducens weakness. The patient frequently complains of blurring of vision at near or occasionally of diplopia, but no neurological signs are elicited except the apparent underaction of nerve VI. The apparent underaction of the abducens nerve is explained when one observes the pupillary contraction in lateral gaze when the patient begins to complain of diplopia. It is the result of convergence in lateral gaze. Voluntary nystagmus may be superimposed. These patients are managed with weak cycloplegic solutions or by increasing the minus sphere in their glasses prescription. Other common disorders frequently confused with abducens nerve palsy are: (1) thyroid myopathy; (2) ocular myasthenia gravis; (3) orbital fracture with entrapment; (4) Duane's retraction syndrome (generally unilateral, widened lid fissure on attempted abduction, narrowed lid fissure on attempted adduction, retraction of globe on adduction); and (5) old esotropia.

Oculomotor Palsy

The eight anatomical types of third nerve palsy are listed in Table 17–7.[7] The two most common causes for paralysis of nerve III are trauma and aneurysm. Trauma may or may not be associated with an identifiable skull fracture. Exact localization of the site at which the nerve is damaged may be difficult. One should look diligently for a fracture line at the base of the skull. Aneurysms causing complete paralysis of the oculomotor nerve are usually located at the junction of the internal carotid artery and the posterior communicating artery. Two less common causes for paralysis are tumor and lues; others are listed in Table 17–8. Diabetes mellitus as a cause for third nerve palsy most often presents in the elderly patient who has had the disease for years. It is distinctly rare in the young diabetic. The paralysis starts suddenly and is often accompanied by headache. The pupil is usually spared. Such paralyses have an ischemic vascular etiology. The circulatory

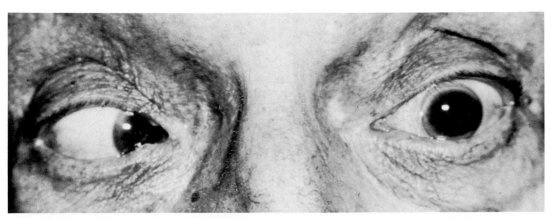

Figure 17–11 Palsy of the left sixth cranial nerve. The patient is attempting to look to the left.

TABLE 17–7 EIGHT ANATOMICAL TYPES OF OCULOMOTOR NERVE PALSIES*

Nuclear	Isolated involvement of an ocular muscle innervated by III, due to disease in the orbit in 99% and the nucleus 1% of the time
Dorsal fascicular	Homolateral paralysis of III with a contralateral hemitremor
Ventral fascicular	Homolateral paralysis of III with contralateral hemiplegia
Root type	Same as ventral fascicular but due to lesion extrinsic to the mesencephalon May be operable
Basal type	Very common type of paralysis of III related to fractures at the base of the skull, tumor, herniation of the uncus with increased intracranial pressure, and aneurysms of the internal carotid artery and posterior communicating artery
Cavernous sinus type	Dysfunction of III usually accompanied by underaction of IV and VI. If the anterior portion of the sinus is involved, the first division of V is commonly affected In disease of the posterior or middle cavernous sinus both the first and second divisions of V are affected Proptosis frequent
Superior orbital fissure	Same as anterior cavernous sinus If lesion is at the fissure, VI cannot be spared when there is total paralysis of III
Orbital apex	Usually have simultaneous involvement of IV, VI, first division of V, and optic nerve with paralysis of III Proptosis common

* After Kestenbaum, A.: Clinical Methods of Neuro-ophthalmologic Examination, 2nd Ed. New York, Grune & Stratton, 1961.

defect involves the tiny vessels that provide nutrition to the nerve (vasa nervorum). The course is one of gradual clearing to complete recovery in two to three months. The causes of isolated internal ophthalmoplegias are listed in Table 17–9.

Trochlear Nerve Palsy

Severe head trauma is the most common cause of paralysis of the fourth nerve (Fig.

TABLE 17–8 ADDITIONAL CAUSES OF OCULOMOTOR PALSY

Diabetes mellitus
Sphenoid ridge meningioma
Nasopharyngeal carcinoma
Metastatic carcinoma to base of skull
Vascular insufficiency to mesencephalon
Syphilitic and tuberculous meningitis (basilar)
Viral diseases
Sarcoid or amyloid
Herpes zoster
Heavy metal intoxication

TABLE 17–9 CAUSES OF ISOLATED INTERNAL OPHTHALMOPLEGIA

Cycloplegic ocular medications (most common cause)
Adie's syndrome
Nasopharyngeal carcinoma (early)
Diphtheria
Botulism
Viral diseases (mumps, chickenpox)
Increased intracranial pressure
Direct ocular trauma

17–12). It may be a bilateral palsy. This is the only cranial nerve that shows complete decussation, as the nucleus is located opposite the exposed portion of the nerve exiting the midbrain. It is also the most commonly congenitally affected cranial nerve and is often responsible for torticollis in early life. Such patients are not infrequently subjected to myotomy of the sternocleidomastoid, only to have no benefit because a congenital paralysis of the trochlear nerve was overlooked. Other causes of fourth nerve palsy are listed in Table 17–10.

Diseases That Affect the Myoneural Junction

Another important group of diseases affects ocular motility directly at the muscle or the neuromuscular junction. Three diseases are of importance: myasthenia gravis, thyroid myopathy, and chronic progressive external ophthalmoplegia.

The eye is often the first organ affected by myasthenia gravis. The patient generally has intermittent ptosis, characteristically better in the morning when he is rested and worse at night. This is usually the first ocular sign of the disease. Later there is diplopia that is usually worse in the evening. Any of the external muscles of the eye may be affected, but the pupillary and accommodative functions are left intact. The patient may have other systemic signs of myasthenia or it may affect the eyes alone, in which case the term "ocular myasthenia" is used. In either case, the edrophonium chloride (Tensilon) test will be positive. Fresh Tensilon must be used. For best results, the patient should look upward until upper lid fatigue is at the maximum and then 1 ml of Tensilon should be given rapidly intravenously. The eyes should be maintained in up gaze for at least two minutes after the drug is given in order to eval-

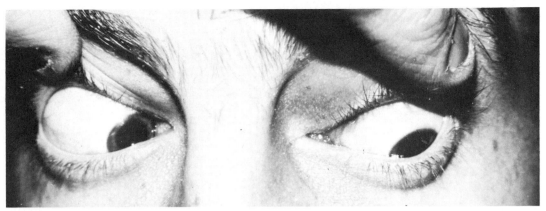

Figure 17–12   Right fourth nerve palsy following severe closed head trauma. Note the higher position of the right eye in gaze down and to the left. The deviation was greatest with the right eye fixing.

uate its effect. A significant number of patients will have other endocrine disturbances associated with myasthenia. Every patient with myasthenia should be evaluated for thyroid disease and diabetes mellitus. It remains axiomatic that any patient who has an unexplained ocular muscle imbalance should have a Tensilon test. Ocular myasthenia deserves a trial of medical management, as does systemic myasthenia. Systemic steroids have recently been advocated in the treatment of ocular myasthenia gravis.[3]

Thyroid ocular disease is described in part in the section on external diseases of the eye. Regardless of whether the patient has laboratory confirmation of thyroid disease, the diagnosis of ocular disease related to disturbed thyroid metabolism is clinical. Monocular limitation of up gaze is the hallmark of thyroid ocular myopathy. This is due to chronic inflammation of the oribtal tissues. An outpouring of mucopolysaccharides is followed by infiltration of all orbital tissues with lymphocytes and plasma cells. Swelling of orbital fat is said to be the cause of proptosis; inflammatory changes in the region of the inferior rectus and inferior oblique muscles result in severe limitation

TABLE 17–10   ADDITIONAL CAUSES OF TROCHLEAR NERVE PALSY

Postinfectious—diphtheria or Guillain-Barré
Vascular—especially upper stem ischemia
Intracavernous carotid aneurysm
Migraine
Diabetes mellitus
Mesencephalic neoplastic—pinealoma, glioma
Postoperative temporal lobectomy or temporal lobe intra-
  cerebral hematoma

of upward gaze. It may be bilateral, and usually is, but is often asymmetrical. Motility is much the same as that seen in the patient with an orbital floor fracture. The eye does not move up well, but moves down almost fully. The horizontal excursions are often normal. The patient appears to have an underaction of the superior rectus muscle. Operation on the ocular muscles can be of help in managing patients with diplopia on this basis.

Another form of severe, progressive damage to the ocular muscles is progressive dystrophy of the external ocular muscles described by Kiloh and Nevin.[8] The preferred term for this disorder is chronic progressive external ophthalmoplegia. The main clinical features are: (1) it usually begins before age 30; (2) frequency is the same in males and females; (3) there is a family history of either ptosis or ophthalmoplegia or both in over 50 per cent of patients (Fig. 17–13); (4) diplopia is the earliest symptom and ptosis the earliest sign; (5) onset is progressive and insidious; (6) exacerbations and remissions are not common; (7) advance of the disease may be halted temporarily or permanently at any stage; (8) pupils are normal, unlike those in myotonic dystrophy, with light-near dissociation of the pupils; (9) there is loss of facial expression; and (10) the temporalis and masseter muscles are often involved, as are those of the upper spinal segments (10 per cent of cases). There is no associated baldness, cataract, or testicular atrophy with this disease. The basic change is fibrillary degeneration of the striated muscle fibers with some inflammatory cell infiltration and fat deposition in a patchy arrangement. A

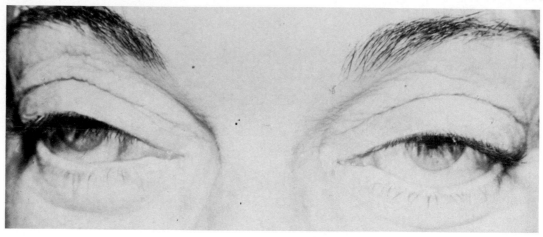

Figure 17–13   Bilateral ptosis in patient with advanced Kiloh-Nevin syndrome. Previously thought due to degeneration of the cranial nerve nuclei, the disease is now considered muscular degenerative.

few patients with chronic progressive external ophthalmoplegia will have retinitis pigmentosa–like retinal changes and fit the diagnostic group of Refsum's syndrome. A very few may also have significant difficulty with an associated heart block and should have an electrocardiogram.

Cranial Nerve Regeneration

Significant damage to the peripheral segments of a cranial nerve may produce initial degeneration of nerve fibers followed by haphazard regrowth, so that muscles of the face and eyes are incorrectly innervated (Fig. 17–14). The ocular signs found in the misdirection syndrome of nerve III, listed in Table 17–11, are explained by the mass firing effect of misdirected nerve fibers.[1] For example, the eye is unable to move up or down fully because the nerve fibers originally destined for the superior rectus and levator are partly supplying the inferior rectus and medial rectus and inferior oblique muscles. When the patient attempts to look up, the superior rectus and inferior oblique and inferior rectus muscles are all fired simultaneously, and the eye is unable to move. The signs of misdirection of the third nerve are important to recognize, as they imply old disease. Over three months are required to obtain significant signs of misdirection in most cases. Diabetes alone never causes misdirection of nerve III. A diabetic with misdirection of the oculomo-

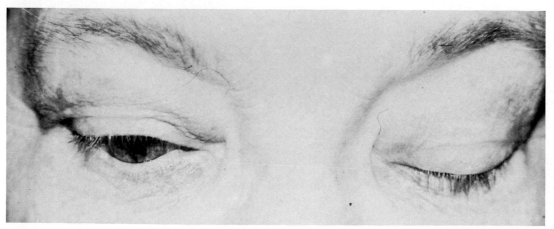

Figure 17–14   The pseudo-Graefe sign in misdirection of oculomotor nerve. The right upper lid retracts in downgaze.

TABLE 17–11 OCULAR SIGNS OF MISDIRECTION OF CRANIAL NERVE III

Pseudo-Graefe lid sign	As eye attempts to move downward upper lid retracts (Fig. 14–15)
Pseudo-Argyll Robertson pupil	Minimal or no response to light, but diameter may vary with direction of gaze
Horizontal gaze lid dyskinesis	Diameter of lid fissure varies with direction of gaze
	As eye is adducted the fissure widens, and the fissure narrows as eye is abducted
	This sometimes best seen in downgaze if misdirection is minimal
Difficult vertical gaze	Eye moves poorly in vertical plane
	Adduction on attempted vertical gaze
Monocular opticokinetic responses	As vertical opticokinetic targets are presented, the eye with misdirection moves little if at all

tor nerve needs either a very good history of prior trauma that accounts for the observation or an arteriogram to rule out a previously undisclosed aneurysm.

Misdirection of the motor division of the fifth cranial nerve produces the Marcus Gunn jaw winking phenomenon. It is characterized by ptosis of the ipsilateral eye, which changes to lid retraction as the patient opens the mouth or moves the jaw to the opposite side. It is a unilateral process and is usually more of a cosmetic detriment than a functional one. The pathways implicated by the clinical findings are afferent ones beginning with the external pterygoid muscle supplied by the motor division of nerve V. The mesencephalic root of the trigeminal nerve, which supplies the external pterygoid, is linked to the muscles of the oculomotor nerve and finally to the levator of the upper eyelid, forming the efferent arc.

Misdirection in regeneration of the seventh cranial nerve may involve the motor and secretory pathway for lacrimation. Peripheral damage to the facial nerve due to any cause will produce misdirection if it is severe. If only the motor function is involved in misdirection, an interfacial synkinesis is produced. When the patient attempts to close the eye, synchronous movements of the upper and lower face occur. This is often quite subtle and may be missed unless specifically searched for in the examination. Paroxysmal lacrimation (crocodile tears) is the secretory correlate of regeneration of nerve VII. It may be congenital and bilateral. In the adult it usually follows Bell's palsy and is often unilateral.

It is rather common in the Möbius syndrome of childhood with bilateral paresis of nerves VI and VII as the major findings.

Opticokinetic Nystagmus

The value of opticokinetic nystagmus (ON) in the investigation of patients with disease of the hemisphere or brain stem is generally underestimated. To evaluate opticokinetic nystagmus carefully only two simple pieces of equipment are required— an opticokinetic tape with 12 to 14 2-by-2-inch squares of red felt sewed to a strip of white felt and an opticokinetic drum (House of Vision, Chicago, Ill.), which is advantageous in subtle opticokinetic dissociation. A cloth tape measure can be useful but requires a vision of at least 20/70 in order to elicit responses.

In lesions involving the cerebral hemispheres, the opticokinetic response is positive in deep parietal lobe disease and negative with lesions elsewhere. Poor opticokinetic nystagmus is found with a deep parietal lobe lesion when targets are moved toward the ipsilateral side. By comparison, moving targets away from the side of the lesion should produce crisp opticokinetic nystagmus. Although a hemianopia (homonymous) should be present with parietal lobe damage that is sufficiently deep to produce a positive opticokinetic nystagmus sign, this sign must not be considered a test for hemianopic visual field loss.

The vertical opticokinetic nystagmus response is useful in localizing certain brain stem lesions. In the normal patient, a crisp sustained vertical response can be elicited with ease. With aging, the vertical responses may be slightly depressed, as compared with the horizontal responses. Adequate responses are never produced without encouragement. The patient should count the targets to himself as they are presented. It is necessary to test a large number of patients to become familiar with the limits of the normal opticokinetic response.

Abnormal Vertical Responses

Vertical Opticokinetic Nystagmus Dissociation

Horizontal responses are symmetrical, but a gross asymmetry exists between the responses obtained with targets moving vertically (up better than down or vice versa). This is found with regularity in Parkinson's disease, brain stem and cerebellar neoplasms, familial nystagmus, multiple sclerosis, and postoperative stereotaxic lesions. The responses to vertical targets are better in one direction. Spontaneous vertical nystagmus is often present or can be elicited with vertical gaze in patients who have vertical opticokinetic nystagmus dissociation.

In brain stem disease, some patients will show poor horizontal responses, but excellent responses to vertical targets. This suggests a lesion at the pontine level. One would expect other neurological signs consistent with pontine damage. These would include slowing or loss of conjugate gaze movements, internuclear ophthalmoplegia, spontaneous nystagmus, Horner's syndrome, and underaction of nerves VI or VII or both. In children, opticokinetic testing can be helpful in differentiating congenital from acquired nystagmus. It can also serve to distinguish whether the patient's vision is severely reduced when congenital nystagmus is present. Horizontal opticokinetic responses are markedly decreased or absent in most patients with congenital nystagmus, regardless of the severity of visual loss. If useful vision is present, though, opticokinetic nystagmus can be superimposed upon congenital nystagmus when vertical opticokinetic targets are used. The examiner will see vertical nystagmus or an accentuation of horizontal nystagmus. A child who fails to show these responses to vertically moving opticokinetic targets has a poor visual prognosis.

Maintenance of horizontal nystagmus in vertical gaze is essentially diagnostic of congenital nystagmus.

Loss of Rapid Phase

This is sometimes found in vertical opticokinetic testing. It is due to the same mechanism in any case—destruction of the corticifugal pathways from the cerebrum to the nuclear masses of the stem. The cause is the same as that for loss of the rapid phase in any form of acquired nystagmus. Sustained slow phase is called the Roth-Bielschowsky deviation.

Monocular Vertical Responses

This is found in the syndrome of misdirection of nerve III as previously described. For practical purposes, this is the only condition causing such responses. It occurs because of mass firing of the vertically acting muscles innervated by the oculomotor nerve when vertical movements are attempted.[1]

Poor Vertical and Intact Horizontal Responses

This dissociation of opticokinetic responses is particularly common in patients with disease at the mesencephalic level. This is because the locus for vertical ocular movements is at this level. The selective depression or complete absence of vertical responses with intact horizontal responses strongly suggests the upper brain stem as the site of involvement. It can be produced with lesions outside the stem from simple pressure effects, as with pinealomas or meningiomas and increased intracranial pressure with brain stem compromise. In this latter circumstance, control of intracranial pressure will rapidly restore normal vertical ocular movements. It can also be seen with intrinsic stem disorders such as gliomas, hemorrhage, arteriovenous malformation, infarction, and inflammatory or degenerative disease. Retraction nystagmus is also found with lesions in this area.

Nystagmoid Movements of the Eyes

Opsoclonus

This dramatic neurological disorder consists of ataxic conjugate movements of the eyes. It has a sudden onset generally following an episode of low-grade fever and upper respiratory disease. Approximately seven days later, the ocular signs of ataxic chaotic conjugate movements begin. The movements are rapid and of large amplitude. There is no diplopia because the movements are conjugate. The patient may close one eye or cover an eye with his hand in an attempt to reduce the amplitude of movement. The movements persist during sleep, but are less violent. Myoclonic jerks of the extremities, face, neck, and trunk are often present. The sensorium is generally clear, and the neurological examination is usually negative except for the myoclonus. The cerebrospinal fluid is normal or shows a slight pleocytosis. The majority of patients have normal hearing, yet cold caloric testing produces no nystagmus. The prognosis is good, with complete recovery occurring within four months. Opsoclonus is currently classified as a sign of cerebellar system dysfunction.

Oculopalatopharyngeal Myoclonus

This unusual ocular movement disorder appears much like nystagmus, but the movement, though rhythmic, lacks a definite slow phase. It is also synchronous with movements of the palate, pharynx, tongue, face, larynx, and eustachian tube orifice, which may cause the patient to complain of clicking in the ear. It may also be associated with arrhythmic movements of the diaphragm, abdomen, and extremities. These movements are thought to be related to a disturbance of the myoclonic triangle (dentate nucleus of the cerebellum, inferior olive, and red nucleus). The common antecedent causes are multiple sclerosis, trauma, vascular accident of the stem, degenerative disease (olivopontocerebellar degeneration), and severe inflammatory disease of the brain stem. Once developed, it tends not to remit.

THE VISUAL FIELDS

Several techniques are available for evaluation of the visual fields. The most commonly employed is the confrontation method. The neurosurgeon should, however, be capable of using techniques other than confrontation in the diagnosis of visual field defects.

Confrontation Testing

The usual confrontation test is performed by having the patient cover one eye and look into the examiner's open eye. The patient is then asked to tell the examiner when an object is in motion and when it is not. This method of testing the visual field leaves much to be desired in both accuracy and sensitivity. A much better method is the "three-stage confrontation technique." One must be certain that the covered eye is completely occluded. The patient is then asked to fix his gaze on the examiner's nose. The examiner then presents the extended fingers of one hand in the various quadrants of the visual field, asking the patient to count the number of extended fingers. The number of fingers presented on each occasion is varied. This requires that the patient remain alert. The speed of presentation will vary according to the patient's ability to respond; great care must be exercised in visual field testing so as not to exceed the patient's reaction time. Visual field testing is particularly difficult in a patient with dysphasia. If he is encouraged to mimic responses, rather than to verbal-

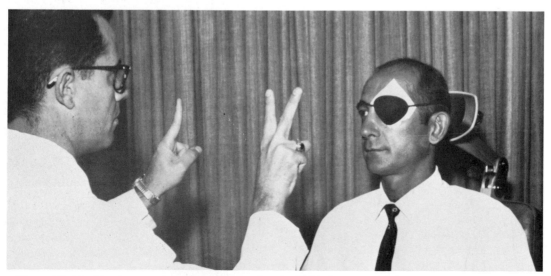

Figure 17–15 The three-stage confrontation test for visual field function. The examiner is in the second stage of the method—double simultaneous stimulation of the half-fields.

ize, some useful information about visual field function may be gained. The most useful numbers are one, two, five, and none.

In the second stage of the confrontation test, fingers are presented simultaneously in the two half-fields (Fig 17–15). The patient is asked to count the total number of fingers he sees. This "double simultaneous stimulation" of the right and left half-fields is particularly helpful in detecting subtle hemianopias.

In the third stage, the examiner's hands are waved in the two half-fields and the patient is asked to "point to the clearest hand." If the patient is unable to recognize any difference in the clarity of the examiner's hands, the visual field is judged normal. This method is of value in detecting the most subtle visual field defects that may be missed on first- or second-stage testing.

Projector Light Testing

This method has two major advantages over the confrontation and standard tangent screen examination: The presentation of the test target can be fully randomized, and the target size and intensity can be varied at will. The field can be quickly screened in less than five minutes. The examiner stands behind the patient during the test and repeatedly checks fixation by localization of the blind spot (Fig. 17–16). This method is adequate for neurosurgical diagnosis. If more detailed quantitation is needed, an ophthalmologist is usually consulted.

The visual field of each eye is recorded as the patient sees it with the fixation point represented anatomically by the macula and the field reversed relative to the visual pathways. Thus, the nasal retina sees the temporal field and the upper retina the lower field. The blind spot represents the visual field projection of the optic disc. The visual field can be divided into four quadrants by drawing an imaginary line vertically through the macula to divide the field into a right and a left half (Fig. 17–17). A horizontal line through the macula then divides the field into four quadrants. The same anatomical relationship of reversal of field to neural pathways (upper retina represents lower field) holds from the retina to the occipital lobe of the brain. In the occipital lobe, the major part of the cortex is devoted to representation of the macula.

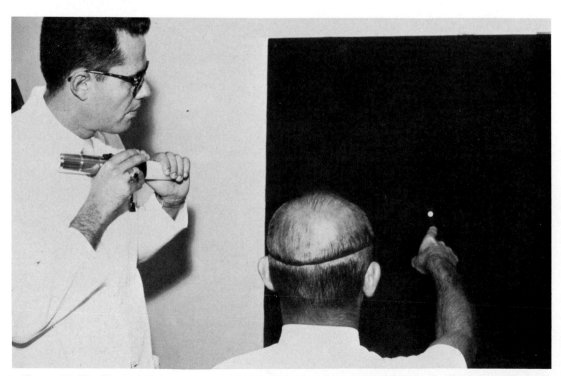

Figure 17–16 The projector light in visual field examination. The patient points to the light as a check on his responses.

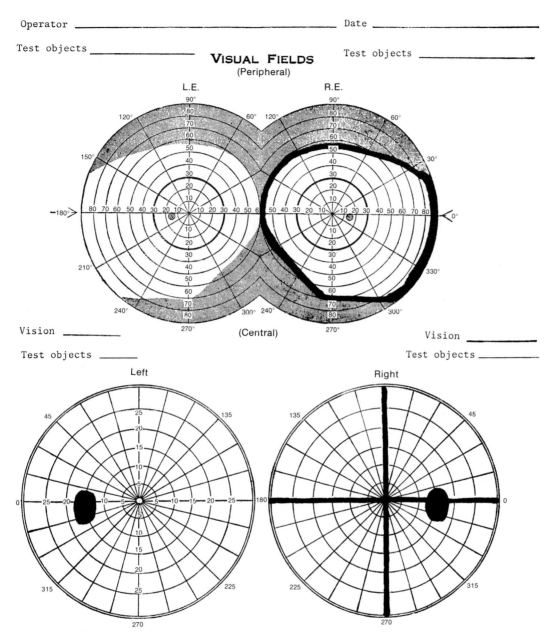

Figure 17-17 *Top,* Outline for peripheral (perimetric) visual field study. *Bottom,* The visual field may be divided into four quadrants as shown on the right. Normal blind spot size is shown also on central field plot (tangent screen).

Definition of Terms

Full field—the normal extent of the field of vision is: nasal = 60 degrees, temporal = 100+ degrees, superior = 60 degrees, and inferior = 70 to 75 degrees (Fig. 17–17). Tested at the tangent screen, with the patient 1 m from the screen, the blind spot is 15 degrees temporal to fixation and measures 132 by 96 mm with the 6/1000 white target.

Scotoma—a defect in the visual field that is surrounded by normal or relatively normal functioning field. The best example of a scotoma is the blind spot. It is a dense scotoma because it may be found even with large-diameter test objects, so long as they do not exceed the visual angle of the blind spot. Scotomas may be dense or relative (subtle).

Hemianopia—a defect in function of one half of the visual field. This includes those

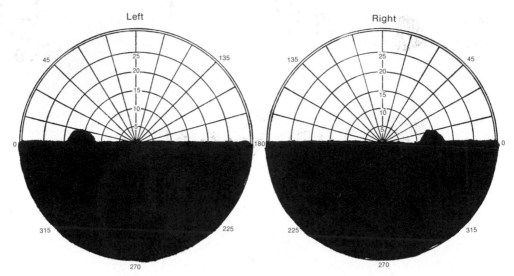

Figure 17–18 Bilateral altitudinal hemianopias.

types of visual field defects that involve the upper or lower half of the field of each eye, the so called altitudinal hemianopias (Fig. 17–18). If the field loss is homonymous, the lesion must be posterior to the chiasm. Bitemporal or binasal field loss is characteristic of lesions of the chiasm. The bitemporal type is most common.

Depression—the most common form of visual field dysfunction. It may be dense or relative, generalized or localized. Generalized depression of field function is commonly due to opacities of the ocular media (corneal scar, cataract) or weak stimulus intensity.

Congruous—a visual field defect that is essentially a carbon copy of another in the same half of visual space. The defects are called congruous in contradistinction to the defect seen in bitemporal hemianopia in which the field defects are "mirror images." Homonymous hemianopias tend to become more congruous as the lesion producing the defect moves toward the occipital cortex. Occipital lobe hemianopias tend to be extremely congruous. Congruity cannot be judged if the defect is a full hemianopia; some part of the half-field must be spared for the assessment of congruity.

Macular sparing—a much overrated sign for localization of the lesion producing the field defect. Classic teaching states that the further posterior a lesion is placed in the visual radiations, the more likely the chance that the field defect will spare fixation. In

the author's experience, even most occipital lobe hemianopias split fixation.

Field Loss as Related to Anatomical Location

Retina and Optic Nerve

Unilateral lesions of the retina and optic nerve produce disturbances of visual field only in the field of vision and of the involved eye. It the contralateral visual field is also involved there must be more than one lesion or the lesion, if only one exists, is posterior to the optic nerve. An altitudinal field defect in one eye often suggests retinal detachment or vascular optic nerve damage. Retinal detachment is usually preceded by subjective manifestations of flashing lights, a shower of dark spots, and finally the onset of a shade or veil before the involved eye. This may occur suddenly or over a matter of days. A common ocular manifestation of carotid ischemic disease is the transient ischemic attack. The patient complains of sudden loss of vision in the ipsilateral eye. The onset of the visual loss is often altitudinal, as is the recovery. The episode lasts only 5 to 15 minutes, and the patient may or may not note the simultaneous occurrence of crossed motor or sensory signs with the attack. Ophthalmic migraine and ischemic optic neuritis may also produce altitudinal visual field impairment.

The visual field defects produced by glaucoma are common, usually accompanied by significant glaucomatous optic atrophy, and when they are advanced, should be followed with the perimeter rather than the tangent screen.

Congenital anomalies of the optic disc may produce visual field disturbances. These lesions include tilting of the optic disc, coloboma, myopic temporal crescent, myelinated nerve fibers, and hyaline bodies of the optic nerve. Tilting of the disc and coloboma of the optic nerve and choroid are important, as they can produce bitemporal hemianopias on visual field examination. Hyaline bodies of the optic nerve head are a frequent cause of pseudopapilledema and often are associated with a defect in the inferior nasal field and enlargement of the blind spot (Fig. 17–19).

Several important causes for visual field loss are the nontoxic causes of optic nerve dysfunction. Multiple sclerosis frequently gives rise to optic neuritis. This typically presents as a retrobulbar neuritis with a tendency for rapid spontaneous remission and a central scotoma as the characteristic visual field defect (Fig. 17–19). Papilledema commonly causes enlargement of the blind spot and on rare occasions may have an associated central scotoma. This is seen only in severe choking when edema fluid leaks into the macular area and the central scotoma occurs. More commonly, a central scotoma follows papilledema when secondary optic atrophy is severe. When serial measurements of the blind spot diameter are used to follow the course of papilledema, at least a 6/1000 white target must be used. Ischemic optic neuropathy usually leaves visual acuity relatively spared, as compared to other forms of optic neuritis, and the common visual field defect is the inferior altitudinal type that is connected to the blind spot. Neuromyelitis optica generally presents as an acute bilateral papillitis with dense large-diameter central scotomas. Visual acuity is often reduced to bare light perception. Full remissions are not so common as in the retrobulbar neuritis of multiple sclerosis. Schilder's disease is a demyelinizing neurological process of children and young adults who have progressive visual loss, deterioration of mentation, and spastic paraplegia. Visual field loss, due to progressive optic atrophy or papilledema followed by atrophy, is often generalized with more profound effects seen in the central field early. Total blindness occurs late in the disease, and most patients do not live over two years. The hereditary optic atrophy of Leber is a disease of young males, although females are occasionally affected, that begins in the 15- to 20-year age group with sudden loss of central vision in one or both eyes. Central or cecocentral scotomas are found. Complete blindness may occur. The ophthalmoscopic appearance of the optic nerve and surrounding retina (pseudoedema, microtelangiectasia and lack of disc staining on fluorescein fundus photography) is virtually diagnostic of this disease.

Syphilitic optic neuritis is an infrequent

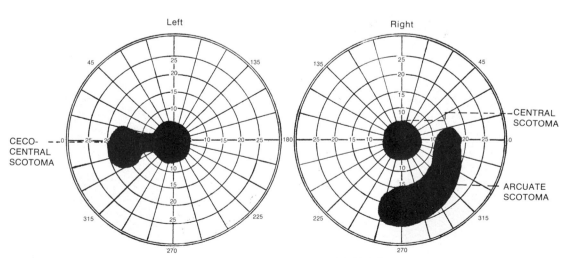

Figure 17–19 Optic nerve type of field defects.

cause of optic nerve disease and consequent visual field loss. Visual field defects may be produced as follows: (1) concentric peripheral contraction, (2) localized peripheral field wedge-shaped scotomas, (3) central and cecocentral scotomas (Fig 17–19), (4) central scotomas combined with peripheral defects, (5) altitudinal defects, and (6) field changes arising in the absence of any ophthalmoscopic evidence of optic nerve disease with defects arising at the blind spot. Peripheral damage to the optic nerve fibers is histologically more common than axial involvement, but central scotomas are seen in 53 per cent of patients with optic nerve injury from this cause.

Optic Chiasm

The classic visual field defect found in diseases affecting the chiasm is the bitemporal hemianopia (Fig. 17–20). Bitemporal hemianopias may be scotomatous or nonscotomatous. The former are more common with lesions in the area of the posterior chiasm; there may be a bitemporal paracentral scotoma. Kearns and Rucker described nerve fiber bundle defects and peripheral midzonal arcuate defects with chromophobe adenomas.[5] In the nonscotomatous type of defect only the peripheral field is influenced. Bitemporal field loss tends to progress clockwise in the right field and counterclockwise in the left field. Altitudinal deficits are rarely seen in chiasmal lesions. Unexplained optic atrophy should al-

ways arouse suspicion of disease in or about the chiasm.

Optic Tract

Primary lesions of the tract are rare. Visual field defects associated with tract dysfunction are most often the result of encroachment upon the tract by disease in surrounding structures. The close relationship of the circle of Willis, pituitary gland, and temporal lobe of the brain account for the majority of tract-induced visual field defects. These visual field defects are characterized by homonymous hemianopia, incongruity, variable density, and some macular sparing, and finally a complete loss of tract function results in a full hemianopia with splitting of fixation (Fig. 17–21).

Temporal Lobe

Because the temporal lobe carries the lower fibers of the visual radiations in its anterior segment, the Meyer's loop, an early lesion of the temporal lobe usually produces an upper quadrantic visual field defect opposite the side of the lesion. This may progress to full hemianopia. The main features of field defects associated with lesions of the temporal lobe are: homonymous hemianopia, incongruity, variable density, early defect starting along the vertical meridian, and early fixation encroachment (Fig. 17–22). Temporal lobe disease producing a defect in visual field function is

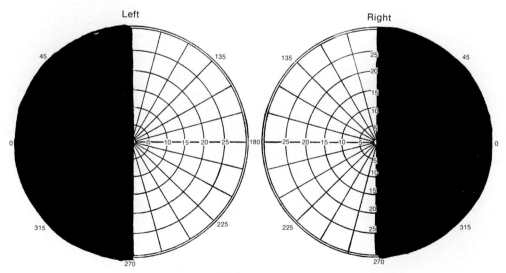

Figure 17–20   Full bitemporal hemianopia, dense.

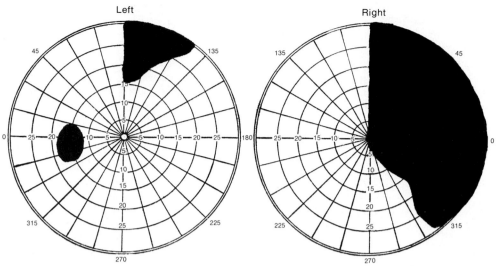

Figure 17–21 Incongruous right homonymous hemianopia (tract hemianopia).

often associated with symptoms of formed visual hallucinations, auditory or olfactory hallucinations, and teleopsia.

Parietal Lobe

The parietal lobe carries the majority of the visual radiations coming from the upper portion of the lateral geniculate body. An early lesion of the parietal lobe tends to produce a homonymous hemianopic visual field loss that is denser below than above. This may progress to a full hemianopia, just as can occur with extensive damage to the temporal lobe, lateral geniculate body, or optic tract. Parietal lobe field loss is more congruous than that of temporal lobe origin (Fig. 17–23). It is less so than that due to disease in the occipital lobe.

Occipital Lobe

The usual occipital lobe of visual field defect is homonymous hemianopic and congruous, and splits fixation (Fig. 17–24). Density varies markedly in these visual field disorders. Because the calcarine cortex is divided into an upper and lower bank, the visual field deficit may occupy only a quadrant. Ischemia of the upper bank of the

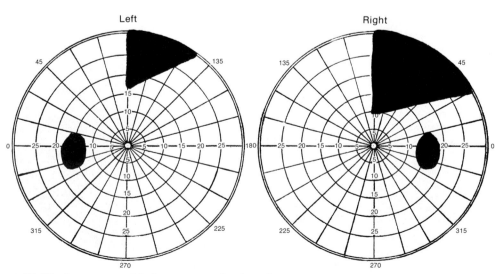

Figure 17–22 Incongruous right homonymous hemianopia upper quadrant defect of the temporal lobe type.

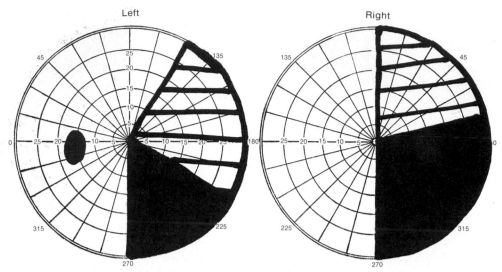

Figure 17–23   Right homonymous hemianopia, denser below than above, of the parietal lobe type.

left occipital lobe produces a right lower quadrant hemianopia. If the lesion is located very near the tip of the occipital pole, the visual field defect will tend toward a paracentral hemianopia. Lesions placed anteriorly in the occipital cortex classically produce the "monocular temporal crescent" type of field loss. The most anterior part of the occipital cortex receives the visual fibers from the peripheral retinae. The right anterior occipital lobe cortex, for example, takes the fibers from the temporal periphery of the right eye and the nasal periphery of the left eye. A lesion in that area of the occipital lobe would cause early loss

of the temporal field of the left eye, which would be impossible to find without the perimeter because only the extreme temporal field is lost. In fact, this type of visual field defect is rare with lesions of the occipital lobe.

If bilateral damage to the occipital lobe cortex occurs, the patient may develop cortical blindness. This is seen with severe ischemia due to saddle emboli of the basilar artery, most often, or with trauma to the occiput. Such blindness has been described in children with relatively minor trauma, but then it is generally of short duration. Cortical blindness has the following clinical

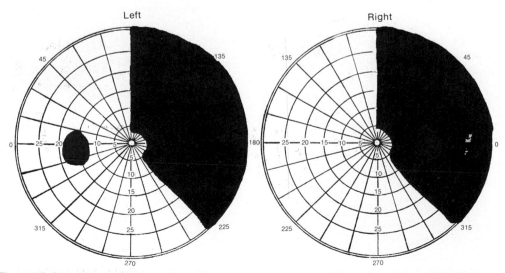

Figure 17–24   Congruous right homonymous hemianopia with macular sparing of the occipital lobe type.

characteristics: (1) bilateral homonymous hemianopias, (2) total blindness with intact pupillary responses, (3) denial of blindness, (4) visual hallucination, (5) confabulation as in Korsakoff's psychosis, (6) amnestic amnesia—loss of recent memory, (7) often no other localizing neurological signs, and (8) allochiria in which sensation from stimuli applied to one limb is localized by the patient in the opposite limb. Such blindness may follow ventriculography, but in these instances there is a much better prognosis for return of visual function than in the usual patient with cortical blindness. Homonymous hemianopias may follow arteriography, especially with direct carotid punctures. This also has a good prognosis for functional recovery.

OPHTHALMOSCOPY

The appearance of the optic disc is of major concern to the neurosurgeon, and this section confines itself entirely to discussion of that structure.

The normal optic nerve head usually appears larger in the myopic eye and smaller in the hyperopic eye. The myopic disc is often rather pale on the temporal side, suggesting optic atrophy. The hyperopic disc, especially in eyes with refractive errors of more than 4 diopters, may mimic papilledema. It is helpful to look at the patient's glasses to decide whether he is myopic or hyperopic. Myopic lenses minify objects viewed through them and hyperopic lenses magnify.

Papilledema, Pseudopapilledema, and Papillitis

Papilledema is the swelling of the tissues of the optic disc, usually because of an increase in intracranial pressure. The rise in pressure within the cranial vault is transmitted to the subarachnoid space around the optic nerves, as this space is continuous with the intracranial subarachnoid cavity. A rise in pressure within this space causes slowing of axoplasmic flow, which produces swelling of the optic nerve head. Vascular congestion of the disc produces transient ischemia that is subjectively realized as transient obscurations of vision. More prolonged ischemia with chronic papilledema may lead to atrophic degeneration of the optic nerve. The clinical signs of papilledema are (1) loss of a previously seen spontaneous venous pulse; (2) elevation of the disc; (3) blurring of the disc margins (especially temporally, as slight nasal blurring is normal); (4) overfilling of the retinal veins; (5) hemorrhages on the surface of the disc and later in surrounding retina; (6) concentric folds surrounding the disc, owing to edema fluid leaking from the disc; and (7) cystic elevation of the macula in chronic papilledema.

Papilledema requires several hours to develop. When it is well developed, it requires weeks to clear. Papilledema usually occurs in both eyes except in special circumstances. Pre-existing optic atrophy may mask the onset of disc swelling. Greatly increased spinal fluid pressure without papilledema means that there has been a false reading, not enough time for papilledema to develop, pre-existing optic atrophy, or a spinal subarachnoid block. Loss of the previously seen spontaneous venous pulse on the central retinal vein is the *earliest ophthalmoscopic sign of papilledema*. It is the first to return when intracranial pressure becomes normal. Transient obscurations of vision are common in patients with papilledema. They describe them as brief periods (seconds) of blurred, fuzzy, or hazy vision followed by instantaneous complete clearing of vision. Transient obscurations may occur hundreds of times per day and they may be unilateral or bilateral. Chronic papilledema may occur in patients with increased intracranial pressure over long periods of time. The ophthalmoscopic picture differs in this circumstance from that seen in the more typical onset of papilledema. Hemorrhages are less conspicuous, the surface of the disc appears dry, and the degree of elevation is often exceptional—4 diopters plus with the direct ophthalmoscope (Fig. 17–25).

The causes of pseudopapilledema include high hyperopic refractive errors, hyaline bodies of the optic nerve head, myelinated nerve fibers, and ischemic optic neuritis. In patients with hyperopia of more than 4 diopters, the disc is often elevated with some blurring of both the nasal and temporal margins. This is thought to be the result of crowding of nerve fibers as they enter the optic nerve in a small eye. The elevation of the disc is usually rather sym-

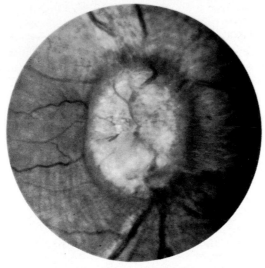

Figure 17–25 Chronic papilledema. Note the crenated surface of the disc, the marked elevation, and the concentric folds in the peripapillary retina.

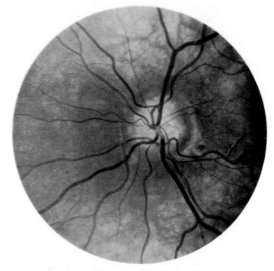

Figure 17–27 Hyaline bodies of the optic nerve located deeper in the substance of the disc.

metrical between the two eyes, the physiological cup is small to nonexistent, a spontaneous venous pulse is usually present, and there are no hemorrhages on the surface of the disc. The blind spot is small.

Hyaline bodies (drusen) of the optic nerve are developmental lesions and are often familial (50 per cent). They are round, laminated, translucent structures. They usually occur bilaterally, but may be very asymmetrical (Figs. 17–26 and 17–27). They are known to increase slowly in size,

but even though they may produce visual field defects, the patient rarely loses significant visual acuity. Although hyaline bodies are said to occur with increasing frequency in patients with tuberous sclerosis and neurofibromatosis, evidence now suggests that the hyaline masses seen at or near the disc in these diseases are astrocytic hamartomas and not simple products of secretion from the neuroglial structure in the nerve. Differentiation from papilledema may be difficult at times.

Myelinated nerve fibers usually occur at the margin of the disc (Fig. 17–28). My-

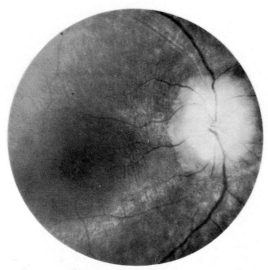

Figure 17–26 Hyaline bodies of the optic nerve. Note the irregular surface of the disc and the small cup.

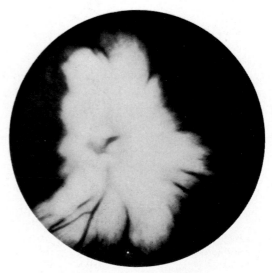

Figure 17–28 Myelinated nerve fibers.

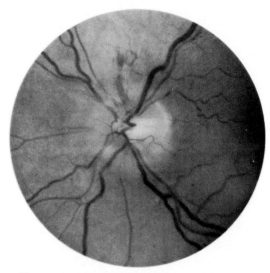

Figure 17-29 Ischemic optic neuritis. Blurred disc margins and flame hemorrhage at the edge of the disc mimic papilledema.

elination normally ends at the cribriform plate of the optic nerve. Occasionally it continues into the eye for variable distances, producing a patch of white on the surface of the retina. Its configuration is characteristic in that the patch has a "feathered edge" especially noticeable in the peripheral portion of the lesion. It may obscure parts of the retinal vessels, and vice versa, proving its superficial location. These are essentially stable deposits; they may be found in the peripheral retina also. They rarely produce a field defect except for a very relative scotoma. They may regress if the patient develops optic atrophy for any reason. These lesions are most often confused with exudates at the margin of the disc and are occasionally mistaken for evidence of papilledema.

Ischemic optic neuropathy is sometimes confused with papilledema (Fig. 17-29). It occurs in patients of 50 to 60 years. They often have pre-existing vascular disease (angina, claudication, myocardial infarction). The common complaint is sudden loss of visual field. Visual acuity is often good. The ophthalmoscopic findings are elevation of the disc, some degree of pallor, and one or more small flame hemorrhages at the edge of the blurred disc margin. The visual field deficit is characteristically inferior altitudinal. The process tends to be bilateral, but the attacks are usually separated by months or years. A patient who has had a previous bout of ischemic optic neuropathy will have primary optic atrophy as the residual. The eye with a fresh ischemic lesion of the nerve will show a picture much like papilledema. This has caused confusion in the past with the Foster Kennedy syndrome (primary optic atrophy ipsilateral to sphenoid wing meningioma with contralateral papilledema) (Fig. 17-30). The Foster Kennedy syndrome is very rare, whereas ischemic optic neuropathy is common. These patients deserve a careful work-up to identify diabetes mellitus, hypertensive cardiovascular disease, collagen vascular disease, lues, and cranial arteritis. Repeated measurement of the blood pressure in *both arms*, a carefully done three- to four-hour glucose tolerance test, erythrocyte sedimentation rate determination, and ophthalmodynamometry should be done in all such patients. If the sedimentation rate is over 30 mm per hour, a temporal artery biopsy should be obtained. Large amounts of systemic steroids or anticoagulation or both may be of value in gaining some return of visual function or preventing further ischemia. Women with a past history of migraine or other vascular disease should avoid using conjugated estrogens, as there is evidence that use of these medications may predispose the patient to ischemic disease of the optic nerve.

Papillitis is an ophthalmoscopic classification for optic neuritis in which the optic nerve involvement is located relatively far

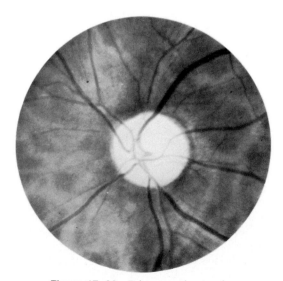

Figure 17-30 Primary optic atrophy.

anteriorly, producing elevation of the disc. The disc is usually more pink than normal owing to increased circulation through the capillaries on the surface. The physiological cup may be smaller than normal. The central retinal vessels are generally normal to somewhat full. There may be frank hemorrhage, and the surrounding retina is not infrequently involved. The process is then called neuroretinitis. It is more often unilateral than bilateral and may look like papilledema. The major distinguishing features are: (1) unilaterality, (2) marked acute loss of vision and visual field function, (3) "cells" in the vitreous, and (4) Marcus Gunn pupil. A partial list of the causes of optic neuritis is seen in Table 17–12.

Retrobulbar optic neuritis is another ophthalmoscopic class of optic neuritis in which the disc appears perfectly normal in the acute stage of the disease and often the only residual is some pallor of the temporal disc. There is often a profound loss of visual acuity in an eye that is ophthalmoscopically normal. It has the same causes as papillitis, but tends to suggest a diagnosis of demyelinizing disease when it is unilateral. Pain on motion of the eye is common. The attacks of retrobulbar optic neuritis associated with multiple sclerosis are generally unilateral, rarely bilateral, and almost never bilateral and simultaneous. The visual prognosis for the first attack is good in multiple sclerosis, which rarely occurs under the age of 10 years. Neuromyelitis optica, however, usually presents a bilateral simultaneous optic neuritis, and the visual prognosis is much less satisfactory.

Optic Atrophy

Four ophthalmoscopic classes of optic atrophy are: primary, secondary, glaucomatous, and consecutive. No cause is implied except in the case of glaucomatous atrophy.

Primary optic atrophy is, except for glaucomatous atrophy, the most common. It leaves the margins of the disc sharp, the central retinal vessels in their normal position, and the color of the disc "bone white." Loss of the exact outline of the physiological cup is frequent. Primary optic atrophy has causes as listed in Table 17–13.

Secondary optic atrophy is characterized by a generalized change of color of the disc

TABLE 17–12 CAUSES OF OPTIC NEURITIS (PARTIAL LIST)

Post-traumatic—direct ocular trauma or orbital trauma
Intraocular inflammatory—uveitis with bacterial, viral, fungal, or idiopathic etiology
Meningitis—due to any cause
Metabolic—diabetes mellitus, thyroid disease, nutrition (alcohol, tobacco, diet) related
Familial—Leber's optic neuritis
Toxic—drugs or heavy metals (Chloramphenicol, lead)
Demyelinizing disease—disseminated sclerosis, Schilder's disease, Devic's disease
Postinfectious—viral
"Septic foci"—teeth, sinuses, etc.
Idiopathic

from pink to a dirty gray. There is an associated proliferation of glial elements over the surface, often obscuring the physiological cup and making the margins of the disc difficult to outline. This type of atrophy follows on the heels of papilledema, regardless of cause, or papillitis.

Glaucomatous optic atrophy is recognized by enlargement and undercutting of the edge of the physiological cup, shifting of the central retinal vessels to the nasal side of the cup, and progressive loss of nerve substance at the temporal edge of the cup. Such changes are usually seen in those persons who have a definite increase in the intraocular pressure above normal limits (12 to 22 mm of mercury). In some the intraocular pressure may be normal or low, and yet a progressive loss of visual field and steady increase in atrophy occurs. These are the so-called "low-tension glaucoma" patients and they should be suspected of having carotid arterial insufficiency if the intraocular pressure is normal when measured repeatedly by applanation and if the atrophy is unilateral.

TABLE 17–13 SOME CAUSES OF PRIMARY OPTIC ATROPHY

Intoxication (alcohol, tobacco, diet)
Intracranial mass lesions (aneurysm, sphenoid wing meningioma, pituitary tumor, suprasellar mass, dilated third ventricle with internal hydrocephalus)
Compression from intraorbital mass lesion (meningioma, dermoid, pseudotumor, thyroid orbital disease, severe orbital hemorrhage)
Direct invasion (glioma of optic nerve)
Trauma (contusion, laceration associated with fracture of optic canal)
Demyelinizing disease
Vascular accidents of the optic nerve
Inflammatory disease of the nerve (tuberculosis, lues) may produce this type of atrophy rather than the usual form of postinflammatory atrophy

Consecutive optic atrophy follows disease of the retina or the choroid and retina. Extensive damage to the retina is needed to produce significant consecutive atrophy. Central retinal artery occlusion causes consecutive optic atrophy because of degeneration of the internal layers of the retina following the occlusion. It is also common in retinitis pigmentosa.

REFERENCES

1. Bender, M. B., and Fulton, J. F.: Factors in functional recovery following section of the oculomotor nerve in monkeys. J. Neurol. Psychiat., 2:285, 1939.
2. Cogan, D. G., and Victor, M.: Ocular signs of Wernicke's disease. A.M.A. Arch. Ophthal., 51:204–211, 1954.
3. Fischer, K. C., and Schwartzman, R. J.: Oral corticosteroids in the treatment of ocular myasthenia gravis. Neurology (Minneap.), 24:795–798, 1974.
4. Glaser, J. S.: Myasthenic pseudo-internuclear ophthalmoplegia. Arch. Ophthal. (Chicago), 75:363–366, 1966.
5. Kearns, T. P., and Rucker, C. W.: Arcuate defects in the visual fields due to chromophobe adenoma of the pituitary gland. Amer. J. Ophthal., 45:505–507, 1958.
6. Kernohan, J. W., and Woltman, H. W.: Incisura of the crus due to contralateral brain tumor. Arch. Neurol. Psychiat., 21:274, 1929.
7. Kestenbaum, A.: Clinical Methods of Neuro-ophthalmologic Examination. 2nd Ed., New York, Grune & Stratton, 1961.
8. Kiloh, L. G., and Nevin, S.: Progressive dystrophy of the external ocular muscles. Brain, 74:115–143, 1951.
9. Smith, J. L., and David, N. J.: Internuclear ophthalmoplegia. Two new clinical signs. Neurology (Minneap.), 14:307–309, 1964.
10. Thompson, H. S., and Mensher, J. H.: Adrenergic mydriasis in Horner's syndrome. The hydroxyamphetamine test for diagnosis of postganglionic defects. Amer. J. Ophthal., 72:472–480, 1971.

18

NEUROTOLOGY

The otorhinolaryngological subspecialty of neurotology deals with the anatomy, physiology, and abnormalities of the three cranial nerves that traverse the temporal bone—the cochlear, vestibular, and facial nerves—and with the specific tests of their functions. The facial nerve is discussed in Chapter 67.

ANATOMY OF THE INNER EAR

The eighth cranial, or vestibulocochlear, nerve consists of two distinct components, the cochlear and the vestibular nerves. The latter originates in the sensory cells of the vestibular labyrinth, while the cochlear (or acoustic) nerve arises in the cochlea.

To best understand the functions of the eighth cranial nerve, the reader should be familiar with the complex structure of both the vestibular and the auditory systems.

In the young embryo, the neurosensory portions of the vestibulocochlear system are derived from ectoderm. With growth and development, these neurosensory epithelial structures become incorporated within the petrous portion of the temporal bone and are enclosed in the otic capsule. At the same time, the middle ear space develops as an invagination from the first (pharyngeal) pouch and comes to lie lateral to the otic capsule. Meanwhile, the external ear develops from the overlying epithelium and the fundus of its canal abuts the middle ear space at the tympanic membrane.

The adult form of the vestibulocochlear labyrinth consists of a continuous complex of bony spaces within the petrous bone, enclosed in the otic capsule. This is the bony labyrinth. It is filled with perilymph (cerebrospinal fluid), and suspended within it is an almost true, miniature replica of the bony spaces—the membranous labyrinth. The labyrinth is filled with endolymph (Fig. 18–1).

It is convenient to divide the vestibulocochlear labyrinth into cochlear and vestibular components. The vestibular labyrinth lies posterior to the cochlea.

The Cochlea

The cochlea (Gr., "snail") is made up of a spiral hollow tube that is coiled two and one half times. The bony center, around which the spiral is coiled, assumes the shape of a tapered screw (L., modiolus) if the outer parts of the bony spiral are removed. The long axis of the modiolus has a sloping anterolateral orientation in the head, its base abutting the anterior part of the fundus of the internal acoustic meatus. Fine canals within the modiolus house the branches of the cochlear nerve and their bipolar cell bodies, which constitute the spiral ganglion.

The most basal turn of the bony tube of the cochlea forms a distinct promontory on the medial wall of the mesotympanum (middle ear) and is the only part of the cochlea that is visible during operations on the middle ear. The rest is enclosed within the petrous bone. At the posterior aspect of the promontory there are two windows: the oval window above, which faces laterally and houses the footplate of the stapes; and the round window below, which is contained within a niche and faces posteriorly. The fundus of this niche contains a fine membrane—the secondary tympanic (round window) membrane.

The inner structure of the cochlea may best be appreciated if the bony canal were

L. BERNSTEIN, D. J. KIENER, AND C. A. McMURTRY

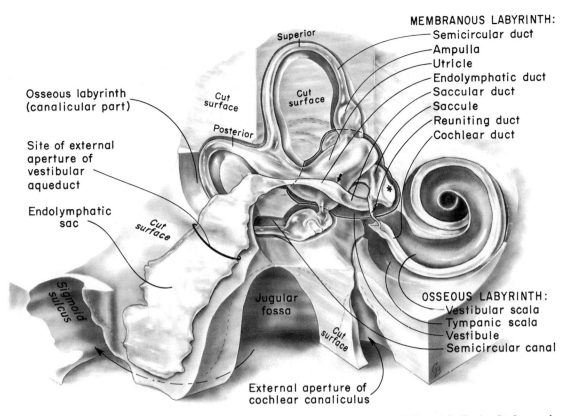

Figure 18–1 Bony and membranous labyrinths. (From Paparella, M. M., and Shumrick, D. A.: Otolaryngology. Vol. I. Philadelphia, W. B. Saunders Co., p. 93. Reprinted by permission.)

to be imagined as a straight tube (Fig. 18–2). A longitudinal section through this unfurled cochlea shows that the tube is divided into upper and lower compartments by the basilar membrane. The two compartments communicate with each other at the apex through a hole (the helicotrema) at the tip of the basilar membrane. At the base of the upper compartment, called the scala vestibuli, is the oval window, and at the base of the lower compartment, the scala tympani, is the round window. These two scalae contain perilymph.

The basilar membrane has resting on it a somewhat complex structure that is best appreciated in cross section. Its upper surface and a thin, sloping membrane above it form a tube that is sealed at the helicotrema. This tube is called the scala media, or cochlear duct, and its overlying sloping roof is Reissner's membrane. It contains endolymph (Fig. 18–3). Stretching along the entire basilar membrane, like a ribbon, is the spiral organ of Corti. This contains the sensory epithelium of the cochlear nerve. Viewed from above, the organ of

Figure 18–2 Graphic representation of uncoiled cochlea, shown in longitudinal section. Note the stapes fitting into the oval window and communicating with the perilymph of the scala vestibuli, while the round window membrane seals the base of the scala tympani. The horizontal party wall represents the cochlear duct, which contains the basilar membrane and the organ of Corti.

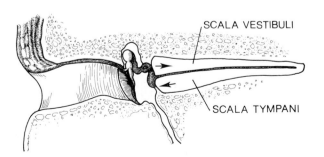

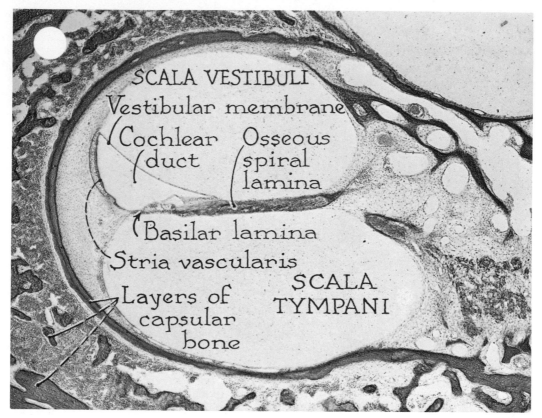

Figure 18–3   Section through one coil of a cochlea in a fetus of 23 weeks. (From Anson, B. J., and McVay, C. B.: Surgical Anatomy. Vol. I. Philadelphia, W. B. Saunders Co., 1971, p. 22. Reprinted by permission.)

Corti is widest near the helicotrema and narrowest at the base. Consequently, reception of the high frequencies is located near the base, while that of the low frequencies is at the apical turns.

The organ of Corti, shown in Figure 18–4, consists of an outer and an inner row of sensory cells, called hair cells because of the filamentous neural fibrils that take origin in them. The two rows of hair cells slope against each other, forming a canal between them, which is triangular in cross section. This is the tunnel of Corti. An apparently cantilevered rooflike structure extends outward in the scala media to hover over the hair cells and is called the tectorial membrane.

From the base of the modiolus, bundles of the cochlear nerve fibers enter the fundus of the internal auditory meatus and almost immediately fuse into a single nerve trunk. The nerve traverses the anteroinferior part of the meatus and enters the pons to synapse in the ventral and dorsal cochlear nuclei in the floor of the fourth ventricle. The nuclei partly encircle the inferior cerebellar peduncle at the junction between the pons and the medulla oblongata. The dorsal cochlear nucleus forms an eminence, the acoustic tubercle, on the most lateral part of the floor of the brain stem.

The foregoing is a rather simplistic description of the cochlea. A more detailed description of the vestibulocochlear labyrinth can be found in appropriate textbooks.[3,12]

The Vestibular Labyrinth

The vestibular labyrinth consists of an expansion that is continuous with the basal turn of the cochlea, the vestibule, and three semicircular bony canals. The canals are at exact right angles to each other, each representing a dimension in space. Thus, there is a horizontal, or lateral, canal and two verti-

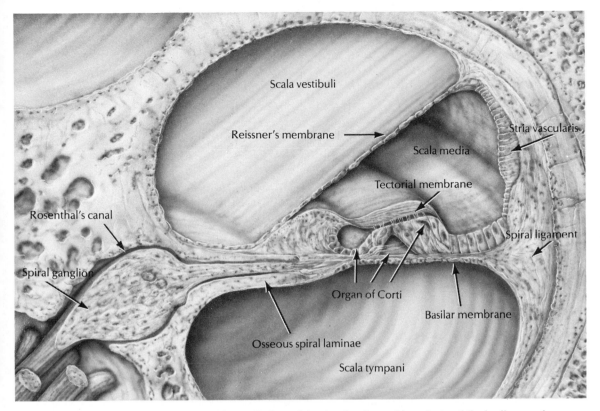

Scala vestibuli

Reissner's membrane

Scala media

Stria vascularis

Tectorial membrane

Rosenthal's canal

Spiral ligament

Spiral ganglion

Organ of Corti

Basilar membrane

Osseous spiral laminae

Scala tympani

Figure 18–4 Section through a cochlear coil of an adult, showing the cochlear duct and the basilar membrane with the organ of Corti. (From English, G. M.: Otolaryngology. New York, Harper & Row, 1976, p. 22. Reprinted by permission.)

cal canals, one termed superior and the other posterior (see Fig. 18–1).

Each canal originates from the lateral aspect of the vestibule and has its return insertion into the vestibule at a more medial location. While the lateral semicircular canal has its own insertion, however, the vertical canals join into a common crus prior to joining the vestibule. Near the origin of each canal, there is a globular expansion within it, known as the ampulla.

Within the bony vestibular labyrinth is a hollow, membranous replica of the system, approximately one quarter its size. Thus, there are three semicircular ducts, each with a distention at the bony ampulla. The distended area houses the neuroepithelium of the respective duct. Within the vestibule proper there are two baglike distentions, the utricle and the saccule, collectively termed the otolith organs. Each otolith organ contains a mass of neural epithelium. As stated previously, the membranous labyrinth is bathed in perilymph, while its own cavities are filled with endolymph.

Each membranous ampulla contains within it a flame-shaped, gelatinous structure called the cupula, which sits on a bony crest, the crista ampullaris (Fig. 18–5). This organ has embedded within it the neuroepithelial cells and their fine hairlike neurofibrils. These are the peripheral beginnings of the vestibular nerve.

The neuroepithelium of the otolith organs is similar in composition to that of the cupulas, although the cells are squat and occupy wider areas; they are termed maculae. The saccular and utricular maculae are distinguished by the very fine sandlike granules (otoconia) that cover their surface, hence "otolith."

From each neuroepithelial area, the vestibular nerve fibrils converge to form fine vestibular branches. These perforate the fundus of the internal acoustic meatus, where they join their cell bodies, the latter forming Scarpa's ganglion. Proximal to the cell bodies, the nerve fibers combine to form two vestibular branches, and these soon join to form the main vestibular nerve.

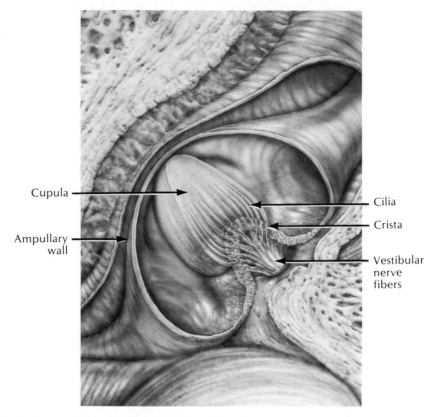

Cupula

Ampullary wall

Cilia

Crista

Vestibular nerve fibers

Figure 18–5   Cutaway illustration of the ampulla of a semicircular canal. (From English, G. M.: Otolaryngology. New York, Harper & Row, 1976, p. 77. Reprinted by permission.)

The nerve enters the pons where its fibers synapse within the four vestibular nuclei in the floor of the fourth ventricle: the superior nucleus of Bekhterev, the lateral nucleus of Deiters, the medial nucleus of Schwalbe, and the inferior nucleus of Roller.

The supranuclear connections in the vestibular system are important, and familiarity with them is necessary to an understanding of the system (Fig. 18–6). The medial longitudinal fasciculus joins the vestibular nuclei to all of the other cranial nerve nuclei, and of particular interest are the connections with cranial nerves III, IV, and VI as well as X. There are also the important vestibulocerebellar tract and the vestibulospinal tract, which connects the vestibular nuclei with all the striated muscles of the body. Fibers also connect these nuclei with the cortex of the temporal lobe. Additional connections involve the autonomic system.

Blood is supplied to the membranous lab-yrinth via a very thin labyrinthine branch of either the basilar artery or the anterior inferior cerebellar artery. This divides into two terminal branches, cochlear and vestibular rami.

The contents of the internal auditory meatus are not only diagnostically valuable but the relationships of the structures to each other are of paramount importance for proper orientation in performing translabyrinthine operations. These features are illustrated in Figures 18–7 and 18–8.

THE VESTIBULAR SYSTEM

Physiology of the Vestibular System

Propulsion and orientation of the body in space is dependent on the vestibular system, on vision, and on the muscle-joint system. Most persons can manage with only two of these systems, but not with one. Accordingly, a patient with a vestibular dis-

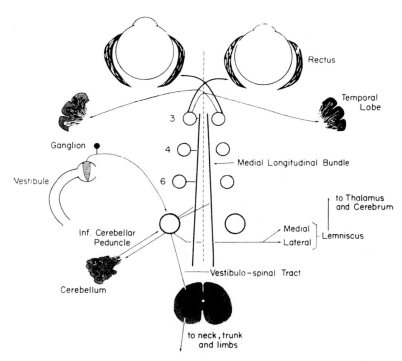

Figure 18-6 Diagrammatic scheme of central connections of the vestibular nuclei. Numbered circles represent cranial nerve nuclei. (From Bernstein, L.: The etiology and diagnosis of vertigo. Arch. Otolaryng., 76:330, 1962. Reprinted by permission.)

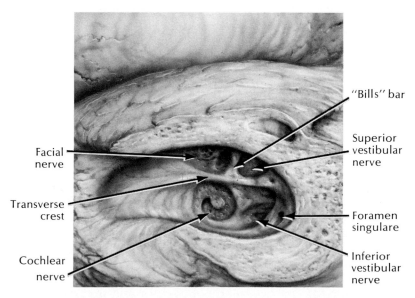

Figure 18-7 Internal auditory meatus of right temporal bone. (From English, G. M.: Otolaryngology. New York, Harper & Row, 1976, p. 25. Reprinted by permission.)

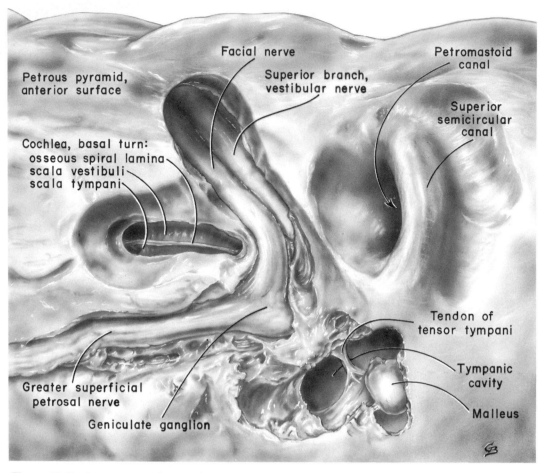

Figure 18–8   Arrangement of nerves in right internal auditory meatus. (From Anson, B. J., and Donaldson, J. A.: Surgical Anatomy of the Temporal Bone and Ear. Ed. 3. Philadelphia, W. B. Saunders Co., 1981, p. 655. Reprinted by permission.)

turbance may have trouble moving about in the dark, where he is deprived of vision also.

The vestibular system, through its peripheral neuroepithelial elements and their various connections, constantly signals the position of the head in space and effects a continuous adjustment of the musculature of the body. More specifically, it signals acceleration and deceleration of motion. The otolith organs are capable of signaling only linear acceleration or deceleration, whereas the neuroepithelial elements within the semicircular ducts are able to signal angular acceleration or deceleration. Constant motion cannot be signaled by the vestibular system.

The registration of accelerated motion is brought about by movement of the endolymph, which in turn displaces the neuro-epithelium. The shearing force exerted on the cells presumably acts as the stimulus. The resting discharge from the crista of a semicircular duct is greatly increased when the neuroepithelium is displaced toward the opening of the ampulla into the vestibule, an ampullopetal displacement, whereas the discharge from a reverse (ampullofugal) displacement is much less. The explanation for this may be that an ampullopetal displacement is probably more physiological than an ampullofugal displacement. It is consequently reasonable to think of the two vestibular systems as being protagonists— the one system propelling its half of the body toward the other side, the vector being a forward propulsion.

Normally, this bilateral system is constantly at work, receiving signals and passing them on to regulate posture and movements of the body, limbs, and eyes. Under normal circumstances, the vestibular stimulus is minimal and more or less equal bilaterally. Consequently, conscious perception of this vestibular activity occurs rather rarely, and then only in association with disease or abnormal stimulation. This abnormal perception is manifested as vertigo, which is the only symptom of vestibular dysfunction. Abnormal perception of vestibular function usually results from unequal stimuli of the paired vestibular system, as may happen when one side is stimulated by an irritating disease, or when it is suppressed by a process such as ischemia, or when one ear is being subjected to a caloric irrigation; or during the irregular and uneven assault on both organs in vehicular travel that may manifest itself as motion sickness.

Vertigo is defined as a hallucination of movement in any plane or direction. That is to say, the senses of the subject are deceived so that he feels himself move or else sees abnormal movement of his surroundings.

The vestibular system may best be studied when only one side is stimulated. If the cupula of a horizontal semicircular canal is displaced forward, it causes the eyes to deviate to the opposite side. A center, thought to be in the midbrain, then signals a return of the eyes to the neutral position. The vestibular stimulus produces a relatively slow movement of the eyes, while the central stimulus produces a rapid return. This is the basis for vestibular nystagmus, which may be defined as an abnormal spontaneous or an induced involuntary, sustained, rhythmic, coupled movement of the eyes consisting of a slow (vestibular) phase in one direction followed by a quick (central) return in the opposite direction. Unfortunately, the direction of the nystagmus has erroneously been established according to the fast component—which may lead to some confusion.

Nystagmus may also be termed according to its degree. First degree: present only when the gaze is in the direction of the quick component. Second degree: present with the gaze straight ahead; accentuated when looking in the direction of the quick component; absent when looking in the opposite direction. Third degree: present in all directions of gaze, but progressively more accentuated as the gaze turns toward the direction of the quick component.

Spontaneous vestibular nystagmus may also be classified as irritative and destructive. An irritating lesion will produce nystagmus with the quick component to the same side, indicating stimulation of a viable vestibular organ. Once the irritating process has gone on to destroy the vestibular function, the nystagmus is reversed so that the quick component is now toward the good ear, indicating lack of function in the diseased vestibule.

As stated earlier, nystagmus, the only sign of a vestibular disorder, may be spontaneous or induced. Spontaneous nystagmus is usually associated with some disturbance of the vestibular system, although it may be found in 5 to 10 per cent of normal subjects. On the other hand, nystagmus may be induced as a test of vestibular function.

Tests of Vestibular Function

The methods of inducing vertigo and nystagmus consist of subjecting the vestibular system to warm or cold stimuli, and positional testing. Other methods consist of spinning and swinging the body, subjecting it to centrifugal and gravitational insults, and stimulating the vestibular nerve with a galvanic current; however, these tests are not discussed here. Nystagmus alone can also be induced by opticokinetic stimuli.

The Caloric Test

If an external auditory canal is irrigated with water above or below body temperature, this sets up eddy currents in the endolymph of the lateral semicircular duct due to the induced change in its specific gravity. The resultant infinitesimal movement of the endolymph is sufficient to bring about a shearing stimulus to the cupula within the ampulla of that semicircular duct.

The caloric test is done with the patient supine and the head elevated 30 degrees. Because the lateral semicircular canal is at 30 degrees to the horizontal plane in the erect position, this places it in the vertical plane. Thus, it is equally sensitive to both warm (ampullopetal) and cold (ampullofugal) stimuli.

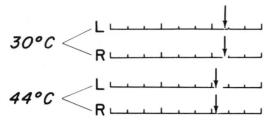

Figure 18–9 Normal response to bithermal caloric test.

The test is done by irrigating the external ear canal with either a given quantity of water at a set temperature, or with a quantity of water at a given temperature for a set period of time. The induced nystagmus is timed from the beginning of the irrigation until the nystagmus ceases. In the presence of a perforated tympanic membrane, the caloric test may be performed with cooled or warmed air or both.

Two varieties of tests are available. The cold caloric test employs 5 ml of ice water. If no response is elicited, then 10 ml of ice water is used, and so on until a stimulus is obtained or a decision is made that the vestibule is not responsive.

The other test—devised by Fitzgerald, Hallpike, and Cawthorne, and known as the bithermal caloric test—employs irrigations at 30°C and 44°C, both being equidistant from normal body temperature and, hence, an equal stimulus in both the ampul-

lopetal and the ampullofugal directions.[8] Each ear is irrigated for 30 seconds with at least 250 ml of water.

A normal response lasts about 2.0 minutes (Fig. 18–9). Abnormal responses are recorded as either canal paresis (hypofunction), or as directional preponderance (Fig. 18–10). Longer periods of caloric-induced nystagmus are usually associated with central lesions. Thus, directional preponderance of caloric nystagmus may assist in localizing a lesion of the temporal lobe on the side of the prolongation.

Electronystagmography

Certain individuals can suppress induced nystagmus, especially by fixing the eyes. Thus, a skater is able to stop suddenly from a rapid spin and have neither nystagmus nor vertigo, as long as he keeps his eyes open; however, if he were to close his eyes after a spin, he would immediately lose his balance. To overcome the patient's ability to fix his gaze, the caloric test is sometimes done with Frenzel's lenses over his eyes. A better method yet is electronystagmography (ENG), which takes advantage of the retinocorneal electrical potential and is done with the patient's eyes closed. The additional advantages of electronystagmography are that it provides a permanent record of the eye movements and it also facilitates accurate measurement of the velocity

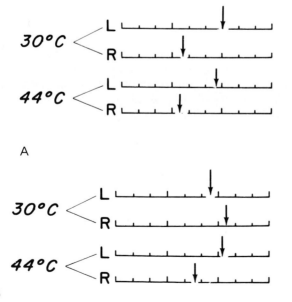

Figure 18–10 Basic abnormal responses of bithermal caloric tests. *A*. Canal paresis (hypofunction) on right side. *B*. Directional preponderance on left.

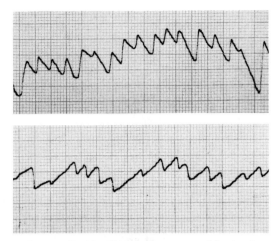

Figure 18-11 Electronystagmographic tracings showing the response of the right ear to cold stimulation (above) and to warm (below). The sloping stroke represents the slow vestibular component. By measuring its slope, its speed may be determined in degrees per second.

of the slow phase of the nystagmus as well as its duration.

In clinical practice, electronystagmographic recordings are usually obtained for spontaneous nystagmus, during positional testing, and with caloric stimulation. Nystagmic rhythms are identified as a sustained saw-tooth pattern, which slopes one way or the other, the sloping stroke representing the slow vestibular component of the nystagmus. It is this slope that is measured to obtain the velocity in degrees per second (Fig. 18-11).

Positional Tests

Positional tests may be done with the eyes open, so that the eyes may be observed for nystagmus; or they may be done with electronystagmography with the eyes closed. In one type of test, the supine subject's head is merely placed alternately in the straight ahead and first one and then the other lateral position.

The second, and more relevant, test consists of suddenly placing the patient's head in one of three positions. The subject is seated with his feet on an examining table so that, if he were supine, his head would hang over the edge of the table. His head is turned toward the examiner, who holds it between his hands—the thumbs just under the lower lids to keep them open, if no recording is being made. The subject is then suddenly placed in the supine position so that the head hangs slightly over the edge of the table. The examiner bends down with the subject and watches the eyes for positional nystagmus (Fig. 18-12).

After the nystagmus has ceased and the patient has been given a brief rest, he is suddenly sat upright and his eyes are again observed for nystagmus. The test is repeated with the head turned in the opposite lateral direction and then with the head straight ahead.

Two types of abnormal responses may be seen. Type 1: There is immediate nystagmus, which may change its direction with or without changing the position of the head. Being of central etiology, this variety is also referred to as malignant. It is not adaptable and may not be accompanied by vertigo. Type 2: After the head is placed in the critical position, there is a latent period of about 10 seconds. The nystagmus, which may be rotary, usually has a very intense onset and dies off in about 20 seconds. It is always accompanied by vertigo and its direction does not change. On repeating the test, the subsequent responses are progressively diminished, and they may not appear at all after two or three tries. Usually, however, it will again be demonstrable after a period of two to three hours. This nystagmus is of the peripheral variety and is referred to as benign.

Opticokinetic Nystagmus

This phenomenon is also known as railroad nystagmus. As the passenger looks

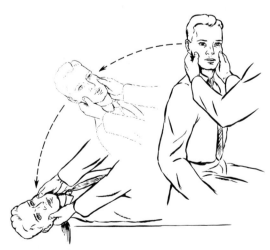

Figure 18-12 Positional testing for nystagmus.

out from the train window, the nystagmus is induced by his looking at the objects that are being passed. Clinically, it may be induced by having the subject watch a rotating drum with vertically oriented stripes on it, or a carpenter's tape while it is being pulled from its spool. The quick component will be in the direction opposite to the motion of the drum or the tape.

Opticokinetic nystagmus is normally equal bilaterally, and its suppression on one side is a valuable localizing sign. Thus, suppression on one side is indicative of a lesion in the opposite parietal lobe. The optico-kinetic test is also of value in differentiating between vestibular and ocular nystagmus—it will accentuate a spontaneous vestibular nystagmus but will have no effect on nystagmus of ocular origin.

The Differential Diagnosis of Vertigo

In attempting to establish the diagnosis of vertigo, it is most essential to obtain an accurate and detailed history. In most instances, this will prove to be the most significant aspect of the work-up and should give a good indication of the diagnosis in most cases.

In obtaining the history, it is very important that the patient be encouraged to describe his symptoms. The word "dizzy" should not necessarily be accepted without a detailed description. Vertigo may best be defined as a hallucination of motion of any kind and in any direction. "Objective" vertigo implies the hallucination of movement of objects or of the environment, and "subjective" applies to the patient himself. There is no clinical difference between the two terms; they are merely used to confirm the symptoms. The definition of vertigo does not include lightheadedness, nausea, a feeling of faintness, or a feeling that the subject may fall.

In addition to the standard examination of the ear, nose, and throat, a routine neurological examination of the head and neck is carried out. The corneal reflex should not be neglected, since its diminution is often the first additional sign in tumors of the cerebellopontine angle.

Examination of the ears is of particular value. Mild vertigo may be caused by impacted cerumen, foreign bodies in the external canal, retraction of the tympanic membrane, and trauma of the middle ear. Cholesteatoma as well as suppurative otitis media should always be suspect as a cause of the vertigo.

Labyrinthine Fistula Test

In the presence of a perforated tympanic membrane in a patient with vertigo, the labyrinthine fistula test should always be performed. It should also be noted that a positive fistula test with an intact tympanic membrane may be encountered in patients who have had fenestration or stapedectomy operations, or with syphilis of the central nervous system.

The fistula test is performed routinely in any patient with vertigo whose tympanic membrane is perforated or to whom the foregoing conditions apply. The air in the external auditory canal is compressed with a pneumatic otoscope. A positive result leads to transient conjugate deviation of the eyes to the opposite side. Negative pressure will cause deviation to the affected ear. A positive fistula test in chronic suppurative otitis media implies the presence of an erosion of the otic capsule down to the endosteum of the labyrinthine cavity. For the test to be positive, the involved vestibule must be viable.

A rare offshoot of a labyrinthine fistula is the Tullio phenomenon. In such cases, the patient is literally thrown off balance by the sudden application of a loud sound to the affected ear.

At the completion of the physical examination, tests for stance, gait, and position are performed. Vestibular and audiometric tests are then carried out. Radiographs of the temporal bones are usually ordered when the diagnosis is not clear. These may be supplemented by special radiographic procedures—such as tomography, angiography, and posterior fossa myelography, depending on the differential diagnosis.

Differentiating Between Central and Peripheral Lesions

When a patient presents with vertigo as a major complaint, one of the earliest differentiations that needs to be made is between an abnormality of the peripheral neuron and a lesion of the supranuclear connections of the vestibular system. In a peripheral lesion, vertigo of any significance is accompanied by nystagmus and the two are usually directly related. Furthermore, spontaneous vertigo and nystagmus of peripheral origin rarely last longer than three weeks. Also, because of the close anatomical relationship of the peripheral vestibular and cochlear systems, the presence of concomitant auditory symptoms suggests a peripheral lesion.

On the other hand, in central lesions, the vertigo and nystagmus are not usually proportional. In fact, the patient may present with gross nystagmus without complaining of vertigo. Because of the location and progression of most central lesions that cause vertigo, there are usually other symptoms and signs that should alert the physician to the correct diagnosis.

Although in most instances of vertigo the routine physical examination may be negative, attention should be directed to the often present phenomenon of spontaneous nystagmus. This is of greatest significance in the primary position of gaze with the eyes straight ahead. Spontaneous nystagmus on lateral gaze is often physiological and not of importance, unless excessive or unusual in type. Spontaneous vertical or diagonal nystagmus is usually diagnostic of a central nervous system lesion, as is the case when nystagmus in different directions exists in the two eyes or when the nystagmus tends to change its direction from time to time.

In positional testing, if the nystagmus is preceded by a latent period and the phenomenon shows adaptability, it is most probably a peripheral lesion. This is also supported by the fact that the direction of the nystagmus stays constant. On the other hand, the changing direction of the nystagmus and the lack of a latent period and of adaptability are more characteristic of a central cause of the condition.

Vertigo of Central Origin

As stated previously, on being confronted by a patient suffering from vertigo, one of the most important things to do is to exclude the possibility of any disorder within the central nervous system. This, in spite of the fact that 9 out of 10 cases of vertigo are likely to be caused by a lesion of the peripheral neuron of the vestibular nerve.[4] Although only few of the peripheral causes of vertigo may be dangerous to health, most of the factors responsible for central vertigo may not only be associated with serious disease, but may also be life-threatening. We shall, therefore, first of all consider those conditions of the central nervous system that cause vertigo.

Even though vertigo may be a prominent symptom in these patients, often there are other features that indicate a lesion within the central nervous system. Therefore, the complaint of vertigo may well be overlooked. It should also be remembered that spontaneous nystagmus due to involvement of the central vestibular pathways in the brain stem may persist indefinitely, even though the vertigo may not be in proportion to the nystagmus; or, it may not even be a symptom any longer.

Epilepsy

Any patient who loses consciousness during a vertiginous disturbance should be suspected of having epilepsy. Suspicion is usually strengthened with repeated episodes. The diagnosis may be confirmed by electroencephalography, which usually shows some focal activity in these cases. This condition may have to be differentiated from orthostatic syncope, which is also usually preceded by vertigo.

Two types of presentations may be encountered. On the one hand, vertigo may occur as an aura in about 16 per cent of cases of epilepsy.[9] A vertiginous aura may precede petit mal, grand mal, or psychogenic seizures. As such, it constitutes no diagnostic problem, since it is followed by the typical features of an epileptic seizure.

On the other hand, vertiginous epilepsy, though rare, is characterized by recurrent attacks of transient vertigo accompanied by momentary loss of consciousness. The latter may be obvious to an observer, but may be unknown to the patient himself. There is no fall and no other associated symptoms. Often there is amnesia for the duration of the attack. The diagnosis is usually heavily supported by positive electroencephalographic findings.[2]

Multiple Sclerosis

Vertigo may be the first and, for some time, the only symptom in many cases of multiple sclerosis.[11] Most commonly there are other symptoms of central nervous system involvement. It is interesting to note that, by the time a diagnosis is made, the vertigo is hardly an important complaint, although gross spontaneous nystagmus may be present.

Vascular Accidents

If an intracranial blood vessel ruptures or becomes thrombosed, sudden vertigo may be an early feature; however, this is soon overshadowed by other, more serious, symptoms. In fact, a leaking aneurysm in the cerebellopontine angle may present symptoms resembling Ménière's disease for some time before the true diagnosis is even suspected.[11]

When the anterior inferior and posterior inferior cerebellar arteries become thrombosed, a definite syndrome may be produced owing to involvement of the brain stem and the cerebellum.[1,7] In addition to the signs of cerebellar injury, this usually consists of vertigo—often associated with nausea and vomiting—deafness, and tinnitus as well as involvement of other cranial nerves, notably the facial. A homolateral Horner's syndrome and diminished sensation of pain, temperature, and touch may be elicited on physical examination.

Tumors of the Posterior Cranial Fossa

These tumors can give rise to marked and persistent vertigo, which may be the only symptom for some time. It should be noted, however, that the acoustic neuroma, which is by far the most common neoplasm of the posterior fossa, does not have vertigo as its prominent feature (see Chapter 93).

In children, the possibility of a cerebellar glioma should be borne in mind and, in later life, secondary neoplastic deposits, especially from a bronchial carcinoma.

Vertigo of Peripheral Origin

The following entities, to be considered in the differential diagnosis of vertigo of peripheral origin, are discussed in the order of their frequency of incidence.

Vertebrobasilar Artery Insufficiency

Since the vestibule is supplied by the labyrinthine end-artery, a branch of the basilar artery, spasm of the vertebrobasilar artery may induce transient vertigo. The condition affects males more than females, from about 45 years of age onward.

The vertigo comes on immediately following a sudden change in the head position and lasts only several seconds, although it may seem much longer to the patient. There are no accompanying symptoms.

Physical examination is usually normal; however, many of the patients may suffer from atherosclerosis. Presbycusis may be an incidental finding in this age group. Positional tests are usually negative.

Ménière's Disease

Ménière's disease, Ménière's syndrome, or endolymphatic hydrops, is an idiopathic condition of the membranous labyrinth that is characterized by spontaneous bouts of prolonged vertigo, fluctuating hearing loss, and tinnitus. It affects primarily adults between the ages of 30 and 60, and is somewhat more common in females. The condition is unilateral in close to 90 per cent of the patients, and when it is bilateral, the second ear usually becomes affected within three years of the first episode.[6] By far the commonest pattern of involvement is that of both the vestibular and the cochlear labyrinths; however, in very rare instances, the disease may produce either vestibular symptoms only or be manifested by episodes of hearing loss only. In these uncommon presentations, the other portion of the labyrinth will eventually become symptomatic as the disease progresses.

The vertiginous episodes last anywhere from 15 minutes to several hours. The pattern of occurrence of the spells varies. Some patients exhibit long remissions between attacks, while others show a clustering of attacks with long symptom-free periods in between. On an average, a patient may experience about three episodes a year.

A classic spell is usually preceded by an aura consisting of pressure on the side of the head on the affected side, tinnitus, and hearing loss. In patients with existing tinnitus and hearing loss, the symptoms become exaggerated. The spell then comes on suddenly, with severe whirling vertigo accompanied by diaphoresis and nausea. In the early stages of the disease, the nausea may progress to vomiting. Head motion usually accentuates the symptoms.

The hearing loss is characterized by a distortion of sound, which is termed "recruitment." This distortion may also be present between spells, especially when the volume of sound is raised. The patient may experience a different pitch perception in the two ears, usually higher on the affected side, termed diplacusis. Loud sounds may be so intolerable as to even be painful. In the intervals between spells, the hearing loss may fluctuate considerably, especially in the early stages of the disease before much destruction of the cochlear labyrinth has taken place.

The general physical examination is invariably normal, so the diagnosis has to depend on an accurate history and on the results of audiometric and vestibular tests.

Pure-tone audiometry usually shows a sensorineural loss in the affected ear, with a flat or rising curve (Fig. 18–13). Fluctuation in hearing level will be elicited on repeated testing at intervals of time. Speech audiometry will invariably demonstrate a drop in discrimination, out of proportion to the level of the sensorineural loss. The alternate binaural loudness balance (ABLB) test for recruitment is uniformly positive in unilateral disease. A large majority of the patients will show recruitment on the short increment sensitivity index (SISI) test.

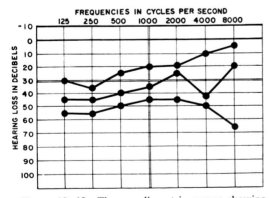

Figure 18–13 Three audiometric curves showing the more common sensorineural losses found in Ménière's disease. Note the involvement of the lower frequencies. (From Bernstein, L.: The etiology and diagnosis of vertigo. Arch. Otolaryng., 76:332, 1962. Reprinted by permission.)

Audiograms performed before and after ingestion of 1.2 ml of glycerol per kilogram of body weight often show an improvement in speech reception threshold and word discrimination in patients with Ménière's disease.

It should also be noted that tuning fork and whisper tests can corroborate the sensorineural nature of the loss and can also demonstrate the discrimination problem, diplacusis, and recruitment.

Tests for vestibular function during quiescence usually demonstrate hypofunction on the affected side on caloric stimulation. Subjectively, the caloric test duplicates the spontaneous episode, although it may be less severe.

DIFFERENTIAL DIAGNOSIS. The most difficult to differentiate from Ménière's disease, in its early stages at least, is an acoustic neuroma or other cerebellopontine angle tumor. These may not only cause vertiginous episodes but may also produce auditory abnormalities similar to those found in Ménière's disease.

Secondary Endolymphatic Hydrops

Endolymphatic hydrops with associated vertiginous symptoms may also be seen in otosclerosis, Cogan's syndrome, and congenital syphilis.

Typical symptoms of endolymphatic hydrops develop in a small percentage of otosclerotic patients. These patients usually respond well to medical treatment.

Cogan's syndrome is nonsyphilitic interstitial keratitis associated with vestibular and cochlear deficits. It is characterized by the appearance of eye pain, failing vision, vertigo, tinnitus, and hearing loss that usually appear within a few weeks of each other and frequently follow a recent viral infection or vaccination. An associated systemic disease, such as periarteritis nodosa, is often present. Prognosis is usually not good for hearing or vestibular function, but the keratitis responds fairly well to topical steroids. Large doses of parenteral steroids are recommended early in the course of the disease to suppress the inflammatory reaction in the labyrinth.

Late congenital syphilis may closely mimic Ménière's disease. In contradistinction to Ménière's disease, however, syphilis affects both ears. Syphilitic hearing loss also has an earlier age onset and may give a positive fistula test in the presence of an intact tympanic membrane. Large doses of systemic steroids can evoke a good transient improvement in hearing.

Vestibular Neuronitis

This condition is characterized by a sudden onset of sustained and severe vertigo, made worse with head movements. The condition usually affects subjects in early to middle age and is usually unilateral. It presents in varying degrees of severity.

Thought to be caused by a viral infection of Scarpa's ganglion, the condition often is preceded or accompanied by an obvious viral infection and may affect several individuals in a community at the same time, hence the term "endemic vertigo" or "endemic labyrinthitis." It has also been called acute viral labyrinthitis and labyrinthine apoplexy.

The condition lasts from one to three weeks and is characterized by an improvement of the symptoms from day to day, although they may be made worse by sudden movements of the head. There is no accompanying deafness or tinnitus, and the central nervous system is normal. The spontaneous nystagmus has its fast component to the opposite side (destructive nystagmus), and the caloric response in the affected ear is either reduced or absent.

Although the vertigo subsides after three weeks, in certain instances it may still be provoked by sudden movements of the head. As a general rule, however, compensation after three weeks is usually the rule, with complete recovery from any symptoms, especially in the younger age groups. Thus, while some patients go to complete resolution, others may be left with permanent hypofunction detectable by the caloric test in the affected ear, although this deficit is invariably asymptomatic.

Benign Peripheral Paroxysmal Positional Vertigo

In this entity, the vertigo is brought on by turning the head into a particular position, but the symptoms last only several seconds. In most cases, this is the only symptom and it is inconsistent at that. A good observer may volunteer that repeated movements of the head into the critical position either bring on vertigo of progressively lesser severity or that this may lead to a symptom-free period of several hours' duration. In many instances, careful questioning may elicit a history of a recent mild head injury.

Routine clinical and audiometric examinations are usually normal. The only vestibular test that may be abnormal, and which is characteristic of this entity, is the positional test. A typical positive response, on suddenly placing the patient's head in the critical position, is a latent period of approximately 10 seconds, followed by gross vertigo and nystagmus that peters out rapidly and ceases after about 20 seconds. The nystagmus persists in the same direction when the test is repeated or if the head position is changed (type 2). Repeating the test may produce a similar response but of lesser severity and of lesser duration until, after the second or third time, it may not be reproducible; however, it may again be induced after one or two hours. This adaptability is characteristic of the disease. It is considered that the condition is due to a mild injury of the otolith organ of the utricle in the ear to which the side of the head is turned in the critical position.[5,7] The symptoms usually subside spontaneously after about a year.

DIFFERENTIAL DIAGNOSIS. If the nystagmus changes direction on repeating the test or in response to changing the head position (type 1), this is more characteristic of a central lesion. Furthermore, a gradual fatigue and cessation of the nystagmus in response to the positional testing suggest a peripheral cause, while persistence of the nystagmus is more likely to be due to a central lesion. Also, a short latent period (time between assumption of the critical position and the onset of the nystagmus) is usually seen with peripheral lesions, but with many central lesions there is immediate onset of the nystagmus.

Labyrinthitis

Serous Labyrinthitis

This condition represents an irritation of the inner ear without bacterial or viral invasion and is usually secondary to direct trauma or to adjacent infection. A classic example is vestibular irritation following an operation on the labyrinth, such as stapedectomy or fenestration, or accompanying acute suppurative otitis media, in which diffusion of toxic products of the infection is thought to occur across the round window membrane. In either instance, recovery is the rule, although hypofunction may persist in response to caloric stimulation.

In serous labyrinthitis, vertiginous symptoms may be constant and they last for hours or for several days. The hearing may be decreased, but usually not severely. The accompanying nystagmus is of the irritative type and may last for days. The response to caloric testing may be diminished but is not lost.

Circumscribed Labyrinthitis

This condition is considered to be present whenever a fistula test is positive in the presence of chronic suppurative otitis media. Compressing the air in the external auditory canal leads to transient conjugate deviation of the eyes to the opposite side, while negative pressure causes deviation toward the affected ear. In this condition, a cholesteatoma or an inflammatory process has eroded bone of the otic capsule down to, but not through, the endosteum of the labyrinth. Invariably this takes place over the lateral semicircular canal. Consequently, compression of the air of the external auditory canal leads to compression of the membranous semicircular duct, thus causing the nearby cupula to be deflected toward the utricle. This ampullopetal deflection causes the eyes to deviate to the opposite side.

A labyrinthine fistula may be symptom-free, but when vertigo is present, the patient may describe it as periodic waves of mild dizziness. Occasionally, the patient may complain of a bizarre gait, in which he feels himself being displaced in the direction opposite to the involved ear. This may signify the erosive process of the cholesteatoma.

These cases require prompt operative removal of the cholesteatoma or the source of the infection or both before the condition progresses to acute suppurative labyrinthitis.

Acute Suppurative Labyrinthitis

Bacterial invasion of the labyrinth always results in total loss of both auditory and vestibular functions. In modern times, it is more likely to follow chronic rather than acute suppurative otitis media.

The condition is characterized by sudden prostration with violent vertigo, nausea, vomiting, and nystagmus. The crisis is usually ushered in with a febrile course. Initially, the hearing may still be present and the quick component of the nystagmus is toward the affected ear (irritative nystagmus). Hearing is gradually lost over a period of hours, and the direction of the nystagmus changes to the opposite side (destructive nystagmus).

Treatment consists of large intravenous doses of appropriate bactericidal antibiotics and must be followed by a labyrinthotomy to prevent intracranial spread of the infection. Postoperatively, the destructive nystagmus continues toward the opposite side until compensation occurs within about three weeks.

Toxic Injury to the Labyrinth

The most frequent and serious cause of toxic change to the inner ear is produced by a group of ototoxic drugs, which consists mainly of various antibiotic, chemotherapeutic, and diuretic agents. Damage from heavy metals or from quinine is now seldom seen. Table 18–1 lists some of the more common agents.

The best clinical, pathological, and experimental information has come from studies of the aminoglycoside group of antibiotics—streptomycin, dihydrostreptomycin, neomycin, kanamycin, and gentamicin—because of the magnitude, frequency, and irreversibility of the end-organ damage they produce in the labyrinth. Ototoxicity is usually dose-related, and since they are excreted by the kidneys, the plasma level of

TABLE 18–1 OTOTOXIC DRUGS AND SITES OF DAMAGE

DRUG	SITE OF DAMAGE		
	Cochlea	Vestibule	Kidney
Dihydrostreptomycin	x	x	
Ethacrynic acid	x	x	
Gentamicin	x	x	x
Kanamycin	x		x
Neomycin	x		x
Nitrogen mustard	x	x	
Streptomycin salts		x	
Vancomycin	x		x
Viomycin	x	x	x

the drug reflects renal function. These drugs are concentrated in the labyrinthine fluids and persist there at a much higher concentration and for a longer duration than in the plasma.

The aminoglycosides cause striking pathological changes in the sensory elements of the inner ear. In the vestibular labyrinth, there is a dramatic loss of hair cells in the ampullary cristae and the utricular and saccular maculae. There is also a change in the number and size of otoconia. Neural degeneration occurs and is presumed to be secondary to hair cell loss. In the organ of Corti, outer hair cells are destroyed in all turns, especially in the first and second rows of the basal turn. Inner hair cells may also be destroyed at the apex. Other changes have been observed in the cochlea that are not unlike those seen in renal tubular cells after administration of similar toxic drugs and may reflect a disturbance of the ionic equilibrium.

Other antibiotics known to cause severe end-organ damage include vancomycin and the tuberculostatic agent, viomycin.

Nonantibiotic ototoxic agents include nitrogen mustard in large doses, which produces cochlear damage while it injures the vestibular organ to a lesser extent. Transient and permanent sensorineural hearing losses have been reported following the administration of ethacrynic acid, and only transient losses with furosemide.

Tinnitus usually precedes noticeable hearing loss or discrimination drop and should be viewed with alarm. Because this heralds significant cochlear damage, the drug should be discontinued at this point if at all possible. Audiometrically, losses are first noted in the upper frequencies, but they soon involve the lower ones as well. Discrimination ability is impaired, and progression may be very rapid.

There may be no warning of impending or early damage in the vestibular systems because of symmetrical damage to both end-organs. With the eyes closed, however, marked disequilibrium will be noticed, because normal equilibrium is dependent upon proprioception and visual cues in addition to vestibular information. As a result, a subject can easily ambulate with two of the three senses intact, but not with only one. Consequently, periodic gait and posture tests should be performed during therapy with these drugs. Electronystagmographic recordings with caloric stimulation can also demonstrate the bilateral decrease in function. If possible, the drug should be stopped at the first evidence of decreased response. The following guidelines may be helpful in the use of ototoxic drugs:

1. Use the drug only for life-saving measures. Prophylactic use is not justified.

2. Inform the patient at the outset of the ototoxic potential of the drug and warn him of the early symptoms of intoxication.

3. Administer the drug on a milligram per kilogram basis.

4. Reduce the dosage in the presence of impaired renal function and in the elderly.

5. Keep the patient well hydrated.

6. Avoid using more than one ototoxic drug at a time.

7. Avoid ototoxic drugs in those with existing end-organ disease.

8. Have the patient evaluated before therapy to establish baselines for: hearing (clinical and audiometric tests), vestibular and statokinetic systems (gait, stance, and caloric tests), and renal function (blood urea nitrogen and creatinine clearance tests).

9. Evaluate during therapy with the same tests: daily clinical hearing evaluation and inquiry about tinnitus, weekly audiometry; weekly renal studies, more often if abnormal; biweekly vestibular and statokinetic tests.

10. Discontinue the drug at the onset of intoxication.

Cervical Vertigo

Vertigo may also follow neck injury. It is usually associated with positional changes and may be accompanied by spasm and tenderness of the cervical musculature, limitation of cervical motion, and some loss of the cervical lordosis.

The mechanism of the vertigo is not quite clear. Considered hypotheses include alteration of the tonic neck reflexes, irritation of cervical nerve roots, involvement of the sympathetic nervous system, and compression of the vertebral artery from osteoarthritis.

Treatment usually consists of rest, traction, a cervical collar, muscle relaxants, and analgesics.

THE COCHLEAR SYSTEM

Physiology of Hearing

For a clearer understanding of the various types of hearing loss, it is important to understand the mechanism of transmission of sound to the neural receptors.

Air vibrations impinge on the tympanic membrane, causing it and the malleus to vibrate. This physical vibration is transmitted via the incus to the stapes and by way of its footplate to the fluids of the labyrinth. The fluid vibrations in turn produce a stimulus along the basilar membrane, which activates the organ of Corti. Hence, impulses are transmitted through the cochlear nerve endings to the cochlear nuclei in the midbrain. The impulses then continue to the auditory areas of the cortex.

The Transformer Mechanism of the Tympanum

The pars tensa of the tympanic membrane and its attached malleus are set into motion by sound; the motion is then continued to the oval window. Since the effective vibratory area of the tympanic membrane is about 17 times as large as the area of the footplate of the stapes, and because the manubrium of the malleus is 1.3 times as long as the long process of the incus, the ratio of amplification from tympanic membrane to stapedial footplate is about 22:1.

Because fluid is incompressible, the secondary tympanic membrane in the round window acts as a compensating membrane to accommodate the vibrations of the stapedial footplate. Thus, if sound vibrations were to reach the oval and round windows at the same time, a certain amount of cancellation of the sound would take place. This does not normally happen because of the phase difference between the windows, which is facilitated as follows: (1) The intact tympanic membrane protects the round window from direct sound impingement. (2) The tympanic membrane is connected to the oval window through the ossicular chain, making faster direct transmission by this route. (3) The round window membrane faces backward, at right angles to the plane of the tympanic membrane, and is recessed within the niche. These factors delay the impingement of sound onto the round window membrane.

As a consequence of these phenomena, a sizeable perforation of the tympanic membrane will result in a 30- to 35-db hearing loss by air conduction, whereas dislocation of the ossicular chain with an intact tympanic membrane will produce an air conduction loss of about 55 to 60 db.

Transmission in the Labyrinth

As stated previously, high frequencies are received near the basal portion and low frequencies near the apical part of the basilar membrane and its organ of Corti. Beyond this, the actual mechanism of sound perception is still quite theoretical, controversial, and incompletely understood.

Hearing Tests

There is still room for assessing a patient's hearing by means of the old-fashioned whispered voice, although admittedly this is a crude test. Tuning forks will help to differentiate between conductive and sensorineural losses. Modern audiometric instruments, however, permit us not only to perform a battery of highly sophisticated tests with a very high degree of accuracy, but the test results may be accurately recorded according to internationally agreed standards.

Tuning Fork Tests

The classic method of diagnosing the type of hearing loss is by noting the patient's response to vibrating tuning forks. The most commonly used tests are the Rinne, the Weber, and the Schwabach.

Rinne Test

This test differentiates between conductive and sensorineural hearing loss.

ADMINISTRATION OF TEST. Standard procedure calls for use of three tuning forks of 256, 512, and 1024 Hz (cycles per second). The vibrating tuning fork is held close to the patient's external ear. When the patient reports that he can no longer hear the sound produced by the fork, the base of the instrument is placed against his mastoid process and he is asked if he can again hear the sound. The method of administration may be reversed—the fork first placed over the mastoid and then shifted to the external ear.

The test may also be done by alternately placing the tuning fork over the mastoid process and at the external auditory canal. The patient is then asked to indicate at which location he hears the fork louder or better.

REPORTING TEST RESULTS. If the patient reports hearing the fork longer (or louder) by mastoid placement (bone conduction) than by external ear placement (air conduction), the result is said to be Rinne negative, indicative of a conductive lesion. If the patient reports hearing the fork longer (or louder) by air conduction than by bone conduction, the result is Rinne positive, indicative of a sensorineural lesion or of normal hearing.

With significant unilateral sensorineural impairment, results of the Rinne test may be misleading because of the participation of the opposite ear during bone conduction testing. When the fork is placed on the mastoid of the poorer ear, the fluid of both inner ears is stimulated. Therefore, it is necessary to prevent the participation of the better ear by introducing a "masking noise" to that ear while testing the poorer ear. This may be done by rubbing a piece of paper rapidly on the opposite auricle.

Weber Test

This test differentiates between conductive and sensorineural impairment in cases of unilateral hearing loss.

ADMINISTRATION OF TEST. A vibrating tuning fork is placed on the midline of the skull. The patient is asked to determine in which ear he hears the tone.

REPORTING TEST RESULTS. If the patient reports that the tone lateralizes to his poorer ear, a conductive impairment is indicated. If he hears the tone in his better ear, sensorineural impairment is indicated. If there is no difference in the sensitivity of the two ears, the tone will be heard equally in the two ears or it will be reported to be heard in the "middle of the head."

Schwabach (Absolute Bone Conduction) Test

Determines the patient's baseline of hearing by bone conduction as compared with that of the examiner ("normal").

ADMINISTRATION OF TEST. The vibrating fork is applied to the patient's mastoid process while the external ear canal is closed by pushing the tragus over it. The patient is instructed to indicate the instant that he no longer hears the fork. At that moment the fork is transferred to the examiner's mastoid process, while he closes his canal by compressing the tragus.

REPORTING TEST RESULTS. The examiner assumes himself to have normal hearing and reports the result as being worse or better than his own. The test may be refined further by recording the number of seconds by which the examiner hears the sound longer than the patient.

This is a crude way of comparing the patient's bone conduction with that of the examiner and assumes the examiner has normal hearing. It may be a useful screening test as well as a means of establishing deterioration of hearing in cases in which previous test results obtained by the same examiner are available.

Audiometric Testing

Tuning fork tests provide information about a patient's hearing that is primarily of a qualitative nature. Quantitative, as well as qualitative, information about hearing may be obtained with an electronic audiometer. The audiometer can generate essentially "pure tones" of various frequencies. The intensity of these tones can be accurately varied from levels so soft as to be inaudible to levels so loud as to be uncomfortable for most people. With more sophisticated audiometers, it is also possible to measure the patient's hearing for speech and to perform site-of-lesion audiological tests.

Pure-Tone Audiometry

Pure-tone audiometric test results are plotted on the audiogram. Parameters are frequency of the tone in cycles per second, or hertz (Hz), on the horizontal axis and intensity in decibels (db) on the vertical axis.

The human ear can perceive sounds over a wide range of frequencies (from as low as 16 Hz to as high as 30,000 Hz). Clinical audiometry is primarily concerned with testing frequencies in the range from 250 to 8,000 Hz. Speech sounds are mainly confined to the midfrequency range of 500, 1,000 and 2,000 Hz. These three frequencies, referred to as the "speech frequencies'' or the ''pure-tone average,'' are used to estimate hearing loss for medicolegal and rehabilitative purposes.

The human ear is able to hear over a wide range of intensity. The loudest sound that is bearable is 100 trillion times the softest audible sound. Because of this wide range of intensity that can be perceived, measuring sound level in absolute values becomes unwieldy. Therefore, the intensity of sound is customarily measured in relative terms using the decibel scale. The zero point on the decibel scale is the intensity that can barely be heard. The value was derived by testing a large population of young adults with no history of ear disease. The average softest level heard by this group at each frequency was then designated as 0 db for that frequency. The decibel scale is a logarithmic scale to the base of 10. Thus, a sound intensity of 10 db is 10 times as intense as 0 db; a sound intensity of 20 db is 100 times as intense as 0 db; and so on. An average whisper at 4 feet produces a level of approximately 20 db; normal conversation at 3 feet, about 60 db. A riveter produces a sound intensity of 100 db at 35 feet.

Hearing thresholds in the 0- to 20-db range are considered to be within normal limits; 20 to 40 db, mild hearing loss; 40 to 55 db, moderate hearing loss; 55 to 70 db, moderately severe loss; 70 to 90 db, severe loss; and above 90 db, profound loss.

Air Conduction Testing

Air conduction testing is performed with earphones placed on both ears. It is a test of the entire hearing mechanism. Hearing loss noted in air conduction testing may result from a lesion anywhere in the auditory system.

The test is conducted in a soundproof room. The patient is instructed to respond to the presentation of the tone by raising his hand or pushing a button. The softest sound to which the patient consistently responds (his threshold) is determined for each test frequency for each ear. Air conduction thresholds are recorded on the audiogram with a red O for the right ear and a blue X for the left ear at each frequency tested.

Bone Conduction Testing

Testing by bone conduction is performed by presenting tones through a vibrator placed on the mastoid process of the temporal bone. In this way the inner ear is stimulated directly, bypassing the outer ear canal and the middle ear. A direct measure of sensorineural hearing acuity is thus obtained.

The test procedure is the same as for air conduction testing, except that the vibrator must be placed separately on each mastoid process. Results are recorded on the audiogram by placing a red > for the right ear and a blue < for the left ear at the hearing threshold for each frequency.

In the presence of hearing loss, if air conduction and bone conduction thresholds are equal at each frequency, the loss is said to be sensorineural in nature and is the result of cochlear or auditory nerve disease or both.

If bone conduction thresholds are normal and hearing loss is indicated by air conduction, the loss is said to be conductive and is the result of a lesion peripheral to the inner ear. If hearing loss is present by both air conduction and bone conduction, but hearing is better by bone than by air, a mixed hearing loss is indicated in which there are abnormalities in both the conductive and sensorineural hearing mechanisms.

Masking

BONE CONDUCTION.   Although the bone vibrator is placed on one mastoid process at a time, both inner ears are stimulated simultaneously by the signal. Unless the patient has an equal bilateral sensorineural hearing loss, it becomes necessary to isolate the test ear from the non-test ear during bone conduction testing. This is accomplished by presenting an adequate level of masking noise through an earphone to the non-test ear. The masking prevents it from participating in the test, while the test signals are being presented through the bone vibrator to the opposite ear in the usual manner.

AIR CONDUCTION.   While the earphones cover both ears, sound will not be heard in the non-test ear until it reaches a level of approximately 50 to 60 db above the threshold for that ear. Accordingly, in air conduction testing, it is customary to mask the opposite (better) ear when there is a difference of 40 db or more in the hearing acuity of the two ears. The examiner then knows that he is obtaining the actual

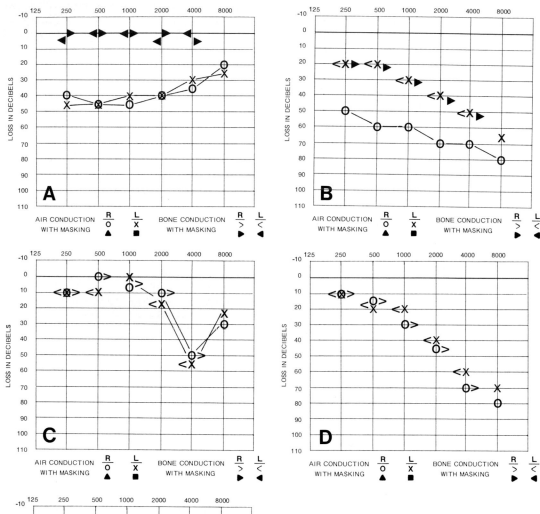

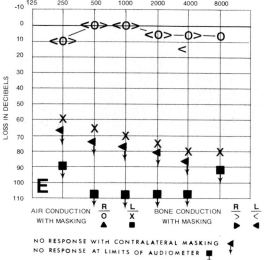

Figure 18–14 Representative pure-tone audiograms. *A.* Typical bilateral conductive hearing loss. *B.* Mixed loss on right and sensorineural loss on left side. *C.* Bilateral high-frequency sensorineural loss, peaking at 4kHz— acoustic trauma pattern. *D.* Bilateral sloping high-frequency sensorineural hearing loss due to aging (presbycusis). *E.* Profound hearing loss on left with normal response on right.

thresholds for the poorer ear, rather than a "shadow curve" of the better ear.

Representative examples of masked and unmasked thresholds are shown in Figure 18–14.

Speech Audiometry

With certain audiometers, it is possible to obtain a direct measurement of a patient's hearing for speech. Speech may be presented by tape or phonograph record, or by live voice through a microphone. The intensity of the signal may be accurately controlled as in pure-tone testing. Two measures of hearing for speech are usually obtained: (1) the softest level of speech that can be heard (speech reception threshold), and (2) how well speech is understood (discrimination score).

SPEECH RECEPTION THRESHOLD. A measure of how soft a level of speech a patient can hear is obtained by presenting a series of spondee (two-syllable) words at progressively softer levels until the patient can only repeat 50 per cent of the words correctly. This is his speech reception threshold (SRT) and should correlate within ±5 db of his pure-tone thresholds for the speech frequencies of 500 to 2000 Hz.

SPEECH DISCRIMINATION TESTING. Speech discrimination ability is evaluated by presenting lists of phonetically balanced words well above the patient's speech reception threshold. Each list contains 50 monosyllabic words chosen to represent speech sounds in the same proportion that they occur in normal speech.

A person with normal hearing, or with a conductive hearing loss, will usually obtain a score nearly 100 per cent correct. Patients with sensorineural hearing loss usually demonstrate decreased speech discrimination ability even when words are delivered at the optimal intensity level for them. This is especially true with lesions of the auditory nerve, in which case speech discrimination scores may be severely depressed despite relatively mild pure-tone hearing loss.

Site-of-Lesion Testing

In sensorineural hearing losses, particularly of a unilateral nature, it is often neces-sary to determine whether the site of the lesion is cochlear or retrocochlear. Pure-tone testing cannot provide this information; however, a battery of special audiological tests can often aid in determining the site of the lesion.

TESTS FOR RECRUITMENT. Recruitment is defined as an abnormal sensitivity to sound increment. A patient with hearing loss and associated recruitment will be unable to hear soft sounds, but will be extremely sensitive to loud sounds. Recruitment is associated with lesions within the cochlea and is usually absent in retrocochlear abnormalities.

ALTERNATE BINAURAL LOUDNESS BALANCE TEST. The alternate binaural loudness balance (ABLB) test is used to determine recruitment with unilateral sensorineural loss. The test consists of comparing the intensity levels at which a given pure tone sounds equally loud to the good ear and the poor ear. Loudness balance judgment responses are obtained at various intensity levels above threshold. In cases of recruitment, tones of the same intensity level may be judged equally loud in the good and in the poor ear at higher sensation levels. In a nonrecruiting ear with hearing loss, the sensation of loudness will never "catch up" with the good ear. Again, the presence of recruitment is associated with a cochlear lesion.

MONAURAL LOUDNESS BALANCE TEST. The monaural loudness balance (MLB) test is used to determine recruitment in a bilateral sensorineural hearing loss in which the high frequencies are more affected than the lower frequencies. The loudness sensation at the impaired frequencies is compared with that of the normal frequencies at various levels above thresholds.

SHORT INCREMENT SENSITIVITY INDEX. Patients with recruitment are not only more sensitive to loud sounds but are also able to detect smaller increases in loudness than people with normal hearing or with hearing loss not characterized by recruitment. The short increment sensitivity index (SISI) test consists of presentation of a continuous pure tone of 20 db above the patient's threshold, with 1-db increments in intensity superimposed upon the steady tone at periodic intervals. The ability to detect these small 1-db increments is largely restricted to patients with cochlear abnormalities. These individuals are able to detect most of the superimposed short bursts of sound, which they are asked to count. Conversely, this ability is invariably absent in patients with normal hearing and in those with conductive or retrocochlear hearing losses. They merely hear the continuous base tone of 20 db.

Tests for Tone Decay

Tone decay may be defined as the decrease in threshold sensitivity resulting from the presence of a barely audible continuous sound.

TONE DECAY TEST. A standard audiometer is used. The patient is instructed to raise his hand as long as he hears the tone and lower it when the tone is inaudible. Starting at the patient's threshold level, the tone is presented for a total of 60 seconds. If the patient indicates that he cannot hear the tone before the minute is over, the intensity is raised by 5 db without interrupting the tone. The test is continued in this manner until the end of the minute. The amount of tone decay from the initial threshold level is determined in decibels.

A patient with normal hearing or with a conductive loss will usually demonstrate little or no tone decay. Patients with a lesion of the cochlea will often demonstrate mild to moderate tone decay (10 to 25 db), while patients with a retrocochlear site of lesion will usually demonstrate marked tone decay (30 db or more.)

BRAIN STEM EVOKED RESPONSE AUDIOMETRY. The most recent advance in the evaluation of the auditory system is brain stem evoked response audiometry (BERA). In 1970, Jewett and co-workers described recording electrical potentials from scalp electrodes in response to auditory stimuli.[10]

Five waves have been observed to be time-locked to the sound stimulus. Those noted during the first 10 msec reflect activity within the auditory nerve and brain stem. Wave I is the eighth cranial nerve action potential, and the wave IV–V complex is related to electrical activity in the inferior colliculus. Waves II and III are related to electrical generators in the area of the cochlear and superior olivary nuclei; the specific origin of these waves remains obscure.

The test resembles electroencephalography. To record the evoked potentials, one electrode is placed over the vertex and one over each mastoid process. These areas are first prepared with an abrasive to decrease electrical resistance. The test is performed in a quiet and dark room in order to minimize extraneous stimuli and consequent artifacts. Young children and infants may be sedated or anesthetized, if necessary, without affecting the results. Adults rest their heads on a pillow to decrease myogenic activity. Earphones are used to deliver monaural short square-wave clicks at various intensities ranging from 10 to 100 db above threshold. Clicks are delivered at a rate of 5 to 70 per second, with a stimulus duration of 1 to 4 msec. At least 2000 clicks are used at each intensity.

The resulting waves are passed through a 100- to 3000-Hz filter, amplified, and averaged by a computer to eliminate electrical activity unrelated to the click stimuli. The averaged responses produce a recording at levels within 10 db of actual hearing levels from which the latency of each wave may be measured (Fig. 18–15). A latency-intensity curve is plotted, which may fall into the normal range or be specific for a given category of hearing loss (Fig. 18–16).

Brain stem evoked response audiometry is currently used to evaluate hearing and auditory pathway integrity in several clinical situations. Thus far, this form of testing has been used mainly to analyze the threshold in infants. Prior methods were notoriously unreliable, so it was difficult to decide which child might benefit by a hearing aid. Brain stem evoked response audiometry is now recommended for all children believed to be "at risk" for hearing impairment because of factors such as prematurity and meningitis. Results must be compared with established standards, since individual wave latencies decrease during the first year of life as a result of auditory pathway maturation. Because the test is noninvasive, is without risk, and requires minimal cooperation from the patient, it is becoming a primary tool for screening large groups of children.

Brain stem disorders may cause a delay in conduction of sound-evoked responses from the cochlea to the cortex. Wave I to wave III and wave III to wave V intervals have been studied most in this regard. It is

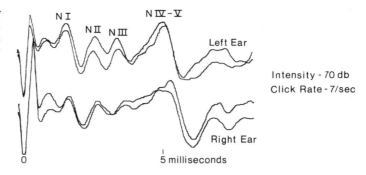

Figure 18–15 Normal tracing of brain stem evoked response audiometry. Note that latency decreases with increasing intensity. In N IV–V latency is between 5.0 and 6.3 m per second.

common to find a patient with a demyelinating disease or brain stem tumor who has normal threshold levels but a delay in central conduction, as evidenced by increased latencies or absence of all waves after NI.

This test is also used to assist in the early diagnosis of acoustic neuroma. Selters and Brackmann listed several abnormalities that were observed in their groups of patients with acoustic neuroma. They included loss of all waves subsequent to NI, increased latency on the involved side, and interaural latency differences. By adjusting results for various degrees of high-frequency neurosensory hearing loss, they have lowered their false-positive rate to 8 per cent while

approaching a 96 per cent tumor detection rate. This has virtually eliminated their use of electronystagmography and tone decay tests in the evaluation of patients for the presence of cerebellopontine angle tumors.[13]

In summary, brain stem evoked response audiometry is an outstanding addition to the modalities for identifying auditory disease. As the apparatus becomes more available and less expensive, it will eliminate existing methods for screening infants. Along with improved computed tomography, it has become a major tool in the diagnosis of acoustic tumors. It can demonstrate hearing levels in people who could not previously be tested. Additionally, it is an excel-

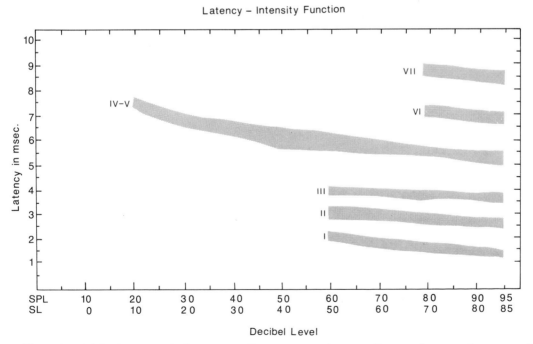

Figure 18–16 Brain stem evoked response audiometry. Normal ranges of latency of generated waves as related to intensity of stimuli.

lent method for detecting threshold shift in experimental animals subjected to drugs, noise, and other agents.

Impedance Audiometry

Impedance audiometry measures the physical characteristics of the middle ear system. More specifically, it records the acoustic resistance (impedance) to vibratory motion of the tympanic membrane and the middle ear structures. It is not a true hearing test in the strict sense of the word. Rather, the information obtained from this test allows certain conclusions to be made regarding the functions in the hearing mechanism of the tympanic membrane, the tympanum and its ossicular chain, and the eustachian tube. In contradistinction to most other clinical audiometric tests, which require a subjective response, impedance audiometry is an objective test.

A small, rubber-tipped acoustic probe is inserted into the external ear canal. The probe has three openings: one for introducing a sound signal (probe tone), a second for monitoring the amount of this signal that is reflected within the ear canal (sound pressure level), and a third to permit changes in air pressure within the ear canal. All measurements depend on detecting changes in sound pressure level within the external auditory meatus.

There are two important tests that are performed with the impedance audiometer: tympanometry and the acoustic reflex.

TYMPANOMETRY. Tympanometry records the elasticity, or compliance, of the middle ear as air pressure is altered in the external ear canal. It can determine the cause of a conductive hearing impairment. Pressure changes will vary with the compliance of the tympanic membrane, the air pressure in the middle ear, and the mobility of the ossicles.

From the tympanogram, one may arrive at a diagnosis of ossicular fixation, ossicular dislocation, middle ear fluid, and eustachian tube dysfunction.

ACOUSTIC REFLEX TEST. A tone of 70 to 100 db will cause a reflex contraction of the stapedius muscle. This stiffens the ossicular chain and the tympanic membrane, which results in less sound being transmitted. This is detected by the acoustic probe as a change in sound pressure level within the external ear canal.

The acoustic reflex test can help differentiate between conductive and sensorineural deafness. This reflex may be absent or show tone decay in about 90 per cent of cases with acoustic neuroma. It is also helpful in evaluating the topography of the lesion in facial paralysis.

REFERENCES

1. Adams, R. D.: Occlusion of the anterior inferior cerebellar artery. Arch. Neurol. Psychiat., 49:765, 1943.
2. Alpers, B. J.: Vertiginous epilepsy. Trans. Amer. Laryng. Rhinol. Otol. Soc. 27. Laryngoscope, 70:631–637, 1960.
3. Anson, B. J., and Donaldson, J. A.: Surgical Anatomy of the Temporal Bone and Ear. 3rd Ed. Philadelphia, W. B. Saunders Co., 1981.
4. Bernstein, L.: The etiology and diagnosis of vertigo. Arch. Otolaryng., 76:329, 1962.
5. Cawthorne, T., and Hallpike, C. S.: A study of the clinical features and pathological changes within the temporal bone, brain stem and cerebellum of an early case of positional nystagmus of the so-called benign paroxysmal type. Acta Otolaryng (Stockholm), 48:89, 1957.
6. Cawthorne, T., and Hewlett, A. B.: Ménière's disease. Proc. Roy. Soc. Med., 47:663, 1954.
7. Dix, M. R., and Hallpike, C. S.: Pathology, symptomatology and diagnosis of certain common disorders of the vestibular system. Proc. Roy. Soc. Med., 45:341, 1952.
8. Fitzgerald, G., and Hallpike, C. S.: Studies in human vestibular function. Brain, 65:115, 1942.
9. Gowers, W. R.: Epilepsy. 2nd Ed. London, J. & A. Churchill, Ltd., 1901, p. 67.
10. Jewett, D., Romano, H., and Williston, J.: Human auditory evoked potentials: Possible brain-stem components detected on the scalp. Science, 167:1517–1518, 1970.
11. Levy, L., and O'Leary, J. L.: Incidence of vertigo in neurological conditions. Ann. Otol., 56:557, 1947.
12. Paparella, M. M., and Shumrick, D. A.: Otolaryngology, Vol. 1. Philadelphia, W. B. Saunders Co., 1973.
13. Selters, W. A., and Brackmann, D. E.: Brain-stem evoked response audiometry in acoustic tumor detection. In House, W. F., and Luetje, C. H., eds.: Acoustic Tumors. Baltimore, University Park Press, 1979, pp. 225–236.

19

PSYCHOLOGICAL TESTING
IN NEUROLOGICAL DIAGNOSIS

EVOLUTION OF MODERN CLINICAL NEUROPSYCHOLOGY

In 1796, Maskelyne, the royal astronomer at the Greenwich Observatory, dismissed Kinnebrook, his assistant, because the assistant recorded the times of stellar transits nearly a second later than he did. Twenty years later Bessell, the astronomer at Königsberg, read of the Kinnebrook incident and began a study that involved measuring what came to be known as the "personal equation" of different observers.[3] Bessell collected data on several trained observers, and subsequently published his findings. They were too late to help Kinnebrook, but in time to represent the first public record of quantitative data on individual differences. Early experimental psychologists, mostly physiologists interested in behavior, addressed themselves to the study of determinants of the personal equation, under the rubric "reaction time." Their original experiments compared two individuals' simultaneous performance of the same task. The introduction of chronographs in the latter half of the nineteenth century enabled them to measure the reaction time of one observer without reference to another observer.[19]

The interest aroused throughout most of Europe by Broca's paper concerning the localization of speech functions in the left hemisphere, published in 1865, stimulated research into the relationship of brain behavior for the remainder of the century. Yet, when the first laboratory of experimental psychology was established in 1879 by Wundt in Leipzig, its focus was on the development of refined procedures for measuring such processes as visual sensation, auditory sensation, and reaction time rather than anything specifically related to mental functioning.[20,78]

Francis Galton was the first to attempt to use sensory processes as indicators of the subject's intellectual level. By 1883 he had devised numerous tests and measures such as the Galton whistle for pitch discrimination and the Galton bar for visual discrimination of length. He established a laboratory in which he tested large numbers of people.[39] From his extensive research he concluded that it was possible, using a comprehensive range of sensory discrimination measures, to differentiate between idiots and the more intellectually able. In recognition of his contribution to science he was knighted.

In 1890, the term "mental test" was first used by Cattell to describe a battery of such measures as muscular strength, speed of movement, pain sensitivity, memory, and reaction time.[22] Similar test batteries were developed by Ebbinghaus and Kraeplin.[32,68] Binet and Henri criticized these tests for laying too much emphasis on the sensory sensations and, in 1895, proposed a new series of tests covering such mental processes as comprehension, memory, and attention.[11] Binet's work was recognized as relevant to educational planning. Subsequently he was commissioned by the French Minister of Public Instruction to prepare a scale to give an index of general mental function. By 1905, Binet and Simon had developed a series of empirical observations of typical abilities of normal children at ages ranging from 3 through 13 years. They also developed a test battery in which items were

---

L. C. HARTLAGE AND P. L. HARTLAGE

grouped by age level and an individual child's score was expressed in terms of his mental age.[12,14]

The Binet-Simon test attracted attention around the world. Psychologists responded to its use of clearly defined test stimuli that were presented in a controlled manner with specific criteria for levels of adequate performance. Physicians recognized its value as a diagnostic test that could distinguish normal from mentally subnormal patients. Its use of mental age as a measurement unit provided at once a useful theoretical construct and a practical means of classifying children according to ability. By 1916, Terman had revised and extended a translation of the Binet scale and published it as the Stanford Revision of the Binet Scale, or Stanford-Binet test.[99,100] It was this scale that introduced the Intelligence Quotient, or ratio between mental age and chronological age, expressed by the formula $IQ = MA/CA \times 100$.

In 1917, on the entry of the United States into World War I, the Army requested a test of intelligence to screen more than a million recruits. Psychologists developed two intelligence tests that could be given in groups: The Army Alpha was designed for general use; the Army Beta, a non-language scale, was designed for illiterates and foreign born draftees who were not sufficiently familiar with English to take a written test.[116] The success of the Army tests demonstrated that psychological tests could be adapted to meet a wide range of practical needs. Following World War I, considerable attention was given to the development, validation, and refinement of psychological tests.[25,102] Although most test developments were based on the concept of a general intellectual factor common to the performance of all mental tasks, psychologists became increasingly aware that a single global measure of intelligence did not necessarily encompass the full domain of mental functioning.[95,96] For example, an individual with a high IQ could do very poorly on tasks involving art or music, just as an otherwise dull or even mentally retarded individual, e.g., idiot-savant, could have remarkable ability in a specific skill such as calculation or memory.[104] In 1928, Kelley published a critical analysis of the data on which the concept of a single general intellectual factor was based. He proposed that mental tests needed to be composed of measures of such discrete mental abilities as spatial relationships, mental speed, and memory, and differential measures of facility with numbers and language.[62] This list of mental ability components of intelligence was expanded by Thurstone in 1938 to include approximately 12 "primary mental abilities," such as verbal fluency, verbal comprehension, perceptual speed, and inductive reasoning, as well as Kelley's original measures.[103] Development of these concepts culminated in Wechsler's 1939 publication of a scale for the measurement of adult intelligence, which was composed of subtests of performance on tasks not unlike those Thurstone proposed to measure primary mental abilities.[111] Grouped according to whether the tasks involved were verbal or more spatial, the subtests could be summed to produce separate "verbal" and "performance" IQ scores as well as a global or "full scale" IQ.

At approximately the same time that Wechsler was pioneering his approach to mental assessment, the first laboratory for the study of behavioral correlates of brain functions in humans was established in Chicago by Ward Halstead. Halstead's academic background and major prior research had been in animal psychology. In the mid 1930's, he began a program of personal observation of patients with brain damage. To identify how their adjustments differed from those of normal individuals, he studied them in their homes, at their jobs, in recreational activities, and in a variety of other problem-solving situations. From these observations he developed a battery of standardized tests to assess the condition of the brain. By the mid 1940's, these tests had been clinically validated with his neurosurgical colleagues, Dr. Percival Bailey and Dr. Paul Bucy, and had evolved into highly sophisticated and sensitive detectors of cerebral dysfunction.

The majority of neuropsychological approaches to the studying of brain-behavior relationships during the 1940's and 1950's dealt with rather heterogeneous groupings of patients with brain damage and focused on tests that differentiated those who were neurologically impaired from those who were intact. Subsequent refinements have produced assessment procedures that consider much more specific aspects of neurological impairment.[1,8,29,44,83]

In 1951, Reitan, a student of Halstead, opened a neuropsychological laboratory in the section of Neurological Surgery at the Indiana University Medical Center. He first produced psychometric evidence of differential effects of right and left cerebral hemisphere lesions. Subsequently he measured differential behavioral effects of such factors as site of lesion, cause, age at onset, premorbid condition, and severity and extent of lesion.[30,61,63,65,81,86] Benton, at Iowa Medical School, and other pioneers helped to refine the specific psychological test correlates of discrete neurological dysfunctions.[7,9,41,90]

INDICATIONS FOR NEUROPSYCHOLOGICAL ASSESSMENT

A neuropsychological examination is a quantitative and comprehensive evaluation of brain function. It combines techniques employed in intelligence testing with modifications of those elements of the traditional neurological examination that are most correlated with cortical function.

For the neurologically oriented physician concerned with the magnitude of change in the patient's mental status resulting from a disease process, operative intervention, or changes in type or dosage or schedule of medication, the neuropsychological evaluation provides highly refined and sensitive measurements based on standardized and reliable testing procedures. The differences between examiners and the variability of findings on neurological examinations, even by one examiner from one visit to the next, are well known. When treatment is undertaken, examiner bias further complicates matters. Neuropsychological testing under standardized conditions minimizes these problems and also provides a broadly based comprehensive survey of cortical function that may help detect unsuspected changes in specific aspects of higher mental function resulting from a known pathological condition. For example, it may demonstrate a contrecoup dysfunction on the side opposite primary head trauma or may show chronic ischemia in brain areas that are not directly involved with arteriovenous malformation.

In patients with degenerative disease or slowly growing neoplasms in their early stages, alterations in function may be detected well before structural change can be demonstrated by neuroradiological studies. In such cases, it is difficult to differentiate organic from psychiatric disease on the basis of the findings of the traditional mental status examination conducted by the physician or the projective test instruments often used by clinical psychologists. Disturbances in language functions and defects in recent memory would, of course, be obvious in the course of a mental status examination. Subtle disturbances in the perceptual and cognitive functions of the nondominant hemisphere would not be so apparent. Patients with this type of lesion might respond in bizarre fashion to projective tests that rely on the interpretation of stimulus figures because of a defect in visuospatial processing.

Planning for the rehabilitation of the neurologically handicapped patient can be considerably enhanced by the neuropsychologist's determination of residual strengths and deficits. The physician's skill in identifying dysfunction is appropriately and by necessity more developed than his skill in identifying areas of normal or superior function. He has little trouble describing what the patient cannot do, but may encounter difficulty in determining what he can do. The neuropsychological evaluation can help to identify the patient's ability to comprehend different modes of communication involved in retraining, and to predict the longer-term likelihood of his ability to resume old activities or learn new skills.

TECHNIQUES IN NEUROPSYCHOLOGICAL EVALUATION

Current Level of Intellectual Functioning

The cornerstone of a neuropsychological assessment is an individual intelligence test. With adults the test most commonly used is the Wechsler Adult Intelligence Scale (WAIS).[112] This scale consists of 11 subtests, 6 measuring language function and 5 measuring nonlanguage aspects of mental function. The test requires approximately one and one half hours to administer. It gives separate age-corrected mental

WAIS RECORD FORM
Wechsler Adult Intelligence Scale

Name _____

Birth Date _____ Age _____ Sex _____ Marital: S M D W
MO   DAY   YR.   CIRCLE ONE

Nat. _____ Color _____ Tested by _____

Place of Examination _____ Date _____

Occupation _____ Education _____

TABLE OF SCALED SCORE EQUIVALENTS*

Scaled Score	Information	Comprehension	Arithmetic	Similarities	Digit Span	Vocabulary	Digit Symbol	Picture Completion	Block Design	Picture Arrangement	Object Assembly	Scaled Score
19	29	27-28		26	17	78-80	87-90					19
18	28	26		25		76-77	83-86	21		36	44	18
17	27	25	18	24		74-75	79-82		48	35	43	17
16	26	24	17	23	16	71-73	76-78	20	47	34	42	16
15	25	23	16	22	15	67-70	72-75		46	33	41	15
14	23-24	22	15	21	14	63-66	69-71	19	44-45	32	40	14
13	21-22	21	14	19-20		59-62	66-68	18	42-43	30-31	38-39	13
12	19-20	20	13	17-18	13	54-58	62-65	17	39-41	28-29	36-37	12
11	17-18	19	12	15-16	12	47-53	58-61	15-16	35-38	26-27	34-35	11
10	15-16	17-18	11	13-14	11	40-46	52-57	14	31-34	23-25	31-33	10
9	13-14	15-16	10	11-12	10	32-39	47-51	12-13	28-30	20-22	28-30	9
8	11-12	14	9	9-10		26-31	41-46	10-11	25-27	18-19	25-27	8
7	9-10	12-13	7-8	7-8	9	22-25	35-40	8-9	21-24	15-17	22-24	7
6	7-8	10-11	6	5-6	8	18-21	29-34	6-7	17-20	12-14	19-21	6
5	5-6	8-9	5	4		14-17	23-28	5	13-16	9-11	15-18	5
4	4	6-7	4	3	7	11-13	18-22	4	10-12	8	11-14	4
3	3	5	3	2		10	15-17	3	6-9	7	8-10	3
2	2	4	2	1		9	13-14	2	3-5	6	5-7	2
1	1	3	1		4-5	8	12	1	2	5	3-4	1
0	0	0-2	0	0	0-3	0-7	0-11	0	0-1	0-4	0-2	0

SUMMARY

TEST	Raw Score	Scaled Score
Information		
Comprehension		
Arithmetic		
Similarities		
Digit Span		
Vocabulary		
Verbal Score		
Digit Symbol		
Picture Completion		
Block Design		
Picture Arrangement		
Object Assembly		
Performance Score		
Total Score		

VERBAL SCORE_____IQ_____

PERFORMANCE SCORE_____IQ_____

FULL SCALE SCORE_____IQ_____

*Clinicians who wish to draw a "psychograph" on the above table may do so by connecting the subject's raw scores. The interpretation of any such profile, however, should take into account the reliabilities of the subtests and the lower reliabilities of differences between subtest scores.

Figure 19-1 Face sheet of the Wechsler Adult Intelligence Scale. (Courtesy of The Psychological Corporation.)

ability measures (scaled scores) for each of the subtests shown in Figure 19–1.

The first six subtests yield a verbal intelligence quotient, and the second five subtests produce a performance IQ. This division of intellectual abilities has neuroanatomical implications. The verbal IQ reflects language and abstract abilities and has been shown to correlate with left hemisphere function. The performance IQ reflects constructional and spatial abilities and is correlated with right hemisphere function.[80]

The verbal and performance subtests provide a Full Scale IQ, which is an expression of how an individual's global intellectual abilities compare with those of his same-age peer group. Although the same test protocol is used at all ages, fiftieth percentile (or IQ 100) score expectancy levels are changed at different age levels to account for expected accumulation of factual information and possible decrement in some performance functions associated with increasing age.

Prior Level of Intellectual Functioning

Since specific data concerning premorbid or prior functional level usually are not available, an estimate has to be made of how the patient's current mental function compares with his prior level. Such an estimate may be derived by one of three principal methods, the most traditional of which is comparison of ability in areas sensitive to decline in cerebral function with ability in areas comparatively resistant to such decline. The Wechsler Intelligence Scale subtests such as Vocabulary and Information, are regarded as "hold" items. The patient's performance on these items is compared to his performance on matched "don't hold" items such as Digit Span and Digit Symbol.

The comparison gives an index of deterioration.[61,112] Another method involves comparing the patient's fund of old, acquired information measured by academic skill in reading, spelling, and computation with his current functional intellectual levels. If a patient's retention of academic skills, for example, is compatible with an IQ of 100, and his current IQ test scores are in the 80–90 range, this suggests that his mental ability has deteriorated. If he had always functioned at an 80–90 IQ level, he would not likely have been able to acquire academic skills at the higher level. The third, and most sophisticated, method includes elements of the other two methods and adds an assessment of the patient's current capacity to process new material. The new material to be processed may require ability to form new cognitive sets involving reasoning classification, as in the Halstead Category Test; ability to process two serial sets simultaneously, as in part B of the Reitan Trail Making Test; ability to recognize principles, as in the conceptual portions of the Shipley Scale; or ability to form associations, as in the Hunt-Minnesota Test.[45,60,81,92]

Sensory-Perceptual Evaluation

The neuropsychological sensory evaluation quantifies the results of sensory examination techniques used by many neurological surgeons and of a few specialized tests of sensory information processing. An example of a quantified sensory perceptual examination familiar to neurologists and neurological surgeons is fingertip number writing. A set of four numbers preselected for maximum discriminability is written on the patient's palm to demonstrate how each number will be formed. The patient is then blindfolded (or asked to shut his eyes) and the numbers are written, in a predetermined sequence, on each of his fingers. A total of 20 numbers is presented to the fingertips of each hand. Although this quantified approach is a sensitive detector of impairment in symbolic tactile sensory recognition, its primary value is its ability to detect subtle differences in the levels of performance of the two sides of the body. Similar procedures are used in tactile recognition of coins and identification of fingers that have been lightly touched on their dorsal surfaces. Sensory stimuli are presented to each side of the body individually and then to both sides simultaneously to check for suppression. These examinations involve tactile, auditory, and visual modalities. Care is taken to present the stimulation at threshold levels for each side. Special sensory measures include the rate at which stroboscopic flicker is seen as steady light; the ability to recognize rhythmic auditory patterns; the ability to identify correct alternatives from similar sounding nonsense words, the rate at which a formboard puzzle can be assembled blindfolded, and the subsequent ability to draw the board and its blocks from memory.

Motor Evaluation

Two of the tests used in motor system assessment are finger oscillation and grip strength. The finger oscillation test consists of having the patient depress and release a lever with calibrated resistance as rapidly as possible, using the index finger of one hand. After the patient has had a practice period, his rate of tapping per 10-second interval is recorded, either electronically or by means of a calibrated counter on the tapping apparatus. A minimum of five separate trials is done for each hand. As with sensory measures such as fingertip number writing, right and left hand trials are counterbalanced to minimize the effect of such factors as fatigue and practice. Grip strength for the hand is measured by having the patient squeeze a dynamometer in a standardized position at arm's length. The size of the grip is adjusted to fit the hand of the patient. Several trials are done for each hand. The grip strength is recorded for each successive trial and weighted to equalize fatigue. In the motor and sensory portions of the neuropsychological assessment, elements of the traditional neurological examination are easily recognized. The exacting manner in which the same modalities are tested by the psychologist adds to the sensitivity of each portion of the examination, reduces discrepancies introduced by various examiners, and gives quantitative data against which subsequent evaluations can be compared.

Special Function Evaluation

The Reitan-Indiana Aphasia Screening Test measures such deficits as anomia, agraphia, letter and number agnosia and alexia, dysarthria, ideokinetic apraxia, and apraxias of construction and spelling.[114] Short-term memory for geometric figures in various spatial configurations is measured with the Benton Visual Retention Test or the Graham-Kendall Memory for Designs Test.[8,43] Receptive language may be measured with the Peabody or Full Range Picture Vocabulary tests, and ability to copy geometric figures of increasing complexity is measured by such instruments as the Beery Developmental Form Sequence or the Bender Motor Gestalt tests.[2,5,6,31]

The subtests from the Wechsler Intelligence Scales (Wechsler-Bellevue, Wechsler Adult Intelligence Scale, Wechsler Intelligence Scale for Children) provide considerable information about specific aspects of mental function.[111–113] The Digit Span subtests—which measure the patient's ability to repeat, both forward and backward, digits presented at timed intervals—are especially sensitive to short-term memory deficits. The Similarities subtest involves abstracting ability and perception of relationships between classes of events. The Arithmetic subtest involves verbal computation. Picture Arrangement, which requires the patient to arrange cartoon-like pictures in an orderly series, is sensitive to sequencing disturbances. Block Design involves the arrangement of colored blocks to match the design on a stimulus card. It is especially sensitive to construction dyspraxias.

Evaluation of children is considerably more complicated than evaluation of adults. Comprehensive batteries of tests for neuropsychological assessment are not well standardized and relatively few of them have localizing implications for children under 6 years of age. Tests that may have good localizing value in adults do not have the same validity in children because, for example, word recognition, which may have fairly specific anatomical implications in adults, is confounded in children by such considerations as the child's age and the reading instructional approach to which he has been exposed.[50,57]

CHOICE OF ASSESSMENT PROCEDURES

The major consideration in choosing the assessment battery and procedures for any patient is the purpose for which the evaluation is being done. Neuropsychological evaluations are most commonly requested to provide baseline measures for evaluating treatment or determining rate of recovery or decline, to diagnose the presence or extent or type of neurological impairment, and to aid in the planning of rehabilitation.

Baseline Studies

There are two major determinants of the testing procedure used in a baseline study. Most importantly, tests must be selected that will be uniquely sensitive to changes related to the patient's disease process and its treatment.[94] For a patient with Parkinson's disease, for instance, repeated measurements of his intellectual capacity to process new information as well as his performance on timed tests of motor dexterity would be selected. In cases in which the effectiveness of a cerebellar stimulator is to be evaluated, the psychologist would select tests maximally sensitive to motor functions. These might include the sustained rate of finger oscillation; the duration of contact between a hand-held metal stylus and a small disc on a rotary phonograph-type surface; the speed and accuracy of using a stylus between two strips of metal graduated in centimeters; the steadiness with which a stylus can be held into holes of graduated sizes without making contact; the manual or finger dexterity and rate of placing shaped objects into appropriate holes with either one or both hands; and resting involuntary movements as measured with a tremograph apparatus. In cases in which treatment has involved operative intervention in the left temporal area, baseline measures would tend to focus more on definitive assessment of such language-related abilities as letter and word recognition, timed word production according to such criteria as "beginning with B" or "rhyming with red," abstracting ability, rate of learning "new alphabet" types of language, and word definition; and ability to see relationships between classes of events. For another type of condition, baseline measures of the patient's level of alertness are often requested. This type of baseline is most commonly employed when the efficacy of drug therapy is being investigated. It can equally appropriately be used to measure rate of decline with a degenerative mental process or rate of improvement following an operation. Measures included in this baseline are those of reaction time to different types of stimuli, performance on timed tests of various types of problem solving (e.g., the Wechsler Block Design or Digit Symbol subtests), speed and accuracy on maze tests, ability to concentrate on a task in the face of distractions (the Stroop Color-Word Test or the Background Interference Procedure), speed and accuracy in such activities as underlining the letter *e* in pages of specially prepared text, and the rate of rapid finger oscillation over extended periods.

In addition to measuring abilities likely to be affected by the condition being studied, tests must be selected with regard to their potential for use over extended periods of time. Some tests have alternate and equivalent forms. By alternating the forms used in serial evaluations, reliable baseline and follow-up studies can be obtained. The results of some tests, such as the Wechsler scales, show the effects of practice if they are administered at intervals of less than six months. As a consequence, they would not be appropriate for use in cases in which repeated measurements several days or weeks apart were needed. The age of the person being evaluated can also influence the appropriateness of tests for use over extended periods, especially in patients up to around 16 years of age.[40,88] The Wechsler Adult Intelligence Scale, for example, is appropriate at any age over 16 years, but a patient at age 15 would be given the Wechsler Intelligence Scale for Children. Thus changes found in a given profile pattern between the ages of 15 and 17 might possibly be attributable to a change in the test instrument rather than to change in the patient's mental function. Other tests, like the Stanford-Binet, use essentially different test items at each age level so that the test items for age 2½ are entirely different from the test items at age 3½.[101] Thus, although resulting in a single numerical IQ score, these tests may be measuring quite different types of mental processing at different

ages.[56] Scores on still other tests, especially those involving fund of knowledge, may be artificially elevated on retest by the patient's having had opportunity to study for the test. Unfortunately, many studies that report improvement in mental function after surgical or medical intervention may be merely reflecting gains due to practice.

General Diagnostic Evaluations

When assessment is requested to determine the presence, location, or type of neurological impairment, a "successive sieves" type of procedure is usually employed.[112] The initial step investigates whether there is evidence of neurological impairment. To do this, the patient's global mental functioning is compared with normative data for his age, educational and work history, and levels of performance on tasks of progressive sensitivity to neurological deficit. Assessment at this level is most sensitive to false positive types of error. Patterns compatible with neurological impairment may also reflect impairment due to anxiety, depression, or other emotional disturbances.[48,51,72,74,109]

The next step is to look for asymmetry of function of the hemispheres, initially comparing levels of language with spatial aspects of intellectual functioning. Numerous studies have reported lower verbal than performance IQ in patients with unilateral left hemisphere lesions and lower performance than verbal IQ in those with right hemisphere lesions.[27,36,80,82,83,93,108]

Localization, either within a cerebral hemisphere or bilaterally, is approached by means of specific Wechsler subtests and the special sensory and motor components of the neuropsychological test battery.[85] The Wechsler Similarities subtest is uniquely sensitive to left temporal lobe dysfunction, just as the Wechsler Picture Arrangement subtest is sensitive to right temporal lesions.[75] Similar relationships have been found between the Wechsler Digit Span subtest and left frontal lesions, between Block Design and right parietal lesions, and between Arithmetic and left parietal lesions.[70] Although these various subtests do have individual localizing correlations, it is common practice to combine them into specific clusters of factors that relate to given brain loci.[18,34,69,89,115]

Rate of rapid finger oscillation and grip strength provide some measure of fairly simple functions subserved by motor areas. The scores achieved are suitable for comparison with appropriate normal expectancies and for comparison of one hand against the other.[17,91,98] More complex aspects of motor integrative functions are assessed by, for example, the Tactual Performance Test, which measures speed of completing a formboard type of puzzle while blindfolded. The patient solves the puzzle with each hand independently and then with both hands. Evaluation of ideokinetic apraxia and construction apraxia may also involve subtests from the Aphasia Screening Test, speed of name writing with preferred and nonpreferred hands, and reaction time to visual and auditory stimuli.[10,15,26,28,84,97] Functions subserved by specific areas of the sensory cortices are evaluated by measuring the response to individual and simultaneous bilateral visual, auditory, and tactile stimuli; ability to differentiate speech sounds and rhythmic patterns and to estimate time; visual search patterns, short-term memory, dichotic listening, and short-term memory for linguistic and spatial imagery.[4,21,24,42,106]

Although not all these measures will be employed by all neuropsychologists in a general diagnostic evaluation, most will be included in one form or another. To determine the presence, location, and type of neurological impairment, it is necessary to sample the abilities measured by these types of tests to reach a valid estimate of the state of the brain.

Inferences concerning chronicity or acuteness of the disorder are based on comparisons of profiles or patterns derived from the various tests with the patient's prior levels of functioning. Average ability levels on such constructional praxis measures as Wechsler Block Design subtests, copying geometric figures, and short-term spatial memory could be regarded as indicative of little or no impairment in a high-school graduate employed as an office worker. An average score in a surgeon or architect, however, would suggest the possibility of a parietal lobe lesion. These latter individuals could be presumed to have functioned well above average on most mental tasks, especially on those specifically related to their areas of special expertise. The magnitude of discrepancies between levels of performance on different types of tasks offers important clues to the chronicity of impairment. In general the greatest discrepancy is found in patients with the more acute types of lesions.[38,87]

As a final step in the general diagnostic evaluation, the levels of performance of intact and impaired functions subserved by specific brain areas are evaluated with regard to possible causes compatible with the findings. To formulate anatomical and etiological diagnoses, the psychologist must be well versed not only in neuroanatomy but also in diseases of the nervous system. Not surprisingly this sort of skill and experience is in limited quantity. While the neurologically oriented physician relies heavily on the clinical history as well as the results of his examination of the patient, traditional neuropsychological diagnoses are formulated with no history whatsoever and without the neuropsychologist himself even seeing the patient. Psychological test data collected by a trained technician are his only input. The fact that this information can be translated into an anatomical localization and a differential diagnosis is surprising. The following case is an example of how well the tests can work.

A young man presented with recurrent headaches. At admission, the physical examination was reported to be normal. The patient had an extensive neuropsychological evaluation. The test data revealed him to be of normal intelligence. All measures of left hemisphere function were normal. Tests reflecting right hemisphere function showed some impairment. Further analysis revealed the functions of the right motor cortex to be good and the right occipital cortex to be normal. Deficits were localized to the functions served by the right parietal lobe. Chronic dysfunction and superimposed acute dysfunction of right parietal lobe were identified. In view of the patient's youth, the absence of multiple foci of involvement, and the failure of the pattern of mental impairment to fall into an area of the brain served by any of the major blood vessels, cerebral infarction was deemed unlikely. Although the dysfunction was localized and had some acute features, the coexistence of chronic dysfunction made a rapidly growing tumor unlikely. Two diagnoses, meningioma and arteriovenous malformation, were given serious consideration, but the extent of deficit was believed to be more compatible with arteriovenous malformation. The lesion was demonstrated by arteriography.

The initial differential diagnosis by the neurosurgeon also was an arteriovenous malformation. Unlike the neuropsychologist, the neurosurgeon had been guided by the patient's history. The complementary nature of these two approaches to a clinical problem is evident.

Rehabilitation Planning

Diagnostic assessment focuses on areas of deficit or impairment. In contrast, evaluation for rehabilitation planning focuses on areas of relative strengths that may have implications for longer-term medical management programs. One area of special interest in rehabilitation planning is the determination of vocational potential. Although there are some variations, it is generally true that there are minimum levels of intellectual function required for the performance of most jobs. Just as a level of intelligence in the top 5 per cent of the population is necessary for an individual to perform adequately as a practicing physician, a functional level in the top 30 per cent is common for electricians, in the top 50 per cent for barbers, and above the twenty-fifth percentile for truck drivers.[46,71] Indeed, in descriptions of job requirements, the Department of Labor lists the mental levels required to do most jobs.[105] In the case of a patient who has had a significant decline in mental function secondary to some neurological impairment, the evaluation of residual mental capacity may be a primary consideration in determining his potential for resuming some sort of gainful employment. In addition to global mental adequacy, many occupations require competence in a particular skill. A factory assembler, for example, must have a certain level of eye-hand and manual dexterity just as a bookkeeper must have facility in calculation. Not uncommonly, following a cerebrovascular accident or closed head injury, a patient may recover a good degree of global mental function, yet have residual deficits in specific areas that would preclude return to his usual type of work. Although most neuropsychologists are not particularly well versed in the mental requirements for specific jobs, their test data relative to discrete abilities can substantially help a vocational counselor or disability examiner to determine to what, if any, jobs the patient may be able to return.

On a more basic level, it may be of value to determine whether a patient is capable of self-care and how to teach these types of skills. Comprehensive neuropsychological evaluation of several hundred patients has revealed that perceptual and cognitive factors are more important than dysphasia, age, medical condition, or hemisensory deficit in predicting physical rehabilitation.[35]

Neuropsychological evaluation can, likewise, help in the early identification of school problems. As a result, it can help in the development of a management plan that will detect potential learning disorders and provide timely intervention for their prevention or amelioration.[49,54] For example, children with shunts for hydrocephalus often present as highly verbal and apparently intelligent. The authors' neuropsychological evaluation of 54 consecutive patients with shunts, however, revealed that a significantly large number of them had lower nonlanguage than language function.[58] If this condition were not detected before these children were considered ready for school, the heavy dependence on perceptual-motor functions of most kindergarten and first grade curricula would place them at risk for early school failure. Promptly identified, these perceptual-motor deficiencies can be treated before the child is exposed to the demands of school. Occasionally children with left hemisphere deficits are able to function fairly effectively in early school grades, but experience increasing academic difficulty as schoolwork demands increasing reliance on higher-order abstracting skills. Although there may be no specific treatment that can improve the child's level of function, the neuropsychologist and neurologically oriented physician may be able to provide school guidance personnel with data concerning the child's relative strengths and weaknesses and thus help both in formulating reasonable expectancies and in developing instructional methods and curricular objectives most compatible with his nonlanguage strengths.

PRACTICAL CONSIDERATIONS IN THE USE OF NEUROPSYCHOLOGICAL TESTING

Before the practicing physician can judge the value of neuropsychological evaluation or any other ancillary diagnostic procedure he must consider its accuracy, risks, and cost in time and money. The physician should know the general nature of the procedure, what is required of the patient, and the type of information about the patient that can be obtained. Some of these questions have been dealt with in previous sections, e.g., the indications for neuropsychological assessment, but the economic considerations and the validity of the diagnoses in comparison with other neurodiagnostic techniques are worthy of separate attention.

Requirements for Adequate Neuropsychological Examination

A comprehensive evaluation requires that the patient be alert and also able to participate in an examination that may require from 6 to 12 hours, quite possibly spread over several days. Examinations should not be planned to follow procedures that require heavy sedation or in the immediate postoperative period. When the purpose of the evaluation is to assess the effects of surgical or medical treatment, it is mandatory that a baseline evaluation be scheduled prior to the treatment. The test materials and the distraction-free environment needed for valid assessment usually require that the patient be seen in a specially equipped laboratory. Costs of an evaluation approximate those of computed tomography in most areas of the country. Although usually covered by insurance programs when the patient is hospitalized, an examination performed as an outpatient procedure may not be covered. Since most neuropsychological laboratories employ a fairly standard battery of tests, the administration usually is delegated to trained technicians. It is not customary for the neuropsychologist to see the patient personally. It is his task to make an objective comparison of a patient's performance with normative data for the same-age peers.

Validity of Neuropsychological Diagnoses

The ability of the standardized neuropsychological test battery to differentiate persons with brain damage from controls has been demonstrated repeatedly.[23,79,108] Such a battery is sensitive to cerebral disease even in those patients who have not shown abnormalities on the neurological examination.[53,64] Some investigators have reported good agreement between neuropsychological findings and lateralized electroencephalographic abnormalities. The Wechsler Verbal IQ's are lower in patients whose electroencephalograms show left hemisphere abnormalities, and the Performance IQ's are lower in those with right-sided abnormalities. Agreement with these findings has, however, not been unanimous.[52,63]

A number of studies confirm the respective correlations of the Wechsler Performance and Verbal IQ scores with right and left hemisphere lesions, verified by operation, radiologically, or at autopsy.[36,63,80] Other studies attest to the lateralizing value of selected neuropsychological tests.[16,59,114] Removal of brain areas such as one prefrontal cortex or one anterior temporal lobe has been associated with little or no change in performance on neuropsychological tests, however, suggesting that chronic disease in these areas may not always be detected by the neuropsychological test battery.[76,77] There are few adequate data based on comparisons of the performance of patients with organic disease and of those with psychiatric disease on neuropsychological tests. Investigators have commonly classified patients as either "organic" or "psychiatric," without determining whether there might be organic disease in the psychiatric patients or psychiatric disease in patients classified as organically impaired.[47,109,110] One study compared 32 patients with brain damage with an equal number of "pseudo-neurological" patients. These groups were matched for age, sex, and years of education. Individuals with subnormal IQ were excluded. All these patients had been evaluated from both the neurological and the psychiatric standpoint. Tests selected from the Halstead battery showed a significant difference between the groups.[74]

The following case histories illustrate the use of neuropsychological testing and demonstrate its correlation with other diagnostic procedures and the validity of the diagnoses.

Case 1. Young Woman
with Severe Focal Headache
of Several Years' Duration

HISTORY. A 35-year-old right-handed woman had complained of "excruciating" headaches for several years. Usually they were on the right. Electroencephalograms and contrast studies had been performed without demonstrating any lesion. No focal abnormalities were present on the neurological examination, but her physicians felt that some organic problem was present and that the patient had experienced some decline in mental function.

TEST BATTERY. Projective technique: Rorschach. Neuropsychological battery: Aphasia Screening Test; Archimedes Spiral; Babcock Sentence; Critical Flicker Fusion; Finger Oscillation; Memory for Designs; Retinal Rivalry Test; Strong Digit Symbol; Tactual Performance Test; Trail Making; Wechsler-Bellevue Intelligence Scale (Form I); Wechsler Memory Scale (Form I); Weigl-Goldstein Color-Form Sorting.

RESULTS. The patient's performance on several tests sensitive to brain damage was considerably below normal. The Tactual Performance, Retinal Rivalry, and Trail Making tests were all done slowly and poorly. Full Scale, Verbal and Performance IQ's were 102, 104, and 99 respectively, falling on the average range. Estimates of her prior level of function, based on such items as her Vocabulary subtest score of 15, suggested an original Verbal IQ potentially at the 134 level, a full 30 points above her current Verbal IQ. Similar estimate placed her original Performance IQ approximately 22 points higher than her present level. All indices of deterioration pointed to a 20–40 per cent loss of intellectual function.

Other findings established specific subacute brain damage in the right hemisphere, primarily in the posterior temporal and parietal area. Suppression of the left-sided stimulus on simultaneous presentation of auditory and tactile stimuli was noted. While tapping speed was only slightly depressed in the left hand compared to the right, the patient required twice as much time to complete a formboard test blindfolded when using the left hand. Simple shapes were recognized with more difficulty than coins in either hand. The patient demonstrated finger dysgnosia and fingertip writing loss on the left hand. No difficulty was encountered in the Picture Arrangement or Memory for Designs tests, which are related to right posterior frontal and anterior temporal integrity.

FOLLOW-UP. Seven years after this examination a tumor was identified and removed from the right temporal parietal region.

Case 2. Repeated Evaluations of Patient with Arteriovenous Malformation

HISTORY. A 17-year-old right-handed high-school student was referred for neuropsychological studies to determine the extent and nature of intellectual and personality impairment involved in his deteriorating school performance. The patient had been a nearly straight A student through the eighth grade. He received B's in ninth grade, C's in tenth grade, and D's in the eleventh grade.

During the summer following his ninth grade of school, he began to experience occasional focal seizures beginning in the right foot and progressing to involve the right leg. Although conscious and able to hear and comprehend during an attack, he could not speak and had difficulty "finding words" for several minutes after an attack. He was examined by a neurologist who noted no focal or lateralizing signs. He had a soft bruit over the left eye. A left frontal-parietal arteriovenous malformation was subsequently demonstrated by cerebral arteriography. Occasional seizures and progressive school difficulty persisted after an anticonvulsant medication regimen was started. There appeared to be striking fluctuations from day to day in intellectual functioning.

TEST BATTERY. Aphasia Screening Test; Archimedes Spiral; Babcock Sentence; Bender Visual Motor Gestalt (on two separate occasions), Critical Flicker Fusion; Finger Oscillation; Memory for Designs; Retinal Rivalry Test; Seashore Rhythm Test; Strong Digit Symbol Test; Tactual Performance Test, Trail Making; Wechsler-Bellevue Intelligence Scale (Form I); Weigl-Goldstein Color-Form Sorting. A projective test, the Rorschach, was also given.

RESULTS. The patient's test performances gave evidence of impairment in both motor and sensory functions of the left hemisphere. Tapping was performed more slowly by the right hand; a significant number of errors in fingertip number writing were noted on the right. It took the patient six minutes longer to complete the Tactual Performance Test with the right hand. He had trouble perceiving correctly the right-sided of two geometric designs and grasping the concept of sorting shapes by color. Although he had difficulty pronouncing "Massachusetts," no other dysphasic symptoms were elicited.

Equally or perhaps more striking were evidences of right hemisphere dysfunction, particularly in the right parietal lobe. There was an extreme 36-point discrepancy between his verbal symbolic ability (Verbal IQ: 117) and his spatial configurational ability (Performance IQ: 81) on the Wechsler-Bellevue Scale. The subtest scores further indicated that he had once had superior intellectual ability and that deterioration was especially marked in his perception of part-whole and body image items as well as in visual-interpretive and perceptual-motor skills.

Subtest Scaled Scores on the
Wechsler-Bellevue Intelligence Scale

Verbal		Performance	
Information	13	Picture Arrangement	11
Comprehension	12	Picture Completion	7
Vocabulary	13	Block Design	3

Arithmetic	13	Object Assembly	6
Similarities	12	Digit Symbol	11
Digit Span	10		

On the Tactual Performance Test, drawing apraxia was dramatic, e.g., "I can picture a star, tell what it is, recognize it, but I can't draw it."

CONCLUSIONS AND RECOMMENDATIONS Conclusion reached from the test battery: The patient's deterioration in school performance was due to a decline in mental functioning caused by the arteriovenous malformation. The scores were especially low in those functions subserved by the right parietal lobe. Although the malformation was on the left side, it appeared to be stealing circulation from the right hemisphere. The patient was advised to alter his class schedule to replace subjects requiring skills in his weaker areas of function, e.g., geometry, with others more related to his areas of strength, e.g., literature. Supportive psychoeducational counseling was offered and begun.

FOLLOW-UP. By modifying his curriculum, the patient was able to bring his grades up to passing level. Subsequent evaluations were performed at 24 and 29 years of age. They revealed further mild deterioration suggesting that the left arteriovenous malformation continued to steal blood from the right hemisphere.

Case 3. Postoperative Evaluation of a Woman with an Arteriovenous Malformation

HISTORY. A 23-year-old right-handed college graduate underwent operation for arteriovenous malformation in the left occipital-parietal area. She was evaluated 16 days later to estimate her potential for recovery.

TEST BATTERY. Aphasia Screening Test; Categories Test; Tactual Performance Test; Tapping Test; Wide Range Achievement Test; Wechsler Adult Intelligence Scale; Trail-Making Test; Rhythm Test; Speech Sounds Perception Test; Finger Agnosia; Fingertip Number Writing, and Tactile Form Recognition tests.

RESULTS. The patient scored in the borderline range of intellectual ability on the verbal section of the Wechsler Adult Intelligence Scale (Verbal IQ: 81) but was unable to perform some of the performance tests, apparently because of the effects of medications, which is not an uncommon problem in the evaluation of neurosurgical patients. Because of the medication, the Performance IQ of 48 was believed to be meaningless.

Speed of tapping and grip strength were depressed in the right hand compared to the left. The patient failed to perceive a tactile stimulus applied on the right hand when simultaneously stimulated in the left side of the face. Simple figures were copied poorly with either hand.

The patient was able to speak in sentences, but word recognition was at the late first-grade level on the Wide Range Achievement Test. On the Aphasia Screening Test, summarized as follows, she had difficulty in naming common objects, in oral reading, and in writing to dictation, as well as dyscalculia and some left-right disorientation. Both verbal and motor perseverations were noted.

Adult Aphasia Screening Test Responses

1. "Copy this.": (Recognizable but poor square.)
2. "Name it.": "Square."
3. "Spell it.": "S-q-u-a-r-e."
4. "Copy this." (cross): (Recognizable but poor cross.)
5. "Name it.": "Square—I call it a square."
6. "Spell cross.": "C-r-o-s-s."
7. "Copy this." (triangle): (Fair likeness.)
8. "Name it.": "I can't tell you—I know but I can't tell you" (cried). "I used to know it—it upsets me that I don't know."
9. "Spell triangle": "T-r-i-a-n-g-l-e."
10. "Name this." (baby): "A picture of a man."
11. "Write what this is." (face of a clock with Roman numerals, hands indicating eleven o'clock): "A number four" (patient looking at Roman numeral X), (she writes) "N I N V."
12. "Name this." (fork): "You can eat with it."
13. "Read this." (7 SIX 2): "Six, seven and six." (Pointing to 2) "That says six."
14. "Read this." (M G W): "M-G-W."
15. "Read this." (He is a friendly animal, a famous winner of dog shows.): "That is a friendly . . . friendual, friendual, friendual, friendual, -ual, -ual, show."
16. "Read this." (See the black dog): "Something about the black dog."
17. "Repeat triangle.": "Triangle."
18. "Repeat Massachusetts.": "Massachusetts."
19. "Repeat Methodist Episcopal.": "Methodist Episcopal."
20. "Write Square.": "S U N N R R" (she writes).
21. "Read this." (seven): "Seven."
22. "Repeat seven.": "Seven."
23. "Repeat 'He shouted the warning.'": "He shouted the warning."
24. "Explain 'He shouted the warning.'": "If something is wrong you'll shout out so to warn them so they won't get caught or hurt or something."
25. "Write 'He shouted the warning.'" (She writes) "S N N R R."
26. "Compute $85 - 27$.": "He shouted something?"
27. "Compute 17×3: (Patient unable. She answered correctly 3×2 but not 12×4 when verbally presented.)
28. "Name this." (key): "A knife, no, that's a key."

29. "Demonstrate how it is used.": (She does.)
30. (Key drawing was omitted.)
31. "Read this." (Place left hand to right ear.): "Place left hand on—at right ear."
32. "Place your left hand to your right ear.": (Places right hand to right ear.)
33. "Place your left hand to your left elbow.": (Places left hand to left ear.)

SUMMARY AND RECOMMENDATIONS. The impairments that this patient showed seemed to be more generalized than usually seen in a purely focal lesion. The right-sided sensory and motor problems together with the fluent aphasia suggest dysfunction throughout the middle part of the left cerebral hemisphere. On the basis of this evaluation, prognosis would be difficult; however, it seemed probable that within a few months she should score at a near-average level of intelligence, although it could not be stated whether she would achieve a premorbid level of function. Follow-up examination in six months was strongly recommended.

Case 4. Malingering Versus Brain Damage in an Auto Accident Victim

HISTORY. A 59-year-old right-handed rancher was involved in an automobile accident. He was thrown from the car and sustained rib fractures and facial lacerations. He remained unconscious for approximately 24 hours. There was a persistent complaint of left-sided weakness, headaches, and fatigue following the accident. His examining physicians believed him to be fully recovered except for a questionable cervical nerve root irritation and mental depression. Because of pending disability hearings and minimal findings on neurological examination, hysteria or malingering was suspected.

TEST BATTERY. At 6 months and 14 months postinjury, complete neuropsychological reevaluation was made with the same battery used in the prior evaluation, except where alternate forms could be applied or other alterations could be made to reduce any effects of practice. The basic battery consisted of the Wechsler Bellevue Adult Intelligence Scale (Form I); Wechsler Memory Scale (Form I); Finger Oscillation Test; Critical Flicker Fusion Test; Tactual Performance Test; Strong Digit Symbol Test; Trail Making Test; Archimedes Spiral Test; Weigl-Goldstein Color-Form Sorting; Babcock Sentence; Seashore Rhythm Test; Memory for Designs; Retinal Rivalry Test; Color Blind Test; Aphasia Screening Test; Rorschach.

RESULTS. On each evaluation, similar findings suggestive of diffuse brain impairment were found. There was marked scatter in Wechsler subtest scores; evidence of central dysarthria, contructional dyspraxia, suppression of hand on simultaneous face-hand stimulation on the Aphasia Screening Test; and scores falling below the normal cut-offs on the Babcock Sentence test. Also Memory for Designs, Strong Digit Symbol Test, Trail Making B, Tactual Performance Test and Finger Oscillation Test suggested diffuse brain impairment.

There was a highly consistent relationship between performance on the two tests with equivalent forms that were used. This consistency in performance was believed to be impossible to counterfeit. The patient's areas of strength as well as of weakness held steady from one examination to the next. It was concluded that the findings of the two evaluations implied the presence of diffuse brain damage that appeared to be permanent and stable, and effectively excluded malingering.

Case 5. Preoperative and Postoperative Evaluation of a Man with Parasagittal Meningioma

HISTORY. A 52-year-old man's illness was diagnosed as a right parasagittal meningioma. His physicians believed him to be of dull normal intelligence even prior to developing the tumor. Since meningiomas are slow growing and extrinsic to the brain substance and derive their vascular supply from the external carotid circulation, they have been believed by physicians and neuropsychologists alike to have little impact on cortical function. No significant mental change was expected in this patient as a result of operation.

TEST BATTERY. Aphasia Screening Test; Archimedes Spiral; Babcock Sentence; Critical Flicker Fusion; Finger Oscillation; Memory for Designs; Retinal Rivalry Test; Strong Digit Symbol; Tactual Performance Test; Trail Making; Wechsler-Bellevue Intelligence Scale (Form I): Wechsler Memory Scale (Form I); Weigl-Goldstein Color-Form Sorting; Raven Progressive Color Matrices Test.

RESULTS. The preoperative intelligence scores for Verbal, Performance, and Full Scale IQ's respectively were 87, 80, and 83, while the postoperative function was revealed, by alternate and statistically equivalent forms, as 104, 100, and 103. Left hand suppression on face-hand stimulation and left finger dysgnosia noted preoperatively were no longer present. His score on the Raven Progressive Color Matrices Test rose from the tenth to the fiftieth percentile. The Memory for Designs Test, failed preoperatively, was passed after operation.

While the patient failed to pass certain items in the neuropsychological battery both preoperatively and postoperatively, the striking 17-point increase in verbal function, 20-point increase in visual spatial function, and 20-point increase in overall intellectual function was gratifying. It would be expected that the patient would also improve in job performance and daily activities.

Acknowledgments. The authors wish to thank neuropsychologists W. Lynn Smith, Ph.D., Porter Memorial Hospital, Denver, Colorado, who provided protocols for cases 1, 2, 4, and 5, and James Reed, Ph.D., New England Medical Center Hospital, Boston, Mass., who provided case 3. The authors assume responsibility for substantial deletions of both data and findings from the cases. We also thank the Psychological Corporation for allowing reproduction of the face sheet of the Wechsler Adult Intelligence Scale.

REFERENCES

1. Aita, J. A., Armitage, S. G., Reitan, R. M., and Rabinovitz, A.: The use of certain psychological tests in the evaluation of brain injury. J. Gen. Psychol., *37*:25–44, 1947.

2. Ammons, R. B., and Ammons, H. S.: The Full Range Picture Vocabulary Test. Missoula, Mont., Psychological Test Specialists, 1948.

3. Anastasi, A.: Differential Psychology. New York, Macmillan, 1960.

4. Baddeley, A. D., and Warrington, E. K.: Memory coding and amnesia. Neuropsychologia, *11*:159–165, 1973.

5. Beery, K. E.: Developmental Test of Visual Motor Integration. Chicago, Follett Publishing Co., 1967.

6. Bender, L.: A Visual Motor Gestalt Test and Its Clinical Use. New York, American Orthopsychiatric Assoc., 1958.

7. Benton, A. L.: Right-left discrimination and finger localizations in defective children. Amer. J. Orthopsychiat., *10*:719–746, 1940.

8. Benton, A. L.: The Revised Visual Retention Test. New York, The Psychological Corp., 1955.

9. Benton, A. L.: Right-left Discrimination and Finger Localizations. New York, Hoetag, 1959.

10. Benton, A. L., and Joynt, R. J.: Reaction time in unilateral cerebral disease. Confin. Neurol., *19*:247, 1959.

11. Binet, A., and Henri, V.: La psychologie individuelle. Année Psychol., *2*:411–463, 1895.

12. Binet, A., and Simon, T.: Methodes nouvelles pour le diagnostic du niveau intellectuel des anormoux. Année Psychol., *11*:191–244, 1905.

13. Binet, A., and Simon, T.: Les Idees Modernes sur les Enfants. Paris, E. Flammarion, 1909.

14. Binet, A., and Simon, T.: The Development of Intelligence in Children. Baltimore, Williams & Wilkins Co., 1916.

15. Blackburn, H. L., and Benton, A. L.: Simple and choice reaction time in cerebral disease. Confin. Neurol., *15*:327, 1955.

16. Boll, T. J.: Right and left cerebral hemisphere damage and tactile perception: Performance of the ipsilateral and contralateral sides of the body. Neuropsychologia, *12*:235–238, 1974.

17. Boll, T. J., and Reitan, R. M.: Comparative ability interrelationships in normal and brain-damaged children. J. Clin. Psychol., *28*:152–156, 1972.

18. Boll, T. J., and Reitan, R. M.: Motor and tactile-perceptual deficits in brain damaged children. Percept. Motor Skills, *34*:343–350, 1972.

19. Boring, E. G.: A History of Experimental Psychology. New York, Appleton-Century-Croft, 1950.

20. Broca, P.: Sur la faculté du language articulé. Bull. Soc. Anthropol., *6*:493–494, 1865.

21. Butters, N., Samuels, I., Goodglass H., et al.: Short term visual and auditory memory disorders after parietal and frontal lobe damage. Cortex, *6*:440–459, 1970.

22. Cattell, J. Mck.: Mental tests and measurements. Minol, *15*:375–380, 1890.

23. Chapman, L. F., and Wolff, H. G.: The cerebral hemispheres and the highest integrative functions of man. Arch. Neurol., *1*:357–424, 1959.

24. Chedru, F., Leblanc, M., and Lhermitte, F.: Visual searching in normal and brain-damaged subjects. Cortex, *9*:94–111, 1973.

25. Cronbach, L. J.: Essentials of Psychological Testing. New York, Harper & Row, 1960.

26. Dee, H. L., and Van Allen, M. W.: Psychomotor testing as an aid in the recognition of cerebral lesions. Neurology (Minneap.), *22*:845–848, 1972.

27. Dennerll, R. D.: Prediction of unilateral brain dysfunction using Wechsler test scores. J. Consult. Psychol., *28*:278–284, 1964.

28. DeRenzi, E., and Faglioni, P.: The comparative efficiency of intelligence and vigilance tests in detecting hemispheric cerebral damage. Cortex, *1*:410, 1965.

29. Dodrill, C. B., and Wilkus, R. J.: EEG epileptiform activity and neuropsychological performance. Presented at the annual meeting of the American Psychological Association, Washington, D.C., September, 1976.

30. Doehring, D. G., and Reitan, R. M.: Concept attainment of human adults with lateralized cerebral lesions. Percept. Motor Skills, *14*:27–33, 1962.

31. Dunn, L. M.: Peabody Picture Vocabulary Test. Circle Pines, Minnesota, American Guidance Service, 1965.

32. Ebbinghaus, H.: Über eine neue Methode zur prüfung questiger fähigkeiten und ihre anwendung bei schulkindern. Z. Psychol., *13*:401–459, 1897.

33. Eckhardt, W.: Piotrowski's signs: Organic or functional? J. Clin. Psychol., *17*:36–38, 1961.

34. Fedio, P., and Mirsky, A. F.: Selective intellectual deficits in children with temporal lobe or centrencephalic epilepsy. Neuropsychologia, *7*:287–300, 1967.

35. Feigenson, J. S., and Brown, E. R.: A multivariate study of neuropsychological factors affecting outcome in stroke rehabilitation. Int. Neuropsychol. Soc. meeting abstr., 1977, p. 4.

36. Fields, F. R., and Whitmyre, J. W.: Verbal and performance relationships with respect to laterality of cerebral involvement. Dis. Nerv. Syst., *30*:177–179, 1969.

37. Fitzhugh, K. B., Fitzhugh, L. C., and Reitan, R. M.: Psychological deficits in relation to acuteness of brain dysfunction. J. Consult. Psychol., *25*:61–66, 1961.

38. Fitzhugh, K. B., Fitzhugh, L. C., and Reitan, R. M.: Wechsler-Bellevue comparisons in groups with "chronic" and "current" lateralized and diffuse brain lesions. J. Consult. Psychol., *26*:306–310, 1962.

39. Galton, F.: Inquiries into Human Faculty and Its Development. London, Macmillan, 1893.

40. Ghent, L.: Developmental changes in tactual thresholds on dominant and nondominant

sides. J. Comp. Physiol. Psychol., 54:670–673, 1961.

41. Ghent, L., Weinstein, S., Semmes, J., and Teuber, H. L.: Effect of unilateral brain injury in man on learning of tactual discrimination. J.Comp. Physiol. Psychol., 48:478–481, 1955.

42. Goodglass, H.: Binaural digit presentation and early lateral brain damage. Cortex, 3:295–306, 1967.

43. Graham, F. K., and Kendall, B. S.: Memory-For-Designs Test: Revised General Manual. Percept. Motor Skills Monogr. Suppl, 2, 11:147–188, 1960.

44. Green, T. K., and Reitan, R. M.: Brain lesion momentum and behavioral adaptation to human intracranial neoplasms. Presented at the annual meeting of the American Psychological Association, Washington, D.C., September, 1976.

45. Halstead, W. C.: Brain and Intelligence. Chicago, University of Chicago Press, 1947.

46. Harrell, T. W., and Harrell, M. S.: Army General Classification Test scores for civilian occupations. Educ. Psychol. Measmt., 5:231–239, 1945.

47. Hartlage L.C.: Common psychological tests applied to the assessment of brain damage. J. Proj. Tech. Pers. Assess., 30:319–338, 1966.

48. Hartlage, L. C.: Diagnostic profiles of four types of learning disabled children. J. Clin. Psychol., 29:458–463, 1973.

49. Hartlage, L. C.: Neuropsychological approaches to predicting outcome of remedial educational strategies for learning disabled children. Pediat. Psychol., 3:23, 1975.

50. Hartlage, L. C.: Differential age correlates of reading ability. Percept. Motor Skills, 41:968–970, 1975.

51. Hartlage, L. C., and Garber, J.: Spatial and nonspatial reasoning ability in chronic schizophrenics. J. Clin. Psychol., 32:235–237, 1976.

52. Hartlage, L. C., and Green, J. B.: The EEG as a predictor of intellective and academic performance. J. Learn. Dis., 6:42–45, 1973.

53. Hartlage, L. C., and Hartlage, P. L.: Relative contributions of neurology and neuropsychology in the diagnosis of learning disabilities. Presented at the annual meeting of the International Neuropsychology Society, New Orleans, February, 1973.

54. Hartlage, P. L., and Hartlage, L. C.: Classroom correlates of neurological soft signs. Presented at the annual meeting of the American Psychological Association, New Orleans, September, 1974.

55. Hartlage, L. C., and Hartlage, P. L.: The application of neuropsychological principles in the diagnosis of learning disabilities. In Tarnopol, L., ed.: Brain Function and Learning Disabilities. Rotterdam, Rotterdam University Press, 1977.

56. Hartlage, L. C., and Lucas, D. G.: Mental Development Evaluation of the Pediatric Patient. Springfield, Ill., Charles C Thomas Co., 1973.

57. Hartlage, L. C., Lucas, D. G., and Main, W. H.: Comparison of three approaches to teaching reading skills. Percept. Motor Skills, 34:231–232, 1972.

58. Hawkins, J., and Allen, M. B.: Our experience with shunts in 99 consecutive cases of shunting for hydrocephalus. Presented at the annual meeting of the Georgia Neurological Society, Atlanta, Georgia, September, 1974.

59. Heimburger, R. F., and Reitan, R. M.: Easily administered written test for lateralizing brain lesions. J. Neurosurg., 18:301–312, 1961.

60. Hunt, H. F.: A practical clinical test for organic brain damage. J. Appl. Psychol., 27:375–386, 1943.

61. Hunt, W. L.: The relative rates of decline of Wechsler Bellevue "hold" and "don't hold" tests. J. Consult. Psychol., 13:440–443, 1949.

62. Kelley, T. L.: Crossroads in the Mind of Man: A Study of Differentiable Mental Abilities. Stanford, Cal., Stanford University Press, 1928.

63. Kløve, H.: Relationship of differential encephalographic patterns to distribution of Wechsler-Bellevue scores. Neurology (Minneap.), 9:871–876, 1959.

64. Kløve, H.: The relationship between neuropsychologic test performance and neurologic status. Presented at the annual meeting of the American Academy of Neurology, Minneapolis, May, 1963.

65. Kløve, H., and Fitzhugh, K. B.: Relationship of differential EEG patterns to the distribution of Wechsler-Bellevue scores in a chronic epileptic population. J. Clin. Psychol., 18:334–337, 1962.

66. Kløve, H., and Reitan, R. M.: Effect of dysphasia and spatial distortion on Wechsler-Bellevue results. Arch. Neurol. (Chicago), 80:708–713, 1958.

67. Kløve, H., and White, P. T.: The relationship of degree of electroencephalographic abnormality to the distribution of Wechsler-Bellevue scores. Neurology (Minneap.), 13:423–430, 1963.

68. Kraepelin, E.: Der psychologische versuch in der psychiatrie, Psychol. Arbeit, 1:1–91, 1895.

69. Lansdell, H.: The use of factor scores from the Wechsler-Bellevue Scale of Intelligence in assessing patients with temporal lobe removals. Cortex, 4:257–268, 1968.

70. Mahan, H.: Sensitivity of WAIS tests of focal lobe damage. Personal communication, 1976.

71. Matarazzo, J. D.: Wechsler's Measurement and Appraisal of Adult Intelligence. Baltimore, Williams & Wilkins Co., 1972.

72. Matarazzo, J. D., and Phillips, J. S.: Digit Symbol performance as a function of increasing levels of anxiety. J. Consult. Psychol., 19:131–134, 1955.

73. Matthews, C. G., and Booker, H. E.: Pneumoencephalographic measurements and neuropsychological test performance in human adults. Cortex, 8:69–92, 1972.

74. Matthews, C. G., Shaw, D. J., and Kløve, H.: Psychological test performances in neurologic and "pseudo-neurologic" subjects. Cortex, 2:244–253, 1966.

75. McFie, J.: Assessment of Organic Intellectual Impairment. New York, Academic Press, 1975.

76. Meier, M. J., and French, L. A.: Longitudinal assessment of intellectual functioning following unilateral temporal lobectomy. J. Clin. Psychol., 21:3–9, 1966.

77. Milner, B.: Some effects of frontal lobectomy in man. In Warren, J. M., and Akert, K., eds.:

The Frontal Granular Cortex and Behavior. New York, McGraw-Hill Book Co., 1964.

78. Poeck, K.: Modern trends in neuropsychology. *In* Benton, A. L., ed.: Contributions to Clinical Neuropsychology. Chicago, Aldine Publishing Co., 1969, pp.1–29.

79. Reitan, R. M.: An investigation of the validity of Halstead's measures of biological intelligence. Arch. Neurol. Psychiat, *73*:28–35, 1955.

80. Reitan, R. M.: Certain differential effects of left and right cerebral lesions in human adults. J.Comp. Physiol. Psychol., *48*:474–477, 1955.

81. Reitan, R. M.: Validity of the Trail Making Test as an indicator of organic brain damage. Percept. Motor Skills, *8*:271–276, 1958.

82. Reitan, R. M.: The significance of dysphasia for intelligence and adaptive abilities. J. Psychol., *50*:355–376, 1960.

83. Reitan, R. M.: A research program on the psychological effects of brain lesions in human beings. *In* Ellis, N. E., ed.: International Review of Research in Mental Retardation, Vol. I. New York, Academic Press, 1966, pp. 153–218.

84. Reitan, R. M.: Complex motor functions of the preferred and non-preferred hands in brain-damaged and normal children. Percept. Motor Skills, *33*:671–675, 1971.

85. Reitan, R. M.: Methodological problems in clinical neuropsychology. *In* Reitan, R. M., and Davidson, L. A., eds.: Clinical Neuropsychology: Current Status and Applications. New York, Halstead Press, 1974, pp.19–46.

86. Reitan, R. M., and Davidson, L. A., eds.: Clinical Neuropsychology: Current Status and Applications. New York, Halstead Press, 1974.

87. Reitan, R. M., and Fitzhugh, K. B.: Behavioral deficits in groups with cerebral vascular lesions. J. Consult. Clin. Psychol., *37*:215–223, 1971.

88. Rourke, B. P.: Issues in the neuropsychological assessment of children with learning disabilities. Canad. Psychol. Rev., *17*:89–102, 1976.

89. Russell, E. W., Neuringer, C., and Goldstein, G.: Assessment of Brain Damage. New York, John Wiley & Sons, 1970.

90. Semmes, J., Weinstein, S., Ghent, L., and Teuber, H. L.: Somatosensory Changes After Penetrating Brain Wounds in Man. Cambridge, Mass., Harvard University Press, 1960.

91. Shiomi, K.: Relationship between EEG alpha frequency and ability of tapping. Psychologia, *16*:30–33, 1973.

92. Shipley, W. C.: A self administering scale for measuring intellectual impairment and deterioration. New Eng. J. Med., *293*:113–118, 1940.

93. Simpson, C. D., and Vega, A.: Unilateral brain damage patterns of age-corrected WAIS subtest scores. J. Clin. Psychol., *27*:204–208, 1971.

94. Soni, S. S., Marten, G. W., Pitner, S. E., Duenas, D. A., and Powuzek, M.: Effects of central-nervous system irradiation on neuropsychologic functioning of children with acute lymphocytic leukemia. New Eng. J. Med., *293*:113–118, 1975.

95. Spearman, C.: General intelligence objectively determined and measured. Amer. J. Psychol., *15*:201–293, 1904.

96. Spearman, C.: The Abilities of Man. New York, Macmillan Publishing Co., 1927.

97. Spreen, O., and Benton, A. L.: Comparative studies of some psychological tests for cerebral damage. J. Nerv. Ment. Dis., *140*:323–333, 1965.

98. Spreen, O., and Gaddes, W. H.: Developmental norms for fifteen neuro-psychological tests age 6–15. Cortex, *5*:170–191, 1969.

99. Terman, L. M.: The Measurement of Intelligence. Boston, Houghton Mifflin Co., 1916.

100. Terman, L. M., and Childs, H. G.: A tentative revision and extension of the Binet-Simon Scale of Intelligence. J. Educ. Psychol., *8*:61–74, 133–143, 198–208, 277–289, 1912.

101. Terman, L. M., and Merrill, M. A.: Stanford-Binet Intelligence Scale. Cambridge, Mass., Riverside Press, 1960.

102. Thurstone, L. L.: A method of scaling psychological and educational tests. J. Educ. Psychol., *16*:433–451, 1925.

103. Thurstone, L. L.: Primary Mental Abilities. Psychometric Monograph No. 1. Chicago, University of Chicago Press, 1938.

104. Tredold, R. F., and Soddy, K.: A Textbook of Mental Deficiency. Baltimore, Md., Williams & Wilkins Co., 1956.

105. United States Department of Labor: Dictionary of Occupational Titles. Washington, D.C., U.S. Govt. Printing Office, 1965.

106. Vander Vlugt, H.: Dichotic listening in lateralization of brain function. Leiden, Boerhaave Commissie Proceedings, 1975.

107. Vega, A., and Parsons, O. A.: Cross-validation of the Halstead-Reitan tests for brain damage. J. Consult. Psychol., *31*:619–625, 1967.

108. Vega, A., and Parsons, O. A.: Relationship between sensory-motor deficits and WAIS verbal and performance scores in unilateral brain damage. Cortex, *5*:229–241, 1969.

109. Watson, C. G.: WAIS profile patterns of hospitalized brain-damaged and schizophrenic patients. J. Clin. Psychol., *21*:294–295, 1965.

110. Watson, C. G., Thomas, R. W., Anderson, D. and Felling, J.: Differentiation of organics from schizophrenics at two chronicity levels by use of the Reitan-Halstead Organic Test Battery. J. Consult. Clin. Psychol., *32*:679–684, 1968.

111. Wechsler, D.: The Measurement of Adult Intelligence. Baltimore, Md., Williams & Wilkins Co., 1939.

112. Wechsler, D.: The Measurement and Appraisal of Adult Intelligence. Baltimore, Md., Williams & Wilkins Co., 1958.

113. Wechsler, D.: Wechsler Intelligence Scale for Children. Manual. New York, The Psychological Corp., 1949.

114. Wheeler, L., and Reitan, R. M.: The presence and laterality of brain damage predicted from responses to a short aphasia screening test. Percept. Motor Skills, *15*:783–799, 1962.

115. Woo-Sam, J., Zimmerman, I. L., and Rogal, R.: Location of injury and Wechsler indices of mental deterioration. Percept. Motor Skills, *32*:407–411, 1971.

116. Yoakum, S., and Yerks, R. M., eds.: Army Mental Tests. New York, Henry Holt, 1920.

20

ULTRASOUND APPLICATIONS IN NEUROSURGERY

Ultrasonic techniques have developed over many years and in many disparate areas. In 1827, underwater sound velocity was first measured by Colladon and Sturm, who simultaneously rang a bell and flashed a light in and over Lake Geneva in Switzerland. In 1912, a few days after the sinking of the Titanic by an unseen iceberg, Richardson applied for a British patent for ultrasound underwater echo-ranging. In the 1940's ultrasound began to be used to detect flaws in metal castings, where cracks and other defects produce echoes. Finally, during World War II, heavy investment in radar and sonar provided the technical knowledge necessary for Howry and Wild to pioneer two-dimensional ultrasonic imaging—the forerunner of today's B-scan examination.[62]

The first commercial ultrasound devices for clinical use became available in the late 1960's. Since then there have been numerous technological advances in diagnostic ultrasound as the commercial impact of these instruments was realized. Currently, ultrasound B-scan imaging in the abdomen is a routine radiological modality with resolution of 1 to 2 mm. For small, relatively superficial structures such as the carotid artery, specialized scanners are available with resolutions of a few tenths of a millimeter and the ability to noninvasively detect 1-mm atherosclerotic plaques in the artery.

Doppler ultrasound, which is employed for blood flow observations, has developed somewhat independently of B-scan technology. The Austrian physicist Christian Doppler, in 1842, observed that the frequency of an acoustic waveform is altered if there is movement of either the receiver or the sender.[14] A familiar example of this phenomenon is the increase in pitch of a train whistle as the train approaches and the decrease as it passes away—the "Doppler effect." As early as 1954, Doppler ultrasound devices were used to detect blood flow.[41] Subsequent practical application has resulted in the use of continuous-wave ultrasonic Doppler detectors to monitor normal arterial, venous, and cardiac blood flow patterns transcutaneously and to diagnose abnormalities within these vascular channels.

The most common neurosurgical application of Doppler ultrasound is the intraoperative detection of air emboli.[34,36,37,40] Other neurosurgical uses include the detection of extracranial vascular occlusive disease, the monitoring of carotid–cavernous sinus fistulae before and after procedures to obliterate them, the assessment of patency of superficial temporal artery–to–middle cerebral artery anastomosis, the intraoperative evaluation of superior sagittal sinus patency, the determination of cerebral spinal fluid shunt patency, and the determination of cerebral arterial reserve.*

PHYSICAL PRINCIPLES

"Ultrasound" refers to sound at frequencies above the range of human hearing, typically 20,000 cycles per second, or hertz (Hz). For biological imaging or Doppler measurements of blood flow, the frequencies employed are in the range of 1,000,000 to 10,000,000 hertz (1 to 10 MHz).

---

* See references 5–7, 9, 10, 18, 24, 25, 28, 32, 33, 35, 37, 39, 40, 46, 61.

M. H. REID, J. C. MAROON, AND M. S. ALBIN

Ultrasound is produced in a transducer in much the same way as sound is produced by a high-fidelity speaker. In the transducer there is a crystal of piezoelectric material— usually a compound of lead, zirconate, and titanium—which has the property of mechanically changing its shape when an electric voltage is impressed across it. The transducer face is a thin disc of this material with electrodes bonded to the face and rear of the crystal. Electronic circuits impress a short pulse of voltage across the electrodes, and the crystal deforms (like a loudspeaker), producing a high-frequency (1 to 10 MHz) sound pulse. This phenomenon is reciprocal; that is, if a sound wave is incident on the crystal, then an electric voltage is produced across the electrodes, and this voltage can be sensed and amplified by appropriate electronic circuits. For B-scan applications the same transducer functions as a transmitter and receiver of sound. Short pulses of sound are generated about one thousand times per second and the transducer is electronically switched to a listening mode between the sound pulses so that returning echoes may be detected. The mechanical articulated arm of the B-scanner has sensors at the arm pivot points so that the position of the transducer and the direction in which it is pointing are known. Then, because the speed of sound, c, is approximately constant in tissue (1.54×10^5 cm per second), the time delay between generation of a sound pulse and reception of a returning echo is proportional to the distance from the transducer face to the tissue interface that produced the echo. Note that echoes are produced at tissue interfaces of differing acoustic impedance $Z (Z = \rho c$, where ρ is tissue density in grams per cubic centimeter). Therefore, the transducer position and direction in space are known by the B-scanner's cantilevered arm sensors, and the depth of the echoes is known from the time delay of the returning echo. An echo "map," the ultrasound image, can then be produced on a television monitor. "Real-time" ultrasound instruments provide the same type of images as a B-scanner except that the image is automatically and repetitively swept (mechanically or electronically) so that events can be viewed in real time much as in x-ray fluoroscopy. The tissue resolution of current real-time instruments is inferior to that of a mechanical-arm B-scanner, but this situation may not pertain for very many more years. Eventually, it is expected that real-time ultrasound instruments will replace the articulated-arm B-scanner.

Doppler instruments for blood flow and motion detection can be made in either of two general formats: continuous-wave or pulsed and range-gated. In either case, when the ultrasound beam is directed through tissue, the frequency of the reflected ultrasound is shifted if the reflection is returned from moving tissue such as red blood cells, vascular walls, or cardiac structures.

Doppler ultrasound devices detect velocity of moving tissues. Therefore, to measure blood flow quantitatively it is necessary to know the vessel diameter, the angle between the vessel and sound beam, and the velocity profile across the vessel. Most Doppler instruments available for medical use give only qualitative measurements of blood flow. Quantitative measurements are possible with specialized instrumentation.[51]

The acoustic impedance differences between tissues govern the strength of returning echoes. For tissue interfaces oriented perpendicular to the sound beam the ratio of the intensity of the return sound pulse to transmitted pulse is $R/T = [(Z_1 - Z_2)/(Z_1 + Z_2)]^2$ where "1" and "2" are the two tissues. A short calculation will show that, if Z_1 is blood and Z_2 is air, R/T is approximately equal to 1.0 and all of the transmitted signal is returned. This phenomenon is easily demonstrated in a swimming pool; those under water and those above water cannot hear each other because the water-air interface reflects all of the sound. The importance of this phenomenon to neurological surgery is that minute amounts of free gas in moving blood are easily detected by Doppler ultrasound because of the large reflection coefficient of the gas bubbles.

Originally, Doppler instruments were developed to supplement auscultation and to be used much like a stethoscope. The auscultatory principle, however, is entirely different. With a continuous-wave Doppler device, the signal heard is produced by ultrasound reflected primarily from moving red blood cells and secondarily from moving vascular walls, myocardium, and heart valves when sound is directed through those structures. This audible signal, of course, is different from the sounds generated by turbulence and valve closure that are detected with a standard stethoscope. Furthermore, the frequency of the audible sound from a Doppler unit is proportional to the flow velocity in the vascular channel.[19,52] The higher the frequency of the audible signal, the higher the velocity of blood flow. It is this characteristic that has led to the ultrasonic detection of peripheral arterial and venous occlusive disease.[52,57,58] In addition, by using an appropriate signal processing system, one can graphically record velocity flow patterns for a permanent record.[59]

Echoencephalography utilizes the most basic and simple form of ultrasound, namely, echo-ranging. Although intracranial imaging is prevented by the skull (bone), it is possible to observe the major echo arising from the falx–brain–cerebrospinal fluid interface when a transducer is placed at the side of the head and directed medially, perpendicular to the falx. Knowing that the sound pulse transit time from transducer to falx to transducer is proportional to the distance therefore permits a measure of the falx-skull distance. If this is done for both sides of the head, the falx can be checked for midline position. The examination is simple to do and is innocuous,

and the equipment is inexpensive. Clinical examples of this technique are given in Chapter 7.

The safety of both B-scan imaging and Doppler flow detection ultrasound devices has been examined extensively in in vitro and in vivo studies. It is clear that high levels of ultrasound intensity can disrupt cells and their molecular framework, but only a few reports of cellular changes at diagnostic ranges of ultrasound intensity (5 to 20 milliwatts per square centimeter average, 5 to 10 watts per square centimeter peak) are available.[15,64] At these low intensities of ultrasound energy, the in vitro effects that have been noted are: probable partial unwinding of deoxyribonucleic acid double-helix strands without breaking them, loss of cellular contact inhibition in cell cultures, loss of cellular attachment to surfaces in cell cultures, and inhibition of DNA synthesis.[3,31,54,60] The in vivo effects that have also been noted are decreased mitotic indices in rat liver and reduced transplantability of mouse lymphosarcoma.[3,54] In extensive clinical reviews of obstetrical patients, no evidence could be found of human fetal or maternal injury secondary to ultrasound. In summary, there has been no

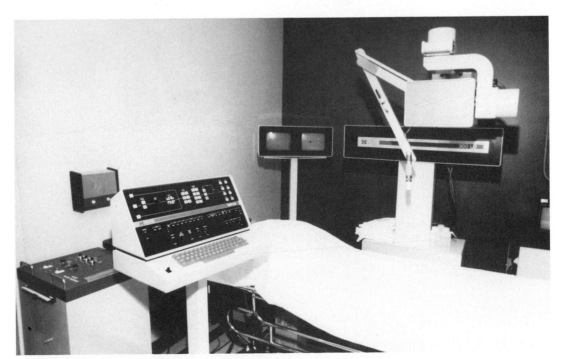

Figure 20–1 Typical ultrasound B-scanner. From left to right: image recording camera, control panel, TV monitors for viewing scans, articulated scanning arm with ultrasound transducer, patient couch.

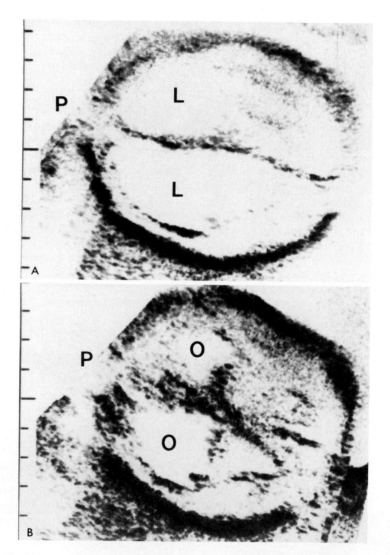

Figure 20–2   Fetal hydrocephalus as a chance finding in an otherwise apparently normal pregnancy of 31 weeks' gestation. *A*. Lateral ventricles (L). *B*. Occipital horns (O). Scan plane is approximately the same as that used in computed tomographic examinations. P, posterior; scale in centimeters.

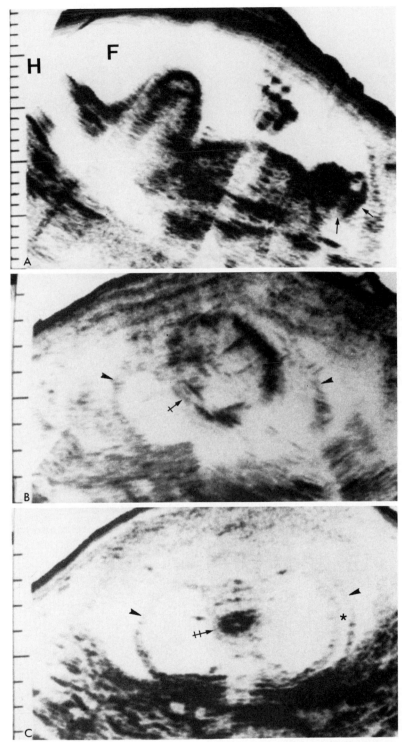

Figure 20–3 A. Fetal anencephaly with associated polyhydramnios. Obstetrical ultrasound examination was performed because the mother was "too large for dates." Fetal head is incomplete superiorly and posteriorly (*arrows*). Orbit, body, and limbs are easily identified. *B* and *C*. Fetal encephalocele as a chance finding in an otherwise apparently normal pregnancy of approximately 22 weeks' gestation. A large fluid-filled sac (*arrowheads*) surrounds the deformed fetal head (*barred arrow*) in *B* and the cervical spine (*double-barred arrow*) in *C*. Note edema in the skin of the sac (*), which was also present in the fetal thorax and abdomen. F, amniotic fluid; H, direction of mother's head; scale in centimeters.

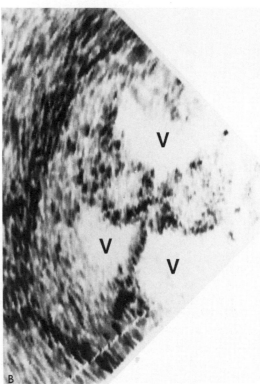

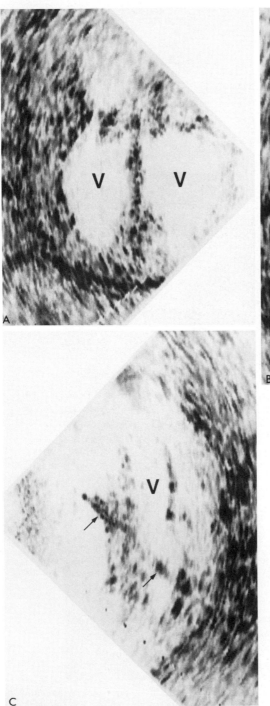

Figure 20–4 Two-week-old infant with hydrocephalus and Arnold Chiari type II malformation. *A* and *B*. Images obtained during the real-time examination demonstrate dilated ventricles (V) before ventricular shunting. *C*. After shunting. The shunt tube could be easily seen during the real-time examination but is poorly demonstrated on the static image obtained from the real-time scanner (*arrows*).

Illustration continued on opposite page

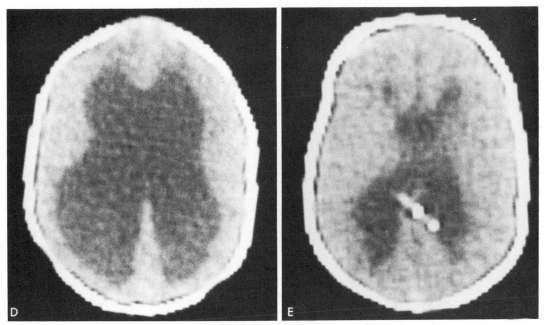

Figure 20–4 (*continued*) *D* and *E*. CT scans corresponding to *A* and *C*. Ultrasound images are in approximately the same scan plane as the computed tomographic examination.

detrimental effect demonstrated in vivo in mammalian tissues from diagnostic ranges of ultrasonic energy.

B-scan ultrasound imaging is generally performed by a radiologist, and a minimum of six months of training is required to achieve competence in obtaining and interpreting images. Specialized "small part" real-time scanners are available that may be particularly useful in imaging carotid arteries. Because of the real-time feature and their limited anatomical applicability, much less training may be necessary to be proficient with such an instrument.

Figure 20–1 shows a typical B-scan instrument. Doppler units are available in a variety of sizes with varying specifications. They range from small pocket-size models with stethoscope earphones to direction-sensing units with frequency meters to determine direction of blood flow and to modified obstetrical units for detecting air embolism.

B-SCAN ULTRASOUND IMAGING

Fetal and Neonatal Cranium

B-scan ultrasound has been widely used in obstetrics to evaluate fetal age and position, placental integrity, and the like, and it has been noted that intrauterine fetal neurological anomalies may be detected.* Unfor-

---

* See references 11, 13, 17, 22, 23, 29.

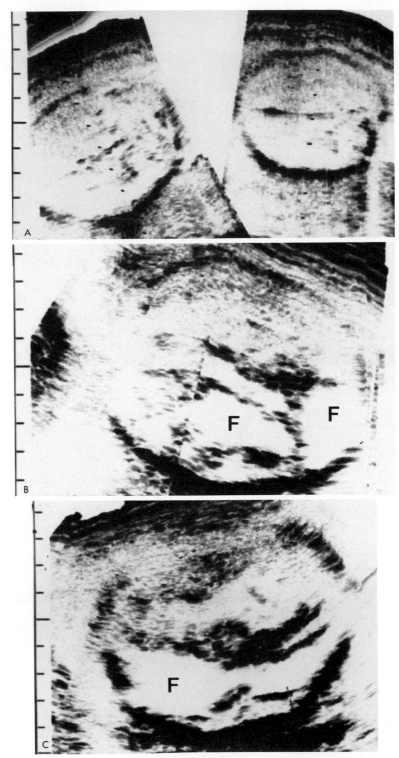

Figure 20–5   Routine obstetrical examination performed because the mother was "too large for dates." *A.* Normal twin pregnancy showing both fetal heads at 24 weeks' gestation. *B* and *C.* Routine re-examination at 31 weeks' gestation now demonstrates abnormal ventricular dilatation and fluid-filled cystic intracranial spaces (F), some of which may represent the ventricles.

Illustration continued on opposite page

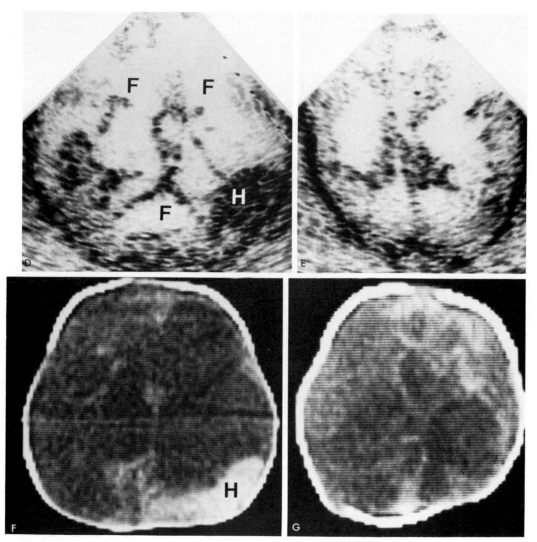

Figure 20–5 (*continued*) *D* and *E*. Real-time ultrasound images. *F* and *G*. Corresponding CT scans of neonates again demonstrate large intracranial cystic spaces (F) and areas of tissue and hemorrhage (H). During the real-time study, strands of fibrinous material could be seen floating in the cystic areas. Ultrasound images are in approximately the same scan plane as that of the computed tomographic examination. Scale is in centimeters.

tunately, the detection of neural tube defects is usually not possible until the third trimester of pregnancy. Both B-scan mechanical-arm scanners and real-time instruments have been used. Typical lesions that are easily identified in utero are anencephaly, microencephaly, encephalocele, meningomyelocele, hydrancephaly, and hydrocephalus. Often there are associated findings such as polyhydramnios or fetal death. In the authors' experience, B-scan ultrasound has been more definitive than real-time ultrasound because of better resolution of intrauterine structures. Real-time observations are an important method of evaluating fetal limb, respiratory, and cardiac motion. Figure 20–2 shows a hydrocephalic fetus. Normally, only a hint of the ventricles is obtained, but a dramatic intracranial pattern is noted in hydrocephalus. For comparison, see Figure 20–5A for the image of an ultrasonically normal (twin) fetal head. Examples of fetal neural tube defects are shown in Figure 20–3. The associated polyhydramnios is the reason for which the greatest number of these patients are referred for ultrasound examination; they are "too large for dates." Fetal death is often present as well, and loss of fetal movement or heart sounds is the second main reason for referral to the ultrasound laboratory.

Intracranial anatomy in the neonate and infant is also amenable to ultrasound imaging.* This may be a useful procedure for following infants (for example, to evaluate ventricular shunt function by ventricular size) when repeated examinations are needed and computed tomography would result in an unacceptable radiation dose. The infant skull is thin enough to allow reasonable intracranial ultrasound images up to 12 months of age and in some children perhaps up to 18 months. Cranial B-scanning can be quite difficult in an infant. The curvature of the head and the presence of hair make skin contact with the transducer hard to achieve, and additionally, it is difficult to produce an aesthetic image without scanning artifacts. Therefore, the authors have employed a phased-array real-time instrument to image the infant head.† The transducer face is approximately 25 mm square, and skin contact is easily achieved.

* See references 20, 27, 30, 42, 43, 55, 63.
† EMI Corporation, Ultrasound model 4500.

The sector image requires that the head be scanned from both sides to visualize the entire brain. The scanning plane is angled approximately 25 degrees to Reed's baseline, i.e., in the same orientation as CT brain scans. If desired, additional sagittal, coronal, or any oblique scans may be obtained. Figures 20–4 A and B are the scans of a 2-week-old infant with hydrocephalus, and Figure 20–4C demonstrates the improvement following ventricular shunting. The shunt was easily seen during the real-time examination, but unfortunately, was poorly visualized in the static image. Figures 20–4 D and E are corresponding CT scans of the same child.

Figure 20–5 illustrates the in-utero diagnosis of large intracranial cystic spaces and hydrocephalus in twins. The neonatal scans were obtained a few days after birth. These static images do not show the "strands" of tissue or fibrin that were seen floating in the cystic spaces in both the in-utero and the neonatal real-time examinations of these infants who had extensive brain destruction secondary to massive intrauterine (viral?) infection.

Figure 20–6 shows a 14-month-old child with a posterior fossa "mass" that did not fill at ventriculography. Ultrasound examination confirmed the fluid (echo-free) nature of this noncommunicating posterior fossa arachnoid cyst.

Figure 20–7 presents the computed tomographic, ultrasound, and angiographic studies in a neonate thought to have either a Dandy-Walker (or variant of Dandy-Walker) cyst or a posterior fossa arachnoid cyst. The CT examination demonstrates the cerebellum and normally shaped fourth ventricle, thus excluding a Dandy-Walker cyst and indicating a better prognosis for the patient. Ultrasound examination was performed to evaluate the efficacy of this modality. As shown, it is clear that the ultrasound images closely match the computed tomographic study and demonstrate the posterior fossa cyst widening and displacing the tentorial notch. The sagittal ultrasound scan can be compared with the vertebral angiogram to confirm the position of cerebellum, clivus, and cyst. The implication of these results is that ultrasound examination might replace computed tomography and angiography in specialized clinical situations.

Some components of intracerebral vas-

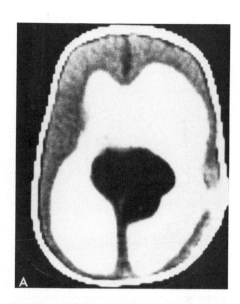

Figure 20–6 Fourteen-month-old infant with hydrocephalus. *A*. Contrast ventriculogram CT scan. *B*. Realtime ultrasound image in near-coronal plane demonstrating ventricular dilatation (V) and a fluid-filled (echo-free) posterior fossa cyst (C) that did not communicate with the ventricles at ventriculography.

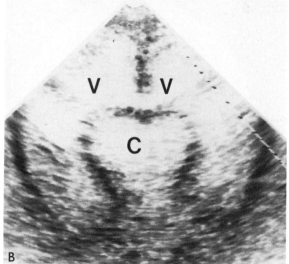

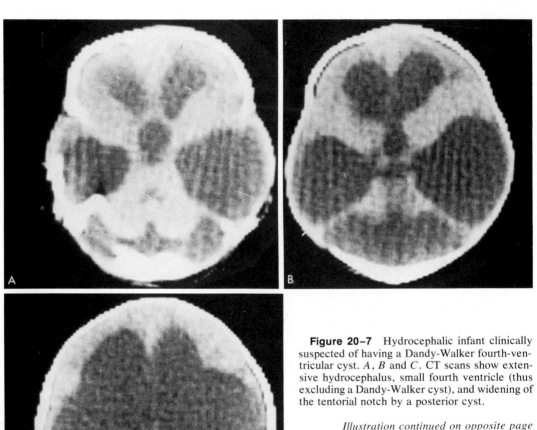

Figure 20–7 Hydrocephalic infant clinically suspected of having a Dandy-Walker fourth-ventricular cyst. *A*, *B* and *C*. CT scans show extensive hydrocephalus, small fourth ventricle (thus excluding a Dandy-Walker cyst), and widening of the tentorial notch by a posterior cyst.

Illustration continued on opposite page

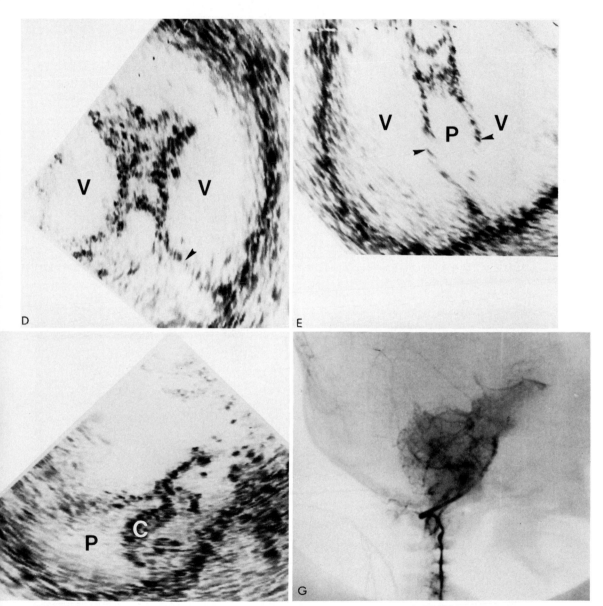

Figure 20–7 (*continued*) *D* and *E*. Corresponding real-time ultrasound images. *F*. Real-time sagittal ultrasound scan. Dilated ventricles (V), tentorium (*arrow*), cerebellum (C), and posterior fossa cyst (P) widening and superiorly displacing the tentorial notch are demonstrated. *G*. Lateral view of vertebral angiogram to compare with *F*. Scale is in centimeters.

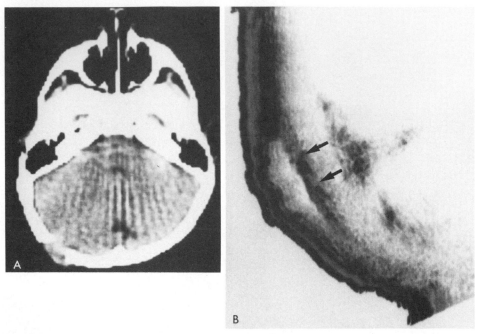

Figure 20–8 A palpable skull defect in a 20-month-old child. *A*. Computed tomogram. *B*. Ultrasound image demonstrates the dural margin (*arrows*) and confirms that there is no intracerebral extension of lesion (a proved eosinophilic granuloma).

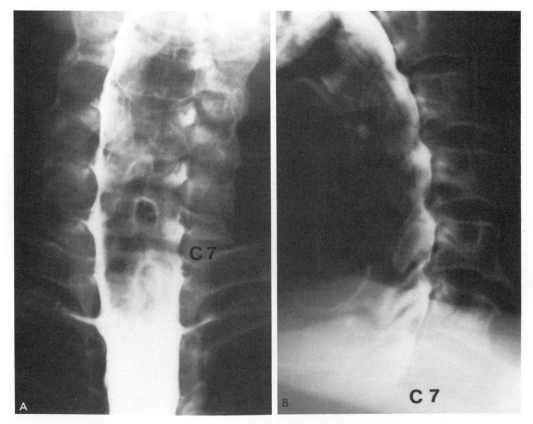

Figure 20–9 *A* and *B*. Myelogram demonstrating a widened cervical cord.

Illustration continued on opposite page

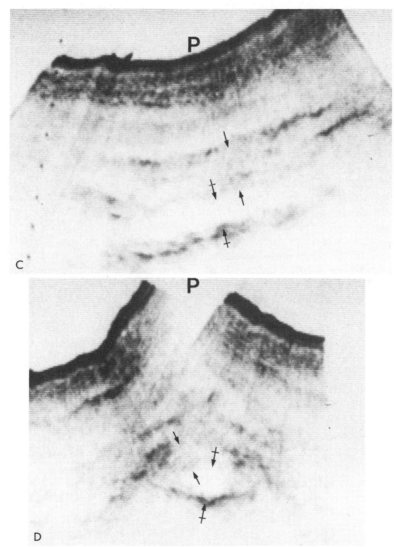

Figure 20–9 (*continued*)   *C* and *D*. Longitudinal and transverse ultrasound scans of the cervical cord (*arrows*) demonstrating a fluid component (*barred arrows*) in the anterior aspect of the spinal cord. P, posterior skin margin of neck; scale in centimeters.

cular anatomy can also be demonstrated easily with real-time ultrasound. The middle cerebral and basilar arteries can usually be recognized and pulsations within them noted. This is quite important for unequivocal definition of the brain stem, clivus, and cerebellum, for example.

Adult intracranial ultrasound examination does not appear possible with current technology because of the attenuation and dispersion properties of the skull, which preclude adequate intracranial image resolution. The authors have not had an opportunity, as yet, to study a patient with a craniotomy defect in whom the limitations of sound transmission through bone would not pertain.

Occasionally, a palpable cranial defect will correspond to findings on a skull radiograph or CT scan of the brain, and such accessible subcutaneous lesions are approachable by ultrasound. Because these types of lesions are quite superficial, it is usually necessary to employ specialized "near focus" transducers or interpose a few centimeters of a water path between the transducer and the skin. Figure 20–8 is the ultrasound image of an erosive lesion of the skull in a young child in whom computed tomography revealed no evidence of intracranial extension. Because the parents were certain that the lesion increased in size whenever the child cried, the possibility of a small meningocele was initially considered. Ultrasound is exquisitely sensitive to fluid-solid differences, and therefore the subcutaneous lesion was examined ultrasonically. No intradural extension of the homogeneous solid-tissue lesion (an eosin-ophilic granuloma) was demonstrated; thus the possibility of a meningocele was excluded.

Spine

Ultrasound imaging of spinal canal lesions has not been widely reported, although one of the authors (M.R.) has examined a number of patients with cervical and thoracic spinal cord cysts, intramedullary tumors, and extradural fluid collections. The presence of bone (posterior spinal elements) limits the evaluation of the spinal canal; but with persistence, patience, and oblique transverse scans through the intralaminar spaces with specialized narrow-beam transducers, useful images can be obtained.

A case of low-grade intramedullary cystic astrocytoma that was examined with conventional iophendylate (Pantopaque) myelography, air myelography, and ultrasound has been reported.[49] In this case, ultrasound was invaluable in detecting the presence of fluid, localizing its anterior position, and confirming that the lesion was not a syrinx (Fig. 20–9). A similar fluid collection is seen in Figure 20–10. Figure 20–11 demonstrates another type of fluid collection (pseudomeningocele) resulting from a dural defect secondary to a meningioma resection. A cystoperitoneal shunt was placed and is visible in the cyst in Figure 20–11. This cystic collection, followed for some months, did not change as the patient's neurological status slowly improved.

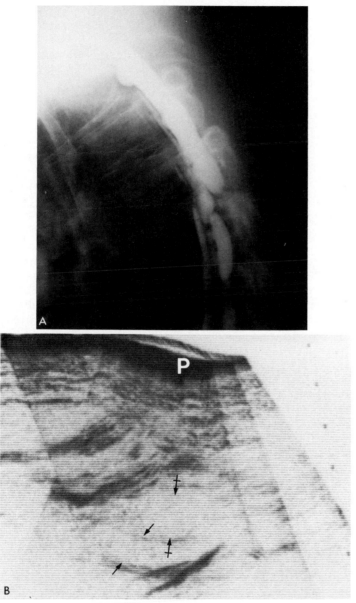

Figure 20–10 *A* and *B*. Myelogram and transverse ultrasound scan of the upper thoracic spine illustrate an arachnoid cyst (*barred arrows*) lying posterior to the spinal cord (*arrows*). P, posterior skin margin of the thorax; scale in centimeters.

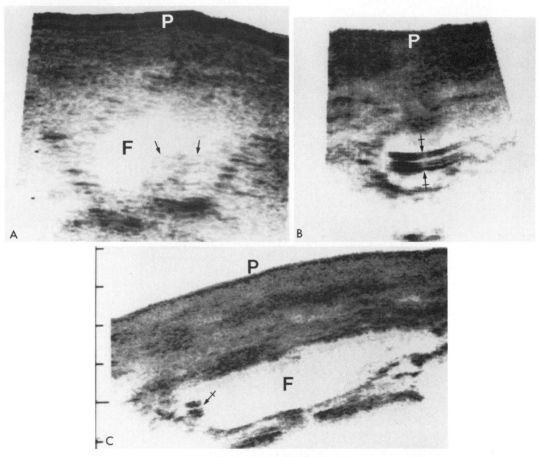

Figure 20–11   Ultrasound scans of upper thoracic spine in a patient who has had a spinal cord meningioma resected. *A*. Transverse scan shows fluid (F) and anterolaterally displaced cord (*arrows*). *B* and *C*. Transverse and longitudinal images demonstrate cystoperitoneal shunt catheter (*barred arrows*) within the cyst. P, posterior skin margin of thorax; scale in centimeters.

Carotid Artery

The usefulness of ultrasound in carotid imaging has been demonstrated.[12,16,21] These studies have employed real-time scanners specifically designed to provide high-resolution images of anatomical structures within a few centimeters of the skin surface. Resolution of 1-mm or larger atherosclerotic plaques is possible either with one of the specialized real-time scanners or with a B-scanner combined with a special focused transducer.[50] Real-time imaging is faster, and it is a simple matter to visualize the carotid bifurcation in longitudinal section to show both internal and external carotid arteries on the same scan. With a B-scanner, longitudinal images in the plane of the internal and external carotid arteries are difficult to obtain because of the mechanics of the scanning procedure. Longitudinal images of the internal, external, and common carotid arteries can, however, be separately formed. Transverse images of the arteries are routine. Figures 20–12 and 20–13 show carotid arteriograms and ultrasound images of patients with atherosclerotic disease of the carotid artery near the bifurcation. Ultrasonic evaluation of the carotid arteries over a distance of a few centimeters superior and inferior to the bifurcation is easily accomplished.

Ultrasound imaging of the extracranial vessels is in its infancy, but it can reasonably be expected to become an important imaging modality for evaluating carotid artery disease. With real-time scanners, only

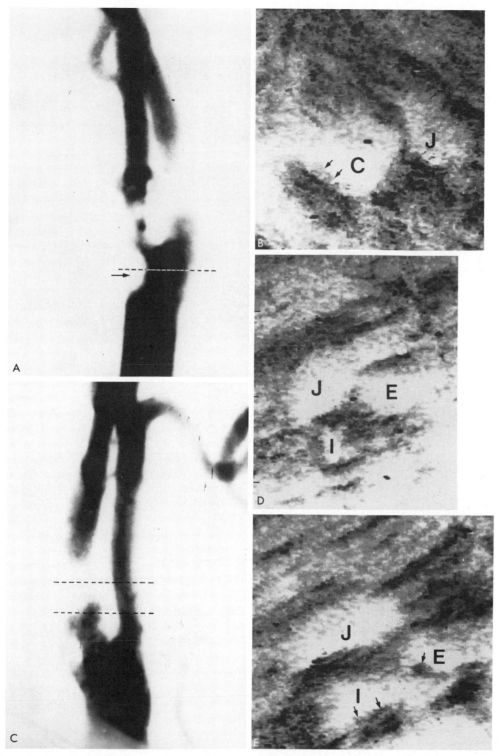

Figure 20–12 *A*. Anteroposterior left carotid angiogram demonstrates narrowing of the common carotid artery secondary to an atherosclerotic plaque (*arrow*). *B*. Transverse ultrasound scan of the left side of the neck taken at the position indicated by the dashed line in *A* again shows the 1- to 2-mm thick plaque (*arrows*). *C*. Lateral right carotid angiogram demonstrates marked narrowing of the proximal internal carotid artery. *D* and *E*. Transverse ultrasound scans of the right side of the neck taken, respectively, at the upper and lower positions indicated by the dashed lines in *C*. Marked narrowing and atherosclerotic plaque disease (*arrows*) in both the internal and external carotid arteries are again demonstrated. C, common carotid artery; I, internal carotid artery; E, external carotid artery; J, jugular vein; scale in centimeters.

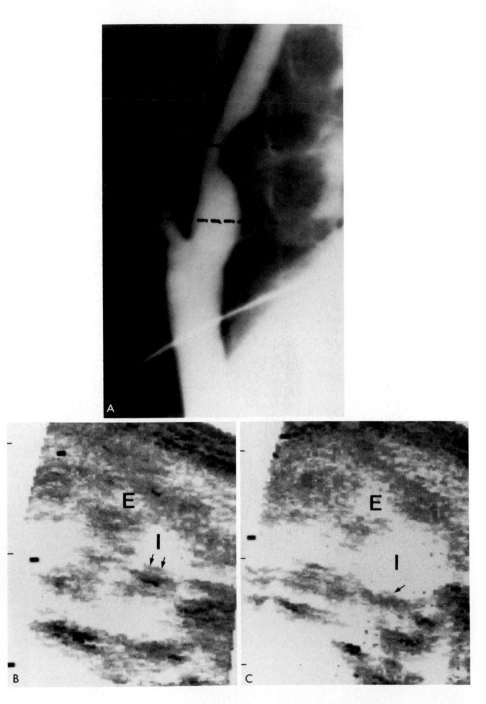

Figure 20–13 *A*. Lateral left angiogram demonstrates atherosclerotic narrowing of both the internal and external carotid arteries. *B* and *C*. Transverse ultrasound scans of the left side of the neck taken at the upper and lower positions respectively indicated by the dashed lines in *A*. Atherosclerotic plaque disease is indicated by the arrows.

Illustration continued on opposite page

minimal training is necessary for the physician, and therefore one can envision this type of screening becoming a standard office or vascular clinic procedure. The examination is innocuous, requires only a few minutes to do, and may (although this is not yet certain) provide the same accuracy as an arteriogram in detecting vascular disease in and around the carotid bifurcation. Carotid Doppler blood flow evaluation and Doppler imaging are discussed later.

Miscellaneous Applications Related to Neurosurgery

Ultrasound is exquisitely sensitive in distinguishing solid from cystic lesions.

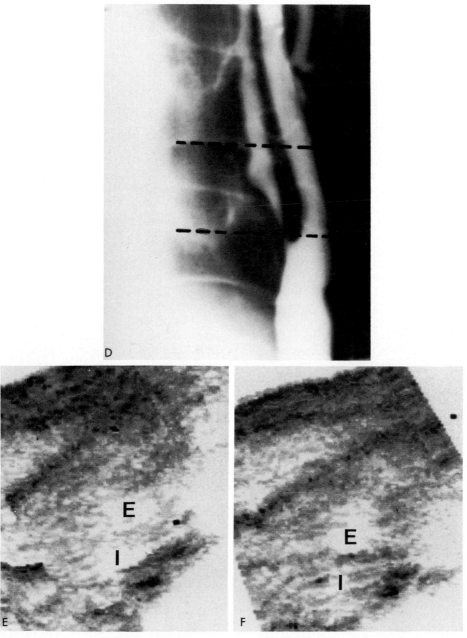

Figure 20–13 (*continued*) *D, E,* and *F.* Corresponding study of the right carotid artery. Marked arterial narrowing is noted bilaterally. I, internal carotid artery; E, external carotid artery; scale in centimeters.

Therefore, any paraspinal (abdominal, retroperitoneal, external) mass may be ultrasonically investigated to differentiate cysts (meningocele) and solid lesions (e.g., tumors such as neurilemoma, neurofibroma, paraspinal sarcoma, meningomyelocele, lipoma). As noted earlier, scans are limited by interposed bone and gas, and this should be kept in mind if an ultrasound examination is contemplated.

DOPPLER ULTRASOUND

Air Embolism

Doppler cardiac auscultation is a sensitive method for detecting air embolism. Laboratory studies comparing the Doppler technique with esophageal and precardiac auscultation, electrocardiographic monitoring, changes in blood gases, and alterations in arterial and venous pressures clearly show the Doppler method to be the only one that detects air directly before any pathological changes occur in the cardiopulmonary system.[38] Recall the aforementioned exquisite sensitivity of ultrasound to the detection of small gas bubbles in fluid.

Prior to the introduction of this means of intraoperative monitoring, air embolism was considered a rare complication of intracranial procedures.[26] Subsequent clinical studies have, however, revealed that air embolism occurs in approximately 25 per cent of patients operated on in the upright position and is a potential hazard in the prone and supine positions if the head to heart gradient is greater than 10 cm.[1,34,36,40,57] With such a gradient, negative venous pressure occurs, and air is aspirated into noncollapsible venous channels such as diploic veins and dural sinuses. If untreated, air embolism's hemodynamic consequences include hypotension, cardiac arrhythmias, pulmonary capillary obstruction, and finally cardiopulmonary arrest.[1,40,53]

When intravascular air passes through a Doppler ultrasound field, characteristic audible signals are heard. The nature of the signal depends on the size of the embolus and the time it remains in the ultrasonic field. A small 0.25- to 1.5-cc embolus may be heard only as a fleeting "chirp." A larger embolus produces a characteristic raucous static similar to the noise heard when a phonograph needle scrapes across a spinning record.[1,36,40,57] This sound occurs because an air-blood interface is a much better acoustical reflector than red blood cells alone. The Doppler shifted signal is therefore much louder than the signal arising from the background motion of red cells. The raucous sound is due to turbulent flow, which is normally not heard unless small gas bubbles are present to provide adequate reflection of sound to be sensed by the Doppler receiver.

For monitoring blood flow in the right side of the heart with a Doppler air embolism detector, the patient is first placed in the final upright position for operation and acoustic gel is applied to the skin over the lower parasternal area in the third and fourth intercostal spaces. The transducer of the Doppler detector is then placed in the same area and positioned so that the cardiac blood flow is optimally heard (Fig. 20–14). The characteristic dull snapping sound produced by movement of the myocardium and the clicking sound of the heart valves should also be heard superimposed on the high-pitched swooshing sound of the intracardiac blood flow.[1,34,36,40,57]

After the appropriate audible signal is detected, the transducer is firmly fixed in position with a suitable adhesive or circumferential chest strap. To confirm the correct position, a bolus of 5 ml of normal saline is injected into one of the peripheral intravenous catheters. The dissolved microbubbles of gas in the saline are immediately detected by the Doppler unit and correct positioning is confirmed. At this point, earphones that automatically eliminate the sound from the instrument's loudspeaker may be used so that only the anesthesiologist monitors the cardiac sounds, or the instrument may be set so that the surgeon too can hear the cardiac sounds continuously.[34] The latter arrangement is valuable for both the surgeon and the anesthesiologist because both can immediately discern changes in cardiac rate and rhythm. This early detection is especially important when the surgeon is working in the posterior fossa near or on sensitive brain stem structures.

Doppler cardiac auscultation does not quantitatively measure the amount of air that is embolized. One can, however, obtain a general idea of the size of an embolus by the intensity of the reflected ultrasonic

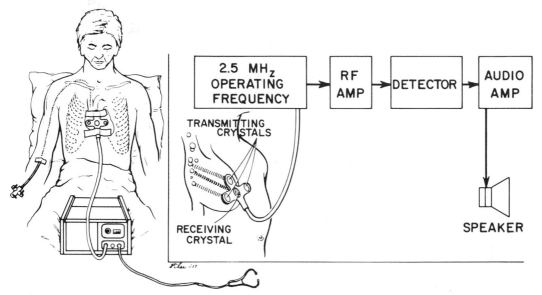

Figure 20–14 Doppler cardiac blood flow and air embolism detector.

signal and the length of time the air remains or continues to accumulate in the heart. The larger the embolus the more raucous the static and the longer it persists.

At the first "hearing" of an embolus, the anesthesiologist immediately withdraws blood from the right atrial catheter. Such an intravenous catheter should be inserted in every patient who is operated on in the upright position. It is not unusual to aspirate 50 to 200 cc of air in this manner.[1,34,40,57] The surgeon immediately applies bone wax, physiological saline, and wet packs, if necessary, to the operative wound. Nitrous oxide is discontinued because of the expansion of gas bubbles with this agent.[45] Jugular compression may be used to increase intracranial pressure and post–end-expiratory pressure can be applied to the endotracheal tube to increase the intrathoracic pressure. It may be necessary to treat cardiac arrhythmias with appropriate drugs such as lidocaine. It rarely is necessary to move the patient from the sitting position, but one should be prepared to do so if air continues to accumulate or if cardiac arrhythmias or hypotension or both supervene.

Several companies now produce ultrasonic instruments that can be used for cardiac auscultation and air embolism detection. Most of the units sold for this purpose are essentially those used for fetal monitoring in obstetrics. For optimal air embolism detection, however, several equipment modifications are required. The most important specifications are concerned with the transducer frequency and mechanical design, the zone of sensitivity, the depth of ultrasonic penetration, and the electronic circuitry for eliminating static.

Because of the variability of the distance of the heart from the anterior chest wall, a transducer frequency and configuration are required that will detect intracardiac blood flow and air emboli in the thin (near) as well as the very large (deep) patient. The button-type transducer most commonly used for such purposes, although adequate in many cases, is not the best. A cloverleaf design is much more effective. The zone of sensitivity begins at a depth of 2.5 cm, and the area of ultrasonic illumination is much greater (Fig. 20–15). This configuration makes initial placement easier and monitors a larger area of cardiac blood flow. Flooding of the intracardiac blood by the ultrasound beam is required rather than a narrow collimated beam as in B-scan imaging.

Another technical problem is the disconcerting static produced by electric cautery devices and the amplification of the static by the audio portion of the Doppler unit. This noise can be eliminated by a commercially available cut-off circuit that automatically switches the Doppler unit off during

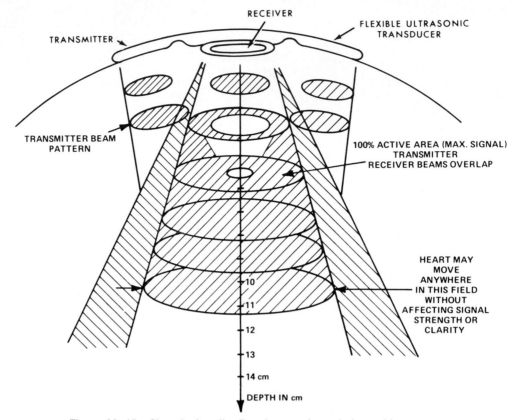

Figure 20–15   Cloverleaf cardiac Doppler transducer design and beam pattern.

actual use of the cautery. Although theoretically an embolus could be missed if the cautery were used continuously (thus keeping the sound turned off), in practice, this has not been a problem. With improved shielding it may be possible in the future to provide continuous monitoring despite the use of electrocautery devices.

Additional discussion of the detection and treatment of air embolism is given in Chapter 30.

Blood Flow Monitoring

A Doppler ultrasonic blood flow detector was first used clinically to localize noninvasively the sites of vascular occlusions in arteries in the extremities.[19,59] Unfortunately, when attempts were made to detect extracranial occlusive lesions directly, it proved impossible to differentiate internal from external carotid artery flow patterns reliably or to identify the carotid bifurcation. The technique was disappointing when recording was done directly over the cervical portion of the carotid arteries. In 1969, however, an indirect technique was devised in which ophthalmic artery blood flow was monitored. Subsequently modified, this method has proved quite accurate in the ultrasonic detection of hemodynamically significant carotid occlusive disease.*

Orbital Doppler Evaluation

In an acute occlusion of the common or the internal carotid artery there is an immediate decrease in the ophthalmic artery blood flow and pressure; hence the physiological basis for ophthalmodynamometry. Soon thereafter, however, collateral channels open between the ophthalmic artery and the external carotid and its branches. The superficial temporal, infraorbital, and facial arteries all may contribute to cerebral perfusion by retrograde ophthalmic artery blood flow.

_____

* See references 5, 32, 33, 35, 37, 44, 47, 61.

To detect this retrograde flow pattern, a 5 to 10 MHz pencil-type Doppler transducer probe is placed over the closed eyelid to monitor blood flow in the ophthalmic artery or its terminal supraorbital branch. The probe is coupled to the skin with a small amount of acoustic gel and is angled to obtain the maximum audible signal. Permanent recordings may be obtained by displaying the frequency component signal on an appropriate recorder. A suspected acute carotid occlusion may be verified by comparing a very diminished ipsilateral signal with the normal contralateral ophthalmic artery flow pattern.

If the audible ophthalmic flow signals are generally the same bilaterally, which is usually the case, the main accessible collateral arteries are then serially occluded digitally while ophthalmic artery blood flow is recorded. If retrograde flow is present, compression of the superficial temporal, facial, or infraorbital arteries would immediately dampen or obliterate the reflected ophthalmic artery or supraorbital artery signal. Retrograde flow, therefore, is a sign of carotid obstruction proximal to the origin of the ophthalmic artery (Fig. 20–16).

It is emphasized that the Doppler orbital-supraorbital examination is useful only in hemodynamically significant carotid disease. It is of no value in the detection of sources of emboli such as plaques that do not significantly compromise the vascular lumen.[9,35] Furthermore, false-negative results may occur when severe ipsilateral internal and external carotid disease is present or when a single high-grade stenotic lesion is present in the common carotid artery.[33] False-positive results can be caused by excessive transducer pressure and by inappropriate positioning. Despite its limitations, the Doppler technique is a safe, noninvasive method that has a degree of accuracy comparable to if not better than such methods as ophthalmodynamometry, ocular plethysmography, thermography, and ophthalmometry. The Doppler method is useful in the evaluation of the asymptomatic carotid bruit, the determination of operative priority in bilateral carotid lesions, the rapid detection of postendarterectomy thrombosis, and the assessment of nonhemispheric cerebral vascular symptoms.

Directional Doppler Scanning of Extracranial Carotid Arteries

Although the aforementioned indirect techniques are effective, it is still preferable to scan the common and internal carotid arteries in the neck because of the high incidence of extracranial atherosclerotic disease. Recent technical advances have made it possible to separate the internal from the external blood flow patterns by linking a Doppler directional flow probe with a position-sensing arm. In this manner one may noninvasively obtain ultrasonic angiograms of subcutaneous arteries.

The equipment for producing these ultrasonic angiograms consists of a sharply focused Doppler ultrasound pencil probe connected to a mechanical scanning arm. An image storage oscilloscope is used with a signal processing unit that receives the directional Doppler flowmeter signals. A monitor oscilloscope and strip chart printout record the analog directional blood flow signal. By repeatedly passing the probe over the extracranial carotid vessels, a two-dimensional picture of the blood channel is built up on the oscilloscope screen. The image thus formed is similar to the morphological display of a radiographic arteriogram or a longitudinal ultrasound B-scan, but represents a functional projection of local blood flow velocities (Fig. 20–17).

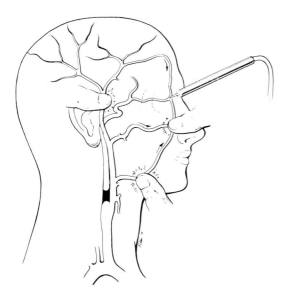

Figure 20–16 Assessment of carotid artery blood flow by ophthalmic artery Doppler flow observations with sequential digital compression of collateral arteries.

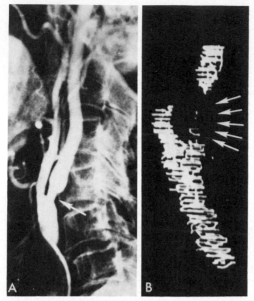

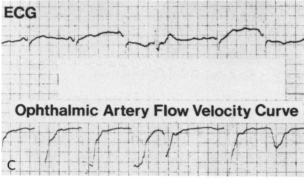

Figure 20–17 Carotid flow profile as observed with a scanning CW Doppler instrument. *A*. Carotid angiogram. *B*. CW Doppler flow profile. *C*. Corresponding Doppler tracing of ophthalmic artery flow.

The anatomical resolution of this type of Doppler scan is not as good as those of the B-scan or real-time devices already discussed.

Several clinical studies using this method have clearly demonstrated internal carotid artery stenosis and also have detected calcified plaques in the absence of complete arterial occlusion.[5,7,8,56] Xerography, when used with Doppler scanning, is particularly effective in identifying intravascular calcification.[61] Incorrect localization of lesions, however, may be a problem. In some patients the level of a stenosis has been thought to be in the region of the internal or external carotid artery when in fact it was found by angiography or operation to be in the distal common carotid artery itself.[7] Such cases, however, were errors in the localization of a lesion and not in the detection of its presence. Also, it was found that in patients with extremely constricted arteries, the width of the vascular lumen might be smaller than the Doppler instrument could detect.[56] In such a case, because of reversal of flow in the ophthalmic artery, a false impression of complete occlusion of the common carotid is possible.

Despite these limitations, with further refinements in instrumentation and techniques, ultrasonic angiography with directional sensing Doppler probes holds great possibilities for screening patients with suspected carotid artery disease.

Pulsed Doppler Examination

The continuous-wave Doppler instrument just described senses blood flow everywhere in the transmitted and reflected ultrasonic beam. A pulsed Doppler device

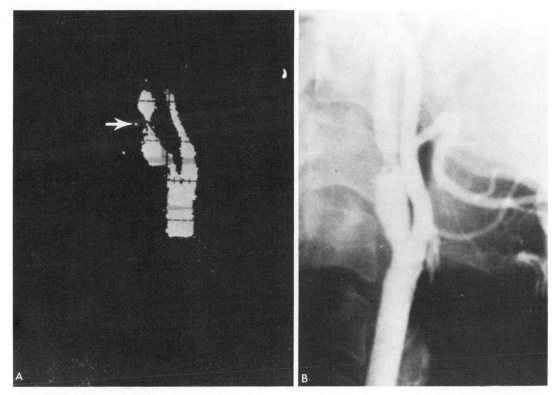

Figure 20–18   Carotid flow profile as observed with a range-gated pulsed Doppler instrument. *A*. Doppler flow profile. *B*. Corresponding carotid angiogram.

emits periodic short pulses of ultrasound and samples the Doppler frequency shift of the return signal after the delay corresponding to the transit time of the sound to and from the region of interest.[2,4,48] With such a system, it is possible to examine discrete points along an ultrasonic beam and thereby develop an ultrasonic system for blood flow imaging. By moving a pulsed Doppler transducer across the skin surface over the carotid arteries one can obtain a cathode ray picture of the cross section of the blood flow. Preliminary studies indicate that totally occluded carotid arteries can be documented with ease, and stenosis of more than 20 per cent of the cross-sectional diameter may also be clearly visualized (Fig. 20–18).[5,24]

Present pulsed Doppler systems still do not show the detail of carotid angiography. Calcification in the arterial wall may interfere with sound transmission and mimic complete occlusion. Nonetheless, noninvasive visualization of the arterial lumen is possible, and further refinements in resolution and technique should make it a reliable screening procedure for extracranial cerebrovascular disease.

REFERENCES

1. Albin, M. D., Babinski, M., Maroon, J. C., and Jannetta, P. J.: Anesthetic management of posterior fossa surgery in the sitting position. Acta Anaesth. Scand., *20*:117–128, 1976.
2. Baker, D. W.: Pulsed ultrasonic Doppler blood flow sensing. I.E.E.E. Trans. Sonics Ultrasonics, *17*:170–185, 1970.
3. Baker, M. L., and Dalrymple, G. V.: Biological effects of diagnostic ultrasound: A review. Radiology, *126*:479–483, 1978.
4. Barber, F. E., Baker, D. W., Nation, A. W. C., et al.: Ultrasonic duplex echo-Doppler scanner. I.E.E.E. Trans. Biomed. Eng., *21*:109–113, 1974.
5. Barnes, R. W., Russell, H. E., Bone, G. E., and Slaymaker, E. E.: Doppler cerebrovascular examination: Improved results with refinement in technique. Stroke, 8:468–471, 1977.
6. Barnes, R. W., Bone, G. E., Reinertson, J., Slaymaker, E. E., Hokanson, D. E., and Strandness, D. E.: Noninvasive ultrasonic carotid angiography: Prospective validation by contrast arteriography. Surgery, *80*:328–335, 1976.

7. Blackwell, E., Merory, J., Toole, J. F., and McKinney, W.: Doppler ultrasound scanning of the carotid bifurcation. Arch. Neurol. (Chicago), 34:145–148, 1977.

8. Bloch, S., Baltaxe, H. A., and Shoumaker, R. D.: Reliability of Doppler scanning of the carotid bifurcation: Angiographic correlation. Radiology, 132:687–691, 1979.

9. Bone, G. E., and Barnes, R. W.: Limitations of Doppler cerebrovascular examination in hemispheric cerebral ischemia. Surgery, 79:557–580, 1976.

10. Brawley, B. W.: Determination of superior sagittal sinus patency with an ultrasonic Doppler flow detector in parasagittal meningioma. Technical note. J. Neurosurg., 30:315–316, 1969.

11. Campbell, S.: Early prenatal diagnosis of neural tube defects by ultrasound. Clin. Obstet. Gynec., 20:351, 1977.

12. Cooperberg, P. L., Robertson, M. D., Fry, P., and Sweeney, V.: High resolution real time ultrasound of the carotid bifurcation, J.C.U., 7:13–17, 1979.

13. Cunningham, M. E., and Wells, W. J.: Ultrasound in the evaluation of anencephaly. Radiology, 118:165, 1976.

14. Doppler, C.: Über das farbige Licht der Doppelsterne und einiger anderer Gestirne des Himmels. Abh. Kgl. Böhm Ges Wissensch. (Prag.), 465 482, 1842.

15. Dunn, F., and Pond, J. B.: Selected non-thermal mechanisms of interaction of ultrasound and biological media. In Fry, F. J., ed.: Ultrasound: Its Applications in Medicine and Biology. Part 2. New York, Elsevier-North Holland Publishing Co., 1978.

16. Dunnick, N. R., Schuette, W. H., and Shawker, T. H.,: Ultrasonic demonstration of thrombus in the common carotid artery. Amer. J. Roentgen., 133:544–545, 1979.

17. Fleischer, A., and Brown, M.: Hydramnios associated with fetal hydrancephaly. J.C.U., 5:41, 1977.

18. Flitter, M. A., Buchheit, W. A., Murtagh, F., and Lapayowker, M. S.: Ultrasound determination of cerebrospinal fluid shunt patency. Technical note. J. Neurosurg., 42:728–730, 1975.

19. Franklin, D. L., Schlegel, W. A., and Rushmer, R. F.: Blood flow measured by Doppler frequency shift of backscattered ultrasound. Science, 132:564, 1961.

20. Garrett, W. J., Kossoff, G., and Jones, R. F. C.: Ultrasonic cross-sectional visualization of hydrocephalus in infants. Neuroradiology, 8:279–288, 1975.

21. Gooding, G. A.: Gray-scale ultrasound detection of carotid body tumors. Radiology, 132:409–410, 1979.

22. Haber, K., Wachter, R. D., Christenson, P. C., et al.: Ultrasonic evaluation of intracranial pathology in infants: A new technique. Radiology, 134:173–178, 1980.

23. Herzog, K. A.: The detection of fetal meningocele and meningoencephalocele by B-scan ultrasound: A case report. J.C.U. 3:307, 1975.

24. Hokanson, D. E., Mozersky, D. J., Sumner, D. S., McLeod, F. D., and Strandness, D. E.: Ultrasonic arteriography. A noninvasive method of arterial visualization. Radiology, 102:435–436, 1972.

25. Hopman, H., Gratzl, O., Schmeidek, P., and Schneider, I.: Ultrasonic Doppler technique for microvascular bypass. Neurochirurgia (Stuttgart), 19:190–196, 1976.

26. Hunter, A. R.: Air embolism in the sitting position. Anaesthesia, 17:467–469, 1962.

27. Johnson, M. L., Mack, L. A., Frost, M., Rumack, C., and Rashbaum, C. L.: B-mode echoencephalography of intraventricular hemorrhage and hydrocephalus in high risk infants. In White, D., and Lyons, E. A., eds.: Ultrasound in Medicine. Vol. 5. New York, Plenum Press, 1979.

28. Kindt, G. W., Youmans, J. R., and Conway, L. W.: The use of ultrasound to determine cerebral arterial reserve. J. Neurosurg., 31:544–549, 1969.

29. Lee, T. G., and Newton, B. W.: Posterior fossa cyst: Prenatal diagnosis by ultrasound. J.C.U. 4:29, 1976.

30. Lees, R. F., Harrison, R. B., and Sims, T. L.: Gray scale ultrasonography in the evaluation of hydrocephalus and associated abnormalities in infants. Amer. J. Dis. Child., 132:376–378, 1978.

31. Liebeskind, D., Bases, R., Elequin, F., Neubort, S., Leifer, R., Goldberg, R., and Koeningsberg, M.: Diagnostic ultrasound: Effects on the DNA and growth patterns of animal cells. Radiology, 131:177–184, 1979.

32. Lye, C. R., Summer, D. S., and Strandness, D. E.: The accuracy of the supraorbital Doppler examination in the diagnosis of hemodynamically significant carotid occlusive disease. Surgery, 79:42–45, 1976.

33. Machleder, H. I., and Barker, W. F.: Stroke on the wrong side. Use of the Doppler ophthalmic test in cerebral vascular screening. Arch. Surg. (Chicago), 105:943–947, 1972.

34. Maroon, J. C., and Albin, M. S.: Air embolism diagnosed by Doppler ultrasound. Anesth. Analg. (Cleveland), 53:399–402, 1974.

35. Maroon, J. C., Campbell, R. L., and Dyken, M. L.: Internal carotid artery occlusion diagnosed by Doppler ultrasound. Stroke, 1:122–127, 1970.

36. Maroon, J. C., Edmonds-Seal, J., and Campbell, R. L.: An ultrasonic method for detecting air embolism. J. Neurosurg., 31:196–201, 1969.

37. Maroon, J. C., Pieroni, D. W., and Campbell, R. L.: Ophthalmosonometry: An ultrasonic method for assessing carotid blood flow. J. Neurosurg., 30:238–246, 1969.

38. Maroon, J. C., Goodman, J. M., Horner, T. G., and Campbell, R. L.: Detection of minute venous air emboli with ultrasound. Surg. Gynec. Obstet., 127:1236–1238, 1968.

39. Matjasko, M. J., Williams, J. P., and Fontanilla, M.: Intraoperative use of Doppler to detect successful obliteration of carotid-cavernous fistulas, Technical note. J. Neurosurg., 43:634–636, 1975.

40. Michenfelder, J. D., Miller, R. H., and Gronert, G. A.: Evaluation of an ultrasonic device (Doppler) for the diagnosis of venous air embolism. Anaesthesiology, 36:164–167, 1972.

41. Miyazaki, M., and Kato, K.: Measurement of cerebral flow by ultrasonic Doppler technique: Haemodynamic comparison of right and left carotid artery in patients with hemiplegia. Jap. Circ. J., 29:383–386, 1954.

42. Morgan, C. L., Trought, W. S., Rothman, S. J., and Jimenez, J. P.: Comparison of B-scan ultrasound and computerized tomography in evaluating infantile hydrocephalus. *In* White, D., and Lyons, E. A., eds.: Ultrasound in Medicine. Vol. 5. New York, Plenum Press, 1979.

43. Morgan, C. L., Trought, W. S., Rothman, S. J., and Jimenez, J. P.: Comparison of gray-scale ultrasonography and computed tomography in the evaluation of macrocrania in infants. Radiology, *132*:119–123, 1979.

44. Muller, H. R.: The diagnosis of internal carotid artery occlusion by directional Doppler sonography of the ophthalmic artery. Neurology (Minneap.), *22*:816–823, 1972.

45. Munson, E. S.: Effect of nitrous oxide on the pulmonary circulation during venous air embolism. Anesth. Analg. (Cleveland), *50*:785, 1971.

46. Nishimoto, A., Shimada, H., Ueda, S., and Yagya, Y.: Ultrasound placement of cardiac tube in ventriculoatrial shunt. Technical note. J. Neurosurg., *33*:602–604, 1970.

47. Nuzzaci, G., Briani, S., Mennonna, P., and Evangelisti, A.: The Doppler ophthalmic test. Report of a study on its value in diagnosis of internal carotid artery insufficiency. J. Neurosurg. Sci., *19*:129–137, 1975.

48. Peronneau, P. A., and Leger, F.: Doppler ultrasonic pulsed blood flowmeter, Proceedings of 22nd Annual Conference on Engineering in Medicine and Biology, Session 10.11, 1969. New York, Institute of Electrical and Electronics Engineers, 1969.

49. Reid, M. H.: Ultrasonic visualization of a cervical cord cystic astrocytoma. Amer. J. Roentgen., *131*:907–908, 1978.

50. Reid, M. H.: Improved ultrasound image detail using ultrafocused transducers. Radiology *136*:473–478, 1980.

51. Reid, M. H., Mackay, R. S., and Lantz, B. M. T.: Noninvasive blood flow measurements by Doppler ultrasound with applications to renal artery flow determination. Invest. Radiol., *15*: 323–331, 1980.

52. Satomura, S.: Study of flow patterns in peripheral arteries by ultrasonics. J. Acoust. Soc. Amer., *15*:151, 1959.

53. Shenkin, H., and Goldfedder, P.: Air embolism from exposure of posterior cranial fossa in prone position. J.A.M.A., *210*:726, 1976.

54. Siegel, E., Goddard, J., James, E., and Siegel, E. P.: Cellular attachment as a sensitive indicator of the effects of diagnostic ultrasound exposure on cultured human cells. Radiology, *133*:175–179, 1979.

55. Skolnick, M. L., Rosenbaum, A. E., Matuzuk, T., Guthkelch, A. N., and Heinz, E. R.: Detection of dilated cerebral ventricles in infants: A correlative study between ultrasound and computed tomography. Radiology, *131*:447–451, 1979.

56. Spencer, M. P., Reid, S. M., Davis, D. L., and Paulson, P. S.: Cervical carotid imaging with a continuous-wave Doppler flowmeter. Stroke, *5*:145–154, 1974.

57. Star, E. G., and Fischer, F.: Ultraschall-Uberwachungsverfahren zur Fruhdiagnose von Luftemboliem bie neurochirurgischen Eingriffen. Anaesthesist, *24*:290–293, 1976.

58. Stegall, H. F., Rushmer, R. F., and Baker, D. W.: A transcutaneous ultrasonic blood velocity meter. J. Appl. Physiol., *21*:707–711, 1966.

59. Strandness, D. E., Schultz, R. D., Sumner, D. S., and Rushmer, R. F.: Ultrasonic flow detection: A useful technique in the evaluation of peripheral vascular disease. Amer. J. Surg., *113*:311–320, 1967.

60. Toombs, B. D., Kolodny, G. M., and Strandberg, M. W. P.: Synergistic biological effects of ultrasound and ionizing radiations evaluated in vitro. Radiology, *132*:731–734, 1979.

61. Turnipseed, W. D., Berkoff, H., and Barriga, P.: Doppler scanning and xerography: A screening procedure for high-risk carotid lesions in surgical patients. J. Surg. Res., *22*:683–686, 1977.

62. Urick, R. J.: Principles of Underwater Sound. 2nd Ed. New York, McGraw-Hill Book Co., 1975, pp. 2–7.

63. Weinstein, P. R.: A new technique for visualization of intracranial pathology in infants. Paper No. 24, Proceedings of Western Neurological Society Annual Meeting, Scottsdale, Arizona, 1979.

64. Wells, P. N. T.: Biomedical Ultrasonics. Chapter 9. New York, Academic Press, 1977.

21

CEREBRAL DEATH

For ancient and medieval man, death was an experience cloaked in mystery and fear. Because of its universal and irreversible nature, the subject has been treated extensively in the literature of philosophy, theology, and science from ancient times to the present. The role of the physician in this drama was to prevent death through treatment and, if this was not possible, then to determine when death had occurred. Thus, various criteria for the determination of death arose, including cessation of respirations and heart beat, lack of pupillary action, rigor mortis, hypostasis, and relaxation of the anal sphincter. However, since even deep coma might be reversible in the rare case, the only incontrovertible sign of death for the ancients was the onset of tissue decay.

The lack of a reliable criterion for distinguishing actual from apparent death caused a universal concern that it might be pronounced prematurely. Indeed, in previous centuries this fear was not unfounded. Numerous instances of individuals who were thought to be dead but had cataplexy, trance states, hysteria, hypothermia, and coma from a variety of causes were reported even in the late nineteenth century.[66] Writing in 1896, Montgomery reported on the condition of bodies removed from a military cemetery. He states:

We found among these remains two that bore every evidence of having been buried alive. The first case was that of a soldier that had been struck by lightning. Upon opening the lid of the coffin we found that the arms and legs had been drawn up as far as the confines of the coffin would permit. The other was a case of death resulting from alcoholism. The body was slightly turned, the legs were drawn up a trifle and the hands were clutching the clothes.[52]

He concluded his report by saying

Nearly two percent of those exhumed were, no doubt, victims of suspended animation.[52]

Pamphlets with such titles as "Burying Alive, a Frequent Peril" kept the public concerned by citing cases like that of a 35-year-old man who was supposed to have died of scarlet fever and was buried 48 hours later. The pamphlet stated

The coffin was moved two months later and the glass front was found to be shattered, the bottom kicked out and the sides sprung. The body was reported to lay face downward with the arms bent and in the clenched fist were handfuls of hair.[74]

Such reports gained wide circulation and fueled the universal fear of premature interment. As a result many individuals throughout the world left instructions that their bodies were to be mutilated by such actions as having a sword put through the heart after death was thought to have occurred. According to Walker, as late as 1918 the law in France was that death could be declared only after temporal or radial arteriotomy produced no hemorrhage.[72] This widespread attitude changed little until a more scientific one developed later in this century. Despite the scientific progress, incidents still happen that support the fear of an incorrect diagnosis of death. For instance, in 1967 an American soldier who had failed to respond to the efforts of a resuscitation team for nearly an hour was left for dead and later showed signs of life as he was about to be embalmed.[54] In view of the centuries-old universal fear of incorrect diagnosis of death and premature burial, it is remarkable that during a mere two decades the world's society could accept such

J. R. YOUMANS, T. M. KELLER, AND J. F. ALKSNE

sweeping sociological, philosophical, and legal changes as to even consider the diagnosis of death of the organism by death of a single organ, i.e., the brain.[4]

The background for acceptance of cerebral death as an entity was developed during the last few decades with the gradual acceptance of the idea that death encompasses many factors and evolves in stages rather than being one simple finite cataclysmic event. The definition of death as a cessation of all vital functions in a living organism was enlarged as insight and diverse connotations were applied to it by individuals of various professions and backgrounds. Many amplifying terms were used. They included such terms as "biological death," "brain death," "cardiac death," "cerebral death," "clinical death," "cortical death," "cytological death," "irreversible death," "legal death," "psychological death," "psychosocial death," and "spiritual death."[72] Against this background, the development of modern techniques that permitted prolonged artificial ventilation of apneic patients gave urgency to the quest for criteria for death that recognized the legal, social, medical, and ethical implications of declaring death in a patient who had lost certain vital functions but not all others.

These discussions have led to many definitions of death. One that has been well accepted defines death as ". . . a point at which the deterioration of functions becomes irreversible so that the organism can never again function as an integrated, rational organ."[10] Perhaps, in the statement attributed to him, Justice Holmes best summarized the problem when he said "to live is to function; that is all there is to living."[27]

The question has arisen whether destruction of the cerebral hemispheres or cerebral cortex in a person with preserved respiratory and vasomotor functions could be considered to be adequate evidence to declare that person clinically or legally brain dead. Some writers have argued that cortical death alone is not sufficient to deprive a person of his right to live.[40] The justification for this argument is that some psychic activity may be present in the brain stem. Others have argued that if the cerebrum is irreversibly destroyed bilaterally, the infratentorial portions of the brain do not have psychic activity and make no significant contribution to the continuing function of the total human organism.[43] The issue in this controversy is whether vegetative functions of the body without accompanying cerebral function constitute an adequate basis for declaring the person to be alive. Some authors have qualified the term "cerebral death" and have subdivided it into "neocortical death," which means the destruction of the cerebral mantle, and "brain death," which has been reserved to mean the total destruction of all the intracranial nervous tissue.[44] Although physicians well-informed in neurology can reliably diagnose brain death even with some lower brain stem reflexes present, at present it would seem that a holistic designation is appropriate and that a subdivision of the diagnosis should not be attempted.

A problem arises when the terms "cerebral death" or "brain death" and "irreversible coma" are used loosely. Cerebral death implies total and permanent abolition of brain function so that both volitional and higher-level reflex activity and responsivity are lost. In contrast "irreversible coma" refers to a state in which all functions attributed to the cerebrum that identify the human essence—mind, personality, behavior, and in theological terms, the soul—are lost, but certain functions that regulate respiration, temperature, blood pressure, and lower-level central nervous system activity remain. Patients with irreversible coma fit the so-called appallic state described by Ingvar and Brun, which implies loss of the pallium, the cortical gray matter that covers the cerebral cortex.[36] These patients are in the broad category that includes the persistent vegetative states, coma vigil, and akinetic mutism.[42] In them a variety of vegetative functions including respiration may be preserved so that survival for years is possible.

The well-publicized case of Karen Quinlan fits the category of irreversible coma.[27] For reasons that are unclear, this 21-year-old girl ceased breathing for two 15-minute periods. On her admission to the hospital her temperature was 100°, her pupils were unreactive, and she was unresponsive to deep pain. She was given respiratory assistance via a respirator. When examined by a neurologist three days later she was found to be comatose with evidence of decortication. The respiratory assistance was continued. Tests of the urine disclosed traces of quinine, barbiturates, and diazepam. A brain scan, an angiogram, and a lumbar puncture were normal. Her electroencephalogram was characterized as "abnormal, but it showed some activity and was consistent with her clinical state." The clinical state was a sleeplike unresponsive condition at first, but later she developed sleep-wake cycles. In the waking state she would blink and cry out. She was "totally unaware of anyone or anything around her," and was characterized as being in a "chronic, persistive, vegetative state, and no longer had any cognitive function."[27]

LEGAL ASPECTS

Prior to the evolution of the concept of cerebral death before death of the entire body, the courts of the United States were applying the definition of death from Black's law dictionary, which was

. . . the cessation of life; the ceasing to exist; defined by physicians as a total stoppage of the circulation of the blood, and a cessation of the animal and vital functions consequent thereupon such as respirations, pulsations, etc.[14]

Typical of the legal rulings based on that definition was that of an appeals court, which said in a case determining which of two men had died first,

. . . death occurs precisely when life ceases and does not occur until the heart stops beating and respirations end. Death is not a continuous event and is an event that takes place at a precise time.[67]

As a result of this type of approach by the courts, the physicians making a diagnosis of cerebral death and stopping respiratory assistance to the patient or removing organs for transplantation before cessation of heart beat were at risk of prosecution for malpractice by omission or criminal prosecution for permitting removal of an organ prior to the patient's death. Gradually over several years the concept of cerebral or brain death as representing the actual death of the individual came to be supported in a number of courts and judicial forums.[35,51,59] For example, one early court ruling that supported the new concept of brain death was that

Death is the cessation of life. A person may be pronounced dead if, based on the usual and cus-

tomary standards of medical practice, it has been determined that the person has suffered an irreversible cessation of brain function. . . .[18]

The legal ramifications of defining death are far-ranging. For instance, the situation may exist in which a person is considered dead for one purpose such as transplantation of organs, and alive for another such as inheritance or predecease of another individual or resolution of problems involving estate taxes. The legal complexities have led legislative bodies to vary widely in the degree of specificity that they enjoin in giving legal sanction to the concept of cerebral death. Some states in the United States have been quite specific and others have followed the advice of the House of Delegates of the American Medical Association, which supported the concept of cerebral death but opposed statutory definitions. In the December 1974 meeting of the House of Delegates, the following resolution was passed.

Resolved, That the American Medical Association reaffirm established policies that: "At first statutory definition of death is neither desirable or necessary"; "that state medical associations urge their respective legislatures to postpone enactment of legislation defining death by statute"; "that death shall be determined by the clinical judgment of the physicians using the necessary available and current accepted criteria"; and "permanent and irreversible cessation of function of the brain constitutes one of the various criteria which can be used in the medical diagnosis of death."[72]

MORAL ASPECTS

The potential for error and laxity causes troublesome ethical and moral questions. The remote possibility of error mandates caution and concern in every aspect of making the diagnosis. When appropriate caution and concern have been used, current theological teachings would support the concept of diagnosing cerebral death and taking appropriate action. For example, Pope Pius XII discussed the obligation to use elaborate and expensive means of resuscitation by saying

It is incumbent on the physician to take all reasonable, ordinary means of restoring the spontaneous vital functions and consciousness, and to employ such extraordinary means as are available to him to this end. It is not obligatory, however, to continue to use extraordinary means indefinitely in hopeless cases.[55]

In this regard the definition of extraordinary means has been interpreted as

. . . whatever . . . is very costly or very unusual, or very painful, or very difficult, or very dangerous, or if the good effects that can be expected from it are not proportionate to the difficulties and inconveniences that are entailed.[20]

WORLD ACCEPTANCE

The acceptance of the concept of cerebral death varies in different countries of the world (Table 21–1). The difference in philosophies of the various nations and societies was shown at the 1976 meetings of the Neurotraumatology Committee of the World Federation of Neurological Societies.[72] Two major views were put forth. One was that the criteria for brain death should be based upon clinical considerations with little or no laboratory confirmation. Those holding that view thought that, with a confirmed diagnosis of an untreatable and soon to be fatal brain lesion, the absence of responsivity and spontaneous respirations and cephalic reflexes for a period of 12 to 48 hours was a simple and satisfactory means of determining the death of the brain that could be used by all physicians regardless of their neurological expertise. The other view was that clinical criteria were inadequate and laboratory tests such as electroencephalographic or metabolic studies were needed to confirm the diagnosis. Implied in this second view is the constraint that the diagnosis of cerebral death could be made only in centers equipped for these laboratory studies and by individuals who were adequately trained to interpret and correlate them with the patient's neurological status. This latter approach would not be a significant impediment to organ transplantation, since organs are transplanted in well-equipped hospitals where the instru-

TABLE 21–1   MEDICAL AND LEGAL STATUS OF CEREBRAL DEATH*

| COUNTRY OR REGION | CONCEPT OF CEREBRAL DEATH ACCEPTED | | CRITERIA OF CEREBRAL DEATH |
	Medically	Legally	
Argentine	Yes	Yes	Yes
Australia	Yes	No	Yes
Bolivia	Yes	No	Local
Brazil	Yes	No	Local
Canada	Yes	No	Yes
Chile	Yes	No	Local
Colombia	Yes	No	Local
Czechoslovakia	Yes	Yes	National
Egypt	No	No	No
France	Yes	No	Local
India	No	No	Local
Israel	Yes	No	Local
Italy	No	Yes	Yes
Japan	No	No	Local
Korea	Yes	No	Local
Mexico	Yes	Yes	Yes
Netherlands	Yes	No	National
Pan African	No	No	No
Peru	Yes	No	Local
Scandinavia	No(?)	No	Yes
Spain	No	No	Local
Switzerland	Yes	No	National
Turkey	Yes	No	Local
United Kingdom	Yes	No	National
Uruguay	Yes	No	Local
U.S.A.	Yes	20 States	No
Venezuela	Yes	No	Local
Totals	Yes, 20; No, 7	Yes, 5; No, 22	Local 14 National 10 None 3

* From Walker, A. E.: Cerebral Death. Dallas, Texas, Professional Information Library, 1977. Reprinted by permission.

mentation for making the various studies is available. However, the question of whether to continue costly and needless support of a hopelessly ill patient arises in smaller and less well-equipped hospitals also. Indeed, the need for the decision to be made for economic and humanitarian reasons involving only the patient and his family will arise much more often than it will for organ transplantation.

CHARACTERISTICS OF BRAIN DEATH

Physical Signs

A patient with brain death will have no respirations but may have a pulse and blood pressure. The blood pressure may be normal or unstable, and pressor agents may be required to maintain it. The pulse rate shows no distinctive pattern with cerebral death. If the blood pressure is unstable, shock should be ruled out. The use of pressor agents may cause characteristic arrhythmias, but these are related to cardiac irritability and not to cerebral responsiveness.

Cranial Nerves

A variety of reflex arcs subserved by the cranial nerves or cephalic reflexes are available to evaluate the viability and function of the brain stem. All these reflexes must be absent for the criterion of absence of cephalic reflexes to be met.

The pupillary light reflex is produced by flashing a bright light into one eye and then the other. Subsequent constriction of the pupil that is stimulated constitutes the direct response, and constriction of the other pupil, the consensual response. The light should be directed into the eye for several seconds while the pupillary response is observed closely. Rapid flashing of the light may cause slow or minimal responses of the pupil to be missed. Small pupillary size may make evaluation of the light reflex difficult. With pontine lesions that interrupt the brain stem sympathetic pathways the pupils will be small. In this situation, reactivity is best assessed by using a magnifying glass or the plus 20 lens on the ophthalmoscope. In as-

sessing this reflex, one must remember that damage to the optic nerves, chiasm, or radiation, and a variety of pharmacological agents, can result in nonreactivity of the pupils.

The corneal reflex is mediated through the pons with the trigeminal nerve as the afferent arc and the facial nerve as the efferent arc. It is elicited by drawing a wisp of cotton over the cornea and noting a blink response of the eye. Bell's phenomenon, the bilaterally responsive eyelid closure and upward deviation of the eyes, will be absent also when the corneal reflex is absent. Corneal hyposensitivity due to drying, edema, or corneal anesthetics reduces the validity of the test.

The oculocephalic reflexes are tested by the doll's head maneuver. The head is briskly turned from side to side to evaluate horizontal eye movements, and the neck is flexed and extended to test vertical eye movements.[34] The normal response, turning of the eyes in the direction opposite to that in which the head is moved, reflects function of the vestibular mechanisms. Absence of vertical and horizontal movements implies dysfunction of the midbrain pretectal area and the pontine conjugate gaze centers respectively. In patients who have suffered trauma, the stability of the cervical spine should be assessed before this maneuver is attempted. The test should be done in conjunction with that of the oculovestibular reflex, since similar pathways are being evaluated. The latter test should not be performed until it has been established that the tympanic membrane is intact. Then 200 ml of ice water may be introduced slowly into the external auditory canal until nystagmus or ocular deviation occurs. An induced conduction current is set up in the labyrinthine endolymph of the lateral semicircular canal that alters the balance of the paired vestibular systems and produces tonic conjugate eye deviation toward the same side with cold stimuli or toward the opposite side with warm stimuli.

The pharyngeal, or gag, reflex is a contraction of the constrictor muscle elicited when the posterior part of the pharynx is touched. It may be unreliable in the apneic patient supported by a respirator owing to the presence of an endotracheal tube. The same may be said for the swallow and cough reflexes.

Sensory and Motor Responses

There are no cerebrally mediated sensory reactions or motor movements in patients with brain death. Decorticate or decerebrate movements may be present as long as lower parts of the brain survive, but usually these will be lost by the time that apnea occurs. If not, they will disappear soon thereafter. Muscle tone may be present in the extremities; in the majority of cases, however, it is absent.

Spinal Reflexes

Movements induced by noxious stimuli applied to the extremities after brain death are due to spinal reflexes. In the lower extremity the response is usually a partial flexor reflex, although other spinal reflexes such as the crossed extensor may be present. In the upper extremities, extensor responses such as those characterizing a high spinal cord transection may be induced.

The spinal reflexes manifested by tendon jerks of the arms and legs are poor indicators of the state of the brain. Since the spinal cord may still be viable in the presence of cerebral death, it is not surprising that the tendon reflexes may persist. Pathological reflexes such as the extensor plantar response will be seen more often than the superficial tendon reflexes.

Laboratory Tests

Unfortunately, the clinical findings are not invariably reliable in making the diagnosis of brain death. Indeed, in the 503 patients who had coma and apnea for 15 minutes and were admitted to the Collaborative Study on Cerebral Death, 41 (9 per cent) survived for longer than three months.[3] As would be expected, many of them had various forms of intoxication. A number of laboratory and pathological correlates may be used to corroborate the diagnosis of brain death.

Cerebral Blood Flow

To perform normally, the brain requires a constant supply of oxygen and glucose. Delivery of these substances requires approximately 15 per cent of the cardiac output.[26] Interruption of this blood flow in the human for only 5 to 10 minutes will begin to cause brain damage, and an interruption of 20 to 30 minutes will cause irreversible damage. As a result, the demonstration of an absence of cerebral circulation can be used to diagnose cerebral death.

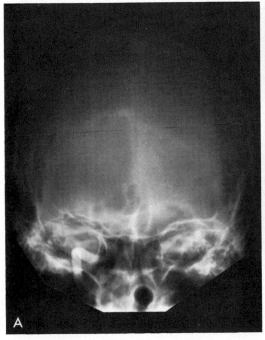
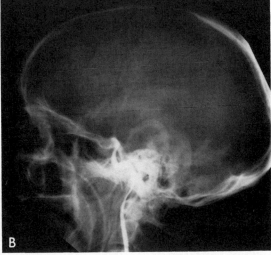

Figure 21–1 Angiogram of a patient with cerebral death due to increased intracranial pressure. The dye does not flow into the intracranial portion of the carotid artery and its branches. *A*. Anteroposterior view. *B*. Lateral view.

Cerebral angiography was the earliest standard technique to assess the status of the cerebral circulation (Fig. 21–1). Mitchell and associates noted the absence of cerebral blood flow in patients with severe intracranial hypertension. The contrast material stopped at the internal carotid artery at the level of the carotid siphon while the external carotid artery and its branches filled normally. At autopsy, patency of carotid vessels was demonstrated, thus confirming that the lack of flow was due to increased intracranial pressure.[50] Greitz and co-workers used aortocranial and carotid angiography in 42 patients with brain death. In them, the contrast media stopped at one of several sites—in the neck close to the carotid bifurcation, in the intradural parasellar part of the internal carotid artery, or intracranially either just distal to the carotid siphon or in the bifurcation of the middle cerebral artery.[31] Angiographic evidence of absence of blood flow is not a sine qua non for the diagnosis of cerebral death, however, because of rare instances in which a therapeutic measure such as ventricular puncture has been successful in relieving the increased intracranial pressure and restoring the cerebral blood flow.[56] Of course, if the elevated intracranial pressure cannot be relieved in a short time, it may be assumed that cerebral infarction and death have occurred.

A noninvasive technique for assessing the cerebral circulation is to inject an isotope such as 2 mc of 99m technetium pertechnetate into an antecubital vein and then to place radioisotope detectors over the head and over the femoral artery. Patients with normal cerebral blood flow show a relatively sharp rise and fall of radioactivity in both cephalic and femoral leads. Patients with hypoperfusion have a small gradual linear increase in activity over the head and normal activity over the femoral artery. This latter pattern occurred in all of Korein and associates' 80 patients who were comatose and apneic.[45] Goodman and co-workers studied more than 500 patients by isotope angiography with the scintillation camera. The cerebral arteries and venous sinuses were visualized in all patients except three who had brain death.[30]

Another technique for evaluating the presence of a cerebral circulation is recording of the pulsatile midline echo of the brain. These recordings are made by using an ultrasonic reflectoscope or echoencephalograph coupled with a device that gives additional processing of the scope's electrical signal so as to show the pulsations of the midline of the brain with each heart beat. This system was tested in 46 patients by Uematsu and colleagues. Three of the patients were in stupor, fifteen in coma, and twenty-eight suspected of having cerebral death on the basis of unresponsiveness, apnea, and electrocerebral silence. One of those who were thought to have brain death and yet had a midline echo pulsation had had a large decompressive craniotomy with removal of the bone flap. It was thought that the persistent midline pulsation might have been transmitted from the external carotid pulsation to the intracranial cavity because of the large decompressive cranial defect.[69] The cause of the midline echopulsations in the other case with presumed brain death is less clear. Perhaps the function of the cortex and electrical activity were lost prior to the total cessation of cerebral flow. In any event, these findings lend credence to the *absence* of the pulsatile midline echo as clear evidence of lack of cerebral flow. Further, when this finding is present for 30 minutes or more, the diagnosis of brain death can be made with confidence.

Electrocardiogram

Electrocardiographic findings may be normal in patients with brain death, but ST-T changes usually are seen in the terminal stages. At necropsy, the heart often has minimal abnormalities such as subendocardial and subepicardial hemorrhages of a nonspecific nature. These changes may be related to anoxia.[25]

CT Scan

CT scans of patients with brain death show no definitive characteristics in spite of the arrest of intracranial circulation as shown by the angiogram.[58] It appears that CT scanning cannot be used to diagnose cerebral death.

Biochemical Changes

As the cerebral function fails in brain death a variety of biochemical changes occur in the brain. It loses the ability to utilize nutrient sources of glucose and oxygen to produce energy through production of high-energy phosphate bonds. Thus, the lack of oxygen consumption is manifest by the diminution in cerebral blood flow and the decrease in the arteriovenous difference of oxygen content across the brain.[61] As less oxygen is used, anaerobic glycolysis begins, and it produces lactic acid. With loss of the brain's normal metabolic integrity there is a depletion of phosphocreatinine, adenosine triphosphate, and adenosine diphosphate in the neurons. They cease to function and become progressively edematous, and the oxidized respiratory enzymes are destroyed.

A variety of tests is available to assess the cerebral metabolic parameters, but they are too complex for routine clinical use.

Electroencephalogram

The electroencephalogram is a valuable aid in evaluating patients who may have brain death. Vestiges of cerebral cortical function may be detected with this test even though the patient is profoundly comatose as judged by the conventional neurological examination. The reliability of the electroencephalogram is shown by the study of the American Electroencephalographic Society's ad hoc committee on electroencephalographic criteria for the determination of cerebral death. They reviewed 2650 cases of coma with presumably isoelectric recordings.[2] Only three patients whose records satisfied the committee's criteria showed any recovery of cerebral function. These three had suffered from massive overdoses of nervous system depressants, two from barbiturates and one from meprobamate. The reported "isoelectric" records of these patients either were, on review, low-voltage records or had been made with techniques inadequate to bring out low-voltage activities.

The distinction should be made between a flat electroencephalogram, an isoelectric electroencephalogram, and electrocerebral silence. The flat electroencephalogram is one that shows no spontaneous activity of higher voltage than 20 μv.[1] The majority of these studies consist of irregular bursts of activity of varying frequency that merge with each other and do not show any constant frequency even during hyperventilation. In rare instances there is almost no spontaneous activity. The flat study is therefore fundamentally one with low voltage and fluctuating frequency. It may be seen in as many as 10 to 13 per cent of healthy persons.[38,48] Further, it is thought that conditions such as advanced age, fatigue, drowsiness, and sleep, and anesthesia increase the number of flat studies.[6,23,29] Diseases such as encephalitis may cause a flat electroencephalogram. Bental and Leibowitz reported the case of a 44-year-old woman with encephalitis who had a flat electroencephalogram for 28 days.[9] Although in their report they speak of her as having "complete absence of electrical activity," it is apparent from review of their publications that she merely had a flat recording and not one that meets the requirements of electrocerebral silence. This patient made a complete clinical recovery, and her electroencephalogram returned to normal.

To avoid confusion, it is recommended that nonphysiological terms such as "isoelectric" or "linear" should not be used to describe the recordings obtained during brain death. The appropriate term is "electrocerebral silence." Electrocerebral silence, or electrocerebral inactivity, is defined as

. . . no electrocerebral activity over 2μv when recording from scalp or referential electrode pairs 10 or more centimeters apart with interelectrode resistances under 10,000 ohms or (impedances under 6000 ohms) over 100 ohms.[2]

The reason for using the term "electrocerebral silence" is that the cardiac action and artifacts from various causes produce electroencephalographic changes (Fig. 21–2). As a result, the recordings are not truly flat or isoelectric.

Once electrocerebral silence has been noted, there is a high degree of correlation with ultimate death; these findings have, however, been present for more than 24 hours and yet some patients recover.[12,32,37,41] Also, a few patients may be deeply comatose, have electrocortical silence, and yet have functioning brain stems.[8,16] In fact, an elderly woman has been reported to have electrocerebral silence and yet to breathe spontaneously.[71]

These reports suggest that although the electroencephalogram is a valuable aid in diagnosing cerebral death, it has to be used in the context of the entire clinical problem or situation and cannot be used as a single

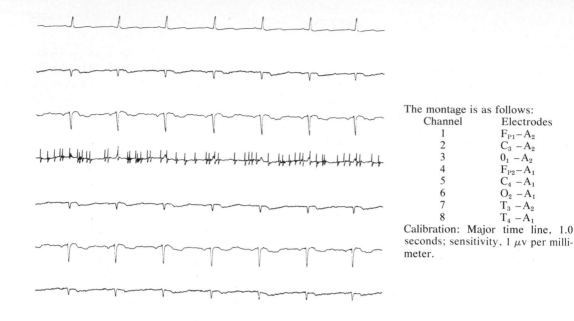

The montage is as follows:

Channel	Electrodes
1	$F_{P1} - A_2$
2	$C_3 - A_2$
3	$0_1 - A_2$
4	$F_{P2} - A_1$
5	$C_4 - A_1$
6	$O_2 - A_1$
7	$T_3 - A_2$
8	$T_4 - A_1$

Calibration: Major time line, 1.0 seconds; sensitivity, 1 μv per millimeter.

Figure 21-2 Electroencephalogram of a 34-year-old man with cerebral death. All waveform changes are related to cardiac or muscle activity. Channel 4 shows muscle artifacts. There is no electrical activity of cerebral origin that is greater than 2 μv. These electroencephalographic findings would confirm the clinical evidence of cerebral death. (Courtesy of Dr. A. Gabor.)

test for it. As Bennett has stated, "in the state of brain death, the EEG is always silent; however ECS does not always mean death."[7]

In order to standardize recordings and to minimize errors in determining electrocerebral silence, the American Electroencephalographic Society has set forth the following recommendations for use in making the recordings.

1. Use of a minimum of eight scalp electrodes and ear lobe reference electrodes.

2. An interelectrode impedance under 10,000 ohms but over 100 ohms.

3. Test of integrity of recording system by artifact potential.

4. Use of interelectrode distances of at least 10 centimeters.

5. Sensitivity increase from 7 μv per millimeter to 2 μv per millimeter during most of the recording with inclusion of appropriate calibrations.

6. Use of time constants of 0.3 to 0.4 second during part of the recording.

7. Use of monitoring devices such as the electrocardiogram and others as needed to detect artifacts emanating from the patient or induced by the surroundings.

8. Use of tests for electroencephalographic reactivity to intense stimuli such as pain (e.g., pinch), loud sound, and (optionally) strong light (stroboscopic if available).

9. Recording time of at least 30 minutes.

10. Recordings to be made only by qualified technologists.

11. A repeat electroencephalogram if doubt exists about electrocerebral silence.

12. Telephone transmission of the electroencephalogram not to be used for determination of electrocerebral silence.[2]

Before the electroencephalogram is performed, the patient should be in a stable state, since shock or hypothermia may depress the amplitude of the recording. Also, it is essential to insure that drugs are not present in sufficient quantities to depress the recording. Drugs that are often associated with electrocerebral silence include barbiturates, methaqualone, diazepam, mecloqualone, meprobamate, and trichloroethylene.* Drugs that can be ingested in toxic quantities and not produce electrocerebral silence as a primary effect include phenothiazides, atropine sulfate, tricyclic antidepressants, nitrazepam, salicylates,

---

* See references 11, 12, 30, 31, 35, 39, 44, 45, 51, 60, 63, 69, 73.

heroin, insecticides, glutethimide, and amanita phalloides (mushroom poisoning). If sedative or intoxicating drugs are present the diagnosis of cerebral death must be delayed until their concentration is below toxic levels.

Evoked Potentials

Another electrophysiological means of evaluating brain function involves the measurement of auditory brain stem responses. The test is an objective method of measuring sensory pathways transversing the brain stem. Starr found that these responses were either absent or markedly attenuated in 27 patients who met the clinical criteria of brain death. In addition, in patients who progressed from mere coma to brain death, a decrease in amplitude and a prolongation of the latency of the later components of the characteristic evoked waveform were noted.[64] The technique can be used as a corroborative test along with the electroencephalogram, especially in evaluation of the brain stem. The American Electroencephalographic Society Ad Hoc Committee on Cerebral Death recommended that an effort be made to evoke potentials by auditory, visual, and tactile stimulation when a patient suspected of having cerebral death is being evaluated.[63]

Atropine Tests

Normally the cardiac activities are under the antagonistic influences of the intracranial parasympathetic system (vagal dorsal nucleus) and the extracranial sympathetic system. In brain stem death the cardiac activities are influenced only by the sympathetic system without regulation from the intracranial centers. As a result the intravenous injection of 2 mg of atropine will not cause an acceleration in the cardiac rate. In a study of 42 successive patients who had cerebral death there were no exceptions to these findings.[57]

Combined Testing

Quaknine reported on 13 types of studies that may be performed antemortem to confirm cerebral death. Forty-two patients were included in the series, and various numbers of patients were given each type of test (Table 21–2).[57] From a study of his findings, it is apparent that cerebral death can be confirmed by a consistent lack of cerebral and brain stem function, absence

TABLE 21–2 TESTS PERFORMED IN 42 PATIENTS IN BRAIN DEATH*

TEST	NO. OF CASES	RESULTS	REMARKS
Electroencephalography	32	Flat tracing even after amplification and stimulation	13 cases under scope only
Atropine test	42	No tachycardia after intravenous injection of atropine (2 mg)	32 cases under ECG
Caloric test	42	No eye movements	With ice water or ethyl chloride into the external auditory meatuses
Electronystagmography	22	Flat tracing	With ice water or ethyl chloride into the external auditory meatuses
Echoencephalography	26	No echopulsations in the scope	Demonstrated in 10 cases by photo with three different exposures
Carotid and vertebral angiographies	26	Circulatory arrest at the base of the skull	Injection under pressure in five cases
Intracranial pressure	7	Very high (>100 mm Hg)	Measured by intraventricular catheter
Brain temperature	6	Brain $T°$ always less than rectal $T°$	Even in cases of hypothermia (ex: $29° < 32°C$)
Cerebral blood flow	8	No significant flow: <10 ml min^{-1} 100 gm^{-1} of brain	Xenon: two cases Hippuran: six cases
Cerebral oxygen consumption	4	<1.5 ml of O_2min^{-1} 100 ml^{-1} of blood	Blood taken from carotid bifurcation and jugular bulb
Brain scanning	12	"Cold brain area" and no appearance of the sup. long. sinus in AP projection	Intravenous technetium
Gamma camera	8	"Cold brain area" and no appearance of the sup. long. sinus in AP projection	Intravenous technetium
Intrathecal injection of radioiodinated serum albumin	6	No cerebrospinal fluid flow	Even after 48 hours
Brain autopsy	28	From cerebral edema to complete lysis of brain	Corresponding to brain death duration (1–7 days)

* From Quaknine, G. E.: Bedside procedures in the diagnosis of brain death. Resuscitation, 4:159–177, 1975. Reprinted by permission.

of cerebral blood flow, brain temperature markedly lower than body temperature, or increased intracranial pressure of a degree that would preclude cerebral blood flow. The test of function of the brain can be accomplished by electroencephalography, the atropine test of heart rate, the caloric test, or electronystagmography. The status of the cerebral circulation may be determined by arteriography or isotope studies. Determination of the brain temperature or the intracranial pressure requires the placement of intracranial probes of an appropriate nature.

Autopsy

At autopsy after brain death, 90 per cent of the brains appear to be abnormal by gross examination.[73] If the patient has required a respirator for more than 24 hours, over 60 per cent will have cortical abnormalities including pericellular edema, necrosis, neuronal loss, hemorrhage, and infarction. About 40 per cent of the cases will have the characteristic findings of the "respirator brain." These findings are a soft brain that is difficult to remove from the calvarium, a gross appearance of generalized swelling, poor fixation, a congested cortex, and a macerated cerebellum of which fragments are found in the spinal canal. Microscopic findings included pyknosis of neuronal cytoplasm in some cells of all sections, little or no inflammation, scattered neuronal changes or loss, and glial, microglial, or vascular alterations at the site of the microscopic findings.

FORMAL CRITERIA OF BRAIN DEATH

Harvard Criteria

In 1968, the need for a better understanding of the concept of cerebral death and the need for obtaining organs for transplantation earlier than at death with cessation of heart beat led the faculty of the Harvard Medical School to appoint an ad hoc committee to study the matter.[22] The goals of this committee were to help identify those patients who had brain death despite sustained heart function and to delete obsolete criteria for definition of death that could lead to controversy and delay in obtaining organs for transplantation. Prior to the pioneering work of this committee, the concept of cerebral death was vague. A large portion of the medical community did not understand or accept the concept, and those who did use it were without legal sanction.

The ad hoc committee recommended that criteria be set up so that the issue of the time of death could be considered solely as a medical one. Further, they emphasized that the patient should be declared dead before the respirator was stopped rather than afterward, since in the latter situation, the physician would be withdrawing respiratory support from a patient who was, under the existing law, still alive. To make the diagnosis of cerebral death safely in a medical and legal milieu in 1968, the committee suggested four criteria to be met in patients in whom hyperthermia or central nervous system depressants such as barbiturates were absent. The criteria were: (1) Unreceptivity and unresponsivity with total unawareness to externally applied stimuli and inner need, with even the most intensely painful stimuli evoking no vocal response, withdrawal of the limb, or quickening of respirations. (2) No movement or breathing over a period of one hour. If the patient was receiving mechanical respiratory support, spontaneous breathing should be totally absent for three minutes after the respirator was removed. (3) The absence of all elicitable reflexes, the absence of postural activity (decerebrate or other), and the presence of fixed and dilated pupils that would not respond to a direct source of bright light. (4) A flat or isoelectric electroencephalogram with the machine run at standard gains of 10 μv per millimeter and 50 μv per 5 mm and at double the standard gain, which is 5 μv per millimeter or 25 μv per 5 mm. All these tests were to be repeated at least 24 hours later with no change. The committee regarded items 1, 2, and 3 as making the diagnosis, the confirmation being made with the fourth item, the electroencephalogram.[22]

The so-called Harvard criteria were a notable advance, but probably were more strict and relied more heavily on the electroencephalogram than was necessary or justified in some cases. In particular, the requirement for re-evaluation in 24 hours often caused needless delays and damage to organs to be transplanted. Later criteria were published by other groups that reduced the period of observation to 12 hours and noted that segmental spinal reflexes such as deep tendon reflexes and triple flexion responses might be present. Further it was noted that the electroencephalogram and cerebral angiography "may provide supportive data and diagnosis of brain death, but they are not essential."[21]

American Association of Neurological Surgeons Guidelines

In the last decade numerous organizations and institutions have set forth criteria for cerebral death based on known physiological principles and observations that were post hoc.[5,13,19,24,39] Among them was the American Association of Neurological Surgeons, which issued the following guidelines for diagnosing cerebral death.

1. Cerebral unresponsivity.
2. Apnea.
3. Absence of cephalic reflexes including the pupillary, audio-ocular, and oculocephalic.
4. Dilated pupil (5.0 mm). In the event that the pupil is less than 5.0 mm, the possibility of a toxic factor is heightened, and determination of blood drug levels or studies of the cerebral circulation or both may be required to eliminate this possibility.
5. Electrocerebral silence. Findings meeting the American Electroencephalographic Society's criteria must be observed for a minimum recording period of 30 minutes at a time when the requisite clinical conditions have persisted for at least six hours. These findings should be re-examined and confirmed on a second occasion at least six hours later. (These criteria may be inapplicable to children under 5 years of age, since there are indications that the immature nervous system can survive significant periods of electrocerebral silence.)[15]

The arguments in favor of the American Association of Neurological Surgeons criteria are: (1) Since brain function is what is being evaluated, only cerebral reflexes are important. (2) The presence of a fixed but nondilated pupil increases the possibility of a toxic factor and therefore requires special consideration. (3) The time frame is shortened because it has been recognized that when the criteria have been met for even a few minutes brain survival is unlikely and

unreasonable measures may be required to maintain cardiovascular function for the 24 hours suggested by the Harvard ad hoc committee. (4) When any question arises about the validity of other findings the demonstration of complete cessation of intracranial circulation verifies brain death.

Evaluation of Criteria

To test the criteria of brain death in a prospective manner, the National Institute of Neurological and Communicative Disease and Stroke supported a collaborative study at nine medical centers distributed geographically throughout the United States.[3] The study collected data on the clinical findings, the electroencephalograms, and the laboratory analyses for drugs of the patients as well as the neuropathological reports on the dead brains. The protocol required that every patient over 1 year of age admitted to the participating medical center hospital in a cerebrally unresponsive state and apneic for 15 minutes be admitted to the study regardless of the cause of these findings. To be considered in the group for a diagnosis of brain death, the prerequisites were absence of sedative drug intoxication, hypothermia, cardiovascular shock, or a remediable primary disorder, and the presence of cerebral unresponsiveness, apnea, and electrocerebral silence.

The combined study demonstrated the practical problems of applying such a protocol in the diagnosis of cerebral death. For instance, in assessing the presence of sedative drug intoxication, it was found that the history of drug ingestion was often unreliable, it was virtually impossible to obtain accurate analysis of toxic agents within a few hours, and it was difficult to evaluate the significance of minimal amounts of drugs in the blood. The determination of normothermia and the absence of cardiovascular shock was less of a problem. Insuring the absence of a remediable lesion often required detailed laboratory studies such as computed tomography or angiography. The average time for obtaining those studies was 7.4 hours. Determining the presence of cerebral unresponsivity was straightforward except in 9 per cent of the cases; in these confusion was caused by spinal reflex movements. Although apnea is easily recognized at the bedside, its determination in this study was imprecise because of the need to maintain artificial respirations. After the diagnosis of brain death had been established by other criteria, removal of the respirator "was rarely followed by any respiratory effort and never by sufficient chest movement to sustain life." Determination of electrocerebral silence was complicated by three factors: technical inadequacies, observer error (misinterpretation in the reading of the record), and the degree of validity of a single recording. There was a 3 per cent disagreement between the panel reviewing the studies and the original interpreter of the recording. Most of the disagreement concerned the confusion of artifact with biological activity. In only 1 per cent of the cases was there disagreement in which the original reader diagnosed electrical cortical silence and the review panel considered that biological activity was present. The report states:

Though on critical analysis some "flat records" may be considered by reviewers who know the complete history of the case as showing biological activity, such varied opinions regarding 1 to 3 per cent of the cases are inevitable at the present state of the art of electroencephalography.[3]

When all drug-induced comas were excluded from the study, no patient in this series recovered after having a 30-minute period of electrical cortical silence.

The cepahlic reflexes—pupillary, corneal, oculoauditory (blink to a clap), oculocephalic (doll's eye), oculovestibular, ciliospinal, snout, cough, pharyngeal (gag), and swallowing—were noted to have varying sensitivity as indicators of brain stem dysfunction. The addition of these reflexes to the basic factors to be considered did not improve the accuracy of the diagnosis of brain death.

Although dilated and fixed pupils have commonly been thought to be present in brain death, they occurred in less than half the patients in this series. Of the 187 patients meeting the three basic criteria for brain death, 128 had dilated, 44 had small, and 15 had unequal pupils. Two patients with drug intoxication had small pupils.

Almost 70 per cent of patients had absence of muscle tone in either arms or legs, and 60 per cent lacked it in both. Another 10 per cent lost their muscle tone sometime before cardiac arrest. In this same group,

abnormal posturing was noted in 14 per cent of cases at the time of the initial examination, but in only half the number at the time of final examination before cardiac arrest.

The spinal reflexes as manifested by tendon jerks with the arms and legs are poor indicators of the state of the brain. Of the 187 patients meeting the basic criteria for brain death, 101 had no reflexes and 71 had active reflexes; the remaining 15 were not examined for their reflexes.

The directors of the combined study concluded that the minimal criteria for diagnosis of cerebral death should be that (1) all appropriate diagnostic and therapeutic procedures have been performed; and (2) the patient is in coma with cerebral unresponsivity and apnea; has dilated pupils, absence of cepahlic reflexes, and electrocerebral silence; and these findings have been present for a period of 30 minutes at least six hours after the onset of coma and apnea. If an early decision about cerebral death is desired and particularly if any of the critical findings are not definitive, it was suggested, a confirmatory test to insure the absence of cerebral blood flow should be made.

Ideal Criteria

The ideal criteria for determination of cerebral death would give unequivocal and reliable results that could be accepted without question by the medical and lay public. Further, they would be simple and clear so that any physician could apply them by merely referring to the list of requirements necessary for making the diagnosis. Unfortunately, criteria that cover all circumstances in the most ideal and expeditious manner do not exist. As a result, the diagnosis of cerebral death should be a medical decision based on the physician's judgment that is made after all factors have been considered. A strict protocol cannot encompass all circumstances that arise, and if one is imposed by institutional policy or legal requirements, needless delays will occur in obtaining organs to be transplanted and needless expenses will be incurred to render treatment that is useless. As a workable, practical, and safe approach to the problem, the authors of this chapter suggest the following factors be considered in making the diagnosis.

1. There should be *cerebral* unresponsivity and unreceptivity. There should be no evidence of a cerebral type of response to intensely painful stimulus, noise, or visual stimuli. Spinal cord or lower brain stem function may be present.

2. There should be no suspicion that the coma is due to depressant drugs. A careful drug history and chemical screening for drug levels is essential in all situations except those with a firm diagnosis of a major intracerebral lesion that is clearly capable of causing brain death.

3. Spontaneous respiration should have ceased. With the blood oxygen tension at normal or higher levels, trials of at first three and then five minutes without the respirator should not produce efforts of spontaneous breathing. To protect against hypoxia, 5 liters per minute of oxygen may be perfused through an intratracheal catheter. If facilities to measure oxygen tension are not present and no organs are to be donated, then the trial without the respirator should be 10 minutes. Since the carbon dioxide tension increases at the rate of approximately 3 mm of mercury per minute, the carbon dioxide build-up should be adequate to stimulate breathing.[60]

4. The patient should have an untreatable brain lesion. This situation may be obvious within hours of a severe head injury, spontaneous intracerebral hemorrhage, or craniotomy. With cardiac arrest, hypoxia, or severe circulatory insufficiency with cerebral anoxia or cerebral embolism, longer periods of observation may be necessary.

5. Primary hypothermia and significant abnormalities of metabolic and endocrine factors should be excluded. It is acknowledged that marked abnormalities of these factors may develop during treatment of the patient over a prolonged time and should not delay the diagnosis of cerebral death if other appropriate factors are present. Whereas *primary* hypothermia should be ruled out, secondary hypothermia develops in a majority of patients with cerebral death. In these patients the temperature may be 96° F or lower.

6. Although a reliable diagnosis of brain death can be made on the basis of the clinical findings and course of events in most cases, additional confirmation may be desirable in other cases. In particular, if there is a question of homicide or other factors that may lead to legal questions the confirmation of brain death by laboratory tests may be particularly desirable. This confirmation can be obtained by several tests or combination of them. Absence of cerebral blood flow may be demonstrated by angiogram, isotope studies, or absence of midline echopulsation. Absence of cerebral blood flow and presumed cerebral infarction may be inferred from persistent intracranial pressure measurements sufficiently elevated over systemic blood pressure to preclude intracranial flow. Electrocerebral silence on the electroencephalogram denotes lack of cerebral function. If suppressant drugs are absent, it is presumptive of cerebral death. Brain stem function and reflexes may or may not be present with electrocerebral silence. If a known structural, untreatable brain lesion of the type that can produce cerebral death is not present, the electroencephalographic electrocortical silence should be confirmed by recordings 24 hours later.

DISCUSSION WITH SURVIVORS

Explaining the concept of brain death to the surviving family and friends requires patience and an understanding of their emotional distress. The question of organ transplantation may be raised by the family, but usually it has to come from the physician attending the patient. When appropriate, the physician should assume a positive role, informing the family of the opportunity to get healthy organs to benefit the victims of chronic disease. After effective communication is established with the family and the criteria for brain death have been met, the declaring of death and removal of the patient to the operating room for the transplantation procedure should cause no difficulty. By arranging this sequence of events, the physician may have aided the family to assuage their grief by helping them to know that the death of their loved one has, through organ transplantation, permitted another person to have an additional gift of life.

Regardless of whether or not organs are to be used for transplantation, the physician and ancillary members of the medical team such as the nurses and social workers must be knowledgeable about the course of events and be willing to explain them, as often as needed, to all members of the family in a kind, calm, and sympathetic manner. Finally, the diagnosis of cerebral death and action based on it, such as discontinuing respiratory assistance, are medical matters. The survivors should not be burdened with the decision about when to stop the respirator. Of course, they should be informed of the plans in a clear, straightforward manner. In most instances they will agree with the suggested course of action. If they disagree, however, then further discussion is in order and the respiratory assistance should be continued until a full understanding is reached or cardiac arrest ensues to settle the matter.

REFERENCES

1. Adams, A.: Studies on the flat electroencephalogram in man. Electroenceph. Clin. Neurophysiol., *11*:35–41, 1959.
2. American Electroencephalographic Society: Guidelines in EEG. Willoughby, Ohio, 1976, 1980.
3. An appraisal of the criteria of cerebral death: A summary statement. J.A.M.A., *237*:982–986, 1977.
4. Arnold, J. D., Zimmerman, T. F., and Martin, D. C.: Public attitudes and the diagnosis of death. J.A.M.A., *206*:1949–1954, 1968.
5. Becker, D. P., Robert, C. M., Jr., Nelson, J. R., and Stern, W. E.: An evaluation of the definition of cerebral death. Neurology (Minneap.), *20*:459–462, 1970.
6. Beecher, H. K., McDonough, F. K., and Forbes, A.: Effects of blood pressure changes on cortical potentials during anesthesia. J. Neurophysiol., *1*:324–331, 1938.
7. Bennett, D. R.: The EEG in determining brain death. *In* Korein, J., Brain Death: Interrelated Medical and Social Issues. Ann. N.Y. Acad. Sci., *319*:110–120, 1978.
8. Bennett, D. R., Hughes, J. R., Korein, J., Merlis, J. K., and Suter, C.: Atlas of Electroencephalography in Coma and Cerebral Death. New York, Raven Press, 1976, p. 244.
9. Bental, E., and Leibowitz, U.: Flat electroencephalograms during 28 days in a case of "encephalitis." Electroenceph. Clin. Neurophysiol., *13*:457–460, 1961.
10. Bergen, R. P.: Legal regulation of heart transplants. Dis. Chest, *54*:352–356, 1968.
11. Bilikiewicz, A., and Smoczynski, S.: Electroencephalographic changes during atropine-induced coma. Polish Med. J., *9*:926–931, 1970.
12. Bird, T. D., and Plum, F.: Recovery from barbiturate overdose coma with a prolonged isoelectric electroencephalogram. Neurology (Minneap.), *18*:456–460, 1968.
13. Black, P. M.: Brain death (second of two parts). New Eng. J. Med., *299*:338–344, 393–412, 1978.
14. Black's Law Dictionary. 4th Ed. St. Paul, Weil Publishing Co., 1968.
15. Board of Directors, American Association of Neurological Surgeons: Brain death guidelines. AANS Newsletter, Vol. 2, No. 1, March, 1976.
16. Brierley, J. B., Graham, D. I., Adams, J. H., and Simpsom, J. A.: Neocortical death after cardiac arrest. Lancet, *2*:560–565, 1971.
17. Brodersen, P., and Jorgensen, E. O.: Cerebral blood flow and oxygen uptake and cerebrospinal fluid biochemistry in severe coma. J. Neurol. Neurosurg. Psychiat., *37*:384–391, 1974.
18. Cal. Sup. Ct., Oakland, Cal., May 21, 1974. Cited in Baylor Law Review, *27*:15, 1975.
19. The Canadian Medical Association statement on death, Nov. 1968. Canad. Med. Ass. J., *99*:1266–1267, 1968.
20. Carroll, T. J., Cerebral death: Theological considerations. Unpublished manuscript, presented at meeting of the American Association of Neurological Surgeons, Cleveland, Ohio, April 15, 1969.
21. Cranford, R. E.: Brain death: Concept and criteria. Minn. Med., *61*:600–603, 1978.
22. A definition of irreversible coma: Report of the Ad Hoc Committee of the Harvard Medical School to examine the definition of brain death. J.A.M.A., *205*:337–340, 1968.
23. Denny-Brown, D., Swank, R. L., and Foley, J. M.: Respiratory and electrical signs in barbiturate intoxication. Trans. Amer. Neurol. Ass., *72*:77–82, 1947.
24. Diagnosis of brain death. Brit. Med. J., *2*:1187–1188, 1976.
25. Drory, Y., Quaknine, G., Kosary, I. Z., and Kellermann, I. J.: Electrocardiographic findings in brain death; description and presumed mechanism. Chest, *67*:425–432, 1975.
26. Ernsting, J.: The effect of brief profound hypoxia upon the arterial and venous oxygen tensions in man. J. Physiol. (London), *169*:292–311, 1963.
27. Foster, H. H., Jr.: Time of death. New York J. Med., *76*:2187–2197, 1976.
28. Frumin, M. J., Epstein, R. M., and Cohen, G.: Apneic oxygenation in man. Anesthesiology, *20*:789–798, 1959.
29. Gibbs, F. A., and Gibbs, E. L.: Atlas of Electroencephalography. Vol. I. Methodology and Controls. Cambridge, Addison-Wesley Press, Inc., 1950, pp. 82–96.
30. Goodman, J. M.; Mishikin, F. S., and Dyken, M.: Determination of brain death by isotope angiography. J.A.M.A., *209*:1869–1872, 1969.
31. Greitz, T., Gordon, E., Kolmodin, G., and Widen, L.: Aortocranial and carotid angiography in determination of brain death. Neuroradiology, *5*:13–19, 1973.
32. Haider, I., and Oswald, I.: Electroencephalographic investigation in acute drug poisoning. Electroenceph. Clin. Neurophysiol., *29*:105, 1970.
33. Haider, I., Matthew, H., and Oswald, I.: Electroencephalographic changes in acute drug poisoning. Electroenceph. Clin. Neurophysiol., *30*:23–31, 1971.
34. Hicks, R. G., and Torda, T. A.: The vestibulo-ocular (caloric) reflex in the diagnosis of cerebral death. Anesth. Intensive Care, *7*:169–173, 1979.
35. Hirsh, H. L.: Brain death. Med. Trial Techn. Quart., *21*:377–405, 1975.

36. Ingvar, D. H., and Brun, A.: Das komplette apallische Syndrom. Arch. Psychiat. Nervenkr., 215:219–239, 1972.

37. Jorgensen, E. O.: The EEG during severe barbiturate intoxication. Acta. Neurol. Scand., 46:suppl. 43: 281, 1970.

38. Jung, R.: Das Elektrencephalogramm. In eds.: von Bergmann, G., Frey, W., and Schweigk, H., Handbuch der Inneren Medizin, Vol. V/1, Berlin, J. Springer, 1953, pp. 1216–1325.

39. Kaufer, C.: Criteria of cerebral death. Minn. Med., 56:321–324, 1973.

40. Kaufer, C., and Penin, H.: Todeszeitbestimmung beim dissoziierten Hirntod. Dentsch. Med. Wschr., 93:679–686, 1968.

41. Kirshbaum, R. J., and Carollo, V. J.: Reversible isoelectric EEG in barbiturate coma. J.A.M.A., 212:1215, 1970.

42. Klee, A.: Akinetic mutism: Review of the literature and report of a case. J. Nerv. Ment. Dis., 133:536–553, 1961.

43. Korein, J.: On cerebral, brain, and systemic death. Stroke, 8:9–14, 1973.

44. Korein, J., and Maccario, M.: On the diagnosis of cerebral death: A prospective study on 55 patients to define irreversible coma. Clin. electroenceph., 2:178–199, 1971.

45. Korcin, J., Braunstein, P., Kricheff, I., Lieberman, A., and Chase, N.: Radioisotopic bolus technique as a test to detect circulatory deficit associated with cerebral death. Criculation, 51:924–939, 1975.

46. Mellerio, F.: EEG changes during acute intoxication with trichlorethylene. Electroenceph. Clin. Neurophysiol., 29:101, 1970.

47. Mellerio, F., Gaultier, M., Fournier, E., Gervais, P., and Frejaville, J. P.: Contribution of electroencephalography to resuscitation in toxicology. Clin. Toxicol., 6:271–285, 1973.

48. Meyer-Michkeleit, V. R. W.: Das Elektrencephalogramm nach gedeckten Kopfverletzungen. Deutsch. Med. Wschr., 78:480–485, 1953.

49. Milhaud, A., Riboulot, M., and Gayet, H.: Disconnecting tests and oxygen uptake in the diagnosis of total brain death. N.Y. Acad. Sci., 315:241–251, 1978.

50. Mitchell, O. C., de la Torre, E., Alexander, E., and Davis, C. H., Jr.: The nonfilling phenomenon during angiography in acute intracranial hypertension. J. Neurosurg., 19:766–774, 1962.

51. The Moment of Death. Medicoleg. J., 30:195–196, 1962.

52. Montgomery, T. M.: In Tebb, W., and Vollum, E. P.: Premature Burial and How It May be Prevented. 2nd Ed., Hadwen, W. R., ed. London, Swan Sonnenschein & Co., Lt., 1905, p. 81.

53. Myers, R. R., and Stockard, J. J.: Neurologic and electroencephalographic correlates in glutethimide intoxication. Clin. Pharmacol. Ther., 17:212–220, 1975.

54. News item. Kansas City Star. November 3, 1978, p. 1.

55. Pius PP. XII: Allocutio: Summus Pontifex coram praeclaris medicis, chirurgis atque studiosis, quaesitis respondit de catholica doctrina quoad anaesthesiam, a Societate Italica de anaesthesiologia propositis. Acta Apostolicae Sedia, 49:129–147, 1957.

56. Pribram, H. F. W.: Angiographic appearances in acute intracranial hypertension. Neurology (Minneap.), 11:10–21, 1961.

57. Quaknine, G. E.: Bedside procedures in the diagnosis of brain death. Resuscitation, 4:159–177, 1975.

58. Rådberg, C., and Söderlundh, S.: Computer tomography in cerebral death. Acta Radiol. Suppl. (Stockholm), 346:119–129, 1975.

59. Renal Transplanation from mortally injured man. Medicine and the Law. Lancet, 2:294–295, 1963.

60. Schafer, J. A., and Caronna, J. J.: Duration of apnea needed to confirm brain death. Neurology (Minneap.), 28:661–666, 1978.

61. Shalit, M. N., Beller, A. J., Feinsod, M., Drapkin, A. J., and Cotev, S.: The blood flow and oxygen consumption of the dying brain. Neurology (Minneap.), 20:740–748, 1970.

62. Silverman, D., Masland, R. L., Saunders, M. G., and Schwab, R. S.: Irreversible coma associated with electrocerebral silence. Neurology (Minneap.), 20:525–533, 1970.

63. Silverman, D., Saunders, M. G., Schwab, R. S., and Masland, R. L.: Cerebral death and the electroencephalogram. J.A.M.A., 209:1505–1510, 1969.

64. Starr, A.: Auditory brain stem responses in brain death. Brain, 99:543–554, 1976.

65. Sternberg, B., Lerique-Koechlin, A., and Mises, J.: Value of the EEG in acute intoxications in children. Electroenceph. Clin. Neurophysiol., 29:101–102, 1970.

66. Tebb, W., and Vollum, E. P.: Premature Burial and How It May be Prevented. 2nd Ed., Hadwen, W. R., ed. London, Swan Sonnenschein & Co., Ltd., 1905.

67. Thomas vs. Anderson, California District Court of Appeals (96 Cal. App. 2nd 371, 211P. 2d 478) 1950.

68. Torda, T. A.: Cerebral arterio-venous oxygen difference: A bedside test for cerebral death. Anaesth. Intensive Care, 4:148–150, 1976.

69. Uematsu, S., Smith, T. D., and Walker, A. E.: Pulsatile cerebral echo in diagnosis of brain death. J. Neurosurg., 48:866–875, 1978.

70. Visscr, S. L.: Nederlandse vereniging voor Elektroencefalografie en Klinische Neurofysiologie: Symposium on the significance of EEG for "Statement of Death." Electroenceph. Clin. Neurophysiol., 27:214–215, 1969.

71. Volavka, J., Zaks, A., Roubicek, J., and Fink, M.: Acute EEG effects of heroin and naloxone. Electroenceph. Clin. Neurophysiol., 30:165, 1971.

72. Walker, A. E.: Cerebral Death. Dallas, Texas, Professional Information Library, 1977.

73. Walker, A. E., Diamond, E. L., and Moseley, J.: The neuropathological findings in irreversible coma. J. Neuropath. Exp. Neurol., 34:295–323, 1975.

74. Wilder, A.: In Tebb, W., and Vollum, E. P., Premature Burial and How It May Be Prevented. 2nd Ed., Hadwen, W. R., ed. London, Swan Sonnenschein & Co., Ltd., 1905. p. 82.

75. Zsadanyi, O., and Molnar, C.: Electroencephalographic analysis of atropine coma. Acta Physiol. Acad. Sci. Hung., 41:63–72, 1972.

IV

PHYSIOLOGY, HOMEOSTASIS, AND GENERAL CARE

22

CEREBRAL METABOLISM

This chapter deals with those aspects of brain metabolism that are of interest to neurological surgeons. More comprehensive accounts of the subject are to be found in texts such as McIlwain and Bachelard's and the Lajtha *Handbook of Neurochemistry*.[64,76] A useful overview is given in *Basic Neurochemistry*, and the physiological aspects of brain metabolism are discussed in recent reviews and in a textbook on brain energy metabolism.[1,108,109,114]

GENERAL CONSIDERATIONS OF CEREBRAL METABOLISM

Although many features of the metabolism of the brain are similar to those of cellular metabolism throughout the body, neurochemistry has, for several reasons, evolved as a separate branch of biochemistry. First, because brain cells have unusually high energy requirements that can only be covered by oxidative metabolism of substrates, much study has been devoted to energy-yielding metabolic pathways and to the supply and utilization of oxygen. Second, the brain possesses specific carrier mechanisms for a variety of substances. Under ordinary circumstances only glucose can support normal oxidative metabolism. The only important exception to this occurs in conditions in which the blood concentrations of ketone bodies (β-hydroxybutyrate and acetoacetate) are increased—primarily starvation and diabetes—in which ketone bodies can supply up to about 50 per cent of the substrate for cerebral oxidation. In vitro, however, brain cells can oxidize a variety of other substrates, including amino acids. The exclusive dependence of the brain on glucose or ketone bodies in vivo is due to the fact that only these substrates attain sufficiently high blood concentrations and are transported from blood to tissue at sufficient velocity. Relatively specific carrier mechanisms exist for a variety of substances that need to be transported between blood and tissue, with the virtual exclusion of others, and their presence is one important feature of cerebral metabolism.[101] Third, since brain cells have a high metabolic rate and constantly require a plentiful supply of oxygen and substrate, cellular hypoxia or hypoglycemia readily induces brain dysfunction. Furthermore, if energy production is curtailed, irreversible cell damage occurs within a relatively short time, and since neurons have a poor capacity for regeneration, the functional consequences are often devastating. Fourth, adequate production of energy is only a very first requirement for normal brain function. Communication between cells also requires the normal synthesis, release, inactivation, and packing of appropriate transmitter compounds. Undoubtedly, transmitter metabolism constitutes one of the most important aspects of brain metabolism. As is discussed later, deficient metabolism of transmitter compounds may be responsible for some of the symptoms observed when the supply of oxygen or substrate becomes insufficient.

From the metabolic standpoint, brain cells are not homogeneous. For example, their sensitivity to hypoxia varies widely. Neurons are the most sensitive, next are oligodendroglia, then astroglia, and finally microglia, which are the least sensitive. Presumably, this difference in sensitivity reflects the fact that neurons are much more active metabolically than glial cells.[45] There are reasons to believe, however, that

---

C. H. NORDSTRÖM and B. K. SIESJÖ

there are also differences in metabolic activity within the neuronal population. Thus, even though some adverse conditions like hypoxia and hypoglycemia may affect all cells, some cells show the phenomenon of "selective vulnerability."[107]

ENERGY PRODUCTION WITHIN THE BRAIN

All cellular work occurs, directly or indirectly, at the expense of energy contained in the adenosine triphosphate (ATP) molecule. When work is done, ATP is degraded to either adenosine diphosphate (ADP) and orthophosphate (P_i) or to adenosine monophosphate (AMP) and pyrophosphate (PP_i).

$$ATP + HOH \longrightarrow ADP + P_i \qquad (1)$$
$$ATP + 2HOH \longrightarrow AMP + PP_i \qquad (2)$$

ATP, ADP, and AMP constitute a pool of adenine nucleotides, the members of which are interrelated via a third reaction, that catalyzed by adenylate kinase (myokinase)

$$ATP + AMP \rightleftharpoons ADP + ADP \qquad (3)$$

Energy production occurs by the reversal of reaction 1, i.e., by rephosphorylation of ADP to ATP. This reversal is achieved in reactions leading to breakdown of substrates. Extensive measurements of cerebral blood flow and arteriovenous differences for oxygen, carbon dioxide, glucose, and other substrates have provided important information on cerebral metabolism. The data in Table 22–1 were obtained in fed subjects by using modern enzymatic techniques for measuring substrate concentrations. As the results show, cerebral blood flow is about 0.5 ml per gram per minute, the rate of cerebral oxygen metabolism ($CMRo_2$) is about 1.5 μmol per gram per minute (about 3 ml/100 gm per minute), that of carbon dioxide metabolism ($CMRco_2$) is similar (i.e., the respiratory quotient is close to unity), that of glucose (CMRgl) is

TABLE 22–1 CEREBRAL BLOOD FLOW, ARTERIOVENOUS DIFFERENCES, AND METABOLIC RATES FOR OXYGEN, GLUCOSE, AND LACTATE IN MAN

	GOTTSTEIN ET AL.* (n = 59)	COHEN ET AL.† (n = 9)
Cerebral blood flow (ml/gm/min)	0.55 ± 0.01	0.45 ± 0.02
Arteriovenous difference (μmol/ml)		
Oxygen	2.99 ± 0.09	3.02
Glucose	0.55 ± 0.02	0.55
Lactate	−0.09 ± 0.01	−0.05
Cerebral metabolic rate (μmol/gm/min)		
Oxygen	1.64 ± 0.04	1.35 ± 0.07
Glucose	0.29 ± 0.01	0.25 ± 0.02
Lactate/glucose index	8	5

* Data from Gottstein, U., Bernsmeier, A., und Sedlmeyer, I.: Der Kohlenhydratstoffwechsel des menschlichen Gehirn. I. Untersuchungen mit substratspezifischen enzymatischen Methoden bei normaler Hirndurchblutung. Klin. Wschr., 41:943–948, 1963.

† Data from Cohen, P. J., Alexander, S. C., Smith, F. C., Reivich, M., and Wollman, H.: Effects of hypoxia and normocarbia on cerebral blood flow and metabolism in conscious man. J. Appl. Physiol., 23:183–189, 1967.

0.25 to 0.27 μmol per gram per minute, and very little lactate or pyruvate is produced. Using the percentage expressions of Cohen and associates, one can interpret the data to show that about 95 per cent of the glucose extracted is oxidized to carbon dioxide and water, the remainder appearing as lactate in the venous effluent ("anaerobic" glycolysis).[17] Results obtained in animals allow the same conclusions, but since venous blood can be sampled from the superior sagittal sinus, animal experiments may give information on cerebral *cortical* metabolic rate. Since the neuron packing density varies inversely with brain size, the rate of cerebral oxygen metabolism is appreciably higher in small animals such as rats.[122] In this species, it has been found that the rate of oxygen metabolism in whole brain is about 75 per cent of that in cerebral cortex.[88]

Figure 22–1 illustrates ATP production from glucose metabolism via anaerobic and

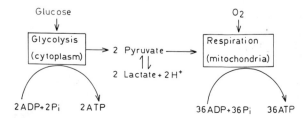

Figure 22–1 Diagram illustrating energy yield of glycolysis and respiration respectively. Under normal circumstances, the contribution of glycolysis to cerebral energy production is negligible. In complete ischemia, no energy can be obtained from respiration, since the oxygen stores are virtually nil, and energy production is then limited to glycolysis, which provides 2 μmol of adenosine triphosphate per micromole of glucose available.

aerobic pathways. The anaerobic metabolism of glucose to two molecules of lactic acid, a series of reactions occurring in the cytoplasm of cells, has a yield of two molecules of ATP (if the substrate of glycolysis is preformed glycogen, three molecules of ATP is formed). When pyruvate is oxidized to carbon dioxide and water by mitochondrial enzymes, another 36 molecules of ATP is formed. The overwhelming part of energy production thus occurs by oxidative reactions. It may be asked whether stimulation of anaerobic glycolysis can substitute for oxygen when that element's supply is short. Results indicate that any effect is marginal, since even if the glycolytic rate is maximally increased to about fivefold, anaerobic production of ATP covers less than 50 per cent of the normal requirements.[73]

As already mentioned, ketone bodies can partially substitute for glucose as substrate for brain metabolism. Owen and co-workers found that in prolonged starvation there was a significant cerebral uptake of β-hydroxybutyrate and acetoacetate.[100] Since part of the glucose extracted was converted to lactate and pyruvate, it could be calculated that ketone bodies accounted for about 50 per cent of the substrate for cerebral oxidation. Animal studies have confirmed these results and have shown that enzyme induction is not a prerequisite.[43,103] Rather, ketone bodies are extracted and oxidized whenever their concentrations in the blood are increased. Transport of ketone bodies between blood and tissue is mediated by a carrier mechanism that achieves translocation of several organic acids, including lactate.[101] Like other carrier mechanisms of similar type (e.g., that transporting glucose and other hexoses) this carrier is passive in the sense that no energy other than that contained in the concentration gradient is required. As a corollary, we may conclude that there is a small loss of lactate from the normal brain only because there is a suitable concentration gradient between tissue and blood. If this gradient is reversed, e.g., by lactate infusion, lactate may be taken up and metabolized by the brain.[87]

ENERGY UTILIZATION WITHIN THE BRAIN

There is no doubt that an appreciable part of the energy produced in the brain is consumed in reactions leading to the coupled extrusion of sodium ion and accumulation of potassium ion. There is evidence that the sodium- and potassium-dependent adenosinetriphosphatase of cell membranes translocates three sodium and two potassium ions for each ATP molecule used:

$$ATP + 3[Na^+]_i + 2[K^+]_e \longrightarrow$$
$$ADP + P_i + 3[Na^+]_e + 2[K^+]_i \quad (4)$$

in which the subscripts i and e stand for intracellular and extracellular, respectively. Thus, utilization of ATP is direct and of the type described by equation 1. The reaction provides one direct link between functional activity and metabolic rate. When cells are

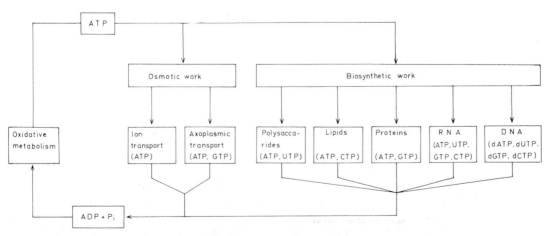

Figure 22–2 Schematic diagram illustrating balance between production and utilization of adenosine triphosphate (ATP). The diagram indicates the nucleotides used in the performance of various types of "osmotic" and biosynthetic work. (From Siesjö, B. K.: Brain Energy Metabolism. London, John Wiley & Sons, 1978. Reprinted by permission.)

active they lose potassium and accumulate sodium ions, changes that automatically trigger increased ATPase activity and lead to ATP hydrolysis. The consequences of this hydrolysis (i.e., decrease in ATP, increases in ADP and P_i concentrations) seem to provide the signal for increased oxidative generation of new ATP.

Although it has been estimated that active transport of ions may account for about 50 per cent of the energy consumed in brain, the actual figures are not even approximately known. Presumably, many cellular constituents have a fast turnover, requiring continuous resynthesis of proteins, phospholipids, and other molecules. Some of these synthetic reactions utilize ATP directly in a manner illustrated by equation 1, others lead to pyrophosphate cleavage as shown by equation 2. A large number of synthetic reactions utilize nucleoside triphosphates other than ATP (e.g., guanosine, cytidine, uridine, and inosine triphosphates [GTP, CTP, UTP, and ITP]). Since these systems are recharged by ATP, the reactions are indirectly driven by ATP energy. (A lucid account of energy-requiring reactions is given by Lehninger.)[65] It should be appreciated that replenishment of cellular constituents may involve transport work. Thus, if molecules or molecular aggregates are synthesized in the cell body but needed in the periphery, it takes energy to achieve translocation over the distances involved ("axoplasmic transport").[54] Current knowledge suggests that ATP and perhaps also GTP are involved.[98]

Reactions leading to energy utilization have been summarized in Figure 22–2, which emphasizes that the various tasks of the cells are associated with utilization of a large number of nucleoside triphosphates but that the whole mechanism is driven by ATP generated in oxidative metabolism.

BALANCE BETWEEN PRODUCTION AND UTILIZATION OF ENERGY

The balance between production and utilization of energy is achieved by metabolic coupling devices of extraordinary efficiency and, when demands are increased or supply of oxygen is curtailed, also by circulatory adjustments. Two major questions arise. First, which are the main cellular mechanisms that retard depletion of ATP whenever its rate of generation becomes limiting, and how can one assess energy failure at cellular level? Second, how tight is the coupling between utilization and production of energy when functional activity is either depressed or enhanced?

Mechanisms Retarding ATP Depletion

Figure 22–3 recapitulates the main reactions leading to utilization and production of ATP and illustrates three reactions that retard its depletion whenever the supply falls below the rate of production. One of these reactions, that catalyzed by creatine kinase, forms ATP at the expense of its storage form, phosphocreatine (PCr). This reaction, like that catalyzed by adenylate kinase, retards both the decrease in ATP and the increase in ADP concentration. The third reaction illustrates the overall result of the various reactions that lead to anaerobic production of lactic acid at the expense of glucose (or glycogen).

The reactions of Figure 22–3 indicate that a precipitous fall in ATP concentration should not occur until the store of phosphocreatine is depleted, and that sensitive indicators of marginal degrees of energy failure may be provided by the decrease in phosphocreatine and the rises in adenosine monophosphate and lactate concentrations. Simultaneously with the increase in lactate concentration there is a rise in the lactate to pyruvate ratio, and this ratio is commonly believed to reflect cellular oxygenation. Given these reactions, one can now inquire into the possibilities of defining an imbalance between production and utilization of energy, or of quantitating its degree. Two facts have been established. First, since both the creatine kinase and the lactate dehydrogenase reactions are pH-dependent, the phosphocreatine concentration may fall and the lactate to pyruvate ratio may rise if cell pH is reduced, even though energy failure is not involved.[111] For this reason, these parameters should be used with some caution. Second, when the level of adenosine monophosphate rises part of it is deaminated to inosine monophosphate and dephosphorylated to adenosine, and the further degradation products include inosine

Energy utilization :

$$ATP + HOH \longrightarrow ADP + P_i + energy$$

Energy production :

$$ADP + P_i + energy \longrightarrow ATP + HOH$$

Emergency reactions, delaying depletion of ATP :

$$PCr + ADP + H^+ \rightleftharpoons Cr + ATP$$

$$ADP + ADP \rightleftharpoons ATP + AMP$$

$$Glucose \longrightarrow 2 \text{ lactate} + 2H^+$$

Energy charge of adenine nucleotide pool :

$$E.C. = \frac{[AT\overline{P}] + 0.5 [AD\overline{P}]}{[AT\overline{P}] + [AD\overline{P}] + [AM\overline{P}]}$$

Figure 22–3 Schematic illustration of the main reactions leading to utilization and production of adenosine triphosphate.

and hypoxanthine.[26,61] Some of these products are diffusible and may be lost to the general circulation. As a consequence, although restoration of oxygen supply leads to rephosphorylation of ADP to ATP, the ATP concentration does not rise to normal values, since the size of the adenine nucleotide pool is reduced (restoration of the pool requires de novo synthesis and is slow). Obviously, if ATP concentration is low in, for example, a postischemic situation, this is not necessarily a sign of mitochondrial failure. One alternative is to use the ATP to ADP ratio. Many, however, prefer to use the adenylate energy charge as a convenient measure of the balance between production and utilization of energy.[6] This expression, which gives the charge of the "energy battery," is not influenced by pH; it takes changes in AMP concentration into account, and it should be a valid measure of energy balance even if the size of the adenine nucleotide pool is reduced.

Relationship Between Rate of Metabolism and Energy Charge

It is well known that the metabolic rate of the brain, e.g., its oxygen consumption, is extraordinarily constant even when there are overt signs of changes in mental activity or behavior such as those occurring during sleep, wakefulness, or performance of mental arithmetic. It is also known, however, that the rate of cerebral oxygen metabolism is depressed in coma, anesthesia, and hy-

pothermia, and increased in hyperthermia and during epileptic seizures.[118] Quantitative relationships have been worked out in some detail in rats. Figure 22–4 shows that when body temperature is reduced by 5°, 10°, or 15°C, cerebral oxygen metabolism is reduced by 25, 50, and 75 per cent, respectively. The depression of oxygen metabolism with a 10°C decrease in body temperature (to about 50 per cent of control value) is similar to that observed during deep anesthesia, e.g., due to barbiturates. In general, the reduction in metabolic rate due to anesthetics is grossly proportional to the degree of reduction in consciousness, but there are important exceptions.[42,116] An increased rate of oxygen metabolism is observed in hyperthermia (roughly, an increase of about 5 per cent for each degree of rise in temperature), during epileptic seizures, and in immobilization stress. The latter finding is in line with the results of some previous investigations in man, which show that infusion of adrenaline leads to a feeling of anxiety and to increases in cerebral oxygen metabolism and blood flow.

The coupling between energy demands and energy production is tight (Fig. 22–5).

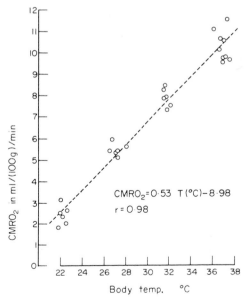

Figure 22–4 Regression line showing temperature dependence of the rate of cerebral oxygen metabolism (CMR_{O_2}) in rat brain. (From Hägerdal, M., Harp, J., Nilsson, L., and Siesjö, B. K.: The effect of induced hypothermia upon oxygen consumption in the rat brain. J. Neurochem., 24:311–316, 1975. Reprinted by permission.)

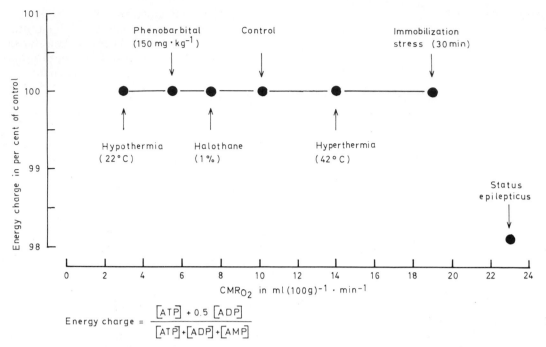

$$\text{Energy charge} = \frac{[ATP] + 0.5\,[ADP]}{[ATP] + [ADP] + [AMP]}$$

Figure 22–5 Relationship between adenylate energy charge and cerebral metabolic rate for oxygen (CMR_{O_2}) of rat cerebral cortex in different conditions. Control animals were anesthetized with nitrous oxide (70 per cent). (From Siesjö, B. K., Carlsson, C., Hägerdal, M., and Nordström, C.-H.: Brain metabolism in the critically ill. Crit. Care Med., *4*:283–294, 1976. Reprinted by permission.)

In fact, the rate of cerebral oxygen metabolism may vary almost tenfold without detectable change in energy charge, and it is only during epileptic seizures, with their tremendously increased energy demands, that the energy charge diminishes (but only by about 2 per cent). It follows from this that as long as the supply of oxygen and substrate is sufficient, the energy-producing pathways adjust to the functional demands. As a corollary, the conclusion must be drawn that it is not possible to improve the energy state of the normal brain by pharmacological means or by changing body temperature. The situation is different when pathological conditions impede normal energy production.

METABOLISM OF TRANSMITTER COMPOUNDS

Established or putative neurotransmitters that achieve communication between neurons within the brain include acetylcholine and the biogenic amines dopamine, noradrenaline, and serotonin, as well as the amino acids gamma-aminobutyric acid, glutamate, and aspartate.[21,63] The pharmacology and biochemistry of these transmitters have been lucidly described in a number of reviews.[20,44,53]

One aspect of the metabolism of neurotransmitters, viz. its relationship to oxygen and substrate supply, could help to explain why neuronal function fails even at relatively mild degrees of energy failure. Acetylcholine, released as a result of synaptic activity in cholinergic neurons, is degraded by acetylcholinesterase to acetate and choline. Resynthesis requires reuptake of choline (or transport from blood to tissue) and a metabolic source of acetate.[101] Although the actual acetate-yielding reaction is not known there is evidence that oxidation of pyruvate by the pyruvate dehydrogenase complex is essential. Thus, conditions that reduce the delivery of pyruvate (hypoglycemia) or its rate of oxidation (hypoxia) lead to a reduced rate of acetylcholine synthesis.[35] Possibly, such reduction may explain at least part of the functional changes observed at moderate degrees of hypoglycemia and hypoxia.

The synthesis of the catecholamines dopamine and noradrenaline, and of the indole amine serotonin, occurs from the amino acids tyrosine and tryptophan in oxygen-requiring reactions. The oxidative reaction involved in catecholamine synthesis, that catalyzed by tyrosine hydroxylase, seems to be the rate-limiting one. The corresponding reaction leading to serotonin synthesis (catalyzed by tryptophan hydroxylase) is not rate-limiting to the same extent, since serotonin synthesis varies with the availability of tryptophan.[128] Since both reactions are influenced by changes in tissue Po_2 around the normal level, however, it seems possible that functional changes occur at moderate degrees of hypoxia (or in hyperoxia) partly because of an influence on the metabolism of biogenic amines.[22]

The metabolism of the amino acids gamma-aminobutyric acid (GABA), glutamate, and aspartate is intimately connected with catabolism of carbohydrates and with ammonia metabolism.[8,102,124] As is discussed later, changes in the tissue concentrations of these amino acids occur in hypoglycemia, hypoxia, and ischemia. These changes take place because endogenous amino acids become important as substrates in hypoglycemia, certain changes in carbohydrate metabolism (notably variations in pyruvate concentration or redox changes or both) induce transamination reactions, and tissue hypoxia influences GABA metabolism. This last influence comes into play because hypoxia interferes with the further metabolism of GABA but does not block its formation via the glutamate dehydrogenase reaction. As a consequence GABA, which is an inhibitory transmitter, accumulates in hypoxia and ischemia. It is of interest that changes in the metabolism of this and other amino acids may persist for relatively long periods after the reoxygenation of tissue following, e.g., ischemia. Conceivably, such changes could contribute to delay in resumption of normal brain function.

HYPOGLYCEMIA

Pronounced hypoglycemia is accompanied by cerebral symptoms ranging from drowsiness and somnolence to convulsions, stupor, and coma. When sufficiently prolonged, hypoglycemic coma leads to irreversible cell damage. The histopathological lesions observed in pronounced hypoglycemia are similar to those occurring in hypoxia and ischemia.[11] It should be noted that ischemia often involves a combination of oxygen and substrate depletion.

The first quantitative measurements of cerebral blood flow and the cerebral metabolic rates for glucose and oxygen during hypoglycemia were reported by Kety and co-workers.[59] These results established that hypoglycemia was accompanied by a reduction in the glucose metabolism rate while cerebral blood flow was at or above control level. Although the results suggested a decrease in the oxygen metabolism rate as well, several subsequent studies have revealed that there is little if any such reduction even when blood glucose concentration is reduced to coma levels.[24] Recently, cortical blood flow and oxygen and glucose utilization rates were measured in lightly anesthetized rats rendered hypoglycemic with insulin.[92] Again, it was found that cerebral blood flow increased when spontaneous electrical activity had ceased (coma) and that there was a pronounced reduction in the rate of glucose metabolism with little if any reduction in that of oxygen metabolism. The results strongly indicate that oxidation of noncarbohydrate substrates must have occurred.

Measurements of cerebral energy metabolites in hypoglycemia indicate that there are no detectable changes in levels of high-energy phosphates in animals with electroencephalographic recordings dominated by slow waves or convulsive polyspike activity.[29,46,68] Possibly, part of the functional aberration is due to changes in metabolism of transmitters such as acetylcholine and amino acids. During long-lasting convulsive activity (20 to 60 minutes), however, clear signs of energy failure develop, and in all animals with an isoelectric electroencephalogram there is pronounced derangement of the cerebral energy state (Table 22–2). Since energy failure develops although oxygen metabolism is close to normal, the results indicate that either the energy demands are higher than normal or the utilization of oxygen is not associated with a corresponding production of ATP (uncoupling of oxidative phosphorylation?).

Available information on changes in glycolytic metabolites, citric acid cycle intermediates, associated amino acids, and am-

TABLE 22–2 CORRELATION OF ELECTROENCEPHALOGRAM AND CONCENTRATIONS OF PHOSPHOCREATINE AND ADENINE NUCLEOTIDES*

ELECTRO-ENCEPHALOGRAM	PHOSPHO-CREATINE	ATP	ADP	AMP
Normal	4.84	3.04	0.299	0.038
	±0.11	±0.02	±0.003	±0.001
Slow waves–polyspikes	4.60	3.04	0.300	0.035
	±0.14	±0.03	±0.008	±0.001
Isoelectric	0.70†	1.13†	0.878†	0.498†
	±0.08	±0.03	±0.022	±0.024
† p < 0.001.				

* The concentrations were determined in animals showing normal, slow wave–polyspike, and isoelectric electroencephalograms; are given in micromoles per gram; and represent means ± S.E.M. †p < 0.001. (Data from Norberg, K., and Siesjö, B. K.: Oxidative metabolism of the cerebral cortex of the rat in severe insulin-induced hypoglycemia. J. Neurochem., 26:345–352, 1976.)

monia indicates that during hypoglycemia endogenous carbohydrate compounds and amino acids are used as substrates. After 5 to 15 minutes of hypoglycemic "coma," the tissue was depleted of glycogen, glucose, and many carbohydrate intermediates.[92] Furthermore, the brain had lost about 10 μmol per gram of glutamate and 4 μmol per gram of glutamine, and had accumulated about 10 μmol per gram of aspartate, and there was a decrease in the pool of available amino acids by about 4 μmol per gram. It is clear that such perturbations of amino acid levels and the associated rise in ammonia concentration should profoundly affect cell function.

The same study has demonstrated that discrepancies in reduction of the cerebral metabolic rates for glucose and oxygen remain when endogenous carbohydrate stores have been depleted and that little further change in amino acid levels occurs.[92] Other results demonstrate that profound hypoglycemia is accompanied by extensive breakdown of phospholipids, indicating that the tissue resorts to its own structural lipids to maintain oxidative metabolism.[47] Probably, when this point is reached irreversible damage occurs to intracellular structures such as mitochondria and endoplasmic reticulum.

HYPOXIA

At tissue level, hypoxia can be defined as a reduction in available oxygen to levels insufficient for maintenance of function, metabolism, or structure. The oxygen availability, i.e., the amount of oxygen that is carried to the tissue at any given moment, may be expressed as

oxygen availability =
$$CBF \times Sa_{O_2} \times [Hb] \times 1.39 \quad (5)$$

where Sa_{O_2} is the percentage saturation of hemoglobin, [Hb] is the hemoglobin concentration, and 1.39 is the amount of oxygen (in milliliters) bound to 1 gm of hemoglobin at full saturation. The term "arterial hypoxia" can be used to describe a reduction in available oxygen in the tissue due to a decrease in either oxygen tension (hypoxic hypoxia) or hemoglobin concentration (anemic hypoxia). Uncomplicated arterial hypoxia is invariably associated with an increase in cerebral blood flow, which serves as an important homeostatic mechanism, allowing the tissue to sustain relatively pronounced hypoxia without energy failure. The third main cause of a reduction in oxygen delivery is a decrease in cerebral blood flow, conventionally called ischemia.

The functional effects of hypoxic hypoxia, as observed in man, are summarized in Figure 22–6. Most of the results were obtained in simulated high-altitude experiments. In order to facilitate comparisons with animal experiments, the figure also shows the inspired oxygen concentrations that would give comparable degrees of hypoxia. It is observed that even relatively moderate hypoxia leads to symptoms of oxygen lack, although arterial oxygen tension must be appreciably reduced to induce unconsciousness. It should be emphasized that arterial hypocapnia, which develops at Pa_{O_2} values of below about 60 mm of mercury, exaggerates tissue hypoxia by reducing cerebral blood flow.[34,99] Nevertheless, the results emphasize the extreme sensitiv-

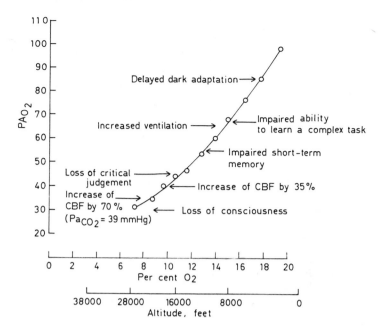

Figure 22-6 Influence of inspired oxygen concentration on alveolar oxygen tension (PA_{O_2}) in man as well as on some symptoms of and physiological responses to hypoxia. The inspired oxygen concentrations given are those equivalent to the altitudes indicated at the bottom. (From Siesjö, B. K., Jóhansson, H., Ljunggren, B., and Norberg, K.: Brain dysfunction in cerebral hypoxia and ischemia. *In* Plum, F., ed.: Brain Dysfunction in Metabolic Disorders. New York, Raven Press, 1974, pp. 75–112. Reprinted by permission.)

ity of the brain to reduced oxygen availability, and they raise the question whether the signs and symptoms of mild hypoxia are caused by energy failure at cellular level. Animal experiments indicate that this is not so. Thus, although there is a progressive lactic acidosis in the tissue at Pa_{O_2} values of below about 50 mm of mercury, indicating that oxygenation is insufficient to maintain normal metabolism, arterial Po_2 may be reduced to 20 to 25 mm of mercury with no significant changes in adenylate energy charge.* Typical results are shown in Figure 22–7. Changes affecting carbohydrate metabolites and amino acids have been discussed comprehensively in three recent communications.[27,90,91]

Obviously, there are symptoms of cerebral oxygen lack at Pa_{O_2} values that do not disrupt the balance between production and utilization of energy. There are two possi-

_____

* See references 7, 27, 40, 74, 110.

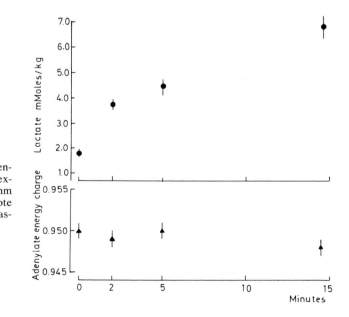

Figure 22–7 Brain tissue lactate concentration and adenylate energy charge in rats exposed to arterial hypoxia (Po_2 = 23 to 24 mm of mercury for 2, 5, and 15 minutes). Note constancy of energy charge in spite of increasing lactate concentration.

ble explanations. First, moderate hypoxia may cause energy failure in a few neurons of key importance for integrated brain function. Alternatively, systems responsible for communication between cells are affected at higher Po_2 values than those responsible for ATP production. It is clear that whole-tissue analyses cannot exclude failure of energy production in a small number of cells. Histopathological studies have, however, failed to reveal damage to cells in animals whose alveolar oxygen tension has been reduced to 20 to 22 mm of mercury for 30 minutes, suggesting that regional anoxia does not occur.[105] There is thus the possibility that hypoxia leads to "transmission failure" by interfering with the metabolism of transmitter compounds.

It is of obvious importance to define those mechanisms that are responsible for energy homeostasis in hypoxia. Although it has been suggested that cellular hypoxia leads to a compensatory decrease in energy utilization, studies in man and experimental animals have failed to show that the rate of cerebal oxygen metabolism is reduced in hypoxia.[17,27,55,57] It therefore seems probable that the main (or sole) compensatory mechanism is the increase in blood flow. This is of considerable clinical interest. Since autoregulation is lost in severe hypoxia, blood flow will vary passively with perfusion pressure. Accordingly, if perfusion pressure is reduced because of hypotension, intracranial pressure, or vascular obstruction, there may be a relative reduction in cerebral blood flow with cellular energy failure.[106,110] If this occurs, irreversible cell damage may develop.[67,105] In this context, it should be emphasized that the brain tolerates even drastic anemic hypoxia under normovolemic conditions. Presumably, this tolerance is due to favorable hemodynamic conditions created by the reduced viscosity.[10,56]

It follows from what has been said that, although relatively severe hypoxia may be tolerated by the brain under optimal conditions, a variety of complicating factors can critically affect tissue oxygenation. Although most of these reduce the effective perfusion pressure, it seems probable that even relatively minor disturbances of the microcirculation (e.g., decreased reactivity due to arteriosclerosis, or trauma from craniotomy and brain retraction) could give the same result. Experimental results suggest that whenever arterial Po_2 cannot be promptly brought to a normal level, tissue oxygenation may be improved by three measures. First, since cerebral blood flow varies with the perfusion pressure, it is essential to counteract hypotension or increased intracranial pressure. Second, since oxygen availability is determined by the arterial oxygen *content*, tissue oxygenation will be improved by measures that increase oxygen content at constant Po_2. In practice, this can be achieved by displacing the oxyhemoglobin dissociation curve to the left by correcting plasma acidosis or by inducing alkalosis. Third, if oxygen availability cannot be further improved, it may be essential to reduce cellular energy requirements. As is discussed later, barbiturate anesthesia protects the brain under conditions of ischemia. Unfortunately, under conditions of arterial hypoxia, barbiturates affect the cardiovascular system and reduce blood pressure. For these reasons, it may be necessary to reduce body temperature. Animal experiments have shown that induced hypothermia dramatically increases cerebral resistance to hypoxic hypoxia.[16] Presumably, the effect is due both to a shift to the left of the oxyhemoglobin dissociation curve and to reduction of cellular oxygen requirements.

ISCHEMIA

Cerebral ischemia, which can be defined as a reduction in cerebral blood flow to levels that are insufficient to maintain normal brain function or metabolism, is one of the most important pathological conditions encountered in neurological surgery. Since the blood flow is determined by the cerebral perfusion pressure (CPP) and by the vascular resistance (CVR), ischemia may theoretically result from either a decrease in perfusion pressure or an increase in resistance. In practice, the cause is usually a reduced perfusion pressure resulting from a fall in arterial pressure, a rise in intracranial pressure, or obstruction of vessels. Exceptions to this rule are conditions in which small resistance vessels or larger arteries are constricted because of, e.g., excessive hyperventilation or spasm. Presumably, increased tissue pressure due to edema or compression by tumor or bleeding obstructs both capillaries and drainage veins. Since cerebral perfusion pressure is usually defined as the difference between arterial and cerebral venous pressures, such conditions cause ischemia both by increasing vascular resistance and by reducing effective perfusion pressure.

In the normal brain, autoregulation secures an unchanged blood flow even if perfusion pressure falls, and ischemia does not occur until the lower limit of the autoregulation range has been reached (see Chapter 23). Although perfusion pressures of 60 to 70 mm of mercury are usually considered adequate for maintaining cerebral blood flow around normal levels, there is no unique pressure below which ischemia occurs.[119] First, at least under certain conditions (e.g., hyperventilation), cerebral blood flow can decrease to about 50 per cent of normal without affecting energy balance to such an extent that irreversible injury results. Second, at any given reduction in blood flow, the metabolic consequences are influenced by the energy demands. For example, deep anesthesia due to barbiturates, or a fall in body temperature of 10°C, reduces energy flow to half normal, with a resulting increase in resistance to ischemia. Third, the tolerance of the brain to a reduction in perfusion pressure is less in patients with hypertension or cerebrovascular disease. Whereas normotensive subjects show signs of cerebrovascular insufficiency when mean blood pressure is reduced to below 35 mm of mercury, such signs may appear at pressures of about 90 mm of mercury in subjects with malignant hypertension.[30] There are also other observations to show that hypertensive patients may show signs of brain ischemia when blood pressure is reduced to normotensive levels.[58] Fourth, there is evidence that perfusion pressure may fall to lower limits without affecting blood flow (or the rate of oxygen metabolism) if the reduction in pressure is due to increased cerebrospinal fluid pressure than if it is caused by arterial hypotension.[39,79]

In the following discussion of cerebral metabolic changes in ischemia, a distinction is made between incomplete and complete ischemia. The last section is devoted to mechanisms of cellular damage and possible measures to ameliorate such damage.

Incomplete Ischemia

Observations in man demonstrate that symptoms of cerebrovascular insufficiency develop at reductions in cerebral perfusion pressure that are not associated with a significant decrease in the metabolic rate for oxygen (cf. sequence of changes in hypoxic hypoxia).[30,58] At even lower pressures, the rate of oxygen metabolism must fall, but available methods do not allow quantification of changes in this rate and in cerebral blood flow, in part because cerebral metabolic changes in ischemia are not homogeneously distributed within the brain.

Analyses of tissue metabolites in rats demonstrate that signs of energy failure in terms of changes in ATP, ADP, and AMP concentrations do not develop until cerebral perfusion pressure falls to 30 to 40 mm of mercury.[111,112] Typical results are shown in Figure 22–8. Histopathological results indicate that when perfusion pressure is reduced below 25 mm of mercury by means of induced hypotension, lesions are preferentially localized to watershed areas, i.e., to areas between the distribution territories of the major cerebral arteries.[13] Subsequent biochemical results have also shown that when parts of cortical tissue that include such a watershed area are taken for analyses, moderate reductions of the adenylate energy charge are observed at perfusion pressures as low as 40 to 50 mm of mercury.[114] Subsequent experiments have elegantly demonstrated the inhomogeneous nature of the metabolic changes.[125] It should be emphasized that such inhomogeneity typically results when ischemia is due to arterial hypotension. When perfusion pressure is reduced owing to increased cerebrospinal fluid pressure, changes in regional cerebral blood flow appear more homogeneous, as would be expected when outflow pressure is elevated.[75]

The cerebral metabolic response in ischemia is qualitatively similar to that observed in hypoxia, since it involves reductions in tissue concentrations of phosphocreatine and adenosine triphosphate and increases in those of adenosine monophosphate and lactate.[97] As usual, changes in lactate content are associated with an increased lactate to pyruvate ratio. Although part of this increase reflects a pH dependence of the lactate dehydrogenase reaction, there is

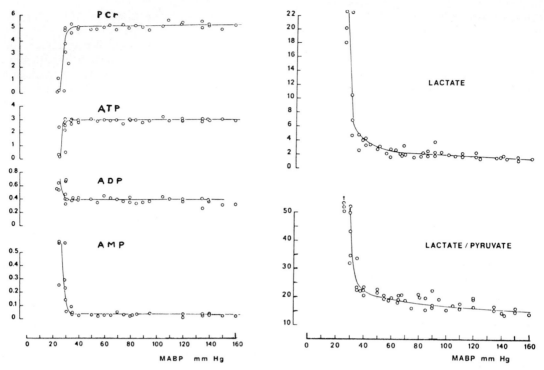

Figure 22–8   The relation between the mean arterial blood pressure (MABP mm Hg) after 20 minutes of hypo-volemic hypotension, and the brain tissue concentrations of ATP, ADP, AMP and lactate (in micromoles per gram) and the lactate to pyruvate ratio. (Data from Siesjö, B. K., and Zwetnow, N. N.: The effect of hypovolemic hypo-tension on extra- and intracellular acid-base parameters and energy metabolites in the rat brain. Acta Physiol. Scand., 79:114–124, 1970.)

also a reduction of oxidation-reduction systems, e.g., the NADH/NAD$^+$ system.[125] As in hypoxia, the continuous supply of glucose via the reduced circulation leads to a progressive lactic acidosis that may become excessive.[28,97] As a result, cell pH may fall from normal values of about 7.05 to below 6.0. When cerebral blood flow is greatly reduced, however, glucose utilization outstrips supply, and glycolytic metabolites become depleted.

The relationship between cerebral blood flow and metabolic state has been studied with models of regional ischemia, using either middle cerebral artery (MCA) ligation in cats or monkeys or ligation of one carotid artery in the gerbil, an animal that lacks a complete circle of Willis owing to absence of posterior communicating arteries.* In general, metabolic results are similar to those obtained with generalized incomplete ischemia. Studies of middle cerebral artery ligation demonstrate that collateral flow

maintains cerebral blood flow at 20 to 50 per cent of normal within the area. Accordingly, there is a gradual change in energy metabolism over hours, and restoration of flow within two to three hours may prevent the development of a permanent lesion.

Recently, results have been published that have a bearing on ischemic thresholds at which functional and metabolic changes occur. Following middle cerebral artery occlusion in the monkey, changes in evoked cortical responses appear at much higher blood flow values, about 35 per cent of control, than are associated with signs of generalized depolarization due to potassium ion massive release.[5] Results in rats in which the metabolic rate was artificially elevated by inducing status epilepticus give comparably separated thresholds for changes in electroencephalographic pattern and potassium ion release. In addition, they showed that lactate accumulates before there is a change in electroencephalographic pattern, that the change in pattern was accompanied by a small change in adenylate energy charge, and that massive

---

* See references 66, 77, 83, 84, 120, 121, 129.

energy failure was at hand at the time of potassium ion release.[89] The combined results indicated that long before a majority of cells show anoxic depolarization, energy failure of only few neurons may disrupt the circuits sustaining integrated electrical activity.

Complete Ischemia

There are many studies of complete ischemia, and changes in cerebral metabolites have been delineated in some detail.[33,36,72,73] Also, many studies of complete ischemia have been performed to gain information on the maximally permissible periods of cell anoxia that can be sustained with full recovery of function (or metabolism). Inherent in this approach is the assumption that complete interruption of oxygen supply represents the maximal insult to cells. As is shown later, there is some doubt that this is necessarily so.

According to classic concepts that are supported by both clinical experience and experimental data, irreversible neuronal damage occurs if the period of ischemia exceeds four to six minutes. Early results showed that somewhat longer periods (seven to eight minutes) are tolerated if measures are taken to prevent damage to the heart during the ischemia.[48] These results and observations have recently been challenged by studies indicating that the inherent resistance of brain cells to anoxia is considerably greater than previously assumed. For example, it was reported by Neely and Youmans that dogs could see, hear, and stand if complete ischemia was induced for up to 25 minutes by means of an increase in cerebrospinal fluid pressure.[85] Relatively long periods during which revival was possible were later obtained in monkeys by Miller and Myers, who reported that one animal sustained 24 minutes of complete ischemia with minimal neurological sequelae.[80] Results reported by Hossmann and collaborators have demonstrated that certain neurophysiological functions return in more than half of the animals even if complete ischemia is maintained for 60 minutes in barbiturate-anesthetized cats and monkeys.[51,52,62,130] In these animals, appreciable metabolic recovery was also seen; lactate concentra-

tion returned to only moderately elevated levels, and the adenylate energy charge recovered to within 93 per cent of the control value. Further data showed that appreciable protein synthesis occurred in the post-ischemic period.

Although it has not been demonstrated that integrated brain function can return after such extended periods of ischemia (i.e., 60 minutes), and although it may be suspected that the barbiturate anesthesia employed could have afforded some protection, the results quoted nevertheless suggest that cerebral neurons do not necessarily suffer irreversible damage if conditions are optimal for revival. Obviously, if extensive brain damage occurs after such short periods as five minutes, complicating factors must come into play.[18] To facilitate discussion of such factors, cerebral metabolic changes occurring during complete ischemia and the recovery of energy metabolism under optimal experimental conditions are described as follows.

Cerebral (cortical) metabolic changes following complete ischemia of 1 to 30 minutes' duration have recently been measured in artificially ventilated rats maintained on 70 per cent nitrous oxide.[33,71,97] Figure 22–9 demonstrates changes in tissue concentrations of phosphocreatine and lactate, and in calculated energy charge. Following interruption of oxygen supply, available glucose and glycogen are anaerobically converted to lactic acid, whose final concentration is set by the preischemic carbohydrate stores.[70] The phosphocreatine store is depleted within one minute, while the charge of the adenine nucleotide pool approaches minimal values after five to seven and one half minutes. Analyses of pyruvate and citric acid cycle intermediates emphasize the drastic change in mitochondrial metabolism (Fig. 22–10). Thus, the tissue contents of pyruvate, α-ketoglutarate, and oxaloacetate are depleted and there is massive accumulation of succinate.[33,36]

Since energy depletion occurs after five to seven minutes of ischemia, a period that was previously thought to be the maximally permissible one, it is tempting to conclude that irreversible damage develops pari passu with the disappearance of ATP. Recovery studies show that this is not so. The data of Figure 22–9 demonstrate that accumulated lactate disappears, phosphocrea-

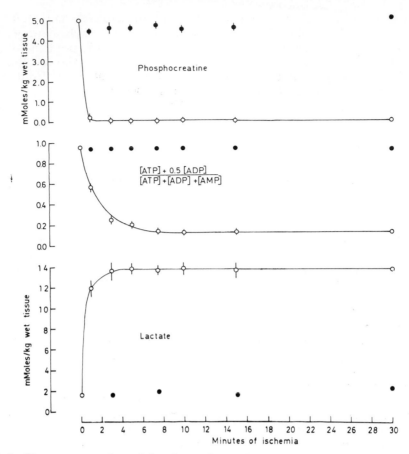

Figure 22–9   Tissue concentrations of phosphocreatine and lactate and calculated adenylate energy charge in rats after 1, 3, 5, 7, 10, 15, and 30 minutes of complete ischemia (*open circles*) compared with control group (70 per cent nitrous oxide). Solid circles indicate animals with ischemic periods according to the time scale but with a subsequent 90-minute period of recirculation before analysis. (From Siesjö, B. K., Carlsson, C., Hägerdal, M., and Nordström, C.-H.: Brain metabolism in the critically ill. Crit. Care Med., *4*:283–294, 1976. Reprinted by permission.)

tine concentration returns to normal values, and the adenylate energy charge returns to within 99 per cent of control values whether ischemia is induced for 5 or 30 minutes. At these periods of ischemia, the ATP concentration is subnormal. This is probably due, however, to the fact that degradation products of AMP (e.g., adenosine, inosine, and hypoxanthine) leave the tissue when recirculation starts, and that resynthesis of purine nucleotides is a slow process.[26,61] In other words, a subnormal value of ATP does not exclude recovery of mitochondrial metabolism, especially since the energy charge is virtually normalized. Analyses of glycolytic metabolites and citric acid cycle intermediates allow the same general conclusion, i.e., that there is extensive recovery of mitochondrial metabolism.[33,97] Furthermore, histopathological examination of brains in which circulation has been restored after ischemic periods of 7.5, 10, or 15 minutes demonstrates that a surprisingly small number of neurons show signs of irreversible damage.[13]

There is a discrepancy between recovery of cerebral energy metabolism and restitution of electrophysiological functions (or integrated brain function). One possible explanation for the slow return of cell function is that ischemia induces a long-lasting perturbation of transmitter metabolism. Figure 22–11 demonstrates that ischemia leads to accumulation of gamma-aminobutyric acid, alanine, and ammonia, and that changes in amino acid levels persist after relatively long periods of recirculation. Possibly, a disturbed metabolism of amino acid transmitters, as well as of biogenic amines, is at least partly responsible

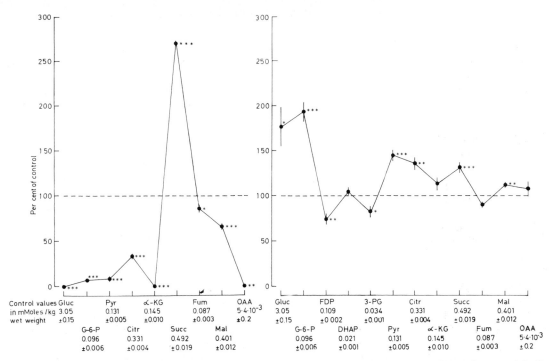

| Control values Gluc
in mMoles/kg 3.05
wet weight ±0.15 | Pyr
0.131
±0.005 | α-KG
0.145
±0.010 | Fum
0.087
±0.003 | OAA
5·4·10⁻³
±0.2 | | Gluc
3.05
±0.15 | FDP
0.109
±0.002 | 3-PG
0.034
±0.001 | Citr
0.331
±0.004 | Succ
0.492
±0.019 | Mal
0.401
±0.012 |

| | G-6-P
0.096
±0.006 | Citr
0.331
±0.004 | Succ
0.492
±0.019 | Mal
0.401
±0.012 | | | G-6-P
0.096
±0.006 | DHAP
0.021
±0.001 | Pyr
0.131
±0.005 | α-KG
0.145
±0.010 | Fum
0.087
±0.003 | OAA
5·4·10⁻³
±0.2 |

Figure 22–10 Changes in some glycolytic (glucose, G-6-P = glucose-6-phosphate; FDP = fructose-1,6,-di-phosphate; DHAP = dihydroxyacetone phosphate; 3-PG = 3-phosphoglycerate) and citric acid cycle intermediates (citrate; α-KG = α-ketoglutarate; succinate; fumarate; malate; OAA = oxaloacetate) after an ischemic period of five minutes' duration (*left*) and at the end of a 15-minute period of recirculation following an ischemic period of five minutes' duration (*right*). The values are given as percentage of controls ($\pm$S.E.M.). The following statistical symbols are used: * = $p < 0.05$; ** = $p < 0.01$; *** = $p < 0.001$. (Data from Folbergrová, J., Ljunggren, B., Norberg, K., and Siesjö, B. K.: Influence of complete ischemia on glycolytic metabolites, citric acid cycle intermediates, and associated amino acids in the rat cerebral cortex. Brain Res., *80*:265–279, 1974.)

Figure 22–11 Changes in the concentrations of some amino acids after an ischemic period of five minutes' duration (*unfilled bars*) and at the end of a 15-minute period of recirculation following an ischemic period of five minutes' duration (*hatched bars*). The values are given as percentage of controls ($\pm$S.E.M.). Glu, glutamate; Asp, aspartate; Gln, glutamine; Ala, alanine; GABA, γ-aminobutyric acid; Aspn, asparagine; NH_4^+, ammonium ion; *, $p < 0.05$; **, $p < 0.01$; ***, $p < 0.001$. (Data from Folbergrová, J., Ljunggren, B., Norberg, K., and Siesjö, B. K.: Influence of complete ischemia on glycolytic metabolites, citric acid cycle intermediates, and associated amino acids in the rat cerebral cortex. Brain Res., *80*:265–279, 1974.)

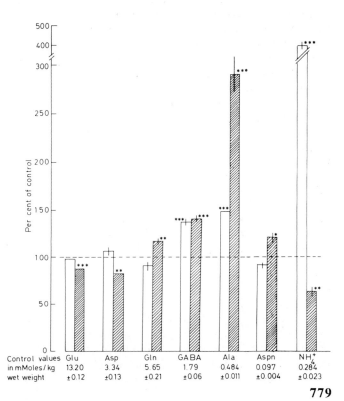

| Control values
in mMoles/kg
wet weight | Glu
13.20
±0.12 | Asp
3.34
±0.13 | Gln
5.65
±0.21 | GABA
1.79
±0.06 | Ala
0.484
±0.011 | Aspn
0.097
±0.004 | NH_4^+
0.284
±0.023 |

for lack of return of function.[14,15] In fact, it is not inconceivable that recovery of integrated brain function requires some remodeling of synaptic connections.

Factors Affecting Postischemic Recovery

The results quoted offer a challenge. Whereas a large body of clinical and experimental experience suggests that irreversible neuronal damage may occur after about 5 minutes of ischemia, other results show that, under optimal conditions, neurons may survive 20 to 30 or even 60 minutes of ischemia. The results raise the question about those factors that limit revival when conditions are suboptimal. The question was posed by Ames and collaborators, who were struck by the relatively pronounced resistance of retinal cells in vitro, as compared to neurons in vivo.[2,3] These authors proposed that revival in vivo was limited by inadequate reflow, and produced evidence that ischemia gave rise to a narrowing of capillary lumina by swelling of endothelial and perivascular glial cells. Subsequent results have not given strong support to the hypothesis of "no-reflow," as originally proposed.[31,32] There is, however, agreement that postischemic hypotension adversely affects the possibility for recovery, and extensive functional recovery has been obtained only when measures have been taken to promote reflow.[51,80] A nice illustration is provided by the results of Safar and co-workers, who succeeded in resuscitating dogs after 12 minutes of cardiac arrest by a combination of increased blood pressure, administration of heparin, and hemodilution.[104]

It has long been known that hypothermia, whether induced by body cooling or by selective brain cooling, prolongs survival following total ischemia in proportion to the reduction in temperature.[4,47,126] There is increasing evidence that certain anesthetics, notably barbiturates, may significantly increase the resistance of the brain to ischemia. In fact, barbiturate anesthesia may double the time in which revival is possible following total ischemia[37,127] Also, it reduces both the size of the infarcts and the severity of the neurological sequelae in experiments with ligation of middle cerebral arteries or other major cerebral vessels.[50,77,82,117] It is of clinical interest that barbiturates afforded significant protection even when given *after* the arteries were clamped. This may not be surprising in view of the fact that the regional ischemia that results from middle cerebral artery occlusion is not complete, and that the ischemia is reversible if flow is restored within two to three hours. It is of considerable interest, however, that a corresponding protective effect is observed in experiments with total ischemia, even when thiopental is infused five minutes after the start of recirculation.[9,86] The significance of this result is discussed in the following section.

Mechanisms of Cellular Damage

Recent results have given new information on the possible mechanisms of irreversible cell damage in the brain. Hossmann and Kleihues noted that recovery was adversely affected if the ischemia was incomplete, i.e., if a trickling flow remained.[51] Subsequent results on rats showed that whereas extensive recovery of cerebral energy metabolism was observed after 30 minutes of complete ischemia, no such recovery was observed if cerebral blood flow was reduced to 5 to 10 per cent of normal (Table 22–3). In this situation of incomplete ischemia, phenobarbital anesthesia afforded marked protection. As noted earlier, metabolic and histological damage is observed after 30 minutes of severe tissue hypoxia. Obviously, a severe reduction in cerebral oxygen availability may have more serious consequences than complete anoxia.

Among possible mechanisms that contribute to the final cell damage following ischemia, inadequate reflow cannot be excluded. If it does play a role, barbiturates may protect by reducing energy requirements to match the inadequate tissue perfusion. There is, however, no strong evidence that this is so, since postischemic cerebral blood flow and oxygen metabolism values are similar in animals anesthetized with 70 per cent nitrous oxide or phenobarbital, during the initial recirculation period following incomplete ischemia.[93] Tentatively, it is assumed that differences in biochemical response are involved.

One possible mechanism of cell damage in ischemia is digestion of intracellular

TABLE 22-3   CORRELATION OF PHOSPHOCREATINE, ATP, ADP, AMP, AND LACTATE LEVELS AND CALCULATED ENERGY CHARGE OF ADENINE NUCLEOTIDE POOL IN CEREBRAL ISCHEMIA*

	PHOSPHO-CREATINE	ATP	ADP	AMP	ENERGY CHARGE	LACTATE
Control (nitrous oxide 70%)	4.48	2.98	0.277	0.039	0.946	1.92
	±0.06	±0.01	±0.006	±0.002	±0.001	±0.20
Complete ischemia 30 min; recirculation 90 min (nitrous oxide 70%)	5.58	2.37	0.263	0.042	0.935	2.36
	±0.21	±0.03	±0.006	±0.002	±0.001	±0.34
Incomplete ischemia 30 min; recirculation 90 min (nitrous oxide 70%)	2.54	1.14	0.370	0.360	0.663	28.9
	±0.50	±0.20	±0.024	±0.040	±0.056	±3.9
Incomplete ischemia 30 min; recirculation 90 min (phenobarbital 150 mg/kg)	5.61	2.61	0.266	0.046	0.938	2.16
	±0.11	±0.06	±0.005	±0.003	±0.003	±0.38

* The concentrations are given in micromoles per gram and represent means ± S.E.M. (Data from Nordström, C.-H. Rehncrona, S., and Siesjö, B. K. : Restitution of cerebral energy state after complete and incomplete ischemia of 30 minutes duration. Acta Physiol. Scand., 97:270–272, 1976.)

structures by hydrolytic enzymes, e.g., those enzymes released from lysosomes.[23] Since the release is enhanced by acidosis, it is tempting to assume that incomplete ischemia (and hypoxia) induces more damage because the lactic acidosis is more severe than that occurring when glucose supply is interrupted. Recent results obtained in hyperglycemic or starved animals favor this possibility.[81] Other results, however, are less consistent with it. First, neuronal damage of a similar type is observed in hypoglycemic coma, a condition that is accompanied by *depletion* of lactic acid. Second, in incomplete ischemia, phenobarbital affords protection, although it does not curtail the lactic acidosis.[95,96]

Since there is indication that lysosomal enzymes are activated late in ischemic processes, alternative mechanisms should be considered for the initial events.[69,123] One such mechanism was proposed by Demopoulos and associates, who have speculated that the damage occurring in regional ischemia is caused by lipid peroxidation due to release of free radicals.[25] This suggestion is supported by measurements showing a decrease in the tissue concentration of a naturally occurring free radical scavenger (ascorbic acid) and by the fact that barbiturates have scavenging properties. It is also of interest that some of the earliest subcellular alterations affect the membranes of mitochondria and endoplasmic reticulum, structures that have a large content of unsaturated fatty acids and that are therefore prone to peroxidative attack.

Whatever the biochemical mechanisms of cell damage under conditions of tissue hypoxia, it seems a distinct possibility that at least some of the final damage is incurred in the reoxygenation period. For example, in studies that have demonstrated that ischemia or hypoxia of 15 to 20 minutes' duration leads to irreversible cell damage, the tissue has been perfusion-fixed for examination after a period of reoxygenation.[12,66,105] Supportive evidence is provided by experiments showing that barbiturates may prolong revival even when given during the recirculation period. There are also results to suggest that, in experiments on total ischemia, disaggregation of polyribosomes does not start until recirculation is begun.[19] Conceivably, a period of hypoxia or ischemia partly interferes with the integrity of vulnerable intracellular membranes, and when reoxygenation occurs, oxidative processes (e.g., those leading to lipid peroxidation) initiate a series of events that ultimately become irreversible.

At present, the mechanisms just discussed must remain somewhat speculative. The possibility that irreversible cell damage requires a relatively long time to develop and involves oxidative processes that are amenable to pharmacological intervention, however, makes these mechanisms of immediate concern to neurological surgeons.

REFERENCES

1. Albers, P. W., Siegel, G. J., Katzman, R., and Agranoff, B. W.: Basic Neurochemistry. Boston, Little, Brown & Co., 1972.
2. Ames, A., III, and Gurian, B. S.: Effects of glucose and oxygen deprivation on function of isolated mammalian retina. J. Neurophysiol., 26:617–634, 1963.
3. Ames, A., III, Wright, R. L., Kowada, M., Thurston, J. M., and Majno, G.: Cerebral ischemia. II. The no-reflow phenomenon. Amer. J. Pathol., 52:437–453, 1968.

4. Anabtawi, I. N., and Brockman, S. K.: Protective effect of hypothermia on total occlusion of the cerebral circulation. Ann. Surg., *155*:312–315, 1962.

5. Astrup, J., Symon, L., Branston, N. M., and Lassen, N. A.: Cortical evoked potential and extracellular K^+ and H^+ at critical levels of brain ischemia. Stroke, *8*:51–57, 1977.

6. Atkinson, D. E.: The energy charge of the adenylate pool as a regulatory parameter. Interaction with feedback modifiers. Biochemistry, *7*:4030–4034, 1968.

7. Bachelard, H. S., Lewis, L. D., Pontén, U., and Siesjö, B. K.: Mechanisms activating glycolysis in the brain in arterial hypoxia. J. Neurochem., *22*:395–401, 1974.

8. Baxter, C. F.: The nature of γ-aminobutyric acid. *In* Lajtha, A., ed.: Handbook of Neurochemistry. New York, Plenum Press, 1970, Vol. 3, pp. 289–353.

9. Bleyaert, A. L., Nemoto, E. M., Stezoski, S.W., Alexander, H., and Safar, P.: Amelioration of postischemic encephalopathy by sodium thiopental after 16 minutes of global brain ischemia in monkeys. Physiologist, *18*:145, 1975.

10. Borgström, L., Jóhansson, H., and Siesjö, B. K.: The influence of acute normovolemic anemia on cerebral blood flow and oxygen consumption of anaesthetized rats. Acta Physiol. Scand., *93*:505–514, 1975.

11. Brierley, J. B., Brown, A. W., and Meldrum, B. S.: The nature and time course of the neuronal alterations resulting from oligaemia and hypoglycaemia in the brain of Macaca mulatta. Brain Res., *25*:483–499, 1971.

12. Brierley, J. B., Ljunggren, B., and Siesjö, B. K.: Neuropathological alterations in rat brain after complete ischemia due to raised intracranial pressure. *In* Lundberg, N., Pontén, U., and Brock, M., eds.: Intracranial Pressure II. Berlin, Heidelberg, New York, Springer-Verlag, 1974, pp. 167–171.

13. Brierley, J. B., Brown, A. W., Excell, B. J., and Meldrum, B. S.: Brain damage in the rhesus monkey resulting from profound arterial hypotension. I. Its nature, distribution and general physiological correlates. Brain Res., *13*:68–100, 1969.

14. Brown, R. M., Carlsson, A., Ljunggren, B., and Siesjö, B. K.: Effect of ischemia on monoamine metabolism in the brain. Acta Physiol. Scand., *90*:789–791, 1974.

15. Calderini, G., Carlsson, A., and Nordström, C.-H.: Influence of transient ischemia on monoamine metabolism in the rat brain during nitrous oxide and phenobarbitone anaesthesia. Brain Res., *157*:303–310, 1978.

16. Carlsson, C., Hägerdal, M., and Siesjö, B. K.: Protective effect of hypothermia in cerebral oxygen deficiency due to arterial hypoxia. Anesthesiology, *44*:27–35, 1976.

17. Cohen, P. J., Alexander, S. C., Smith, F. C., Reivich, M., and Wollman, H.: Effects of hypoxia and normocarbia on cerebral blood flow and metabolism in conscious man. J. Appl. Physiol., *23*:183–189, 1967.

18. Cole, S. L., and Corday, E.: Four-minute limit for cardiac resuscitation. J.A.M.A., *161*:1454–1458, 1956.

19. Cooper, H. K., Zalewska, T., Kawakami, S., Hossmann, K.-A., and Kleihues, P.: The effect of ischemia and recirculation on protein synthesis in the rat brain. J. Neurochem., *28*:929–934, 1977.

20. Cooper, J. R., Bloom, F. E., and Roth, R. H.: The Biochemical Basis of Neuropharmacology. New York, Oxford University Press, 1974.

21. Curtis, D. R., and Johnston, G. A. R.: Amino acid transmitters in the mammalian central nervous system. Ergebn. Physiol., *69*:97–188, 1974.

22. Davis, J. N., and Carlsson, A.: The effect of hypoxia on monoamine synthesis, levels and metabolism in rat brain. J. Neurochem., *21*:783–790, 1973.

23. De Duve, C., and Wattiaux, R.: Functions of lysosomes. Ann. Rev. Physiol., *28*:435–492, 1966.

24. Della Porta, P., Maiolo, A. T., Negri, V. U., and Rosella, E.: Cerebral blood flow and metabolism in therapeutic insulin coma. Metabolism, *13*:131–140, 1964.

25. Demopoulos, H. B., Flamm, E., and Ransohoff, J.: Molecular pathology and CNS membranes. *In* Jöbsis, F. F., ed.: Oxygen and Physiological Function. 60th FASEB Annual Meeting. Dallas, Professional Information Library, 1977.

26. Deuticke, B., Gerlach, E., and Dierkesmann, R.: Abbau freier Nucleotide in Herz, Skeletmuskel, Gehirn und Leber der Ratte bei Sauerstoffmangel. Pfleuger. Arch. Ges. Physiol., *292*: 239–254, 1966.

27. Duffy, T. E., Nelson, S. R., and Lowry, O. H.: Cerebral carbohydrate metabolism during acute hypoxia and recovery. J. Neurochem., *19*:959–977, 1972.

28. Eklöf, B., and Siesjö, B. K.: The effect of bilateral carotid artery ligation upon acid-base parameters and substrate levels in the rat brain. Acta Physiol. Scand., *86*:528–538, 1972.

29. Ferrendelli, J. A., and Chang, M.-M.: Brain metabolism during hypoglycemia. Effect of insulin on regional central nervous system glucose and energy reserves in mice. Arch. Neurol., *28*:173–177, 1973.

30. Finnerty, F. A., Jr., Witkin, L., and Fazekas, J. F.: Cerebral hemodynamics during cerebral ischemia induced by acute hypotension. J. Clin. Invest., *33*:1227–1232, 1954.

31. Fischer, E. G., and Ames, A., III.: Studies on mechanisms of impairment of cerebral circulation following ischemia: effect of hemodilution and perfusion pressure. Stroke, *3*:538–542, 1972.

32. Fischer, E. G., Ames, A., III., Hedley-Whyte, E. T., and O'Gorman, S.: Reassessment of cerebral capillary changes in acute global ischemia and their relationship to the "Noreflow phenomenon." Stroke, *8*:36–39, 1977.

33. Folbergrová, J., Ljunggren, B., Norberg, K., and Siesjö, B. K.: Influence of complete ischemia on glycolytic metabolites, citric acid cycle intermediates, and associated amino acids in the rat cerebral cortex. Brain Res., *80*:265–279, 1974.

34. Gibbs, E. L., Lennox, W. G., and Gibbs, F. A.: Bilateral internal jugular blood. Comparison of A-V differences, oxygen-dextrose ratios and

respiratory quotients. Amer. J. Psychiat., *102*:184–190, 1945–46.

35. Gibson, G. E., and Blass, J. P.: Impaired synthesis of acetylcholine in brain accompanying mild hypoxia and hypoglycemia. J. Neurochem., *27*:37–42, 1976.

36. Goldberg, N. D., Passonneau, J. V., and Lowry, O. H.: Effects of changes in brain metabolism on the levels of citric acid cycle intermediates. J. Biol. Chem., *241*:3997–4003, 1966.

37. Goldstein, A., Jr., Wells, B. A., and Keats, A. S.: Increased tolerance to cerebral anoxia by pentobarbital. Arch. Int. Pharmacodyn., *161*:138–143, 1966.

38. Gottstein, U., Bernsmeier, A., und Sedlmeyer, I.: Der Kohlenhydratstoffwechsel des menschlichen Gehirn. I. Untersuchungen mit substratspezifischen enzymatischen Methoden bei normaler Hirndurchblutung. Klin. Wschr., *41*:943–948, 1963.

39. Grubb, R. L., Raichle, M. W., Phelps, M. E., and Ratcheson, R. A.: Effects of increased intracranial pressure on cerebral blood volume, blood flow, and oxygen utilization in monkeys. J. Neurosurg., *43*:385–398, 1975.

40. Gurdijan, E. S., Stone, W. E., and Webster, J. E.: Cerebral metabolism in hypoxia. Arch. Neurol. Psychiat., *54*:472–477, 1944.

41. Hägerdal, M., Harp, J., Nilsson, L., and Siesjö, B. K.: The effect of induced hypothermia upon oxygen consumption in the rat brain. J. Neurochem., *24*:311–316, 1975.

42. Harp, J. R., and Siesjö, B. K.: Effects of anaesthesia on cerebral metabolism. *In* Gordon, E., ed.: A Basis and Practice of Neuroanesthesia. Vol. 2 in Monographs in Anaesthesiology. Amsterdam, Excerpta Medica, 1975, pp. 83–112.

43. Hawkins, R. A., Williamson, D. H., and Krebs, H. A.: Ketone-body utilization by adult and suckling rat brain in vivo. Biochem. J., *122*:13–18, 1971.

44. Hebb, C.: Biosynthesis of acetylcholine in nervous tissue. Physiol. Rev., *52*:918–957, 1972.

45. Hess, H.: The rates of respiration of neurons and neuroglia in human cerebrum. *In* Kety, S. S., and Elkes, J., eds.: Regional Neurochemistry. Oxford, Pergamon Press, 1961, pp. 200–212.

46. Hinzen, D. H., and Müller, U.: Energiestoffwechsel und Funktion des Kaninchengehirns während Insulinhypoglykämie. Pfleuger. Arch., *322*:47–59, 1971.

47. Hinzen, D. H., Becker, P., and Müller, U.: Einfluss von Insulin auf den regionalen Phospholipidstoffwechsel des Kaninchengehirns in vivo. Pfleuger. Arch., *321*:1–14, 1970.

48. Hirsch, H., Euler, K. H., and Schneider, M.: Über die Erholung und Wiederbelebung des Gehirns nach Ischämie bei Normothermie. Pfleuger. Arch. Ges. Physiol., *265*:281–313, 1957.

49. Hirsch, H., Bolte, A., Schaudig, A., and Tönnis, D.: Über die Wiederbelebung des Gehirns bei Hypothermie. Pfleuger. Arch. Ges. Physiol., *265*:328–336, 1957.

50. Hoff, J. T., Smith, A. L., Hankinson, H. L., and Nielsen, S. L.: Barbiturate protection from cerebral infarction in primates. Stroke, *6*:28–33, 1975.

51. Hossmann, K.-A., and Kleihues, P.: Reversibility of ischemic brain damage. Arch. Neurol. (Chicago), *29*:375–382, 1973.

52. Hossmann, K.-A., and Zimmermann, V.: Resuscitation of the monkey brain after 1 hour's complete ischemia. I. Physiological and morphological observations. Brain Res., *81*:59–74, 1974.

53. Iversen, L. L.: Biochemical aspects of synaptic modulation. *In* Schmitt, F. O., and Worden, F. G., eds.: The Neurosciences. Third study program. Cambridge, Mass., the MIT Press, 1974, pp. 905–915.

54. Jeffrey, P. L., and Austin, L.: Axoplasmatic transport. Progr. Neurobiol., *2*:205–255, 1973.

55. Jóhansson, H., and Siesjö, B. K.: Cerebral blood flow and oxygen consumption in the rat in hypoxic hypoxia. Acta Physiol. Scand., *93*:269–276, 1975.

56. Jóhansson, H., and Siesjö, B. K.: Brain energy metabolism in anaesthetized rats in acute anemia. Acta Physiol. Scand., *93*:515–524, 1975.

57. Kety, S. S., and Schmidt, C. F.: The effects of altered arterial tensions of carbon dioxide and oxygen on cerebral blood flow and oxygen consumption of normal young men. J. Clin. Invest., *27*:484–491, 1948.

58. Kety, S. S., King, B. D., Horvath, S. M., Feffers, W. A., and Hafkenschiel, J. H.: The effects of an acute reduction in blood pressure by means of differential spinal sympathetic block on the cerebral circulation of hypertensive patients. J. Clin. Invest., *29*:402–407, 1950.

59. Kety, S. S., Woodford, R. B., Harmel, M. H., Freyhan, F. A., Appel, K. E., and Schmidt, C. F.: Cerebral blood flow and metabolism in schizophrenia. The effect of barbiturate seminarcosis, insulin coma and electroshock. Amer. J. Psychiat., *104*:765–770, 1947–48.

60. King, B. D., Sokoloff, L., and Wechsler, R. L.: The effects of l-epinephrine and l-nor-epinephrine upon cerebral circulation and metabolism in man. J. Clin. Invest., *31*:273–279, 1952.

61. Kleihues, P., Kobayashi, K., and Hossmann, K.-A.: Purine nucleotide metabolism in the cat brain after one hour of complete ischemia. J. Neurochem., *23*:417–425, 1974.

62. Kleihues, P., Hossmann, K.-A., Pegg, A. E., Kobayashi, K., and Zimmermann, V.: Resuscitation of the monkey brain after 1 hour complete ischemia. III. Indications of metabolic recovery. Brain Res., *95*:61–73, 1975.

63. Krnjević, K.: Chemical nature of synaptic transmission in vertebrates. Physiol. Rev., *54*:418–540, 1974.

64. Lajtha, A., ed.: Handbook of Neurochemistry. New York, Plenum Press, 1969–71.

65. Lehninger, A. L.: Bioenergetics. Menlo Park, Calif., W. A. Benjamin, 1973.

66. Levy, D. E., and Duffy, T. E.: Effect of ischemia on energy metabolism in the gerbil cerebral cortex. J. Neurochem., *24*:1287–1289, 1975.

67. Levy, D. E., Brierley, J. B., Silverman, D. G., and Plum, F.: Brain hypoxia initially damages cerebral neurons. Arch. Neurol. (Chicago), *32*:450–455, 1975.

68. Lewis, L. D., Ljunggren, B., Ratcheson, R. A., and Siesjö, B. K.: Cerebral energy state in insulin-induced hypoglycemia, related to blood

glucose and to EEG. J. Neurochem., *23*:673–679, 1974.

69. Little, J. R., Kerr, F. W. L., and Sundt, T. M., Jr.: The role of lysosomes in production of ischemic nerve cell changes. Arch. Neurol. (Chicago), *30*:448–455, 1974.

70. Ljunggren, B., Norberg, K., and Siesjö, B. K.: Influence of tissue acidosis upon restitution of brain energy metabolism following total ischemia. Brain Res., *77*:173–186, 1974.

71. Ljunggren, B., Ratcheson, R. A., and Siesjö, B. K.: Cerebral metabolic state following complete compression ischemia. Brain Res., *73*:291–307, 1974.

72. Ljunggren, B., Schutz, H., and Siesjö, B. K.: Changes in energy state and acid base parameters of the rat brain during complete compression ischemia. Brain Res., *73*:277–289, 1974.

73. Lowry, O. H., Passonneau, J. V., Hasselberger, F. X., and Schulz, D. W.: Effect of ischemia on known substrates and cofactors of the glycolytic pathway in brain. J. Biol. Chem., *239*:18–30, 1964.

74. MacMillan, V., and Siesjö, B. K.: Brain energy metabolism in hypoxemia. Scand. J. Clin. Lab. Invest., *30*:127–136, 1972.

75. Marshall, L. F., Durity, F., Lounsbury, R., Graham, D. J., Welsh, F., and Langfitt, T. W.: Experimental cerebral oligemia and ischemia produced by intracranial hypertension. Part 1: Pathophysiology, electroencephalography, cerebral blood flow, blood-brain barrier and neurological function. J. Neurosurg., *43*:308–317, 1975.

76. McIlwain, H., and Bachelard, H. S.: Biochemistry and the Central Nervous System. Edinburgh and London, Churchill Livingstone, 1971.

77. Michenfelder, J. D., and Sundt, T. M.: Cerebral ATP and lactate levels in the squirrel monkey following occlusion of the middle cerebral artery. Stroke, *2*:319–326, 1971.

78. Michenfelder, J. D., Milde, J. H., and Sundt, T. M.: Cerebral protection by barbiturate anesthesia. Arch. Neurol. (Chicago), *33*:345–350, 1976.

79. Miller, J. D., Stanek, A., and Langfitt, T. W.: Concepts on cerebral perfusion pressure and vascular compression during intracranial hypertension. Progr. Brain Res., *35*:411–432, 1971.

80. Miller, J. R., and Myers, R. E.: Neurological effects of systemic circulatory arrest in the monkey. Neurology (Minneap.), *20*:715–724, 1970.

81. Myers, R. E., and Yamaguchi, M.: Effects of serum glucose concentration on brain response to circulatory arrest. J. Neuropath. Exp. Neurol., *35*:301, 1976.

82. Moseley, J. I., Laurent, J. P., and Molinari, G. F.: Barbiturate attenuation of the clinical course and pathological lesions in a primate stroke model. Neurology (Minneap.), *25*:870–874, 1975.

83. Mršulja, B. B., Lust, W. D., Mršulja, B. J., Passonneau, J. V., and Klatzo, I.: Post-ischemic changes in certain metabolites following prolonged ischemia in the gerbil cortex. J. Neurochem., *26*:1099–1103, 1976.

84. Mršulja, B. B., Mršulja, B. J., Ito, U., Walker, J.

T., Jr., Spatz, M., and Klatzo, I.: Experimental cerebral ischemia in mongolian gerbils. II. Changes in carbohydrates. Acta Neuropath. (Berlin), *33*:91–103, 1975.

85. Neely, W. A., and Youmans, J. R.: Anoxia of canine brain without damage. J.A.M.A., *183*:1085–1087, 1963.

86. Nemoto, E. M.: Pathogenesis of cerebral ischemia-anoxia. Crit. Care Med. *6*:203–214, 1978.

87. Nemoto, E. M., Hoff, J. T., and Severinghaus, J. W.: Lactate uptake and metabolism by brain during hyperlactatemia and hypoglycemia. Stroke, *5*:48–53, 1974.

88. Nilsson, B., and Siesjö, B. K.: A method for determining blood flow and oxygen consumption in the rat brain. Acta Physiol. Scand., *96*:72–82, 1976.

89. Nilsson, B., Astrup, J., Blennow, G., and Siesjö, B. K.: Cerebral function and energy metabolism at critical thresholds of oxygen availability: A study in rats during status epilepticus induced by bicuculline. Eighth International Symposium on Cerebral Function, Metabolism and Circulation, June 26–July 1, Copenhagen, 1977.

90. Norberg, K., and Siesjö, B. K.: Cerebral metabolism in hypoxic hypoxia. I. Pattern of activation of glycolysis. Brain Res., *86*:31–44, 1975.

91. Norberg, K., and Siesjö, B. K.: Cerebral metabolism in hypoxic hypoxia. II. Citric acid cycle intermediates and associated amino acids. Brain Res., *86*:45–54, 1975.

92. Norberg, K., and Siesjö, B. K.: Oxidative metabolism of the cerebral cortex of the rat in severe insulin-induced hypoglycemia. J. Neurochem., *26*:345–352, 1976.

93. Nordström, C.-H., and Rehncrona, S.: Postischemic cerebral blood flow and oxygen utilization rate in rats anaesthetized with nitrous oxide or phenobarbital. Acta Physiol. Scand., *101*:230–240, 1977.

94. Nordström, C.-H., and Siesjö, B. K.: Effects of phenobarbital in cerebral ischemia. Part one: cerebral energy metabolism during pronounced, incomplete ischemia. Stroke, *9*:327–335, 1978.

95. Nordström, C.-H., Rehncrona, S., and Siesjö, B. K.: Restitution of cerebral energy state after complete and incomplete ischemia of 30 minutes duration. Acta Physiol. Scand., *97*:270–272, 1976.

96. Nordström, C.-H., Rehncrona, S., and Siesjö, B. K.: Effects of phenobarbital in cerebral ischemia. Part two: Restitution of cerebral energy state, as well as of glycolytic metabolites, citric acid cycle intermediates and associated amino acids after pronounced, incomplete ischemia. Stroke, *9*:335–343, 1978.

97. Nordström, C.-H., Rehncrona, S., and Siesjö, B. K.: Restitution of cerebral energy state, as well as of glycolytic metabolites, citric acid cycle intermediates and associated amino acids after 30 minutes of complete ischemia in rats anaesthetized with nitrous oxide or phenobarbital. J. Neurochem., *30*:479–486, 1978.

98. Ochs, S.: Fast axoplasmatic transport of materials in mammalian nerve and its integrative role. Ann. N.Y. Acad. Sci., *193*:43–58, 1972.

99. Otis, A. B., Rahn, H., Epstein, M. A. and Fenn,

W. O.: Performance as related to composition of alveolar air. Ann. J. Physiol., *146*:207–221, 1946.

100. Owen, O. E., Morgan, A. P., Kemp, H. G., Sullivan, J. M., Herrera, M. G., and Cahill, G. F., Jr.: Brain metabolism during fasting. J. Clin. Invest., *46*:1589–1595, 1967.

101. Pardridge, W. M., and Oldendorff, W. H.: Transport of metabolic substrates through the blood-brain barrier. J. Neurochem., *28*:5–12, 1976.

102. Roberts, E., Chase, T. N., and Tower, D. B., eds.: GABA in Nervous System Function. Amsterdam-Oxford, Excerpta Medica, 1976

103. Ruderman, N. B., Ross, P. S., Berger, M., and Goodman, M. N.: Regulation of glucose and ketone-body metabolism in brain of anaesthetized rats. Biochem. J., *138*:1–10, 1974.

104. Safar, P., Stezoski, W., and Nemoto, E. M.: Amelioration of brain damage after 12 minutes' cardiac arrest in dogs. Arch. Neurol. (Chicago), *33*:91–95, 1976.

105. Salford, L. G., Plum, F., and Brierley, J. B.: Graded hypoxia-oligemia in rat brain. II. Neuropathological alterations and their implications. Arch. Neurol. (Chicago), *29*:234–238, 1973.

106. Salford, L. G., Plum, F., and Siesjö, B. K.: Graded hypoxia-oligemia in rat brain. I. Biochemical alterations and their implications. Arch. Neurol. (Chicago), *29*:227–233, 1973.

107. Schadé, J. P., and McMenemy, W. H., eds.: Selective Vulnerability of the Brain Hypoxaemia. Oxford, Blackwell Scientific Publications, 1963.

108. Siesjö, B. K.: Physiological aspects of brain energy metabolism. *In* Davison, A. N., ed.: Biochemical Correlates of Brain Structure and Function. London, Academic Press, 1977.

109. Siesjö, B. K.: Brain Energy Metabolism. London, John Wiley & Sons, 1978.

110. Siesjö, B. K., and Nilsson, L.: The influence of arterial hypoxemia upon labile phosphates and upon extracellular lactate and pyruvate concentration in the rat brain. Scand. J. Clin. Lab. Invest., *27*:83–96, 1971.

111. Siesjö, B. K., and Zwetnow, N. N.: The effect of hypovolemic hypotension on extra- and intracellular acid-base parameters and energy metabolites in the rat brain. Acta Physiol. Scand., *79*:114–124, 1970.

112. Siesjö, B. K., and Zwetnow, N. N.: Effects of increased cerebrospinal fluid pressure upon adenine nucleotides and upon lactate and pyruvate in rat brain tissue. Acta Neurol. Scand., *46*:187–202, 1970.

113. Siesjö, B. K., Folbergrová, J., and MacMillan, V.: The effect of hypercapnia upon intracellular pH in the brain, evaluated by the bicarbonate-carbonic acid method and from the creatine phosphokinase reaction. J. Neurochem., *19*:2483–2495, 1972.

114. Siesjö, B. K., Carlsson, C., Hägerdal, M., and Nordström, C.-H.: Brain metabolism in the critically ill. Crit. Care Med. J., *4*:283–294, 1976.

115. Siesjö, B. K., Jóhansson, H., Ljunggren, B., and Norberg, K.: Brain dysfunction in cerebral hypoxia and ischemia. *In* Plum, F., ed.: Brain Dysfunction in Metabolic Disorders. New York, Raven Press, 1974, pp. 75–112.

116. Smith, A. L., and Wollman, H.: Cerebral blood flow and metabolism. Anaesthesiology, *36*: 378–400, 1972

117. Smith, A. L., Hoff, J. T., Nielsen, S. L., and Larson, C. P.: Barbiturate protection in acute focal cerebral ischemia. Stroke, *5*:1–7, 1974.

118. Sokoloff, L.: Circulation and energy metabolism of the brain. *In* Albers, R. W., Siegel, G. J., Katzman, R., and Agranoff, B. W., eds.: Basic Neurochemistry. Boston, Little, Brown & Co., 1972, pp. 299–325.

119. Stone, H. H., MacKrell, T. N., and Wechsler, R. L.: The effect on cerebral circulation and metabolism in man of acute reduction in blood pressure by means of intravenous hexamethonium bromide and head-up tilt. Anesthesiology, *16*:168–176, 1955.

120. Sundt, T. M., and Michenfelder, J. D.: Focal transient ischemia in the squirrel monkey: Effect on brain adenosine triphosphate and lactate levels with electrocorticographic and pathologic correlation. Circ. Res., *30*:703–712, 1972.

121. Sundt, T. M., and Waltz, A. G.: Cerebral ischemia and reactive hyperemia. Studies of cortical blood flow and microcirculation before, during and after temporary occlusion of middle cerebral artery of squirrel monkeys. Circ. Res., *28*:426–433, 1971.

122. Tower, D. B., and Young, O. M.: The activities of butyryl-cholinesterase and carbonic anhydrase, the rate of anaerobic glycolysis, and the question of a constant density of glial cells in cerebral cortices of various mammalian species from mouse to whale. J. Neurochem., *20*:269–278, 1973.

123. Trump, B. F., Mergner, W. J., Kahng, M. W., and Saladino, A. J.: Studies on the subcellular pathophysiology of ischemia. Circulation, *53*(3 suppl. 1):17–26, 1976.

124. van den Berg, C. J.: Glutamate and Glutamine. *In* Lajtha, A., ed.: Handbook of Neurochemistry. Vol. III. New York, Plenum Press, 1970, pp. 355–379.

125. Welsh, F. A., Durity, F., and Langfitt, T. W.: The appearance of regional variations in metabolism at a critical level of diffuse cerebral oligemia. J. Neurochem., *28*:71–80, 1977.

126. White, R. J., Austin, P. E., Jr., Austin, J. C., Taslitz, N., and Takoaka, Y.: Recovery of the subhuman primate after deep cerebral hypothermia and prolonged ischemia. Resuscitation, *2*:117–122, 1973.

127. Wright, R. L., and Ames, A., III: Measurement of maximal permissible cerebral ischemia and a study of its pharmacologic prolongation. J. Neurosurg., *21*:567–574, 1964.

128. Wurtman, R. J., and Fernstrom, J. D.: Control of brain neurotransmitter synthesis by precursor availability and nutritional state. Biochem. Pharmacol., *25*:1691–1696, 1976.

129. Yamaguchi, T., Waltz, A. G., and Okazaki, H.: Hyperemia and ischemia in experimental cerebral infarction: Correlation of histopathology and regional blood flow. Neurology (Minneap.), *21*:565–578, 1971.

130. Zimmermann, V., and Hossmann, K.-A.: Resuscitation of the monkey brain after one hour's complete ischemia. II. Brain water and electrolytes. Brain Res., *85*:1–11, 1975.

CEREBRAL BLOOD
FLOW IN
CLINICAL
PROBLEMS

The brain constitutes only about 2 per cent of the total body weight yet it receives approximately 15 per cent of the cardiac outflow and utilizes about 20 per cent of the oxygen consumed by the body. This enormous demand for blood and oxygen requires a smoothly functioning delivery system. That system is made up of the heart, major cervical vessels, and intracranial vascular system. An acute major impairment of the delivery system at any level can cause unconsciousness within 20 seconds and the beginning of irreversible central nervous system damage within four to eight minutes.[76] Lesions that develop slowly over months or years, however, can cause a major impairment of function and yet can be tolerated quite well if collateral channels exist or can be developed.

AMOUNT OF CEREBRAL BLOOD FLOW

The original method of determining cerebral blood flow was described by Kety and Schmidt.[185] Their technique utilized the Fick principle, which is based on the law of conservation of matter. As applied to the brain, it means that the amount of a substance taken up by the brain in a given time is equal to the amount of the substance brought to the brain by the arteries less the amount taken away from it by the veins. Kety and Schmidt used nitrous oxide, a highly diffusible inert gas, as the indicator substance. In this method, the gas is introduced into the arterial blood via the lungs. Blood samples are then taken repeatedly from a peripheral artery that is assumed to be representative of the cerebral arteries and from the main venous drainage of the brain, the internal jugular vein. After about 10 minutes, a fair degree of saturation of cerebral tissues with the gas has been obtained. At this point, the venous blood from the brain will have approximately the same level of the gas as the arterial blood and the total uptake of the gas by brain can be calculated. In turn, from these figures, the cerebral blood flow can be calculated. The results are usually expressed as the number of cubic centimeters of blood that flows through a gram of brain tissue in one minute. The results of studies by a number of investigators are given in Table 23–1.

The use of diffusible substances in studying cerebral blood flow is based on the assumption that the substances diffuse in the brain and tissue so rapidly that their concentration is dependent on blood flow rather than on diffusibility. This assumption is supported by the fact that the capillary bed of the brain is extremely rich and the intercapillary distances are small.

Methods that utilize diffusible substances have several potential sources of error. An obvious one is that the cerebral tissues may have different perfusion rates. Another is that the experiment may not be continued until all the cerebral tissues are saturated. Also, the venous return may be contami-

J. R. YOUMANS

TABLE 23–1 MEAN CEREBRAL BLOOD FLOWS OF HUMANS OBTAINED BY INERT GAS TECHNIQUES

AUTHOR	METHOD	ARTERIAL Pco_2 (mm Hg)	CBF (ml/min/100 gm)
Cohen et al.*	[85]Kr	41.4 ± 1.7^a	44.4 ± 5.3^a
Ehrenreich et al.†	N_2O	43.8 ± 2.2	46.3 ± 8.4
Kety and Schmidt‡	N_2O	43 ± 2	53 ± 7
Lambertsen et al.§	N_2O	41.3 ± 3.4	61.7 ± 10.8
Lassen and Lane[‖]	[85]Kr		44.3 ± 6.4
Lassen and Munck¶	[85]Kr	37.6 ± 6.0	52 ± 8.6^a
Mangold et al.**	N_2O	41.3 ± 0.9^a	54.8 ± 4.3^a
Novack et al.††	N_2O	43 ± 5	53 ± 16
Patterson et al.‡‡	N_2O	39.2 ± 4.2	50 ± 8
Wasserman and Patterson§§	N_2O	38.5 ± 1.7	55.1 ± 9.8

[a] Standard deviations as reported by author. All others are calculated from original papers by Reivich, M.: Clin. Neurosurg., 16:378–418, 1968.

* Effects of hypoxia and normocarbia on cerebral blood flow and metabolism in conscious man. J. Appl. Physiol., 23:183–189, 1967.
† Influence of acetazolamide on cerebral blood flow. Arch. Neurol., 5:227–232, 1961.
‡ The nitrous oxide method for the quantitative determination of cerebral blood flow in man: Theory, procedure and normal values. J. Clin. Invest., 27:476–483, 1948.
§ Respiratory and cerebral circulatory control during exercise at .21 and 2.0 atmospheres inspired pO_2. J. Appl. Physiol., 14:966–982, 1959.
[‖] Validity of internal jugular blood for study of cerebral blood flow and metabolism. J. Appl. Physiol., 16:313–320, 1961.
¶ The cerebral blood flow in man determined by the use of radioactive krypton. Acta Physiol. Scand., 33:30–49, 1955.
** The effects of sleep and lack of sleep on the cerebral circulation and metabolism of normal young men. J. Clin. Invest., 34:1092–1100, 1955.
†† The effects of carbon dioxide inhalation upon the cerebral blood flow and cerebral oxygen consumption in vascular disease. J. Clin. Invest., 32:696–702, 1953.
‡‡ Threshold of response of the cerebral vessels of man to increase in blood carbon dioxide. J. Clin. Invest., 34:1857–1864, 1955.
§§ The cerebral vascular response to reduction in arterial carbon dioxide tension. J. Clin. Invest., 40:1297–1303, 1961.

nated with extracerebral blood, and one jugular vein may not be representative of the whole brain. Finally, the brain weight of the person tested is not known, and the total blood flow can be calculated only by assuming brain weights.

The indicator dilution technique is based on the Stewart Hamilton principle that dilution of an indicator in an organ depends on the amount of blood flowing through the organ.[249] The method consists of the injection of a dye into the internal carotid artery and subsequent withdrawal of venous blood from both jugular bulbs. The main difficulty with using this technique is in determining the amount of indicator that recirculates through the organ and alters the results. Studies with the indicator dilution technique indicate that with a single carotid injection, approximately two thirds of the indicator leaves via the ipsilateral internal jugular bulb and one third via the contralateral bulb.[135,284] When flow through the right or the left jugular bulb is calculated separately, it is found that, on the average, the right bulb drains 62 per cent of the cerebral flow whereas the left drains only 38 per cent.

The total cerebral blood flow as determined by several investigators utilizing a variety of techniques is given in Table 23–2.

Regional Cerebral Blood Flow

The term "regional blood flow" may refer to blood flow in a single cerebral lobe, a restricted region of the parenchyma or the cortex, or even a very discrete microregion of the brain. It can be calculated by methods based on extracranial recordings of the uptake and clearance of a radioisotope that is freely diffusible in the cerebral substance.

The technique that has given the best results has been the intracarotid injection of either [85]krypton or [133]xenon.[143,160] These isotopes are freely diffusible and effectively eliminated from the bloodstream through the lungs. Provided the diffusion of the gases is sufficiently rapid to maintain equilibrium between brain tissue and efferent blood, the shape of the clearance curve will depend solely on the dose, the blood flow, and the relative solubility of the isotope

TABLE 23-2 TOTAL CEREBRAL BLOOD FLOW IN HUMANS

AUTHOR	METHOD	CBF (ml/min)
Gibbs et al.[*]	Evans blue	614 ± 215[a]
Hellinger et al.[†]	Indocyanine green	708 ± 96
Kety and Schmidt[‡]	N_2O	756 ± 98[b]
Lewis et al.[§]	[85]Kr	1236 ± 246
Nylin et al.[‖]	Labeled RBC's	915 ± 169[a]
Reinmuth et al.[¶]	[131]I iodoantipyrine	1097 ± 185
Shenkin et al.[**]	Evans blue	986 ± 435[a]
Steiner et al.[††]	Indicator fractionation	709 ± 178

[a] Values are given as calculated from original paper by Reivich, M.: Clin. Neurosurg., 16:378–418, 1968.

[†] Assuming brain weight of 1400 gm.

[*] Volume flow of blood through the human brain. Arch. Neurol. Psychiat., 57:137–144, 1947.

[†] Total cerebral blood flow and oxygen consumption using the dye-dilution method. J. Neurosurg., 19:964–970, 1962.

[‡] The effects of altered arterial tensions of carbon dioxide and oxygen on cerebral blood flow and cerebral oxygen consumpiton of normal young men. J. Clin. Invest., 27:484–492, 1948.

[§] A method for the continuous measurement of cerebral blood flow in man by means of radioactive krypton (Kr[79]) J. Clin. Invest., 39:707–716, 1960.

[‖] Cerebral circulation studied with labelled red cells in healthy males. Acta Radiol., 55:281–304, 1961.

[¶] Total cerebral blood flow and metabolism. Arch. Neurol. (Chicago), 12:49–66, 1965.

[**] Dynamic anatomy of the cerebral circulation. Arch. Neurol. Psychiat., 60:240–252, 1948.

[††] The measurement of cerebral blood flow by external isotope counting. J. Clin. Invest., 41:2221–2232, 1962.

concerned in the brain tissue. To perform the study the isotope is dissolved in sterile saline and injected into the internal carotid artery. The gamma radiation from the isotope is recorded by means of one or more scintillation detectors placed extracranially.

A mere determination of the flow to the brain is not the total picture. As shown by Wollman and co-workers, there is a differential between the blood flow to the white and that to the gray matter of the brain.[414] They did a two-compartmental analysis on young male volunteers. Flow patterns indicating two distinct rates of flow were shown. The white matter was assumed to be the slower compartment, which was found to represent 50.8 per cent of the cerebral tissue. The flow rate in the white matter is 15.9 ml per 100 gm per minute. The faster area, which is assumed to be the gray matter, constitutes 49.2 per cent of the cerebral tissue. It has a flow rate of 64.6 ml per 100 gm per minute. Other studies have shown even greater differences in flow in

the fast and slow compartments. Obrist and associates reported a flow of 74.5 ml per 100 gm per minute in the fast compartment and 24.8 ml per 100 gm per minute in the slow compartment.[287]

As noted, the regional cerebral blood volume may be assessed by radioisotope studies.[152,217] It can also be determined by computed tomography.[202] This latter technique reveals significant regional differences in the volume; the frontal and temporal regions have lower and the occipital region has higher than the mean hemisphere values. The left hemisphere has a greater cerebral blood volume than does the right in most patients.[147] A new noninvasive method for determining flow in an intracranial vessel has been described by Lantz and co-workers.[211] It utilizes a videodensitometer and measures the flow in the vessels as a fraction of the cardiac output. Determinations of flow in the cerebral vessels are easily made, and probably the technique can be utilized intracranially. Further evaluations will have to be made to determine whether it will be a valuable aid in the evaluation of stroke patients.

GENERAL FACTORS AFFECTING BLOOD FLOW

The general laws of hydrodynamics apply to the vascular system; however, they are altered by the properties of blood and the vascular system.

Viscosity

Blood is a non-newtonian fluid. It does not fulfill the rquirement of a newtonian fluid that the velocity gradient be proportional to the applied stress at all velocities. The anomalies of the behavior of blood flow result, in part, from the presence of the cells suspended in plasma. The cells accumulate in the axial portion of the bloodstream. Since fluid moving through a tube normally acts as a series of thin layers slipping against each other and proceeding at different velocities, the accumulation of cells in the axial portion will have the same effect as decreasing viscosity and will increase the velocity of flow.

If water is assigned a viscosity of 1, then

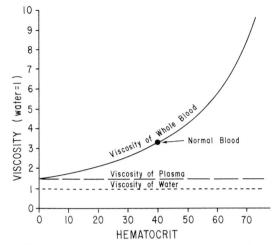

Figure 23–1 Effect of changes of hematocrit on whole blood.

the viscosity of plasma is about 1.5 and the viscosity of normal blood is about 3. Figure 23–1 shows the effect of changing hemoglobin concentration on the viscosity.[113] The lower levels of hemoglobin have only a slight effect on the viscosity; the upper levels, however, have a marked effect.

Vessel Length

As blood flows along a vessel there is friction between the blood and the vessel wall. The longer the vessel, the greater the distance along the wall over which the blood must slip and, therefore, the greater the friction. Consequently, the resistance of the vessel to flow is directly proportional to its length (Fig. 23–2).

Vessels in Series

The resistance of vessels in series is additive and is as though they were one continuous vessel. The only difference is the change of the diameter as the blood progresses from one vessel to another, and hence the change in resistance in the various vessels. The total peripheral resistance caused by vessel length is obtained by adding the resistance of the arteries, the arterioles, the capillaries, and the veins, in sequence (Fig. 23–2). The formula is simply

$$R \text{ (total)} = R_1 + R_2 + R_3. \ \ldots$$

Vessels in Parallel

The effect of vessels in parallel on resistance is quite complicated. As a general approximation, however, it can be stated that the resistance of vessels in parallel is far less than that of any single vessel, and if these vessels are of approximately the same size, the total resistance is equal to the resistance of the vessel divided by the number of vessels in parallel (Fig. 23–3). The formula is

$$\frac{1}{R \text{ (total)}} = \frac{1}{R_1} + \frac{1}{R_2} + \frac{1}{R_3} + \frac{1}{R_4}.$$

This principle is extremely important when one is considering vascular flow in systems in which vessels of approximately the same size are connected in parallel.[419] The cerebrovascular system has numerous examples of such vessels in parallel, beginning with the carotid and vertebral arteries in the neck and continuing intracranially with the major cerebral arteries and small arterioles.

Perfusion Pressure and Vascular Resistance

Circulation through the brain, as through any other organ, depends upon the perfusion pressure and the resistance to flow. Hence, the blood flow is determined by the

Figure 23–2 Effect of changes in vessel length on flow of blood.

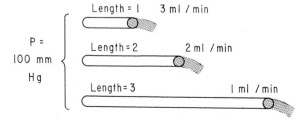

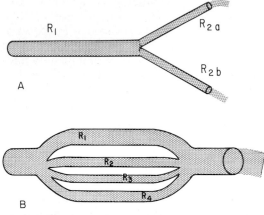

Figure 23-3 *A*. Resistance in each vessel in series is additive. Formula for calculation of resistance is $R = R_1 + R_{2a}$ or $R = R_1 + R_{2b}$.

B. Vessels of various size that are in parallel. Formula for calculating resistance is $\dfrac{1}{R} = \dfrac{1}{R_1} + \dfrac{1}{R_2} + \dfrac{1}{R_3} + \dfrac{1}{R_4}$.

Vascular Diameter

The character of the laminar flow of a fluid is markedly influenced by the diameter of the vessel. The overall effect of the diameter of a vessel with its influence on the resistance to flow is summarized by Poiseuille's law. The formula for Poiseuille's law is complex.* When considering clinical problems, however, one may use a simplified formula without a critical loss of accuracy. In simplified form it may be stated that the velocity of flow in a tube is proportional to the cross-sectional area of the tube.[61,113]

Poiseuille's law is derived from a study performed in rigid tubes, usually glass ones, in which streamline flow occurs. In the vascular system, the vessels are distensible and usually the blood flow is broken by bifurcations or binds that set up considerable turbulence. The overall effect is to increase the resistance above the level that would be present in a streamline flow in glass tubes.

Rigid application of the principles of Poiseuille's law to the circulatory system is not warranted. It does, however, give an approximation of the effect of changing vascular size and emphasizes the fact that change in vascular diameter greatly affects the blood flow. As noted earlier, most of the movement of blood occurs by slippage of successive molecular layers over each other, with the centermost portion of the blood in the vessel flowing rapidly and that nearest the wall flowing more slowly. Since the portions of fluid nearest the wall are impeded more severely than those in the center of the vessel, blood flow in the small vessels is greatly impeded because none of the blood in the vessel is far from the wall.

There is still another cause for increased resistance in small vessels as compared with large vessels. Because of the small cross section of the smaller vessel, the velocity of the flow must increase greatly if the same quantity of blood is to pass through the vessel in a given time.[113] The combined effects of laminar flow, change in vessel size, and viscosity on the resistance

balance between the extracranial or extrinsic factors making the perfusion pressure, and the intracranial or intrinsic factors determining the vascular resistance. Under normal circumstances the cerebral venous pressure is 5 mm of mercury or less and is insignificant. As a result, for practical purposes, the systemic blood pressure represents the perfusion pressure of the brain.

Distensibility of Vessels

The cerebrovascular resistance depends mainly on two factors: the viscosity of the blood and the vascular factors affecting resistance, which are the diameter, length, and interconnections of the vessels. An aspect adding to the complexity of vascular factors determining blood flow is that the blood vessels are distensible. As the pressure is increased, the elasticity of their walls permits the vessels to enlarge and, hence, the vascular resistance is reduced. Conversely, a reduction in pressure causes the vessels to retract and, hence, to increase the resistance. The effect of direct changes in the vessel size from pressure is counterbalanced in part by the effects of the myogenic reflex of the arterioles. This reflex is discussed in the section concerning control of blood low.

---

* Formula for Poiseuille's law: $\Delta P = \dfrac{8L}{\Pi r^4}\ FV$ where ΔP = pressure drop, L = length, r = radius, F = flow, V = viscosity.

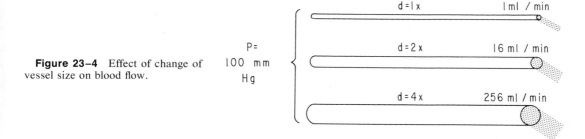

Figure 23-4 Effect of change of vessel size on blood flow.

is summarized in the formula R $\alpha \frac{L \cdot V}{r^4}$, in which R is resistance, L is vessel length, V is viscosity, and r is radius. Again, as a generalization, a simplified formula may be used without marked loss of accuracy. The simplified formula is R $\alpha \frac{1}{r^4}$. The effect of these changes is shown in Figure 23-4, which shows that vessels having a relatively small change in diameter have a markedly altered capacity for carrying blood flow. The great influence of the diameter size on the resistance of a vessel is especially important in the arterioles.

The diameter of the arterioles may vary greatly as they go from maximum relaxation to marked spasm. In fact, the effective radius of the arterioles may become so small that they act as though they were occluded. This means that the resistance to flow may change many hundredfold under different physiological or pathological conditions.

CONTROL OF CEREBRAL BLOOD FLOW

Galen believed that "by the diastole of the brain the spirit of life was sucked in through the cribriform plate and mingled with the vital spirit which ascended by the arteries from the heart."[139] His theory was that the animal spirits were mixed in the cerebral ventricles and were propelled into the nerves and muscles during systole of the brain. Waste products of the activity were excreted through the nose, and if it was blocked the patient might suffer apoplexy.

In 1783 Monro stated that there could be little or no variation in the quantity of blood within the cranial activity. He argued that

. . . the blood must be continually flowing out by the veins, that room may be given to the blood which is entering by the arteries. For, as the substance of the brain, like that of the other solids of our body, is nearly incompressible, the quantity of blood within the head must be the same, or very nearly the same, at all times, whether in health or disease, in life or after death, those cases only excepted, in which water or other matter is effused or secreted from the blood-vessels; for in these, a quantity of blood, equal in bulk to the effused matter, will be pressed out of the cranium.[267]

This view received support from experiments made by Kellie in 1824 and became known as the Monro-Kellie doctrine.[182] The Monro-Kellie doctrine received further support from Hill, who, in 1896, denied the existence of functional vasomotor nerves.[139]

In 1889 the basis for the current understanding of the control of cerebral blood flow was being set by Roy and Sherrington.[329] With extraordinary insight, they postulated an intrinsic metabolic control of the caliber of the cerebral vessels with dilation of these vessels in the presence of metabolites such as lactic acid; however, their ideas were ignored for many years. A basic concept came in 1902 when Bayliss observed,

The muscular coat of the arteries reacts, like smooth muscle in other situations, to a stretching force by contraction. It also reacts to a diminution of tension by relaxation, shown, of course, only when in a state of tone. These reactions are independent of the central nervous system, and are of myogenic nature.[20]

Cow added an important link in our knowledge in 1911 when he observed that carbon dioxide caused vasodilation of a sheep's carotid artery that was suspended in Ringer's solution.[49] Another milestone came in 1937 when Fog confirmed that the

NORMOTENSION

$$\frac{\text{Blood pressure}}{\text{Cerebrovascular resistance}} = \text{Cerebral blood flow}$$

HYPERTENSION

$$\frac{\text{Blood pressure increases}}{\text{Cerebrovascular resistance increases}} = \text{Constant cerebral blood flow}$$

HYPOTENSION

$$\frac{\text{Blood pressure decreases}}{\text{Cerebrovascular resistance decreases}} = \text{Constant cerebral blood flow}$$

Figure 23–5 Formula for autoregulation of cerebral blood flow.

cerebral vessels reacted to pressure changes in a manner similar to that observed in systemic vessels by Bayliss.[90] These observations formed the basis for many studies reported during the following decades that firmly established the influence of the blood pressure and the chemistry of the brain and cerebral vessels on cerebral blood flow.[343,411]

Blood Pressure and Cerebral Blood Flow

Blood pressure is determined by the vasomotor centers of the medulla, which receives input from the baroreceptors in the carotid sinus and aortic arch. Changes in blood pressure are avoided by constant monitoring by the baroreceptors, with appropriate variations in inhibitory impulses to the vasomotor centers. Loss of baroreceptor sensitivity due to arteriosclerosis in the carotid sinus and the aortic arch may cause severe postural hypotension.[335] Normal individuals do not have appreciable changes in cerebral blood flow until the pressure falls to about 50 mm of mercury or below. With chronic hypertension, arteriosclerosis, or occlusion or stenosis of some of the cerebral vessels, the critical level of blood pressure causing symptoms of cerebral ischemia is considerably increased.

Autoregulation

Under normal circumstances the resistance of the cerebral vessels is varied so as to maintain a constant blood flow despite changes in perfusion pressure (Figs. 23–5 and 23–6). This tendency to maintain a constant blood flow is known as the autoregulation phenomenon. The basis for this phenomenon is still a matter of dispute. Several theories have been promulgated to explain

it, among them the myogenic theory, the tissue pressure theory, the neurogenic theory, and the metabolic theory.

Myogenic Theory

This theory is based upon an observation made by Bayliss in 1902.[20] In brief, he observed that if the pressure within a vessel was increased, the vessel contracted to give an increased vascular resistance and thus reduced blood flow to the normal level. If pressure within the vessel is decreased, the vessel wall relaxes and reduces the vascular resistance. The reduced resistance permits the flow to increase again to the normal level.

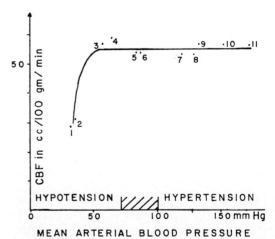

Figure 23–6 Classic diagram of Lassen showing blood pressure and cerebral blood flow of patients with 11 different acute or chronic conditions. The number on the line indicating blood pressure is placed at the mean blood pressure of the particular patient group. The conditions indicated by the numbers are: 1 and 2, drug-induced severe hypotension; 3 and 4, drug-induced moderate hypotension; 5 and 6, normal pregnant women and normal young men; 7, drug-induced hypertension; 8, hypertensive toxemic pregnancy; 9, 10, and 11, essential hypertension. (From Lassen, N. A.: Cerebral blood flow and oxygen consumption in man. Physiol. Rev., *39*:197, 1959. Reprinted by permission.)

Tissue Pressure Theory

This theory ascribes autoregulation to purely mechanical events. An increased arterial blood pressure causes greater outward filtration of fluid, which in turn increases tissue pressure and decreases flow. A lowered arterial pressure decreases the outward filtration fluid, which reduces the tissue pressure and hence permits an increased flow. The speed with which the autoregulation phenomenon can produce changes in cerebral circulation would tend to discredit this theory that tissue pressure is a major basis for the control of cerebral blood flow.

Neurogenic Theory

The anatomical basis of this theory rests on the demonstration of perivascular fibers accompanying the cerebral vessels. In the sympathetic system, postganglionic fibers from the stellate and cervical ganglia form the carotid plexus and supply sympathetic fibers to the vertebral and carotid arteries. These nerves have been followed up the internal carotid artery to the circle of Willis and its major branches.[247] Stimulation of the cervical sympathetic fibers causes a vasoconstriction of cerebral vessels and a minor decrease in cerebral blood flow.[255] Stimulation of parasympathetic fibers accompanying cranial nerves causes a mild dilation of the vessels that is of questionable significance in influencing the cerebral blood flow.[43]

Marked increases in cerebral blood flow have been shown with electrical stimulation of the pontine and midbrain reticular formations, the thalamus, and the hypothalamus.[256] Shalit and associates have suggested that a carbon dioxide–sensitive center exists in the brain stem and regulates the cerebrovascular resistance in the hemispheres via a neurogenic mechanism.[352,353] Their evidence for this hypothesis was that an increased oxygen tension in the cerebrospinal fluid caused an increase in cerebral blood flow despite a constant or lowered carbon dioxide level in the arterial blood and that destruction of the upper part of the medulla, the pons, and the lower part of the mesencephalon abolished the usual cerebral blood flow response to changes in arterial P_{CO_2}.

Evidence against a brain stem center regulating cerebral blood flow is provided by Skinhøj and Paulson.[363] They found that regional cerebral blood flow in the cerebral hemispheres was increased when blood in the internal carotid artery had a high carbon dioxide content but was not increased by an equivalent elevation in Pa_{CO_2} in blood traversing the vertebrobasilar system. Further evidence against a carbon dioxide–sensitive center in the brain regulating cerebral blood flow was presented by Kindt and Youmans.[193] They found that blood flow in *each region* of the brain of the monkey was determined by the P_{CO_2} of the blood perfusing *that region*.[193]

Metabolic Theory

This theory implies that the flow passively follows changes in the perfusion pressure and that these changes in flow lead to alteration in the chemistry of the tissue. The change in the concentration of metabolites induces changes in the caliber of the vessels so as to maintain a relatively constant flow.

Whether there is metabolic control of cerebral blood flow or not, there is no question that increased cerebral activity is accompanied by increased blood flow and oxygen consumption. A correlation can be made with the electroencephalogram, which shows an increased wave frequency with increased blood flow and a decreased wave frequency in conditions that cause a reduction in cerebral blood flow and oxygen utilization. The increased blood flow with increased cerebral activity was confirmed in a classic experiment by Schmidt and Hendrix in which they demonstrated increased blood flow in the striate area of the cat when a small spot of the retina was illuminated.[344]

Much controversy has existed regarding the mechanism for metabolic influences on cerebral blood flow. For years the concentration of carbon dioxide was thought to be the central factor. More recently the pH of the extracellular fluid surrounding the vessels has been thought to be more important. According to current hypotheses, the arteries act like a P_{CO_2} electrode.[215] Carbon dioxide diffuses freely around the endothelial membrane, but hydrogen and bicarbonate ions cannot freely cross this membrane. Hence, it is the intravascular carbon dioxide and the extravascular bicarbonate ion that determine the pH around and presumably inside the smooth muscle cells.[101]

This theory agrees rather well with Severinghaus's idea that cerebrovascular resistance is regulated by the pH of the cerebral extracellular fluid. He states,

Since there are no buffers against CO_2 induced acidosis in this fluid, acute alteration of arterial P_{CO_2} produces large pH changes, which result in the observed readjustments of cerebral blood flow. If the P_{CO_2} remains altered, the pH of the extracellular fluid is restored to normal by active transport processes, probably across glial cells to blood. When this corrected pH reaches the pH sensitive sites of the cerebral vessels, vascular resistance returns to its normal value. When P_{CO_2} returns to its normal level, cerebral blood deviates in the opposite direction, until the reverse correction is completed.[350]

The metabolic theory could explain the intense vasodilation or vasoparalysis that occurs in a region that is reperfused after being ischemic.[157,214] Within these areas, the rate of blood flow no longer follows the demand of the depressed metabolism, but rather it exceeds the need. A pathological condition of hyperoxygenation is established with red venous blood.[80,399] This condition of relative hyperemia has been called red cerebral veins or the luxury perfusion syndrome. In this syndrome, the local arterial pressure is close to the systemic level, with marked vasodilation and sometimes absolute hyperemia. The sequel of cerebral ischemia thus brings about an uncoupling of the normal correlation between blood flow and cortical activity. The luxury perfusion syndrome coexists with depressed cortical activity, a slow electroencephalogram, and decreased oxygen uptake.[154]

Very probably it is unwise to attempt to explain the control of cerebral blood flow by a unified hypothesis that relates all cerebrovascular changes to one mechanism. Undoubtedly, tissue pressure, perfusion pressure, tissue acidosis, the inherent reaction of smooth muscle to stretching, the effects of extra-arterial pH, and other mechanisms that are unknown play a role in controlling cerebral blood flow.

It should be stated that although the autoregulation is well accepted and well proved at this time, some animal studies have been reported in which the isolated cerebral circulations in the animals were perfused and a linear relationship between the cerebral blood flow and the systemic blood pressure was observed.[95,331] The operations used in these experiments involved deep barbiturate anesthesia and extensive operative procedures with the risk of cerebral trauma and anoxia, both of which are known to impair the autoregulation phenomenon.

The autoregulation phenomenon accompanies such diverse conditions as hypertension due to toxemia of pregnancy, essential hypertension, and moderate induced hypertension or hypotension, and fails only with marked hypotension.[195,213] Hypoxia, trauma, infarction of cerebral tissue, vasospasm, and many other factors can alter or prevent the autoregulation of flow. When these conditions occur, the element of the variable cerebrovascular resistance is removed and the blood flow varies directly with the pressure. In all conditions except cerebral vasospasm the vessels become dilated.

EFFECT OF COLLATERAL SYSTEM ON FLOW

The collateral circulatory system of the brain involves the collateral anatomical structures and the physiological changes that allow their most effective use in carrying blood. The high metabolic demands of the brain require that the collateral system be immediately available if a catastrophe is to be averted following a significant impairment of the normal cerebral circulation.

The anatomy of the collateral circulatory system undergoes many changes during its embryological development.[298] The constantly changing embryological circulation gradually sets up a system that permits a reasonably adequate collateral blood supply to all vessels except those penetrating into the midline structures of the brain.[178] These channels of collateral blood supply may be divided into two broad categories: one, the vessels normally present in the mature arterial system; and the other, the congenital anomalies.

Congenital Anomalies

Detailed examination of the cerebrovascular system will reveal a high percentage of anomalies.[8,198,269] Most of these either are insignificant or adversely affect the collateral blood supply. A few anomalies do increase the capacity of the collateral circulatory system; however, their degree of effectiveness usually is a matter of mere speculation. A persistent trigeminal artery occurs in about 1 per cent of patients.[410] It is one of the most frequent of the anomalous vessels that may function as a collateral blood supply. Other examples of anomalies that increase the collateral supply are an ascending pharyngeal–vertebral anastomosis, the otic artery, the hypoglossal artery, vertebral–external carotid anastomoses, and abnormal veins that provide unusual connections to the dural sinuses.[178,279]

Normal Collateral Channels

The congenital anomalies that have potential function as collateral channels can be considered clinically only after they have been demonstrated by angiography. Since their capacity is usually a matter of the most gross speculation, it is more rewarding to consider the usual collateral channels of the normal cerebrovascular system. The normal collateral channels may be divided into three groups: the extracranial collaterals, anastomoses between external and internal carotid arterial systems, and intracranial arterial anastomoses.

Extracranial Collaterals

Carotid and Vertebral Arteries

The main extracranial collateral channels consist of the carotid and vertebral arteries in the neck. If the average cerebral circulation is assumed to be 750 ml per minute and the vertebral arteries to carry 10 per cent of the cerebral circulation as suggested by Hardesty and co-workers, then each carotid artery would be carrying approximately 335 ml of blood per minute.[124,321] The potential for immediate marked increase in the amount of flow in a carotid artery after occlusion of the contralateral vessels has been shown in humans and experimental animals when the carotid flow has more than doubled with occlusion of the contralateral carotid.[195,420] Doppler ultrasonic techniques can be used to obtain a general but not a quantitative assessment of the change in flow in the carotid arteries as a result of the need for increased collateral circulation.[40] In normal circumstances, the combined flow in both vertebral arteries is about 75 ml per minute. When needed, the flow in each vertebral artery can more than double. Retrograde flows up to 120 ml per minute have been shown when an acute subclavian steal is produced experimentally.[318]

Ordinarily, the flow in the vertebral and basilar arteries is quite slow in comparison with that in the carotid arteries.[201] This slower flow may be necessary, since many of the arterial branches of the basilar artery that supply the brain stem leave the parent artery at right angles, and according to Bernoulli's principle, a rapid flow in the parent artery would lessen pressure and flow in these branches. Hence, if the vertebral and basilar system is used as a collateral channel and has a rapid flow through it, ischemia of the brain stem could be induced.

External Carotid Artery

The external carotid artery is an excellent source of collateral blood supply after occlusion of the common carotid artery either by disease or an operative procedure. The collateral flow from this source reduces the mortality rate and the serious morbidity associated with occlusion of the common carotid artery as compared with ligation of the internal carotid artery.[16,246,397] With abrupt occlusion of the common carotid artery and the ensuing prompt reduction in the blood supply to the brain, approximately 40 per cent of the patients use, and probably need, the external carotid artery as a source of collateral blood supply.[389] In these patients, a reversal of the direction of flow in the external carotid artery permits blood to continue to flow through the internal carotid artery and to its dependent cerebral hemisphere.[123,423] The value of the contribution of the flow from the external carotid after ligation of the common carotid is shown by the average increase of internal carotid artery back pressure by 21 per cent.[231] The volume of blood coming from the external carotid artery varies widely and apparently on a basis of cerebral need. When there is great need, as after ligation of the common carotid artery in a patient with a carotid cavernous fistula, as much as 180 ml per minute of blood may come from the external carotid to the internal carotid artery immediately after the common carotid artery is ligated.[389] Undoubtedly, the collateral channels over the face and neck can open up even further over a few hours or days and provide a nearly normal blood supply through the internal carotid artery.

Potential Cervical Collateral Channels

The connections between the vertebral and external carotid artery rarely are seen unless a need for collateral circulation has caused them to enlarge.

Normally, no significant collateral circulation exists between the occipital and vertebral or the vertebral and the carotid arteries.[336] The potential for developing these connections exists in the small and normally insignificant vessels that connect each of them.[298,422] The occipitovertebral anastomoses are large enough to be seen in 1 per cent of normal angiograms.[336]

Anastomosis Between External and Internal Carotid Arterial Systems

Ophthalmic Artery

The ophthalmic artery has received much attention as a source of collateral blood supply, particularly since angiography has come into use.[223,268,397] Anatomically, the ophthalmic artery is rather constant.[98] It is small and an immediate source of only a small collateral supply of blood. When the occlusion of the carotid artery develops slowly, however, and there is time for the ophthalmic artery to enlarge, it can become an important source of collateral supply.

Jackson, among others, has emphasized a valuable function of the ophthalmic artery in conjunction with the external carotid artery in maintaining the cerebral blood supply.[164,226] He reported five cases in which the patient had an abrupt onset of symptoms of cerebral ischemia despite the presence of an obviously long-standing occlusion of the internal carotid artery. At operation, there was an acute thrombus in the external carotid artery. Endarterectomy could not be done in the internal carotid artery where the old clot was fibrosed.

After endarterectomy and removal of the fresh clot in the external carotid artery, there was a retrograde flow from the external carotid. Following the endarterectomy of the external carotid artery, the symptoms of cerebral ischemia were relieved in all five of his patients. He postulated that the occlusion of the internal carotid artery was gradual and did not become symptomatic because of the development of a collateral supply from the external carotid artery to the ophthalmic artery. Only with progression of the plaque at the bifurcation of the carotid in the neck, and finally stenosis or occlusion of the external carotid artery, did the patient begin to have symptomatic cerebral ischemia. These observations and their clinical implications probably deserve greater consideration than they have received thus far.

The value of the ophthalmic artery as an immediate source of supply after acute occlusion is limited, and indeed some reports indicate that when it is seen on angiograms in a patient with an acute stroke, the prognosis is worse than if it were not visualized.[306] Most probably, visualization of the ophthalmic artery indicates an inadequate circle of Willis. Thus, a larger area of cerebral infarction will occur than if the circle of Willis were adequate and the ophthalmic artery did not fill on angiography.

Adequate measurements of the flow through the ophthalmic artery of the human have not been made. In the monkey, with both external carotid arteries ligated, the ophthalmic and other branches of the internal carotid artery have been reported to have an average outflow of 10 to 44 per cent of the blood normally carried by the internal carotid artery.[162,254] It would appear that these figures represent capacity and not the usual flow patterns. Under normal conditions, the external carotid artery would supply most of the tissues being perfused by the ophthalmic artery and other branches in the experimental preparations.

Intracranial Arterial Anastomoses

Circle of Willis

The circle of Willis is undoubtedly the most important collateral channel for circulation in the brain. The circle varies considerably, and the definition of normal has to be somewhat arbitrary.[8,88] It may be assumed that the normal circle of Willis is a closed circuit in which fluid may circulate from any point of entrance to make an entire circle and return to that point of entrance with the component vessels being more than 1 mm in outside diameter and with no unusual vessels or unusually placed vessels making up the circle or its adjacent vessels. By this definition, a study of Alpers and associates reveals only 52 per cent of so-called normal brains to have a normal circle of Willis.[8] The abnormalities, such as accessory vessels and anomalous origins (e.g., embryonic origin of posterior cerebral artery) are not of serious consequence since they do not impair the effectiveness of the circle of Willis as a channel of collateral circulation. Twenty-eight per cent of the patients in the group studied by Alpers and associates did have anomalies that would detract from the adequacy of the circle as a channel for collateral circulation. Almost all the abnormalities of this group consisted of a stringlike vessel or absence of a vessel in some part of the circle. It is important to note that although the stringlike areas had a diameter of 1 mm or less, usually they were patent. Presumably, many of these vessels could enlarge over a period of time if the need for their use arose gradually. Certainly, they can be of little or no benefit in giving an immediate response to increased need for collateral supply.

Indeed, the correlation between the abnormalities of the circle of Willis and symptomatic cerebrovascular disease is striking. Undoubtedly, the abnormalities associated with disease contribute to the severity of the ischemia and hence the production of symptoms. The figures on the percentage of abnormalities in the circle of Willis belie the full significance of these lesions as seen in patients with neurovascular problems.[7] Hypoplasia of a part of the anterior portion of the circle of Willis has been reported in as many as 85 per cent of patients with aneurysms of the anterior communicating artery.[408] Further, the incidence of abnormalities of the circle of Willis is significantly increased in patients who have cerebral softening as a result of a cerebrovascular accident.[17,333]

An estimate of the effectiveness of the circle of Willis can be obtained from studies in the monkey.[162] When the internal carotid artery is occluded just above the entrance of the vessel into the cranium, there is an average increase of 19.7 per cent in the flow in the contralateral carotid and vertebral arteries. If these figures were extrapolated to the human, using a carotid artery flow of 335 ml per minute and a vertebral flow of 37 ml per minute, the flow through the circle of Willis would be 82 ml per minute, or an equivalent of 25 per cent of the normal flow through the carotid.[124,321] Most probably this flow represents the need for and not the capacity for flow.

Leptomeningeal Arteries

These arteries were first described by Huebner in 1874.[137] They occur over the cortex and offer a source of collateral blood supply after occlusion of the proximal portions of the major cerebral or cerebellar arteries. Their function and especially their value as a source of collateral blood supply have been the center of much argument and speculation.[356,395] Despite intensive study, their exact contribution to the collateral supply of the cerebral cortex or the underlying tissues is not known.

Vander Eecken and Adams measured the diameters of the anastomotic vessels between the anterior, middle, and posterior cerebral arteries and the cerebellar arteries in 10 normal brains. The aggregate diameter of the anastomotic vessels between the major vessels over the cerebrum ranged from 200 to 610 microns. The aggregate diameter of the anastomotic vessels between the major vessels over the cerebellum varied from 180 to 543 microns. Further, there was a wide variation in the aggregate diameter of the connections between the cerebral arteries in different brains and, hence, a wide variation in the potential collateral blood supply afforded by these channels.[395]

The clinical significance of the variations in the size of the leptomeningeal anastomoses between the major cerebral arteries is confirmed by studies of patients who have thrombosis of the middle cerebral artery. Patients who had a massive infarction of tissue in nearly the entire anatomical area supplied by this vessel had smaller and less numerous anastomotic loops than normal patients or patients who had smaller areas of cortical infarction. The combined diameter of the anastomotic beds between the middle and the anterior and posterior cerebral arteries in patients with the massive infarctions was 3,000 microns or less. In contrast, in the normal brain and in the patients with smaller infarctions, the combined diameter of the anastomotic bed was 3,600 to 4,200 microns. Vander Eecken and Adams note that occlusive lesions of the supply vessel tend to cause greater infarction of the basal ganglia and brain stem than of the cortex. The difference in size of the occlusion is attributed to the fact that the leptomeningeal vessels supply part of the blood needed by the cortex.[395] Thus the infarction of the cortical tissues is not as large as is seen in the deeper structures where arterial anastomoses are absent or so small as to be ineffective.

The monkey has been used to study the effect of the collateral circulation available through these leptomeningeal vessels.[381] In the monkey, occlusion of the middle cerebral artery causes a reduction in vascular pressure within the middle cerebral field to between 10 and 30 mm of mercury. The pressure changes occur in less than five seconds. Obviously, the collateral circulation through the leptomeningeal vessels is inadequate; otherwise, the pressure would be maintained at a higher and more nearly normal level in the field of the occluded vessel.

From experimental studies, it can be inferred that, in the monkey, the blood going from the anterior cerebral artery to the middle cerebral area after occlusion of the middle cerebral artery varies from 1 to 7.5 per cent of that normally carried in one carotid artery.[162] Extrapolation of these figures to the human is only conjecture, but it is of interest to note that on the basis of a carotid flow of 335 ml per minute, the calculated flows would range from 3.5 to 25 ml per minute. If applicable to humans, these variations in the flow rate give added credence to the theory that the size of the cortical infarction after an occlusion of a major cerebral vessel is determined in large part by the capacity of the leptomeningeal collateral circulation of the area.

The flow changes caused by a proximal occlusion of a middle cerebral artery in the monkey take place in about 30 seconds and thereafter there is no appreciable change. Presumably, this means that the collateral channels open immediately in response to changes in blood pressure in the vessels.[20] Although the blood gas levels and the presence of the products of metabolism continue to influence the vessel size of the collateral circulation, the changes are caused first and to the greatest extent by alterations of intraluminal pressure.

When the occlusion of the cerebral vessel progresses slowly, the leptomeningeal collateral circulation has time to increase and extensive collateral circulatory patterns can be developed.[324,346,404] In these circumstances, a proximal portion of a major cerebral vessel may be occluded and a quite adequate circulation be obtained through the leptomeningeal vessels from the adjacent artery's area of circulation.

Penetrating Vessels of Parenchyma of Brain

The anastomoses between the vessels penetrating into the cerebral hemispheres are even less adequate than the small connections between the leptomeningeal vessels.[178] This is unfortunate since the deeper structures are more vital than the cortical structures of the brain. Indeed, the collateral circulation between these deep penetrating vessels in the thalamus, basal ganglion, and brain stem is so meager that for clinical purposes they may be considered to be end-vessels.

Veins

Blood flow from the venous system to the capillary bed of the brain has been suggested by Owens and his colleagues as being another source for collateral blood supply after arterial occlusion.[12,297] He has presented experimental evidence to show that the infarction of the brain in dogs is smaller if the venous pressure is raised prior to occlusion of the middle cerebral artery.[295] In addition, he has used the technique of jugular vein compression to increase cerebral venous pressure in two patients with symptoms of cerebral ischemia with results that were interpreted to be favorable.[296] Although these studies are quite interesting, it would appear safe to say that, at this time, increasing cerebral venous pressure is an unproved technique for producing flow from veins to the cerebral capillary bed or for improving the collateral blood flow to the ischemic area by enlarging the venous outflow system.

Arteriovenous Shunts

Other anatomical structures with a possible effect on the blood supply to the brain are cerebral arteriovenous shunts. These shunts were described a long time ago, but have gained prominence only in the past 20 years.[129] Injection studies by Rowbotham and Little demonstrated the shunts on the cortical surface to be as large as 160 microns.[327] Hasegawa and associates identified two types of shunts in the cerebral parenchyma.[129] One was a "precapillary thoroughfare channel joining arteriole with venule," that is, 8 to 12 microns in diameter. The other was the "simple type of normal arteriovenous ansastomosis" of Liebow.[229] These latter type shunts were 14 to 25 microns in diameter.

Precapillary arteriovenous anastomoses have been found throughout the body and can be an important factor affecting tissue perfusion.[229,235] For example, in some disease states, the lung can shunt over 50 per cent of the cardiac output from the arterial to the venous system.[113] While cerebral shunts have a relatively much smaller capacity, it is quite possible that they are an important factor in such clinical manifestations as a severe neurological deficit associated with cerebral spasm. They may allow blood to go from arteries to veins and make the brain even more ischemic than would the spasm alone. Also, they may be a factor in necrosis of the cortical tissue even when there appears to be a good arterial circulation as judged by brisk bleeding from the cortex or parenchymal cerebral tissue when it is incised. Further, these shunts may help to explain such findings as red blood in the surface veins of an exposed cerebral hemisphere after an epileptic seizure or operative trauma, variations in circulation time such as are seen in cerebral angiography in normal brains, anomalous cerebral blood flow estimations using the Fick principle, and the combination of intracerebral ischemia with rich surface vascularization; and possibly may be one cause of cerebral arteriovenous angiomas.[327,346]

Since these anatomical connections clearly have the capacity to carry blood from the arteries to the veins, they can influence the blood supply of the cerebral tissue in a negative manner, but it is doubtful that they can influence it beneficially. Studies in rhesus monkeys indicate that, although arterial venous shunts are functional, the amount of blood shunted in the brain probably is relatively small.[328]

Time Factors Influencing Collateral Circulation

There is an immediate increase in collateral flow that occurs within 5 to 10 seconds after the need develops.[162,251,381] This change is too rapid to be effected entirely on a humoral or a chemical basis such as a build-up of metabolic products. Undoubtedly, a major part is due to the Bayliss effect secondary to a lowered arterial pressure in the arteriolar system and a decrease in the peripheral vascular resistance. Following the marked increase in collateral blood flow immediately after an acute need arises, there is a progressive but small increase in flow over the first few days, a noticeable leveling out at about five to seven days, a very small change over the next three to four weeks, and thereafter changes too small to be measured.[162,251,368]

Age

Age is a factor in the ability of a patient to withstand trauma and hypoxia. The younger patient's ability to withstand these injuries is coupled with a greater potential for developing collateral circulation. Observations in the rat reveal that injection of growth hormone markedly increases, whereas cortisone markedly lessens, the development of collateral circulation.[248,325] These studies may explain, in part, the greater ability of the young to develop collateral blood flow.

Arterial Pressure

While the capacity of the collateral system is the prime factor in determining the efficacy of the effort to avert a catastrophe due to ischemia, the pressure gradient above and below the obstruction also is very important.[368]

RESPIRATORY GASES AND DRUGS

Carbon Dioxide

Carbon dioxide is the most potent cerebrovascular dilator that is known.[188] It causes a relaxation of the smooth muscles of the arterioles. In turn, the relaxation of the smooth muscle causes a decreased cerebrovascular resistance, which greatly increases the cerebral blood flow.

With a normal cerebrovascular system and a normal blood pressure, even modest alterations in the carbon dioxide tension are capable of markedly altering the cerebral blood flow (Fig. 23–7 A).[125] The change follows the carbon dioxide level rather closely except in the extreme ranges.

Within the range of 30 to 60 mm of mercury, there is a 2.5 per cent change in blood flow as the PCO_2 increases or decreases 1 mm of mercury. Above or below these levels, the effect per millimeter of mercury of PCO_2 is markedly attenuated.[125,301] As the PCO_2 decreases to about 25 mm of mercury the change is no longer linear. There is a pronounced lessening of the change in cerebral blood flow as the carbon dioxide content continues to decrease until at levels of 15 to 18 mm of mercury the flow becomes steady and there is no further effect from a decreasing PCO_2. Likewise at the extreme high levels of 75 to 80 mm of mercury there is a lessening of change with each increment of increased PCO_2, and levels above approximately 80 mm of mercury cause no further increase in cerebral blood flow.

In moderate hypotension, such as 100 mm of mercury of mean arterial blood pressure, changes in the carbon dioxide tension can cause only moderate changes of cere-

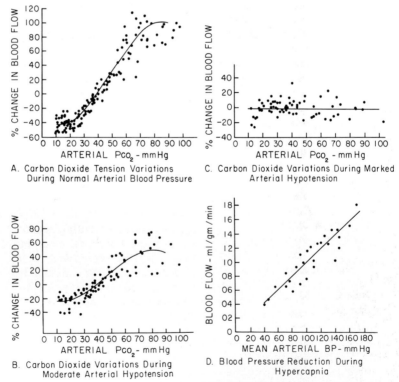

Figure 23–7   Influence of PCO_2 and blood pressure on cerebral blood flow in the canine. *A*. Changes of cerebral blood flow as the PCO_2 is varied during normotension. *B*. PCO_2 is varied during modest hypotension with a mean arterial blood pressure of 100 mm Hg. *C*. The PCO_2 is varied during marked hypotension with a mean arterial pressure of 50 mm Hg. *D*. Changes with alterations of blood pressure during hypercapnia. (From Harper, A. M.: The inter-relationship between aPCO_2 and blood pressure in the regulation of blood flow through the cerebral cortex. Acta Neurol. Scand., *41*:suppl. 14:94–103, 1965. Reprinted by permission.)

bral blood flow (Fig. 23–7B). In frank shock, such as with a mean arterial blood pressure of 50 mm of mercury, changes in the carbon dioxide level have essentially no effect on the cerebral blood flow (Fig. 23–7C). This is true even with PCO_2 in the extreme ranges of 10 to 100 mm of mercury.

When used by the clinician in an attempt to increase cerebral blood flow, 5 to 7 per cent carbon dioxide in oxygen is the gas that is usually used. Inhalation of carbon dioxide at levels of 5 to 7 per cent causes an increase in cerebral blood flow averaging 75 per cent. The cardiac output is not altered significantly. The response is variable; however, there is often an increase in peripheral arterial blood pressure that can be explained by an outpouring of catecholamines from the adrenal glands that is provoked by the carbon dioxide.[348] Thus, indirectly the ventilation with carbon dioxide may cause peripheral vasoconstriction, an effect quite opposite to that exerted on the cerebral circulation. When the PCO_2 is very high the cerebral blood flow is pressure dependent (Fig. 23–7D). When the blood pressure is elevated, a maximal increase in cerebral blood flow is obtained.

The usefulness of inhalation of carbon dioxide in treatment of impending or actual cerebral ischemia has been the subject of controversy for many years. In recent years the procedure has had fewer proponents. As outlined in Table 23–3, the use of carbon dioxide is not the most appropriate means of treating cerebral ischemia. When an area of the brain becomes ischemic, the autoregulation phenomenon causes full re-

laxation of the arterioles of the ischemic area. An elevated carbon dioxide level cannot further enlarge these vessels and thus cannot increase the flow to the area by a further reduction of the cerebrovascular resistance. Only by means of the outpouring of catecholamines and elevation of the arterial blood pressure and, hence, the arterial perfusion pressure, can the increased carbon dioxide tension improve the blood flow to the ischemic area. Obviously the use of vasopressors is a more reliable means of influencing the perfusion pressure than the variable response of catecholamine release due to the elevated PCO_2. Further, there are theoretical reasons to suspect that the use of hypercapnia may have deleterious effects on the blood flow to an ischemic area by creating an intracerebral steal phenomenon, which is discussed later in this chapter.

Caution must be exercised in using carbon dioxide inhalations. Following cessation of carbon dioxide ventilation, blood pressure and cardiac output may fall below preventilation levels and thus cause a posthypercapnic decrease in cerebral blood flow.[48] Also cardiac arrhythmias may follow ventilation with carbon dioxide. Further, since hypercarbia causes systemic and pulmonary arterial blood pressure to rise, special caution must be exercised in patients with systemic or pulmonary hypertension. The increase in cardiac workload during carbon dioxide ventilation could jeopardize the patient with coronary artery disease or congestive heart failure.

Chronic lung disease and other problems creating inadequacy of ventilation may lead to prolonged exposure to elevated carbon dioxide levels. Many factors, including the bicarbonate content of the blood, the oxygen and carbon dioxide dissociation curves, blood calcium, blood potassium, and carbonic anhydrous activity, all combine to aid in adaptation to an elevated PCO_2. Animal studies suggest that there is an adaptation to ventilation with elevated carbon dioxide levels within as few as 14 days.[24]

High levels of carbon dioxide in the inspired air cause discomfort to the awake patient.[348] Levels of 7 to 14 per cent cause the patient to describe the experience as "horrible," "unbearable," "like strangling," or "suffocating." Some patients experience the fear of calamity or a feeling of

TABLE 23–3 EFFECTS OF CARBON DIOXIDE AND BLOOD PRESSURE ON BLOOD FLOW

	CEREBRAL BLOOD FLOW	
	Normal Region of Brain	Ischemic Region of Brain
Elevate Pa_{CO_2} above normal	Increase marked	Steady or may decrease
Elevate BP above normal	Unchanged	Increase marked
Elevate BP plus Pa_{CO_2} above normal	Maximal	Increases, may increase less than with normal Pa_{CO_2}

Pa_{CO_2} is arterial tension of carbon dioxide.
CBF is cerebral blood flow.

impending death. Profuse sweating is common, and severe headaches and auditory and visual hallucinations are not infrequent. At carbon dioxide levels above 80 mm of mercury most patients lose consciousness and may have involuntary movements ranging from tremors and twitching of the fingers to gross movements of the body that require restraint. Plasma concentrations of catecholamines and corticosteroids are increased in every subject during extreme hypercarbia. With moderate hypercapnia, the increase in catecholamines is variable, and this probably explains the variation of response of blood pressure during carbon dioxide ventilation.[348]

A decreased carbon dioxide level produced by active or passive hyperventilation diminishes cerebral blood flow to about one third of the control value.[186] Cardiac output is reduced an average of 11 per cent during passive ventilation, but during active ventilation the cardiac output is maintained by an accompanying tachycardia. Blood pressure is stable or tends to rise slightly. The cerebral arteriovenous oxygen differences invariably increase, with a range of from 41 to 84 per cent and an average of about 58 per cent of the normal values. Cerebral oxygen consumption is consistently and significantly increased during active hyperventilation, with a range 5 to 35 per cent and an average of 15 per cent.[186] The increase in cerebral oxygen consumption during active hyperventilation is attributed to the actual increase in cerebral metabolic activity, since no corresponding change is seen in passive hyperventilation of the same extent. The exact mechanism for the cerebral vasoconstriction resulting from hypocapnia is unresolved. Apparently it is unrelated to arterial pH. With a constant Pco_2, acute change in blood pH has little effect on the cerebral blood flow.[205]

Hyperventilation is frequently used to lower arterial Pco_2. The hyperventilation depletes the entire body of carbon dioxide, and if the patient is abruptly returned to spontaneous hypoventilation he may have apnea or spontaneous hypoventilation. Even with complete apnea, some time may be required for the retained carbon dioxide to restore the total body's content to a normal level. Spontaneous ventilation during the recovery period will cause relative hypoventilation until the body has regained all the carbon dioxide lost during hyperventilation. When the patient is breathing room air, this relative hypoventilation inevitably results in a decrease in alveolar oxygen tension. Animal studies have shown that the alevolar oxygen tension will be as low as 73, 90, and 97 mm of mercury at 10, 30, and 60 minutes after hyperventilation has ceased compared with 101 mm of mercury several hours later.[375]

Following hyperventilation, conscious patients seldom have apnea, although in some instances it does occur in the weak or debilitated.[13,86] It is, however, invariable in patients who have been hyperventilated during general anesthesia.

Since it has been shown that hyperventilation reduces cerebral blood flow, controversy has existed whether cerebral hypoxia is or is not produced. With the frequent use of hypocapnia to reduce brain volume and to improve intracranial exposure for the neurosurgeon, this question has become even more important. An additional question is whether the effects of occlusion or compression of cerebral arteries would be accentuated by the hypocapnia and perhaps even cause infarction, whereas with normocapnia the stress might be sustained with less damage. Studies of the dog by Soloway and associates may give part of the answer.[371] Following occlusion of the middle cerebral artery, infarction was substantially smaller in the hyperventilated animals (6 sq mm) than in the normocarbic animals (15 sq mm), suggesting an apparent protective effect of hyperventilation under these circumstances. Quite obviously the protective effect of the hyperventilation did not result from the decrease in cerebral blood flow. It may be speculated that the presence of ischemia had already maximally dilated the precapillary arterioles and thus increased Pa_{CO_2} could not cause further dilatation.[31] Increase in Pa_{CO_2} would serve only to dilate arteries in the surrounding nonischemic brain and cause a pressure drop in the collateral circulation and decrease in flow through the ischemic cortex. Thus it might be speculated that hyperventilation and hypocarbia might increase flow in the ischemic region by increasing peripheral resistance in the normal brain, thus improving collateral circulation to the ischemic area.

The vascular reactivity to carbon dioxide

is present in all age groups, and there is only gradual reduction of reactivity in the normal aging process.[340] With severe cerebral vascular disease such as arteriosclerosis there is a marked decrease in reactivity to carbon dioxide.

Oxygen

Moderate variations of oxygen tension above and below normal level do not affect the cerebral blood flow. This is probably because the dissociation for oxyhemoglobin is close to horizontal at normal arterial oxygen tensions and causes little change in the arterial blood oxygen and delivery to the brain.

Ventilation with 85 to 100 per cent oxygen for 30 minutes causes a decrease of 13 per cent in the mean cerebral blood flow with no change in cerebral oxygen consumption, carbon dioxide level, or pH of the arterial blood.[188] Cerebrovascular resistance is increased, which indicates that vasoconstriction is the probable mechanism for the reduction of flow. Increasing the arterial P_{O_2} causes constriction of the surface arterioles of a nonischemic brain along with an associated decrease in blood flow. In ischemic cerebral hemispheres, increasing the partial pressure of oxygen has no effect on cerebral blood flow of arterial caliber.

Inhalation of 10 per cent oxygen causes a pronounced fall in arterial oxygen content. The cerebral blood flow increases by 35 per cent despite a significant reduction in the femoral artery arterial pressure.[188] Anoxia of this severity decreases the cerebrovascular resistance to approximately the same degree as inhalation of 5 to 7 per cent carbon dioxide. There is no consistent or significant change in cerebral oxygen consumption. Animal experiments have shown that chronic exposure to 10 per cent oxygen causes cats to have an increased cerebral blood flow for a minimum of one and a maximum of 11 days before response to the lowered oxygen level is lost.[24]

Maintaining a constant arterial carbon dioxide tension and administering only 6.9 to 7.9 per cent oxygen produces a 71 per cent increase in cerebral blood flow.[188] Again there is no change in cerebral oxygen consumption. The glucose metabolism, however, is altered with an increase of glucose uptake and a reduction of aerobic metabolism of glucose.[45] The anaerobic glucose metabolism and lactic acid production is increased. Thus, changes in glucose metabolism appear to be a more sensitive indication of cerebral hypoxia than changes in oxygen consumption. Anaerobic glycolysis yields only one nineteenth as much energy as does the complete oxidation of glucose. Therefore, if the rate of energy production is to remain unchanged, the rate of glucose consumption will be considerably greater than that of oxygen consumption.

With a normal patient, the general circulatory effect of inhalation of 6 to 10 per cent oxygen is a significant increase in cardiac output, which results from an acceleration in the ventricular rate.[188] Despite the increased cardiac output there is a fall in mean arterial blood pressure, which suggests a considerable degree of peripheral vasodilatation.[45]

Inhalation of 10 per cent oxygen causes a degree of hypoxia that results in mental symptoms.[19,45,225] Consciousness is lost when the P_{O_2} of jugular venous blood is around 15 to 20 mm of mercury. The failure to show changes in the oxygen uptake of the brain, except with severe hypoxia, may be related to defects in the measuring technique itself or to some other factor.[213]

Administering oxygen in a hyperbaric chamber causes vasoconstriction and great changes in cerebral blood flow (Table 23–4).[203] The hyperoxic effect may be attenuated somewhat by a concomitant increase in tissue P_{CO_2}. The P_{CO_2} increases as a result of the decreased carbon dioxide absorbing capacity of highly oxygenated capillary blood. Reivich and colleagues demonstrated that the cerebral vasoconstrictor effect of hyperbaric oxygen is present even when it is preceded by hypocarbia.[319]

The mechanisms through which the carbon dioxide levels influence the extremes of cerebral blood flow are unknown. It is, however, reasonable to suggest that during hypoxia the cerebral blood flow increases as a result of anaerobic metabolism and lactic acid and hydrogen ion production by the brain. This hypothesis is supported by the observation that cerebral extracellular fluid hydrogen ion concentration, measured with a pH electrode placed on the surface of the cortex of dogs, decreases progressively as

TABLE 23-4   EFFECTS OF HYPERBARIC OXYGEN ADMINISTRATION ON CEREBRAL BLOOD FLOW

STUDY	SUBJECT	ATMOSPHERES OF OXYGEN	SYSTEMIC ARTERIAL P_{CO_2} (mm Hg)	CEREBRAL OXYGEN CONSUMPTION	DECREASE OF CEREBRAL BLOOD FLOW (%)
Kety and Schmidt*	Man (awake)	1	41	No change	13
Lambertsen et al.†	Man (awake)	1	38	No change	15
		3.5	34	No change	25
Jacobson et al.‡	Dog (anesthetized)	1	38	16% decrease	12
		2	35	38% decrease	21
Reivich et al.§	Man (awake)	2	19	No change	22
		3.5	14.6	No change	27

* The effects of altered arterial tensions of carbon dioxide and oxygen on cerebral blood flow and cerebral oxygen consumption of normal young men. J. Clin. Invest., 27:484–492, 1948.

† Oxygen toxicity: Effects in man of oxygen inhalation at 1 and 3.5 atmospheres upon blood gas transport, cerebral circulation, and cerebral metabolism. J. Appl. Physiol., 5:471–486, 1953.

‡ The effects of O_2 at 1 and 2 atmospheres on the blood flow and oxygen uptake of the cerebral cortex. Surg. Gynec. Obstet., 119:737–742, 1964.

§ Reversal of blood flow through the vertebral artery and its effect on cerebral circulation. The New Eng. J. Med., 265:878–885, 1961.

hypoxemia is maintained.[56] Also, a fourfold increase in cerebral lactate production has been found in healthy human subjects made hypoxic by the inhalation of 6.9 to 7.5 per cent oxygen.[45] At a mean of Pa_{CO_2} of 35 mm of mercury, the amount of glucose taken up by the brain and combined with oxygen decreases by an average of 16 per cent, while the amount of glucose converted to lactate increases by an average of 14 per cent.

Sleep

Cerebral blood flow during sleep varies with the stage of the sleep. Compared with the flow during normal waking state, it is reduced 6 to 14 per cent during slow-wave sleep and increased 3 to 12 per cent during rapid eye movement (REM) sleep.[392] The hypothalamus of research animals has been shown to have a selective increase in blood flow during sleep. Compared with wakefulness, during rapid eye movement sleep the hypothalamic blood flow increases 63 per cent, and during non–rapid eye movement sleep, 25 per cent.[354]

Anesthetics

The effect that any general anesthetic exerts on cerebral blood flow depends upon many factors. If the anesthetic agent reduces cardiac output or total peripheral resistance, then the resultant drop in arterial pressure may alter flow. Central venous pressure may be increased by the anesthetic agent that impairs myocardial contractual force or by the position of the patient on the table, as with the head-down tilt of the operating table or a face-down position with pressure on the thoracic cage. Increasing the central venous pressure effectively reduces the perfusion pressure.[244] If the anesthetic agent causes respiratory depression in a patient who is breathing spontaneously, an increase in Pa_{CO_2} may develop and produce cerebral vasodilatation with a resulting increase in blood flow.

When given in sedative dosages, barbiturates do not alter cerebral blood flow or cerebral metabolic rate.[190] If sleep occurs, however, there is an increase in cerebral blood flow due to a slight rise in P_{CO_2}. During barbiturate anesthesia, the cerebral metabolic rate is reduced approximately in proportion to the depth of the anesthesia, and the cerebral blood flow appears to follow these changes in metabolic rate so that the greatest reduction in flow occurs with the deepest anesthesia.[140] As a result of the reduction of blood flow and the reduction of the metabolic rate, the tensions of oxygen and carbon dioxide in the cerebral vessels are not appreciably altered during barbiturate anesthesia. Also the cerebral vessels retain their sensitivity to changes in arterial P_{CO_2}.

All inhalation anesthetics reduce cerebral metabolism, but the effects are not proportional to the depth of the anesthesia. Rarely is the reduction in the oxygen consumption more than 25 per cent of normal.[414] The leveling off of the effects of inhalation anesthetics at a reduction of about 25 per cent of oxygen consumption is in contrast with the action of barbiturates.[412]

Thiopental is unique among anesthetic drugs in that it is a potent cerebral vasoconstrictor.[304] As a result, it can rapidly reduce intracranial pressure.[355] Further, it has a protective action against the effects of cerebral ischemia.[121,146]

All volatile drugs except perhaps nitrous oxide cause vasodilatation, decrease cerebral vascular resistance, and increase cerebral blood flow.[212,411] Specifically, these changes have been reported for halothane, cyclopropane, chloroform, diethyl ether, trichloroethylene, and methoxyflurane.[3,244] Ketamine given intravenously markedly increases cerebral blood flow by causing vasodilation.[385] Enflurane is an inhalational anesthetic that produces a modest increase in cerebral blood flow.[314]

Dose-response relationships of blood flow to anesthetic concentrations appear to vary according to the depth of anesthesia. There is evidence that very light concentrations of diethyl ether and cyclopropane in man and halothane in the dog produce an initial phase of cerebral vasoconstriction before the vasodilatory effect is encountered at moderate to deep levels of anesthesia.[3,4,412] Chloroform produces a reduction in metabolic rate and an increase in cerebral blood flow ranging from 19 to 62 per cent with the arterial Pco_2 being kept constant. One study has shown that trichloroethylene reduces cerebral oxygen uptake by 20 per cent but does not significantly alter cerebral blood flow.[245]

In most cases the increase in cerebral blood flow that occurs with the volatile agents is compensated for by redistribution of intracranial contents. Unfortunately, however, there is a variability of flow response, and certain patients show a marked rise of cerebrospinal fluid pressure on exposure to the volatile anesthetic drugs.[171] Even a small increase in intracranial pressure may cause harm in a patient with a supratentorial mass lesion. As a result, the difference between the effects of barbiturates and the volatile drugs on the oxygen uptake and cerebral blood flow may be of more than academic interest.

Sodium nitroprusside is often used to lower the systemic blood pressure during craniotomy. Its reported effects on cerebral blood flow are not uniform. Turner and colleagues reported that it caused significant increase in intracranial pressure when the mean arterial pressure was increased moderately.[393] They believe that this was due to an increase in the intracranial blood volume subsequent to cerebral vasodilatation. Ivankovich and co-workers reported that, given to anesthetized and unanesthetized animals in the recommended clinical dose, it produced systemic hypertension but did not significantly alter the cerebral blood flow.[163] In contrast, Crockard and associates noted it to decrease the cerebral blood flow in monkeys by 16 per cent even with only a 5 per cent decrease in mean arterial pressure.[50] In their study, increasing hypertension was associated with a further decrease in cerebral blood flow. Further, these studies have suggested that the evanescent action of nitroprusside produces sudden flucuation in mean arterial pressure, changes which appear to offset the ability of the cerebral circulation to autoregulate its flow. Under these circumstances, sudden alteration in mean arterial pressure, either acute hypotension or acute hypertension, would be associated with significant changes in cerebral blood flow and cerebral volume. These changes are of special significance in the neurosurgical patient. A gradual return to baseline values of arterial pressure at the end of a period of induced hypotension seems advisable, and the prevention of hypertensive episodes in the period immediately after the operation would appear to be desirable.[89] Brown and co-workers showed a small reduction in blood pressure during the administration of nitroprusside, but the cerebral blood flow decreased by 15.9 per cent.[34]

Autoregulation and Carbon Dioxide Tension

With the normal cerebrovascular system the sensitivity to the changes in carbon dioxide level is retained during general anesthesia.[412] Autoregulation of cerebral blood flow is preserved during moderate depths of anesthesia; however, it is impaired by the marked vasodilation that is present during deep anesthesia.[126,367]

The action of anesthetics on abnormal cerebral circulation is complex. The vasodilator effects of most inhalation anesthetics could be expected to dilate the normal portion of the cerebral circulation and thus contribute to an "intracerebral steal" of perfusion from the abnormal portions of the cerebrovascular circulation. This effect probably would be intensified by the anesthetically induced respiratory depression and hypercarbia. Further, any beneficial effects of hypocapnic constriction of normal vessels on the perfusion of ischemic areas would be opposed by anesthetics that dilate the cerebral arterioles. In areas where the autoregulation has been abolished by injury or disease, systemic arterial hypotension, which may be induced by general anesthetics, will reduce the perfusion pressure and thus impair the perfusion of the area. Contrariwise, arterial hypertension during anesthesia may exacerbate cerebral edema formation.

Hyperventilation

Hypocapnic hypoventilation has a profound but probably temporary effect on cerebral blood flow. It produces approximately a 2 per cent decline in flow for each 1 mm of mercury decline in Pa_{CO_2}.[309] This effect appears to be mediated through changes in perivascular pH of the cerebral resistance vessels acting directly on the vessel wall. During prolonged hyperventilation, the blood flow returns toward normal as the pH in the cerebral spinal fluid is restored.

Reduction in the cerebral blood flow by hyperventilation also decreases intracranial pressure. As a result, hyperventilation has been used in the treatment of head injuries with beneficial results in some cases.[51] Since the head injury can abolish cerebral autoregulation, the brain capillaries and veins are exposed to an increased intraluminal pressure that forces fluid into the extracellular space of the brain.[209,347] Hyperventilation has been advocated as a treatment to reduce tissue acidosis, restore autoregulation, and reduce increased intracranial pressure.[173,202]

Cerebral infarction causes a loss of autoregulation in the area affected and in adjacent areas. When generalized vasoconstriction in the brain is produced by hyperventilation, the cerebral blood flow in the affected regions increases at a time when flow elsewhere decreases.[302] Presumably, these paradoxical responses occur because the vessels in the diseased region are maximally dilated and unable to respond to changes in the arterial carbon dioxide tension. As a result, with hypercapnia the resistance in normal vessels falls and blood is shunted away from the ischemic focus, and with hypocapnia the reverse occurs. Some authors have disputed the claim that flow increases in the diseased area following hyperventilation. Meyer and associates observed a reduction of flow in the infarcted hemisphere in all patients during hypoventilation, and on no occasion did they encounter a paradoxical increase in flow. They concluded that hyperventilation should not be used with cerebral infarction because the collateral vessels feeding the ischemic area, although naturally dilated, remained responsive to Pa_{CO_2} and constricted during hyperventilation.[257]

Acute intracranial hypertension is benefited by short-term hyperventilation.[206] This beneficial effect comes from reducing the overall cerebral blood flow. It has been used with hyperventilation to produce arterial carbon dioxide levels of about 15 to 25 mm of mercury during anesthesia for craniotomies. A Pco_2 of 24 mm of mercury will reduce flow through the brain to about 60 per cent of normal. It is generally accepted that under the condition of anesthesia there is not a significant compromise of cerebral oxygenation.[412]

If the Pa_{CO_2} is reduced below 20 mm of mercury, anaerobic metabolism increases and there is an increased conversion of glucose to lactate.[46] Profound hypocarbia produces a marked decrease in cerebral blood flow and a severe alkalosis, which is accompanied by a shift of the oxyhemoglobin dissociation curve. The affinity of oxygen for the hemoglobin is enhanced, and there is less oxygen available for use by the tissues.

Although generally accepted to be safe for the patient, there is still some question about possible untoward effects of prolonged severe hyperventilation, especially in older patients. Doubts about its absolute safety are increased by studies such as those that show a lowered score on the flicker fusion test after hyperventilation.[5] Quite disturbing are the studies by Wollman and Orkin, who tested the preoperative and postoperative reaction time of 37 patients who were hyperventilated during anesthesia for superficial operative procedures.[415] Each patient was anesthetized in a manner that did not alter the cerebral blood flow when the arterial carbon dioxide tension was normal. Hyperventilation was used to reduce the Pa_{CO_2} to levels ranging from 12 to 38 mm of mercury. In 20 patients whose Pa_{CO_2} was 24 mm of mercury or lower, there was prolonged reaction time on a reaction time test. The reaction time of these patients returned to normal in three to six days. Sixteen patients whose Pa_{CO_2} remained above 24 mm of mercury did not have a prolonged reaction time on the test. In the opinion of Wollman and Orkin there were no significant differences in age, sex, duration or type of operative procedure, anesthetic dose, or level of oxygenation in the two groups that could account for the results that they observed. In view of these reports, further controlled studies with physiological and psychometric testing are needed to answer the question completely.

Systemic Drugs

In assessing the action of a drug on cerebral blood flow, great care must be taken to account for changes in levels of the respiratory gases. Many drugs that affect flow do so by altering the respiratory rate and level of consciousness, which in turn alter the carbon dioxide and oxygen content of the blood.

A partial list of the many drugs that have been studied with regard to their effect on blood flow to the brain is given in Table 23–5. Most drugs that alter cerebral blood flow are effective only if given intravenously or intra-arterially. In general, they are effective only during the period of administration or for a very short time thereafter. Stress should be placed on the fact that the results shown in Table 23–5 are transient and not therapeutically useful. In fact, despite great effort being spent in the search, no drug has been found that will give a prolonged and therapeutically useful increase in cerebral blood flow to an ischemic area.

Central nervous system stimulants such as picrotoxin, nikethamide, strychnine, and pentylenetetrazol (Metrazol) in subconvulsive doses do not alter flow.[95,345] With doses that produce convulsions, however, as in epilepsy, the metabolic rate and blood flow are increased markedly.

Reports concerning the catecholamines are conflicting.[92,194] Varying degrees of reduction of cerebral blood flow have been ascribed to direct action on the cerebral vessels or to mild hyperventilation and secondary hypocapnia.[108] Ganglionic blocking agents act mainly on the autonomic ganglia. They produce a peripheral vasodilation that causes the blood pressure to decrease. Cerebral blood flow is unaffected unless the blood pressure falls to shock levels.

Originally, the xanthines were thought to increase cerebral blood flow; however, they have been found to cause mild constriction of the cerebral vessels.[102,364] Peripheral vasodilating agents such as nicotinic acid, cyclandelate, nylidrin (Arlidin), and papaverine have been found to increase cerebral blood flow significantly in laboratory animals, but when they have been used in patients who have cerebral vascular disease, the clinical improvement has been insignificant.[96]

Ethyl alcohol in amounts that produce drowsiness and euphoria does not change the cerebral blood flow or oxygen consumption in normal individuals. The flow is reduced with acute alcoholic intoxication.[18] Some studies of flow in chronic alcoholics have shown normal values.[361] Berglund and Ingvar studied regional blood flow in these patients, however, and found the flow to be reduced in some areas, particularly the temporal lobe in patients over 45 years of age.[22] Interestingly, they found no differences between the alcoholics of the same age who had started drinking excessively while in their 30's or 40's and those who had started earlier. From their studies they concluded:

The reduction of the CBF in the present group of alcoholics was caused by alcohol, since this is the only major factor which could be responsible for these effects in the present patients who lacked a history of brain disorders or serious somatic disease. Since CBF is ultimately regulated by the oxidative metabolism of the neurons, the flow reduction which we have demonstrated most likely represents reduction in cerebral metabolism.[22]

Patients with delirium tremens have a defi-

Text continued on page 813

TABLE 23–5 VASOACTIVE DRUGS AND CEREBRAL BLOOD FLOW

AUTHOR	YEAR PUBLISHED	SUBJECT STUDIED	AGENT STUDIED	METHOD OF ADMINISTRATION	EFFECT DURING OR TRANSIENTLY AFTER ADMINISTRATION
Sympathomimetics					
King et al.[197]	1952	Humans	l-Epinephrine	Intravenous	20% increase of flow
Forbes et al.[92]	1933	Cats	Epinephrine	Topical on pial vessels	Vasoconstriction
Gottstein[102]	1965	Humans	Epinephrine	Intravenous	No significant change of flow
Greenfield and Tindall[108]	1967	Humans	Epinephrine	Intracarotid	No significant change of flow
Fog[91]	1939	Cats	Epinephrine	Topical on pial vessels	Smaller vessels do not constrict ($\downarrow 100\ \mu$) Larger vessels constrict ($\uparrow 100\ \mu$)
Ekstrom-Jodal et al.[70]	1974	Dogs	Noradrenalin	Intravenous	Reduction in flow
MacKenzie et al.[232]	1976	Baboons	Norepinephrine	Intra-cartoid	50% increase in flow
King et al.[197]	1952	Humans	Norepinephrine	Intravenous	8% decrease of flow
Greenfield and Tindall[108]	1967	Humans	Norepinephrine	Intravenous	No significant change of flow
Greenfield and Tindall[108]	1967	Humans	Norepinephrine	Intracarotid	No significant change of flow
Reiss and Rosomoff[316]	1968	Dogs	Nylidrin hydrochloride (Arlidin)	Intravenous or intramuscular	Significant decrease of flow
Winsor et al.[409]	1960	Rabbits	Nylidrin hydrochloride (Arlidin)	Intracarotid	49% increase of flow
Reiss and Rosomoff[316]	1968	Dogs	Isoxsuprine hydrochloride (Vasodilan)	Intravenous or intramuscular	Significant decrease of flow
Ferguson[81]	1956	Humans	Mephentermine (Wyamine)	Intravenous	No significant change of flow
Carey et al.[39]	1969	Dogs	Isoproterenol	Intravenous	70% increase of flow
Moyer et al.[271]	1954	Humans	Metaraminol (Aramine)	Intravenous	9% decrease of flow
Carey et al.[39]	1969	Dogs	Ephedrine	Intravenous	Significant decrease of flow
Carey et al.[39]	1969	Dogs	Phenylephrine (Neo-Synephrine)	Intravenous	Significant decrease of flow
Haggendal[117]	1965	Dogs	Metaraminol (Aramine)	Intravenous 1.5–40 mg/kg	30% decrease of flow
Moyer et al.[271]	1954	Humans	Metaraminol (Aramine)	Intravenous 50 mg/liter	9% decrease of flow
Carey et al.[39]	1969	Dogs	Ephedrine	Intravenous	Significant decrease of flow
Carey et al.[39]	1969	Dogs	Phenylephrine (Neo-synephrine)	Intravenous	Significant decrease of flow
Abreu et al.[1]	1948	Humans	Amphetamine sulfate	Intravenous	20% decrease of flow
Shenkin[357]	1951	Humans	Amphetamine sulfate	Intravenous	No significant change of flow
Dumke and Schmidt[63]	1943	Monkeys	Amphetamine sulfate (Benzedrine)	Intracarotid	Significant decrease of flow
Cholinergic					
Matsuda et al.[242]	1976	Baboons	Acetylcholine	Intravenous	Marked increase in flow
Ganglionic Blocking Agents					
Moyer and Morris[270]	1954	Humans	Hexamethonium	Intravenous	Change of flow related to blood pressure
Moyer and Morris[270]	1954	Humans	Trimethaphan (Arfonad)	Intravenous	Change of flow related to blood pressure
Moyer and Morris[270]	1954	Humans	Azamethonium (Pendiomid)	Intravenous	Change of flow related to blood pressure

Author	Year	Species	Drug	Route	Effect
Ganglionic Stimulating Drug					
Ingenito et al.[153]	1971	Cats	Nicotine hydrochloride	Intraperitoneal	Transient decrease of flow
Miyazaki[206]	1969	Humans	Cigarette smoking (nicotine)	Inhalation	Significant decrease of flow
Skinhøj et al.[366]	1973	Humans	Nicotine	Inhalation and intravenous	Increased flow and decreased arterial venous oxygen difference leaving metabolic rate of oxygen unchanged
Rauwolfia Alkaloid					
Aizawa et al.[2]	1961	Humans	Reserpine	Intravenous and intramuscular	No significant change of flow
Alpha Adrenergic Blocking Agent					
Gottstein[102]	1965	Humans	Tolazoline hydrochloride (Priscoline)	Intravenous	No significant change of flow
Moyer et al.[272]	1954	Humans	Phenoxybenzamine (Dibenzyline)	Intravenous	Change of cerebral blood flow related to blood pressure
Ergot Alkaloids					
Gottstein[102]	1965	Humans	Dihydroergotoxine mesylate (Hydergine)	Intravenous	No significant change of flow
Abreu et al.[1]	1948	Humans	Dihydroergotamine	Intravenous	No significant change of flow
Antihypertensive Drugs					
Hydralazine					
Hafkenschiel[115]	1953	Humans with hypertension	1-Hydrazinophthalazine (Apresoline)	Intramuscular	No significant change of flow
Veratrum Alkaloids					
Aizawa et al.[2]	1961	Humans	Veratrum viride	Intravenous	No significant change of flow
Vasodilator Drugs					
Gottstein[102]	1965	Humans	Nicotinic acid (Ronicol)	Intravenous	No significant change of flow
Aizawa et al.[2]	1961	Humans	Nicotinic acid	Intravenous	No significant change of flow
O'Brien and Veal[286]	1966	Humans	Cyclandelate (Cyclospasmol)	Oral	Significant increase of flow
Géraud et al.[96]	1965	Humans with CVD	CAA 40	Intravenous	No significant change of flow
Gottstein[102]	1965	Humans	Papaverine	Intravenous	10% increase of flow
Autacoids					
Shenkin[357]	1951	Humans	Histamine	Intravenous	Change of cerebral blood flow related to blood pressure
Dumke and Schmidt[63]	1943	Monkeys	Histamine	Intracarotid	Significant increase of flow
Karlsberg et al.[180]	1953	Monkeys	5-Hydroxytryptamine (serotonin)	Intracarotid	Vasoconstriction
Polypeptide					
Greenfield and Tindall[108]	1967	Humans	Angiotensin amide (Hypertensin)	Intravenous or intracarotid	No significant change of flow
Greenfield and Tindall[108]	1967	Humans	Angiotensin amide (Hypertensin)	Intracarotid	No significant change of flow

Table continued on following page

TABLE 23–5 VASOACTIVE DRUGS AND CEREBRAL BLOOD FLOW (*Continued*)

AUTHOR	YEAR PUBLISHED	SUBJECT STUDIED	AGENT STUDIED	METHOD OF ADMINISTRATION	EFFECT DURING OR TRANSIENTLY AFTER ADMINISTRATION
Carbonic Anhydrase Inhibitor					
Kong et al.[200]	1969	Dogs	Acetazolamide (Diamox)	Intravenous	36% increase of flow
Local Anesthetic					
Scheinberg et al.[338]	1952	Humans	Procaine	Intravenous	No significant change of flow
Aliphatic Alcohols					
Battey et al.[19]	1952	Humans	Methyl alcohol (poisoning)	Oral	28% decrease of flow
Battey et al.[19]	1952	Humans	Ethyl alcohol (delirium tremens intoxication)	Oral	32% decrease of flow
Battey et al.[19]	1952	Humans	Ethyl alcohol	Intravenous	No significant change of flow
Central Nervous System Stimulating Drugs					
Xanthines					
Gottstein[102]	1965	Humans	Caffeine	Intravenous	14% decrease of flow
Skinhøj and Paulson[364]	1970	Humans	Aminophylline	Intravenous	Vasoconstriction of normal vessels. Increased flow in cerebrovascular disease
Gottstein and Paulsen[104]	1972	Humans	Aminophylline	Intracarotid	Significant decrease in flow
Magnussen and Hoedt-Rasmussen[236]	1977	Humans	Aminophylline	Intracarotid	21.9% decrease in flow
Gottstein[102]	1965	Humans	Aminophylline	Intravenous	11% decrease of flow
Gottstein[102]	1965	Humans	Theophylline (KGG 158)	Intravenous	7% decrease of flow
Dumke and Schmidt[63]	1943	Monkeys	Theophylline	Intracarotid	Significant increase of flow
Gottstein et al.[105]	1972	Humans	Theophylline	Intravenous	Decrease in flow
Stimulants					
Aizawa et al.[2]	1961	Humans	Methylphenidate hydrochloride (Ritalin)	Oral	Minor increase of flow
Aizawa et al.[2]	1961	Humans	Pentylenetetrazol + nicotinic acid	Oral	No significant change of flow
Schmidt et al.[345]	1945	Monkeys	Pentylenetetrazol (Metrazol)	Intravenous and intra-arterial	No significant change of flow
Schmidt et al.[345]	1945	Monkeys	Picrotoxin	Intra-arterial	No significant change of flow

Reference	Year	Species	Agent	Route	Effect
Schmidt et al.[345]	1945	Monkeys	Nikethamide (Coramine)	Intra-arterial	No significant change of flow
Geiger and Magnes[95]	1947	Cats	Strychnine	Intra-arterial	No significant change of flow
Hormones					
Forbes et al.[92]	1933	Cats	Vasopressin (Pitressin)	Topical on pial vessels or intravenous	Vasodilatation
Dumke and Schmidt[63]	1943	Monkeys	Posterior pituitary extract	Intra-arterial	Change of cerebral blood flow related to blood pressure
Schieve et al.[342]	1951	Humans	Adrenocorticotrophic hormone (ACTH)	Intramuscular	18% decrease of cerebral blood flow
Agents Affecting Volume and Composition of Body Fluids					
Gottstein and Held[103]	1969	Humans	Rheomacrodex	Intravenous	43% increase of flow
Gottstein and Held[103]	1969	Humans	Macrodex	Intravenous	22% increase of flow
Gottstein and Held[103]	1969	Humans	0.9% saline solution	Intravenous	No significant change of flow
Ulano et al.[394]	1970	Dogs	3–6% saline solution	Intracarotid	Transient decrease in flow for 15 sec followed by increase in flow for average of 4 min.
Shalit[351]	1974	Cats	Mannitol	Intracarotid	Transient increase in regional flow
Johnston and Harper[172]	1973	Baboons	Mannitol	Intravenous	Transient increase in flow
Schieve and Wilson[341]	1953	Humans	0.9% saline solution	Intravenous	No significant change of flow
Schieve and Wilson[341]	1953	Humans	2% saline solution	Intravenous	10% increase of flow statistically not significant
Schieve and Wilson[341]	1953	Humans	1.2% sodium bicarbonate	Intravenous	30% increase of flow
Schieve and Wilson[341]	1953	Humans	3% sodium bicarbonate	Intravenous	65% increase of flow
Schieve and Wilson[341]	1953	Humans	0.8% ammonium chloride	Intravenous	20–25% decrease of flow
Opiates					
Abreu et al.[1]	1948	Humans	Methadone hydrochloride (Dolophine)	Intravenous	No significant change of flow
Moyer et al.[273]	1957	Humans	Morphine	Intravenous	No significant change of flow
Opioid Antagonist					
Moyer et al.[273]	1957	Humans	n-Allylnormorphine (Nalline)	Intravenous	No significant change of flow
Group B Vitamins					
Aizawa et al.[2]	1961	Humans	Thiamine (vitamine B₁), cocarboxylase, thioctic acid, pangamic acid, nicotinic acid, nicotinamide, pantothenic acid, and orotic acid	Intravenous	No significant change of flow

Table continued on following page

TABLE 23–5 VASOACTIVE DRUGS AND CEREBRAL BLOOD FLOW (Continued)

AUTHOR	YEAR PUBLISHED	SUBJECT STUDIED	AGENT STUDIED	METHOD OF ADMINISTRATION	EFFECT DURING OR TRANSIENTLY AFTER ADMINISTRATION
Radiographic Contrast Media					
Ulano et al.[394]	1970	Dogs	Meglumine iothalamate (Conray 60%)	Intracarotid	23% increase of flow for average of 2 min
Ulano et al.[394]	1970	Dogs	Methylglucamine diatr-zoate (Renografin 60%)	Intracarotid	30% increase of flow for average of 2 min
Tindall et al.[388]	1965	Humans	Sodium diatrizoate (Hypaque 50%)	Intracarotid	50% increase of flow for average of 2 min
Ulano et al.[394]	1970	Dogs	Sodium acetrizoate (Urokon 70%)	Intracarotid	80% increase of flow for average of 10 min
Kagstrom et al.[176]	1958	Cats	Sodium acetrizoate (Triurol)	Intracarotid	100–300% increase of flow for average of 10 min
Ingvar and Soderberg[156]	1957	Cats	Umbradil	Intracarotid	10–25% decrease of flow
Tranquilizers					
Aizawa et al.[2]	1961	Humans	Chlorpromazine	Intramuscular and intravenous	No significant change of flow
Miscellaneous					
Aizawa et al.[2]	1961	Humans	ATP + 40% glucose	Intravenous	Increase of flow
Aizawa et al.[2]	1961	Humans	ATP + saline	Intravenous	No significant change of flow
Aizawa et al.[2]	1961	Humans	Gamma-amino butyric acid	Oral	No significant change of flow
Aizawa et al.[2]	1961	Humans	Pipradol	Oral	No significant change of flow
Aizawa et al.[2]	1961	Humans	Dimethylamino ethanol	Oral	No significant change of flow
Buyniski and Rapela[37]	1969	Dogs	Adenosine	Intravenous and intracarotid	No significant change of flow
Prostaglandins					
Yamamoto et al.[417]	1972	Dogs	Prostaglandins E_1	Intracarotid	Marked reduction in flow
Yamamoto, et al.[418]	1972	Dogs	Prostaglandins E	Intracarotid	42% decrease
Nakano et al.[276]	1973	Dogs	Prostaglandins F_{2a}	Intracarotid	E_1, E_2, A_1, and A_2 increase in flow
			Prostaglandins E_1 E_2, A_1, A_2, F_{2a}		F_{2a} decrease in flow
Biogenic Amines					
Welch et al.[403]	1973	Baboons	Serotonin	Intracarotid	Marked reduction in flow
von Essen[396]	1974	Dogs	Dopamine	Intravenous	Decrease in flow
Ekstrum-Jodal[71]	1974	Dogs	L-Dopa L-Tryptophan	Intravenous	Initial increase and then decrease in flow

nite change from normal, with a blood flow as low as 34 ml per gram per minute and an oxygen consumption as low as 2.4 ml per gram of brain per minute compared with normal values of 50 ml and 3.1 ml respectively.[19] Methyl alcohol poisoning gives acute changes of blood flow and oxygen metabolism at about the same levels as just given for delirium tremens. As the patient recovers from the acute phase of methanol poisoning, he may have a period of increased cerebral blood flow.

Radiographic Contrast Agents

These drugs are hypertonic. They produce a transient vasoconstriction, which is followed by vasodilatation that lasts about five minutes.[388,394] Sodium acetrizoate (Urokon) has the maximal effect and may increase flow as much as 80 per cent for about 10 minutes.

Infusions

The isotonic solutions do not affect cerebral blood flow. Hypertonic solutions such as 3 to 6 per cent solutions of saline provoke vasodilatation and increased flow when injected intracarotidly or intravenously.[341]

Low molecular weight dextran frequently is used in neurological surgery to improve the rheological characteristics of the blood. It is a nonionic substance that plates the surface of the red blood cells and platelets. By this plating action, it decreases the tendency of the red blood cells to sludge and aggregate in the microvasculature.[405] It also aids in keeping the platelets suspended and reduces prothrombin activation.[62,349] As a result, prothrombin consumption and clot retraction are delayed in the presence of dextran.

When dextran is administered after occlusion of a small cerebral vessel in research animals, the cellular aggregates in the area of the occlusion become smaller and gradually begin to move with increasing speed.[27] Infusion of low molecular weight dextran before an artery is occluded markedly decreases the vascular stasis and sludging of cells in the area of the occlusion and decreases the size of the infarction.[286] After an acute occlusion of the femoral artery of the hind limb of a dog, Dextran-40

has been shown to give a 182 per cent increase in the backflow from the vessel distal to the occlusion.[322] Blood or saline infusion had little effect in the same preparation. In long-term preparations the Dextran-40 had less effect than it did immediately after occlusion, but still it gave significant increases in the backflow from the vessel distal to the occlusion. These effects of dextran are attributed to changes in the rheological qualities of the blood and the vasodilation that are produced.[322]

Patients treated with Dextran-40 have been reported to show a lower mortality rate and to have a better quality of survival following cerebral infarction due to thromboembolism.[99] Finally, it appears that this agent might be of value to patients with ruptured aneurysms accompanied by cerebral vasospasm and other neurological conditions in which stasis and sludging of blood in the microvasculature is a problem.

DISEASE AND ABNORMAL CONDITIONS

Cerebrovascular Disease

Acute focal cerebrovascular lesions of the brain usually are secondary to thrombosis, embolism, or hemorrhage. Often the lesion causes occlusion or spasm of the artery. Distal to the site of the lesion, there is an immediate drop in pressure, and vasodilatation occurs within the ischemic area. The efficacy of the collateral circulation determines whether an infarction of cerebral tissue will occur. If the collateral circulation is severely deficient, the cerebral oxygen level begins to fall in about 10 seconds. Hypoxia with neuronal death follows immediately. The decreasing P_{O_2} and increasing P_{CO_2} both act to cause vasodilatation.

Aging of Vessel Walls

The larger arteries have a variable pulse pressure and a variable pulse volume with each heartbeat. The elastic wall of the normal artery absorbs part of the energy of each heartbeat. This action makes the flow of blood more smooth and steady than it would be if the artery were rigid.

With aging and loss of arterial elasticity, the arteries gradually become more rigid.

Thus, the older, more rigid wall is more and more exposed to the pulsatile pressure-thrust-flow phenomenon. The result is that the extremely rigid arterial wall is subjected to much greater hydraulic forces than the resilient arterial wall. Without the smoothing effect of the elastic action of the healthy arterial wall, the briskness of the pressure changes with each heartbeat causes the flow to become quite turbulent.

As the elasticity of the arterial tube is lost, the tube lengthens and often increases in diameter. The arch of the aorta may be displaced upward, with the cervical vessels being uplifted. The primary changes of aging together with the uplifting of the aortic arch may cause increased curves and kinks in the carotid, vertebral, and basilar arteries (Fig. 23–8). Bifurcation angles of the branches are less acute and more obtuse. Such changes in the arteries lead to increased vascular resistance and slowing of cerebral circulation as shown by high speed angiocinematography.[68] The arteriosclerotic kinking or curving of vessels causes a dynamic lesion that is variable during diastole and systole. The extreme thrust of the arterial flow during systole increases the deformity and can cause significant effects

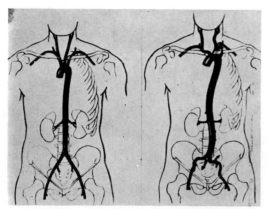

Figure 23–8   The course of the major trunk arteries while they retain full elasticity (*left*), and after the loss of elasticity due to age (*right*). The aorta and its branches increase in length and diameter as their elasticity is lost. The course becomes meandering, a phenomenon that occurs particularly at the branches of the arch of the aorta. Synchronous movements occur with the pulse, and kinking occurs. (From Eichhorn, O., and Schlict, L.: The importance of hydraulic principles in the regulation of cerebral blood flow. *In* Meyer, J. S., Lechner, H. and Eichhorn, O., eds.: Research on the Cerebral Circulation, Int'l Salzburg Conference, 1966, Springfield, Ill., Charles C Thomas, 1969, pp. 332–346. Reprinted by permission.)

on the circulation. Arterial pressure recordings above and below carotid loops have shown a diminution in pressure above the loop of as much as one third of the base pressure during systole.[68] The pressure curve below the loop is dicrotic, whereas above the loop it is more sinusoidal.

Evaluation of the effects of these lesions is most difficult, and great caution should be exercised in attributing cerebral ischemia to them. However, if functional disturbances occur that cannot be explained on any other basis, then the operative correction may be worthy of consideration.[320]

Stenosis of Vessel

Local constriction of an artery causes little change in blood flow until a marked and critical degree of stenosis is reached.[238] Thereafter, further reduction in lumen size beyond the critical stenosis rapidly reduces flow and distal blood pressure. The length of the stenosed area influences the point of critical stenosis.[194] A longer area of stenosis, such as that seen with a long arteriosclerotic plaque, will reach the point of critical stenosis with a smaller decrease in the lumen of the vessel than would be required by a very short plaque. Figure 23–9 shows the change in the point of critical stenosis as the length of the stenosed area is increased from 0.1 cm to 8 cm.

A 70 per cent decrease in diameter and a 90 per cent reduction in cross-sectional area is widely accepted as the degree of stenosis that causes significant clinical problems.[420] If the stenosed area is short, this level of stenosis causes about a 50 per cent reduction of flow.[238]

The effect of a stenotic lesion is influenced by the presence or absence of disease in other vessels.[195,419,420] A stenotic lesion in the collateral circulatory system results in an immediate compensatory increase in flow in the remaining vessels.[381] The increase in flow is secondary to a decreased cerebrovascular resistance and, hence, a greater perfusion gradient. As shown in Figure 23–10, a given amount of stenosis causes a greater change in blood flow when the collateral channels are impaired than when they are normal. This is explained by the fact that when the collateral channels are impaired, a larger and faster flow goes through the vessel in question. As the flow rate increases, turbulence and

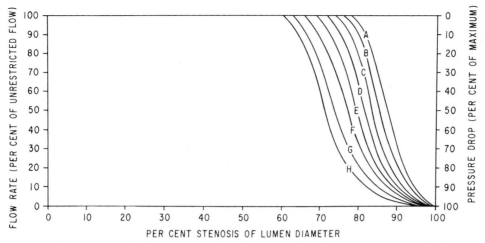

Figure 23-9 Composite graph demonstrating the changes in blood flow and pressure reduction associated with a reduction in the diameter of strictures of various lengths. Note that no change in blood flow or pressure occurs until the constriction increases beyond 60 per cent occlusion, which is the critical arterial stenosis for an 8-cm stricture. A, 0.1-cm length; B, 0.5-cm length; C, 1-cm length; D, 2-cm length; E, 3-cm length; F, 4-cm length; G, 6-cm length; H, 8-cm length. (From Kindt, G., and Youmans, J.: The effect of stricture length on critical arterial stenosis. Surg. Gynec. Obstet., *128:*732, 1969. Reprinted by permission.)

energy loss increases at the point of stenosis. As a result, there is a greater effect by the stenotic lesion than if the collateral channels were open.

Kinks and Coils

Kinking and coiling of the internal carotid artery is thought to lead to cerebrovascular ischemia, but indisputable evidence for this supposition is lacking.[59,334] Coiling of the artery is of embryological origin, whereas kinking or buckling is associated with atherosclerosis. Sarkari reported nine infants with cerebral vascular disease who exhibited unilateral or bilateral looping or kinking.[334] He theorized that the vascular anomaly was responsible for the hemiplegia suffered by these children and he suggested operative correction. These severe neurological deficits in the children that he reported were difficult to explain. Since no pathological studies of the vessels were made, the presence or absence of emboli could not be ascertained. It is possible, however, that a combination of events such

Figure 23-10 Study of the monkey showing carotid artery blood flow during gradual occlusion with the collateral arteries patent and with the collateral arteries occluded. Note that at approximately 87 per cent constriction of the artery there is a 50 per cent reduction in blood flow with the collaterals patent and a 62 per cent reduction with the collaterals impaired. (From Youmans, J., and Kindt, G.: Influence of multiple vessel impairment on carotid blood flow in the monkey. J. Neurosurg., *29*:136, 1968. Reprinted by permission.)

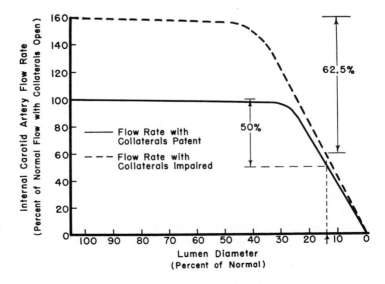

as an obstruction of the neck, neck rotation, and a microembolus could have been responsible for the cerebral ischemia and hemiplegia. Others have reported hemiparesis in children, some of whom were treated by operation on the carotid artery with clinical improvement.[299] Kinking and coiling of the carotid artery has been associated with ischemic vascular disease in adults, but with even less sure correlation as to the etiology.[58,128,308] Again, the results of operative treatment have not been conclusive.

Occlusive Disease

Angiographic evidence indicates that many occlusive processes are transitory.[53] This may be due to disintegration of the thrombus or emboli, or bypassing of the lesion by the collateral circulation. It appears likely that the occlusive process often disappears and hyperperfusion is established in the dilated network of vessels distal to the lesion.

If the ischemic process continues, irreversible metabolic changes occur with an increase of lactic acid and a rapid decrease of energy-rich phosphates.[368] Within minutes, the acid-base milieu is changed within the ischemic region, and a long period of tissue acidosis mainly due to intracellular and extracellular lactic acid production supervenes.[216] The acid metabolites have a vasodilatory action and are less diffusible than carbon dioxide, which normally plays a major role in regulating the cerebrovascular tone. These acid metabolites appear to be responsible for the prolonged states of vasodilatation that may follow even brief periods of cerebral ischemia or anoxia.

Blood flow and oxygen metabolism of the hemisphere with the vascular lesion are reduced in all patients, but the reduction is greater in patients with angiographic evidence of vascular occlusion.[258] Lesions that appear clinically and radiologically to be focal often demonstrate a general reduction of cerebral blood flow that may even involve the healthy hemisphere.[53,69,144] Possibly, the remote effects of the focal lesion, that is, the reduction of cerebral function at a distance from the actual focus, may be caused by interruptions of neural connections. A global depression of all cerebral functions with permanent coma may occur following a lesion of the reticular system.

Usually this condition is accompanied by a marked reduction of cerebral blood flow and decreased metabolism.[160]

Patients with cerebral atherosclerosis have a moderate but definite reduction in cerebral blood flow.[131] In addition, they usually have low cardiac output, low total blood volume, increased systemic and cerebral vascular resistance, and a prolonged circulation time throughout the entire circulatory system. These circumstances considerably reduce the margin of safety that is enjoyed by a normal patient. Even slight changes in any of these factors may be enough to precipitate symptoms of cerebral ischemia. The arteriogram is valuable in assessing the status of occlusive disease of the neck and head; however, regional cerebral blood flow has an even better correlation with the presence or absence of symptoms of cerebral ischemia.

Cerebral Infarction

Acute unilateral cerebral infarction reduces the hemispheric blood flow and metabolism in the healthy hemisphere as well as in the hemisphere with the infarction. This finding is present in patients of all ages. In younger patients, the blood flow and metabolism of the healthy hemisphere show a marked increase within three weeks and approach normal in the ensuing months. In contrast, these values remain depressed in the uninfarcted hemisphere of older patients, probably reflecting diffuse as well as focal cerebral vascular disease. The outcome of the infarction or ischemic attack correlates with the reduction in hemispheric blood flow at the time of the attack. As would be expected, the patients who have a severe permanent neurological deficit have a greater reduction of blood flow than those who have a transient ischemic attack or a prolonged but reversible neurological deficit.

The reduction in regional cerebral blood flow in the hemisphere contralateral to an infarction is uniform in all patients and varies from a mean of 30 to 47 per cent.[221] The depression in the flow is not related to cerebral dominance, previous hypertension, or arterial carbon dioxide levels. Also, it occurs both in patients who are fully alert and in those who have lowering of consciousness, but it tends to be more diminished in the latter group. Apparently, the flow reduction in the nonaffected hemisphere is a part of a general phenomenon that affects the entire brain and is caused by globally reduced cerebral metabolism.

Symptoms of cerebral ischemia and electroencephalographic abnormalities appear when cerebral venous oxygen levels reach 20 mm of mercury.[339] If blood flow is restored within minutes, brain function recovers rapidly. If regional cerebral blood flow is below 18 to 20 ml per 100 gm brain per minute for five minutes or longer, cerebral infarction with permanent neurological deficit is likely to ensue.[10,28,30] This risk is incurred regardless of whether the ischemia is caused by clamping of the carotid artery during an operation or secondary to head injury or intracranial disease. Except in the unusual case of reactive hyperemia or so-called "luxury perfusion" that results from early lysis of emboli or thrombi, patients with recent cerebral infarction have reduced flow in the territory supplied by the vessel and bordering areas of relative hypermia.[84,104,145] In most patients the severity of the reduction of regional blood flow correlates well with the anatomical position of the lesion as determined clinically and by laboratory studies.

The susceptibility of the brain to anoxia is considered to be the limiting factor for resuscitation after transient circulatory arrest. Classic experiments have shown that the upper limit for full recovery is 3 to 4 minutes of circulatory arrest and 8 to 10 minutes of isolated cerebral vascular arrest.[109,141,142,175] Because of the close correlation between the depletion of energy-rich phosphates and irreversibility of brain damage, the high sensitivity of the central nervous tissue to ischemia has been attributed to low reserve in substrates suitable for anaerobic energy metabolism.[312] The time limits for recovery after circulatory arrest are not absolute. Under suitable conditions the nerve cells may survive extended periods of ischemia. For instance, Neely and Youmans had dogs that survived complete arrest of cerebral blood flow secondary to markedly increased intracranial pressure for periods of up to 30 minutes and recovered the ability to eat, stand, and walk within 24 hours.[277] Other investigators have shown in a series of experiments that every function returned to normal in at least a few animals after an hour of normothermic ischemia, but not all functions were fully re-

stored in any one animal.[148] Curiously, the brain seems to survive better when it has total circulatory arrest or is perfused with saline rather than being perfused with severely hypoxic blood that is laden with waste products of metabolism. Hossmann and Kleihues detected no evidence of histological damage after up to 30 minutes when the animals were perfused with saline.[148] Quite probably, the recovery of the animals in the studies of Neely and Youmans and Hossmann and Kleihues was related to the fact that the blood was largely or completely removed from the cerebral vessels during the time of the ischemia, and intravascular clotting was decreased. As a result, the recirculation of blood was less impeded.

Autoregulation is impaired by ischemic strokes. There is a significant correlation between the degree of dysautoregulation and an increase in the cerebral perfusion pressure.[361] An inverse correlation is shown between the degree of dysautoregulation and the duration of the ischemic episode during both hypotension and hypertension. Patients with brain stem lesions, including those with transient ischemic attacks, have a greater impairment of autoregulation than patients with hemispheric lesions. Also, the impairment lasts longer in patients with brain stem lesions.

Conventional wisdom has been that hypertensive episodes cause infarction in the brain. A study by Torvik and Skullerud of patients who were resuscitated after cardiac arrest and died from one to several weeks later revealed that only 5 per cent of the patients had brain infarcts that were probably caused by hypotensive episodes during or after the resuscitation.[391] There was almost no increase in the frequency of recent brain infarctions with an increasing degree of cerebral arteriosclerosis. In contrast, the distribution of old brain infarctions showed a significant correlation with the degree of cerebral arteriosclerosis. They interpreted these findings to suggest that the combination of cerebral arteriosclerotic stenosis and hypertensive episodes is not a major cause of brain infarction in elderly people. Further, they believe that the risk of precipitating brain infarction by lowering blood pressure in hypertensive patients is not much greater in arteriosclerotic than in nonarteriosclerotic patients.

Both hemorrhagic and ischemic infarctions cause reduction of regional cerebral blood flow in the area of infarction. A method of treatment that needs further study is the infusion of glycerol, which has been shown to redistribute blood from the hyperemic areas adjacent to the ischemic areas.[293]

The blood viscosity is increased in patients with recent cerebral infarction.[292] This is true despite the fact that the hematocrit values are normal and, thus, not a reliable guide to the viscosity levels. The increase in blood viscosity may be accounted for by excessive agglutination of red blood cells and elevation of concentrations of lipids or fibrinogen or both.*

Carbon Dioxide

In cats, inhalation of carbon dioxide has no effect on cerebral blood flow in an area made ischemic by occlusion of major vessels.[310] It does cause constriction of the arterioles and decreased regional flow in the nonischemic areas.

Hyperbaric Oxygen

Hyperbaric oxygenation at 2 atm causes an increase in arterial oxygen tension to 1227 mm of mercury and a reduction of intracranial pressure of 30 per cent in dogs that have been exposed to cerebral cold injury.[261] Hyperbaric oxygenation at 3 atm causes arterial oxygen tension to increase to 1891 mm of mercury but fails to reduce intracranial pressure. Apparently, the effect of hyperbaric oxygenation in experimental intracranial hypertension is dependent on the vasoconstrictor tone of the cerebral vessels.[177,275] At least these studies show that when the vessels are no longer responsive to changes in carbon dioxide, reduction of intracranial pressure with hyperbaric oxygenation is also lacking. In human subjects, hyperbaric oxygenation at 2 atm caused a marked reduction of blood flow in the common and internal carotid arteries, but little change in the vertebral arteries.[177] The decreased flow in the carotid areas undoubtedly is responsible for reduction of intracranial pressure that accompanies hyperbaric oxygenation. This reduction in intracranial pressure has been used

in treatment of head injuries and other conditions, but without conclusive results.

Hemorrhagic Disease and Vasospasm

Subarachnoid hemorrhage causes a decrease in the regional cerebral blood flow of the brain near the site of rupture.[133] There is a general correlation between the decrease in flow and the severity of the neurological deficits. Patients with diffuse vasospasm of a severe grade have focal areas of decreased flow to below 30 ml per 100 gm per minute in addition to a reduction of mean cerebral blood flow.[161] Patients with a severe neurological deficit and marked diffuse vasospasm have an increase in regional cerebral blood volume despite the decreased flow.[110] This finding is thought to be due to a massive dilatation of intraparenchymal vessels at the same time that there is a constriction of the large vessels that is visible on the angiogram. The relief of disappearance of vasospasm on the angiogram is followed by an increase in the regional cerebral blood flow in the ischemic focus and a mean increase in the total cerebral blood flow.[161]

The correlation between the presence or absence of spasm on the arteriogram and the clinical condition of the patient is not close in all instances. Indeed, in some series there is no correlation between the existence of spasm and the outcome of treatment. The dynamic brain scan correlates better with the eventual outcome of treatment than the presence or absence of spasm on the arteriogram. As a result, it is suggested that patients in grades I or II neurological condition with normal dynamic scans be operated on early to prevent rebleeding and that patients in grades I or II with abnormal dynamic scans have the operation delayed until the scans return to normal.[183] Nilsson found that alterations in blood flow seemed to precede the change in the patient's clinical condition. Further, he found that the incidence of death or severe morbidity following operative treatment for aneurysm correlated with the preoperative blood flow. With a normal or only slightly disturbed cerebral blood flow in the preoperative period, the rate of death or severe morbidity following operative treatment was estimated at about 8 per cent. With patients who have a preoperative blood flow reduction of more than 40 per cent, the

---

* See references, 55, 60, 130, 252, 285, 377, 405.

morbidity and mortality rates were in the range of about 30 per cent. He suggested that the status of the cerebral blood flow was a diagnostic parameter of great clinical significance and could be used to predict the probable outcome of operative treatment of intracranial aneurysm.[280]

There is dispute concerning the correlation of cerebral vasospasm with the patient's clinical condition and the outcome following subarachnoid hemorrhage from ruptured intracranial aneurysm. Millikan studied 198 consecutive patients with subarachnoid hemorrhage and came to three conclusions.

(1) There is no clinical picture consistently present coincident with known cerebral vasospasm; (2) cerebral vasospasm has no effect on the mortality from subarachnoid hemorrhage due to ruptured aneurysm; and (3) there is no relationship between the frequency and severity of the complications from surgical or conservative treatment and the presence or absence of vasospasm.[264]

A review of these same patients by neurosurgeons in his institution led to the conclusion that vasospasm did have a significant effect on the outcome of treatment. Speaking of vasospasm, they noted

It is the fear of this complication that has caused many experienced neurologists and neurosurgeons to recommend a delay in surgery. This has resulted in a lower surgical mortality figure. . . .[263]

Arteriospasm is frequently seen on angiograms of patients with subarachnoid hemorrhage. This spasm may be focal in the area of the hemorrhage or it may be diffuse and even involve the contralateral hemisphere. Clinically, it has been observed that if patients with subarachnoid hemorrhage have spasm shown by the arteriograms, their prognosis is poor and they have a larger percentage of ischemic lesions than if no spasm is seen. Flow studies reveal close correlation between changes in cerebral blood flow and the presence or absence of arterial spasm.[11,166]

In about half the patients with a ruptured aneurysm, the spasm will be unilateral. Under those circumstances the spasm is on the side of the aneurysm in almost all cases.[379] Occasionally, when the spasm is bilateral, the most severe changes are on the side opposite to the aneurysm. Clearly, when multiple aneurysms are present these events make it difficult to use spasm as a localizing feature to decide which aneurysm has bled. Fortunately, the CT scan usually locates the site of the hemorrhage and lessens the need to depend on spasm as a means of determining which aneurysm has bled.

Often, the arterial spasm is severe enough to produce local ischemia of the cerebral cortex. When this occurs the spasm or blood flow is unaffected by the inhalation of carbon dioxide. If spasm is seen on the angiogram, the transit time of the cerebral circulation may be as much as 26 per cent longer than in comparable patients in whom no spasm is seen.[47] Regional cerebral blood flow studies have been variable, but some reports have shown striking correlations between the spasm and a reduced flow in the area.[85]

When an artery ruptures, several events occur that may play a role in the production of arterial spasm. Mechanical stimulation occurs as the artery is torn. The blood rushes out of the artery and forms a hematoma in the area. As the hematoma is formed, the vessel is displaced and the arachnoidal attachments to the vessel cause traction on it. Although there is no question that mechanical stimulation alone is a sufficient stimulus to cause an artery to constrict, animal research indicates that trauma alone probably does not cause prolonged spasm. Following trauma by stroking with a pledget of cotton or stripping of arachnoid from its wall, the vessel returns to normal size within 15 minutes.[179]

As blood enters the subarachnoid space, vasoactive materials are released into the cerebrospinal fluid. Included in these materials are serotonin, norepinephrine, bradykinin and angiotensin, blood iron products, prostaglandins, and thromboxanes.* From numerous studies, it appears that serotonin is probably the blood agent that is most responsible for the cerebral arterial spasm.[6] Experimental evidence suggests that the vascular spasm is produced by substances acting at the alpha-adrenergic receptor of the vessel wall.[93,179,378] There is an abundance of periarterial nerves in a plexus around the adventitia of the major intracranial vessels. Angiotensin and serotonin

_____

* See references 6, 65, 72, 73, 199, 291, 406.

have been shown to cause constriction of vessels when applied to their outer walls. Kapp and co-workers studied these substances in the cat and noted that when either substance was tested alone in a wide range of concentrations, neither substance produced the degree of vascular constriction that was produced by autogenous blood or lysed platelets.[179] Angiotensin is rapidly destroyed by blood enzymes. Serotonin is more persistent and probably plays a larger role in the production of arterial spasm. When an antagonist to the effects of serotonin on smooth muscles is applied to the adventitia of a normal basilar artery, an immediate dilatation of the vessels results.[93] In this instance, the dilatation is to a far larger than normal diameter and cannot be reversed by subsequent applications of blood, serotonin, or noradrenalin.

Both the experimental and the clinical evidence suggest that there is a two-phase character to the spasm.[11,32] An early phase comes within hours after the hemorrhage and tends to be more acute than the latter phase. The latter phase may represent an initial onset or an exacerbation of the initial phase that was becoming quiescent.

Much evidence supports the conclusion that serotonin release is related to arterial spasm in some way. How it relates to the timing of the onset of the spasm is unclear. With the destruction of blood and cerebral and vascular tissues during the initial hemorrhage, the release of serotonin is easy to understand. The events that occur with delayed spasm are more of a mystery. Perhaps the observations that platelets of the clotted blood absorb serotonin and release it over the succeeding days provide part of the answer.[425]

Prevention and management of cerebral vasospasm has received considerable attention, but the results have been disappointing.[136] Unsuccessful physiological measures have included the inhalation of 7 per cent carbon dioxide and superior sympathectomy, ganglionectomy, or blockade. Rheomacrodex decreases blood viscosity and probably decreases platelet adhesiveness and tendency to rouleau formation and stagnation of blood, but still its effectiveness in treating vasospasm and increasing cerebral blood flow has been disappointing. Further, Rheomacrodex carries a small but significant risk of producing intracerebral hemorrhage in the postoperative patient. The demonstration of its ability to increase regional cerebral blood flow in the ischemic area with hypertension has led to its use in treatment of vasospasm. Although this technique is effective in increasing blood flow to the affected area, it has the disadvantage of increasing the risk of rebleeding during the postoperative period.

Numerous direct smooth muscle relaxants have been found to be only partially effective in the relief of experimental vasospasm. They include papaverine, procaine, cyclandelate (Cyclospasmol), nitroglycerin, isosorbide dinitrate (Isordil), magnesium sulfate, isoxsuprine, and the experimental vasodilator YC-93. Chlorpromazine has a direct relaxing action on vascular smooth muscle and also antagonizes alpha-adrenergic agents and serotonin. Nitroprusside is a powerful direct smooth muscle relaxant and is commonly used in surgical practice to induce systemic hypotension. In dogs it has been shown to reverse cerebral vasospasm produced by intracisternal administration of blood.[136] Its usefulness in humans is to be further demonstrated.

Kindt and associates have used 1 per cent lidocaine topically with promising results in treating postoperative vasospasm after aneurysmal repair.[196] They left a catheter in place so that the vessels in spasm could be irrigated even several days postoperatively. The effectiveness of the treatment was documented both arteriographically and by clinical improvement of the patient.

Salbutamol, a beta²-adrenergic stimulating drug, has been used in treatment of experimental vasospasm produced by induced subarachnoid hemorrhage in rhesus monkeys. The drug was effective in relieving vasospasm in 50 per cent of those animals that developed it.[282] Combinations of Salbutamol and aminophyllin, a phosphodiesterase-inhibiting drug, were effective in relieving spasm in research animals even when Salbutamol alone was ineffective. It is suggested that this combination deserves clinical trial in humans.

Zervas and co-workers studied the effectiveness of reserpine and kanamycin in reducing the incidence of cerebral vascular ischemic complications in patients who had had a recent subarachnoid hemorrhage. The patients in this study had no neurological deficits after the subarachnoid hemorrhage. The presence or absence of spasm was determined arteriographically. Twenty-eight patients were in the treated group, and twenty-six were in the control group and received no treatment. Treated patients received reserpine 0.2 mg subcutaneously four times daily and kanamycin 1 gm orally three times daily until the date of operation. The time between rupture of the aneurysm and operation was variable; however, an angiogram was done preoperatively to ascertain the presence of vasospasm. It was present in eight of the control patients and one treated patient preoperatively. Postoperatively it developed in 4 of 16 control patients who were operated on and in 1 of 22 treated patients. Serotonin values were determined in both groups of patients. They were normal on admission in both groups, but decreased significantly in 48 to 72 hours after treatment began in the treated group. The authors of this study suggest that the reduction in spasm in the treated group may be related to the reduction in blood serotonin.[423] Reserpine is known to reduce the level of circulating serotonin by interfering with the uptake and storage of that compound by platelets and nerve terminals.[239,307] Reserpine also blocks the nerve terminal reuptake and storage of other vasoactive substances such as norepinephrine and dopamine.[274] Kanamycin probably reduces blood serotonin by modifying the bowel flora, thus interfering with the synthesis of pyridoxine, which is necessary as a cofactor in the synthesis of serotonin from tryptophan.[326] It should be noted that the decrease in blood serotonin does not conclusively implicate this agent as an etiological factor in the production of vasospasm, since other changes may be caused by the reserpine and kanamycin. While the study of Zervas and his group was limited to patients in stable condition, and the treatment was not given to those with markedly increased intracranial pressure in neurological impairment, they believe that the treatment should be undertaken in the latter group also.

Arteriovenous Malformations

As would be expected, regional blood flow studies show an increased flow if the lesion is near the surface.[119] If the lesion is deep in the parenchyma of the brain, the isotope studies may be normal despite a lesion of significant size.[288] When regional blood flow is abnormal preoperatively, postoperative changes can be used along with angiograms to determine the efficacy of the operative resection of the lesion.

Psychological testing of patients before and after excision of arteriovenous malformation reveals improvement in the visuomotor function and visual recall.[40] These improvements are thought to be due to the elimination of arteriovenous shunts that are taking blood away from the normal functional tissue.

The effect of an arteriovenous anomaly on the physiology of the surrounding brain is difficult to assess. The exact changes in the blood flow in the affected areas of the brain cannot be measured. Almost surely, the physiological changes are adverse. Clinical observations support this thesis. Patients with large arteriovenous anomalies often show lower intelligence and achievement than their normal siblings.

The adverse change associated with the anomalies may be due to multiple factors. Larger ones can cause a true steal of arterial blood from the adjacent area. Also, the near arterial pressure in the veins reduces the pressure differential from the arterial to the venous end of the capillaries. As a result, the flow through the capillaries may be reduced.

Intracerebral Steal Phenomenon

The term "intracerebral steal" has become popular in recent years. It refers to a situation in which blood is drained from one area because of lowered cerebral vascular resistance in another.[79] Originally it was applied to cases of arteriovenous malformations or vascular tumors in which the flow through the lesion was so great that blood would be taken from the surrounding normal brain. Recently, the term has been used to describe loss of blood flow from an area of ischemia to an area of relatively normal brain that has had its vascular resistance markedly decreased by carbon dioxide, anesthesia, or some other agent that impairs the autoregulation phenomenon.

The mechanism of the intracerebral steal phenomenon is as follows. Prior to the onset of the steal there is autoregulation of flow in the normal brain and a normal vascular resistance. The high resistance to flow in the normal areas of brain increases the total resistance in the intracranial vessels. This increased resistance increases the pressure in the intracranial vessels and consequently the perfusion pressure. The increased perfusion pressure helps the ischemic area. When the autoregulation phenomenon is impaired or lost in the normal brain, the decrease in resistance in the vessels in the normal tissue decreases the perfusion pressure and permits a relative shift or flow from the ischemic area to the normal area.

The intracerebral steal phenomenon may be more than a fancy hypothesis for explaining the events that are observed in the laboratory.[31] Curious developments that are observed clinically may be explained by this phenomenon. For example, after a carotid ligation, a patient may be normal for many days and then develop a hemiparesis despite the absence of vascular occlusion anywhere in the carotid tree or embolus from the ligated vessel being shown on the arteriogram or at autopsy. In these patients the setting for an intracerebral steal phenomenon may be established when the patient develops an increased carbon dioxide tension. The P_{CO_2} may become elevated as the patient suffers impairment of consciousness, develops a chest infection with poor ventilatory function, or perhaps even if he is deeply asleep.[190] In these circumstances, a clinical trial of hyperventilation in an attempt to provoke the "Robin Hood" syndrome that has been described by Lassen and Skinhøj would appear to be indicated.[100,220,379] The hyperventilation would be done in an attempt to increase the focal blood flow by producing vasoconstriction in the surrounding normal brain. This effect can occur around mass lesions such as a brain tumor. Meyer and colleagues studied such a patient and reported that

Five per cent CO_2 inhalation caused an "intracerebral steal" probably as a result of increasing intracranial pressure and "squeezing" or displacing of blood from the hemisphere swollen by tumor into the normal hemisphere.[257]

A carotid-cavernous fistula may cause a "steal phenomenon" that can be made symptomatic by occlusion of the carotid artery that feeds it.[15] For this reason, the patient may show signs of cerebral ischemia if the fistula is not obliterated before the carotid artery is ligated in the neck. Of course, occlusion of the carotid intracranially at a point distant to the fistula would not provoke the "steal phenomenon."

Reversal of blood flow through the vertebral artery can cause cerebral ischemia. This reversal of flow can be caused by occlusion of the subclavian artery proximal to the origin of the vertebral artery. An occlusion in this area causes the so-called "subclavian steal" syndrome.[318] Patients with this syndrome have signs of cerebral ischemia that may be provoked by strenuous exercise of the left arm. Also, exercise of the left arm may cause reduction of regional cerebral blood flow.[234]

Anemia and Polycythemia

Anemia and polycythemia affect blood flow by altering the viscosity and the oxygen-carrying capacity. Lowering of the hematocrit with anemia has relatively little effect on viscosity of the blood (see Fig. 23-1). Apparently, the decrease in oxygen-carrying capacity is a more important factor in producing the increase in cerebral blood flow that has been shown with severe anemia.[138] By the increase in blood flow, the cerebral metabolic need for oxygen is met in all but the most severe cases of anemia.

Increase in viscosity of the blood by elevation of the hematocrit decreases cerebral blood flow. Polycythemia vera may reduce flow by more than 50 per cent.[184] Nevertheless, oxygenation of the cerebral tissue is adequate. The symptoms associated with this disease are attributed to an accompanying high platelet count and a circulatory stagnation with sludging and embolization that accompanies the increased viscosity.

Headache

According to the classic theory, the first or prodromal phase of migraine headaches is caused by ischemia within the internal carotid system and the second phase with the headache by vasodilatation, especially within the external carotid system. Marked decreases in regional cerebral blood flow have been reported in patients with cerebral symptoms accompanying their headaches.[360,383] A patient with aphasia, apraxia, and agnosia had a reduction of 67 per cent from the baseline flow in the brain area that would correlate anatomically with these symptoms. This degree of reduction of flow would appear to confirm the hypothesis that cerebral ischemia is the cause of the neurological changes during the initial phases. The headache phase is accompanied by higher than normal cerebral blood flow.

Cluster headaches are accompanied by marked increases in intracranial flow, with values going as high as 73 to 83 ml per 100 gm per minute.[281,332] The increased flow continues for hours even after drug treatment gives partial or complete relief. The increased flow may cause the headaches or be due to the same factor that causes both the headache and the change in flow, or it may be due to pain alone, since even the application of cutaneous stimulation sufficient to cause pain will produce a significant increase in mean cerebral blood flow.[158]

Increased Intracranial Pressure

Cushing studied the effects of increased intracranial pressure on the arterial blood pressure. From his observations he concluded that

. . . a simple and definite law may be established, namely, that *an increase of intracranial tension occasions a rise of blood pressure which tends to find a level slightly above that of the pressure exerted against the medulla.* It is thus seen that there exists a regulatory mechanism on the part of the vaso-motor centre which, with great accuracy, enables the blood pressure to remain at a point just sufficient to prevent the persistence of an anaemic condition of the bulb, demonstrating that the rise is a conservative act and not one such as is consequent upon a mere reflex sensory irritation.[57]

This phenomenon is called the Cushing reflex. It comes into play when the cerebral perfusion pressure is less than 30 to 50 mm of mercury.[426] Presumably, its basis is ischemia of the brain stem.[330]

For years it was believed that the Cushing reflex prevented cerebral blood flow changes unless the pressure of the spinal fluid was elevated to levels above the arterial pressure.[106] Moderately elevated levels of cerebrospinal fluid pressure were thought to have no significant effect on cerebral flow. Recent studies have shown that a beginning decrease in flow follows acute elevations of cerebrospinal fluid pressure above 350 to 450 mm of water.[107,189]

At first the changes of cerebral blood flow with increasing intracranial pressure are minor. There is a decrease of approximately 4 per cent of the control level of flow when the cerebrospinal fluid pressure is 380 mm of water.[107] When the cerebrospinal fluid pressure is elevated to 920 mm of water, the decrease in blood flow is 25 per cent. The perfusion is the critical factor in maintaining cerebral blood flow. Cerebral perfusion pressures of 70 mm of mercury or more maintain adequate flow.[120] If the perfusion pressure drops to 40 to 50 mm of mercury there is a marked reduction in cerebral blood flow.[240,262]

Changes in intracranial pressure influence the cerebral blood flow through two mechanisms. One is through the general pressure increase, which in turn increases the tissue pressure. The increased tissue pressure is transmitted through the vessel wall to increase the cerebrovascular resistance, which decreases blood flow. The other mechanism is alteration of the transmural pressure gradient. As the intracranial pressure is altered, the pressure gradient between the inside and outside of the vessel wall, the transmural pressure gradient, is increased or decreased. When the transmural pressure is decreased, the myogenic reflex of the smooth muscle wall causes the smooth muscle to relax so that the vessel may enlarge. The vessel enlarges, with the effect that the resistance is reduced to normal again and cerebral blood flow is again normal.

The decrease in the transmural pressure gradient is responsible for the arterial dilatation that has been demonstrated so often in laboratory animals when the pressure is elevated to modest levels.[207] The vasodilation that occurs with increased intracranial pressure is part of the autoregulation phenomenon.

The cerebral arterioles still react to the administration of carbon dioxide even when there is a maximum vasodilatory effect from increased intracranial pressure.[426] The increase in flow with carbon dioxide indicates that a different mechanism may underlie the dilatation of blood vessels during autoregulation and hypercapnia or that hypercapnia has a stronger influence than changes of the transmural pressure gradient on the smooth muscle of the arterioles.

Only with markedly increased intracranial pressure that nears the arterial pressure do the arteries begin to collapse. If intracranial pressure is raised further to the levels of the systolic blood pressure, the cerebral blood flow ceases completely. This has been confirmed angiographically and is called the nonfill syndrome.[207,265]

Animal studies show that if the markedly increased intracranial pressure is relieved after being sustained for some time, flow will be re-established through the larger vessels. However, sludging and massive emboli will prevent re-establishment of flow in the small arterioles and capillaries.[134] After release of the pressure, there is a period of vasoparalysis, hyperemia, cortical hemorrhages, and progressive cerebral edema leading to death.[208]

Continuous monitoring of patients with increased intracranial pressure shows that there are spontaneous increases of intracranial pressure up to 500 to 1000 mm of water.[208] These increases come as pressure waves. Clearly, the height of the pressure at the peak of the pressure wave is enough to affect cerebral blood flow and to produce a degree of cerebral hypoxia. The pressure waves up to 75 mm of mercury cause little change in the blood flow despite some decrease in cerebral perfusion pressures.[174] Repeated pressure waves even at the same level of pressure have a more marked effect in decreasing the cerebral blood flow. Hulme and Cooper studied patients who had moderately increased intracranial pressure in the range of 400 to 500 mm of water. They found that the pressure waves had a marked association with certain stages of sleep as determined by the electroencephalogram. The waves were rarely observed in patients during the waking state or during periods of deep sleep, but rather, occurred most frequently during transition from a period of deep to light sleep as shown by the desynchronization of the electroencephalogram and the appearance of rapid eye movements. They suggest that the increased incidence of the waves during these periods of sleep is a reflection of enhanced cortical activity and, therefore, of carbon dioxide production.[150] The usual retention of carbon dioxide that occurs with sleep plus the increased production that occurs during light sleep may explain the tendency of the pressure waves to occur at that time. The increased frequency of pressure waves during some stages of sleep offers another possible explanation for the familiar observation that clinical deterioration and accentuation of symptoms of raised intracranial pressure often occur during the night.

Patients with benign intracranial hypertension or pseudotumor cerebri have a modest reduction in regional cerebral blood flow (mean of 10 per cent) and a marked increase in regional cerebral blood volume (mean of 85 per cent).[241] These findings support the concept that venous engorgement and increased intracranial blood volume play an important role in the pathophysiology of increased intracranial pressure in these conditions.

Brain Tumors

Brain tumors have direct effects on cerebral blood flow through their influence on the adjacent cerebral tissue and indirect effects by increasing intracranial pressure.[260] The effects caused by increasing intracranial pressure are discussed in the preceding section of this chapter.

The histological character of the tumor markedly influences the circulation time on angiography and the blood flow through the region of the tumor. Obviously, quite vascular lesions have increased flow through the tumor itself, and avascular lesions have decreased flow.

Serial angiography reveals slowing of the cerebral circulation time in patients with brain tumors, particularly those with papilledema. The individual transit times from patient to patient have overlapped so much that it is difficult to assess the significance of a measurement in a particular patient. Indeed, some investigators have not been able to establish any significant difference in cerebral blood flow between normal patients and patients with space-occupying lesions.

By regional blood flow studies, patients with brain tumors can be classified into groups according to whether the blood flow in and around the tumor is unchanged, decreased, or increased. A few patients have a decreased flow in the region of their tumor, while the majority have an increased flow. In most cases an increased flow can be correlated with the presence of arteriovenous shunts and pathological arteries shown on the angiogram.[35]

While the data from various reports are conflicting, it appears that the vascular tumors such as the meningiomas and the very malignant gliomas have a greater flow than normal brain, whereas the metastatic and other avascular tumors have a lower flow than normal brain.[289] The vascular tumor masks the flow in the surrounding tissue. Very probably, the flow in the cerebral tissue surrounding the tumor is decreased with all types of tumors. The tumors that cause edema in the surrounding tissue appear to cause the greatest decrease in flow in the adjacent tissue.

Hyperemic regions with the loss of autoregulation may be seen in sites remote from the tumor.[74] The location of the remote areas of abnormal blood flow seems to depend on the site of the tumor. Frontal and posterior fossa masses cause hyperemic areas in the lower part of the temporo-occipital region, whereas central parietal mass lesions have hyperemia mostly in the frontal region of the brain. These findings may be due to local tissue compression against unyielding anatomical structures such as the falx and tentorium.

Pressure waves accompanying brain tumors are accompanied by marked increases in cerebral blood volume at the same time that there is a decrease in blood flow.[54,243] Matsuda and associates believe that these plateau waves are closely related to the intrinsic vasomotor control of the cerebral circulation and can occur as long as cerebral vasodilating ability is maintained, irrespective of the existence of cerebral autoregulation.[243]

Trauma

Mild cerebral trauma that does not cause a concussion will not affect the cerebral blood flow. More severe injuries cause a loss of autoregulation and an immediate increase in cerebral blood flow. Animal studies have shown that immediately after a significant injury there is a marked increase in blood flow. Measurements of the internal carotid flow have shown an increase to as much as 250 per cent above control levels

at 30 seconds after the injury, the flow gradually returning to normal within 6 to 10 minutes.[35,294] The alteration in flow after the injury is not influenced by cervical sympathectomy or vagotomy and is independent of any rise in systemic blood pressure.[250] Several factors influence the length of time that the cerebral blood flow is increased. One is the severity of the injury. Another is the increase in intracranial blood volume after the loss of autoregulation. Studies in cats have shown that the increase in blood volume after a quite severe head injury can be up to approximately 50 per cent of the volume of the cranial cavity.[228]

At a variable time after the injury, the dilatation phase of the vasoparalysis clears and the cerebral blood flow is reduced. Rather soon after the injury, spasm of the arteries may be seen on the angiograms of some patients.[407] One study found vascular spasm and prolonged circulation time in 33 patients whose injury was serious enough to be fatal.[233] Undoubtedly, there is a degree of arterial spasm in all patients who have had serious head injury, even though their angiograms may be normal. At this time the autoregulation phenomenon is impaired.

Studies of humans without intracranial space-occupying masses have shown a 10 to 15 per cent reduction in cerebral blood flow soon after the injury and a gradual increase in the flow back to normal as the patient regains consciousness.[14,33] If the patient had evidence of an intracranial space-occupying lesion, his decrease in regional cerebral blood flow might be as much as 50 per cent of normal. Interestingly enough, induced arterial hypertension increases regional cerebral blood flow in areas around the lesion, and in some cases hyperventilation is followed by an increase in flow also. This is a hint that therapeutic hyperventilation as discussed in the section on the intracerebral steal phenomenon of this chapter may indeed be useful.

When the intracranial pressure is acutely increased by a balloon and then relieved by rapid evacuation of the balloon, there is a rush of blood through the arteries and veins that were compressed. The intracranial pressure falls to zero during the evacuation, but as the vessels fill with blood the intracranial pressure rebounds within a few seconds to again cause compression of the brain. Cortical hemorrhages frequently are seen after the rapid relief of the increased pressure and the resumption of flow in the area that was being compressed.[210] These observations fit with clinical experiences in which evacuation of a large hematoma causing marked compression of the brain has been followed by swelling of the brain, hemorrhages in the adjacent area or even throughout the brain, and prolonged increased intracranial pressure.

A study of cerebral blood flow in patients who have prolonged symptoms after head injury has been made by Skinhøj. He studied patients with the typical postconcussion syndrome of headaches, dizziness, inability to concentrate, irritability, fatigability, and emotional and vegetative instability. Their clinical neurological examinations, electroencephalograms and pneumoencephalograms were normal. The psychological tests showed no sign of organic dementia, but did show neurotic and neuroasthenic disturbances of the post-traumatic type. Of seven patients who originally were thought to have only a cerebral concussion, all had normal cerebral blood flow except one patient. In retrospect, it was realized that he had an undetected skull fracture and possibly a cerebral contusion. His flow was moderately reduced. An additional seven patients with cerebral contusion or cerebral laceration diagnosed at the time of the injury were studied. Only one of these seven had recovered completely, and he had a normal cerebral blood flow and metabolic rate for oxygen utilization. Two patients had subjective sequelae and, although their neurological examinations, electroencephalograms, and pneumoencephalograms were normal, they had significant reduction of cerebral blood flow and cerebral metabolic rate. Four patients who had severe clinical signs of a brain lesion including dementia, motor disturbances, abnormal electroencephalograms and cerebral pneumoencephalograms all showed markedly reduced cerebral blood flows and metabolic rates.[362]

Repeated studies have shown an improvement in cerebral blood flow and oxygen utilization in patients as they improve clinically after an injury. When taken in context with the time after the injury, it appears that the cerebral blood flow and metabolic rate for utilization of oxygen are important indicators of the patient's clinical status and progress. While the prognosis for an individual patient cannot be given, prognosis does correlate well with outcome in large groups of patients.[36]

Effort

The concept that increased cerebral activity causes increase in cerebral blood flow is an old one. In 1889 Roy and Sherrington wrote that

the chemical products of cerebral metabolism contained in the lymph which bathes the walls of the arterioles of the brain can cause variations in the caliber of blood vessels.[329]

In 1928 Fulton noted that the occipital lobe became more vascular during visual activity.[94] Despite these observations, it was not possible to confirm an increase in cerebral blood flow by using techniques such as the Kety-Schmidt method for measuring average intracranial blood flow. In recent years the techniques for regional cerebral blood flow measurements have enabled investigators to confirm the concept. Ingvar and Schwartz use these techniques to study the effects of speech and reading on the dominant hemisphere of the the brain. They report:

Dominant hemisphere speech and reading cause a change in resting blood flow pattern which is mainly augmentation of the flow in a Z-like figure including the premotor, the middle and lower rolandic, as well as the anterior and middle sylvian regions. This Z-like figure corresponds rather closely to the upper speech cortex, the hand, arm-face-tongue-area of the sensorimotor region, as well as the anterior (Broca) speech cortex, and the middle sylvian region.[155]

Stereognostic testing causes an increase in the regional cerebral blood flow in the corresponding contralateral sensorimotor region and a focal area in the premotor part or frontal lobe.[323] Also, the general level of alertness may influence the cerebral blood flow. Increased alertness or increased effort causes modest increases in flow.[305]

Effect of Aging

Advancing age is an insignificant cause of change in cerebral blood flow and oxygen utilization unless it is accompanied by vascular disease. Sokoloff made a study of young and elderly volunteers who were not part of a hospital population.[370] Those in the elderly group were 65 years or more of age. Among the patients who were asymptomatic and had no evidence of disease on physical examination, there was no statistically significant difference in the cerebral circulatory functions of the normal young and normal elderly patients despite the fact that there was approximately a 50-year difference in their mean ages. Of patients who had asymptomatic vascular disease, hypertension, or arteriosclerosis, there was a small but significant decline in cerebral blood flow below the level of normal young subjects. The cerebral venous P_{CO_2}, which was thought to indicate the level of oxygen tension in the cerebral tissues, tended to be slightly reduced in the normal elderly group and somewhat more so in the subjects with asymptomatic vascular disease, although in both the change was insignificant. The cerebral oxygen consumption was not reduced, which indicates that although there was a degree of circulatory insufficiency in the asymptomatic group with disease, it was not sufficient to limit the metabolism of the brain. He concludes that

. . . declines in cerebral blood flow and oxygen consumption are not the inevitable consequences of chronological aging or duration of life per se. When these changes occur in otherwise apparently healthy, or at least asymptomatic, elderly individuals, they are probably the results of vascular disease, arteriosclerosis in particular.[370]

Dementia

Along with the decrease in gray matter there is a decrease in cerebral blood flow to both hemispheres in senile and presenile dementia.[329,361] Hagberg and Ingvar performed regional flow studies in demented patients and found that there was

. . . a rough proportionality between the cognitive reduction and a decrease in the cerebral blood flow (especially the flow in the gray matter). In addition, certain regional flow abnormalities correlated with specific cognitive functions in a manner resembling the cognitive defects found in focal brain lesions in the same area. Thus, patients who showed only memory distur-

bances demonstrated a focal flow reduction in the temporal region. More severely affected patients with reduction of verbal ability and signs of agnosia, showed very low flows in occipito-tempero-parietal parts of the hemisphere.[116]

In contrast, the cerebral blood flow and oxygen uptake levels in alcoholics with Korsakoff's psychosis of long standing are normal.[22,132,361]

Not all studies show decrease in cerebral blood flow with primary dementias. Hachinski and co-workers found the flow to be normal with primary degenerative diseases causing dementia, but lower than normal in those who were demented owing to multiple infarcts.[114] The cerebral blood flow of patients with dementia due to cerebral atrophy and those with normal-pressure hydrocephalus have been studied.[111] The flow and cerebral oxygen utilization were decreased to a mild extent in both groups and no characteristics could be distinguished to help differentiate between the two conditions.

Position of Head

When a person moves from the recumbent to the standing position, profound changes occur in the circulatory system. Orthostatic pressure exerted vertically from head to foot causes 300 to 800 ml of blood to pool in the legs, resulting in a decreased cardiac output.[25] Furthermore, the hydrostatic pressure affects the columns of fluid in the carotid and vertebral arteries, jugular veins, and subarachnoid space. If these effects were not immediately counterbalanced by an adjustment of arterial tone in the extremities by the autonomic nervous system and local autoregulation of the cerebrovascular bed, the reduction in cerebral blood flow would be serious. Despite these adjusting mechanisms, moving from a recumbent to a standing position causes a temporary reduction of cerebral blood flow of about 20 per cent.[300] If and how rapidly it fully returns to baseline values is unknown.[66,359]

Patients with cerebral vascular insufficiency often note that a particular head position may precipitate their symptoms.[38] This influence of head position on the patient's symptoms has been attributed to a stimulation of the carotid sinus reflex mechanism or to local anatomical factors that permit a more effective compression of the sinus when the head is rotated.[75,82] Indeed, these mechanisms may cause a reduction in cerebral blood flow. There is, however, evidence that the position of the head also influences cerebral blood flow by compression of the cervical vessels. Toole and Tucker studied cadavers varying in age from newborn to 78 years. In every cadaver, at least one vessel was found to have no flow at some point when the head was moved through a range of motions that could be considered normal. The vertebral arteries were more readily occluded than the carotids, but flow in the latter occasionally ceased also. In general, the older the patient, the more readily was flow occluded by change in head position.[390] Undoubtedly the increased effect of change of head position in the elderly is related to arteriosclerotic plaques, the loss of vascular elasticity, and cervical osteoarthritis with osteophytes projecting from the apophyseal and uncovertebral joints into the lumen of the transverse foramen. These protuberances produce vessel distortion and compression that vary during movement of the cervical spine.[151,278]

With the patient under anesthesia, turning the head to one side causes a decrease of flow in the opposite carotid artery ranging from 10 to 27 per cent.[122] The mechanism by which the carotid flow is altered by head rotation is unknown. However, the transverse process of the first cervical vertebra appears to cause compression of the artery as the head is rotated, and this has been postulated as the cause of the change in blood flow.[26] Since the head is frequently turned when the patient is positioned for a neurosurgical procedure, the influence of head position on the vertebral and carotid flows should be considered in every patient. Clearly, the largest and most dependable cerebral blood flow is obtained with the head aligned with the body in the midline position.

The Trendelenburg position has long been used in the treatment of operative and neurogenic shock. The rationale for using this position is to increase cerebral blood flow by increasing the orthostatic pressure. The perfusion pressure is increased transiently. However, studies in animals indicate that if the carotid sinus reflex mecha-

nism is intact, there is a rapid onset of a significant decrease in pressure and flow in the carotid arteries.[112] This correlates with the experimental studies in rats showing that the head-down position does not have any beneficial effect in the treatment of severe hemorrhagic shock.[402] Since the head-down position causes a decrease of 15 to 20 per cent in the vital capacity, it should be used with caution.[9,41] Elevation of the legs would appear to give the desired result of increasing the blood available for circulation to the head without the deleterious effects of the head-down position.

Miscellaneous Diseases

Many techniques have been used to study the effects of a wide range of neurological disorders on cerebral blood flow. Oldendorf and Kitano utilized radioisotope studies of the turnover of the brain's blood as an index to the brain circulation.[290] They studied 517 patients with various neurological disorders (Fig. 23–11). Shortening of the turnover time of the brain's blood is evidenced in patients with arteriovenous malformations and headaches. The turnover time was normal in patients with idiopathic epilepsy, alcoholic epilepsy, noncerebral neurological disease, and major hypertensive disease of the extracranial arteries. Slight prolongation of the turnover time was shown in patients with post-traumatic seizures, transient cerebral ischemic disease, and hypertensive cerebral infarctions. Patients with alcoholic encephalopathy, extracranial major arterial disease, and brain tumor had a prolongation of the turnover time. A marked prolongation of the turnover time was seen in patients with post-traumatic encephalopathy, degenerative neurological disease, and normotensive cerebral infarction.

As would be expected, there is an increase in cerebral blood flow during epileptic seizure.[149,222] Regional flow measurements show an increase in flow in the area of the epileptic focus during the seizure and a decrease in the focus area during the interictal period. These changes are so marked that the determination of the regional cerebral blood flow is said to be a better method for localizing the epileptic focus than is the electroencephalogram.

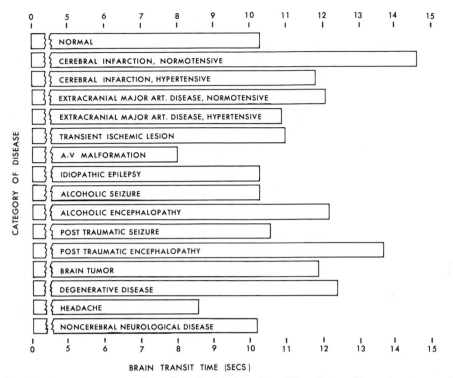

Figure 23–11 Average turnover time of the brain's blood in 517 patients with various types of disease. (Adapted from Oldendorf, W. H., and Kitano, M.: Radioisotope measurement of brain blood turnover as a clinical index of brain circulation. J. Nucl. Med., 8:578, 1967.)

Hougaard and colleagues studied 10 patients with seizures and reported

The localization of the cortical epileptic focus by the rCBF method was more precise than the crude localization by the EEG. A hyperemic focus was found in all ten cases, while a well defined EEG focus was present only in two cases.[149]

Bromide psychosis with a serum bromide level of 45 mMol per liter causes a reduction in blood flow of about one third of normal.[23] The regional flow pattern is also abnormal with low flows in the frontal and parieto-occipital regions. As the bromide is removed by metabolism or hemodialysis, there is overall improvement in the flow, which progressively becomes normal.

Diabetes of long standing impairs autoregulation of cerebral blood flow.[21] The blood flow is pressure dependent to a much greater extent than is normal. The cause of the impaired autoregulation in these patients is believed to be diffuse or multifocal dysfunction of cerebral arterioles due to diabetic vascular disease.

Polycythemia can significantly reduce cerebral blood flow. Lowering of the hematocrit by venesection markedly improves the flow and reduces the old blood viscosity.[386]

CLINICAL METHODS OF INCREASING FLOW

When faced with the need to increase cerebral blood flow to an ischemic area, the physician has relatively few effective techniques at his disposal.

Lowering of Intracranial Pressure

Increased intracranial pressure increases the cerebrovascular resistance and increases tissue pressure, which impedes the outflow of nutrients from the vessels to the cells. Although only marked elevations of intracranial pressure cause serious derangements of blood flow, an effort should be made to maintain the intracranial pressure at a normal level.[107]

Blood Viscosity and Rheology

The effectiveness of the blood's ability to carry oxygen should be maintained by preventing anemia. Excessive dehydration with marked increase in viscosity will impede cerebral blood flow, but probably does not cause cerebral anoxia. When dealing with any form of ischemia, and particularly that due to cerebral spasm, dextran may be useful in improving the rheological qualities of the blood.[322] Dextran decreases the tendency of the blood to sludge and form emboli. It markedly improves flow through collateral circulation, and fortunately it can be used for prolonged periods. High molecular weight dextran should be avoided, however, since it increases blood viscosity and reduces blood flow without the redeeming feature of increasing oxygen-carrying capacity as occurs with polycythemia or ordinary dehydration.[118]

Hyperventilation

Hyperventilation to increase blood flow to an ischemic area is predicated on laboratory observations and theoretical considerations. Basically, it is an application of the principle of increased perfusion pressure. An increase in the resistance in the normal brain increases the pressure and, hence, the perfusion pressure throughout the intracranial arterial system. Since the hyperventilation does not affect the ischemic area, the overall effect is to increase perfusion pressure for this area and possibly to increase perfusion of it.

Its usefulness may be limited, but moderate successes have been reported with it in treatment of focal ischemic lesions. Further trials and evaluations are warranted.[379]

Head Position

When possible, the head should be in a normal midline position with the body. Marked turning or other abnormal positions may occlude one or more of the cervical vessels supplying the brain.[122,390] The sitting position should be avoided during operations on patients with arteriosclerotic cerebrovascular disease or cardiopulmonary problems that may cause hypotension or hypoxia.

Carbon Dioxide

This agent is useful in increasing flow to the nonischemic brain. When the brain is ischemic, the autoregulation phenomenon is abolished, and as a result, the vessels are fully dilated and carbon dioxide is unable to increase blood flow.[192] Further, as outlined in the section on intracerebral steal in this chapter, the use of carbon dioxide may even reduce flow to a focal ischemic area.

Some clinicians have observed improvement of patients who were suffering with an ischemic episode and were treated by carbon dioxide inhalations. This inconstant beneficial result of carbon dioxide inhalations is best explained by the elevation of blood pressure that occurs in some patients who have been given carbon dioxide inhalations.

Oxygen

A normal arterial oxygen tension of 95 mm of mercury should be maintained. If the Po_2 is low, the first effort should be to increase the efficiency of the ventilatory system by reducing airway obstruction and suctioning out the tracheobronchial tree. Impediments to adequate respiratory excursion should be eliminated by the appropriate means. These impediments may be a painful fractured rib, a flail chest, or a face-down or head-down position that reduces respiratory excursion. If these measures do not give the desired results, then inhalation of a higher oxygen content by mask or tube may be used.

Hyperbaric oxygen produces a marked increase in the oxygen tension, which will maintain adequate oxygenation of the brain with a reduced cerebral blood flow. The reduced blood flow helps to reduce intracranial pressure. It is claimed that it will give striking relief of symptoms in patients in coma from raised intracranial pressure.[374] This is ascribed to reduction in intracranial pressure secondary to cerebral vasoconstriction. When 2 atm of oxygen was used as a prophylactic measure during carotid endarterectomy it was reported to offer little benefit.[169] In view of the problems inherent in the technique of administration with the hyperbaric chamber, its overall usefulness with any neurological problem is questionable.

Drugs

Numerous drugs act on the cerebrovascular system and give a transient increase in blood flow. Almost universally, they act by altering the autoregulation phenomenon of the normal cerebral tissue. Since the autoregulation phenomenon already is absent in a focal ischemic area, they cannot increase flow to that area. Unfortunately, no drug has proved to give a sustained and clinically useful effect.

Nerve Block

The cerebrovascular system has a nervous supply that is demonstrable; however, its effectiveness in altering the cerebral blood flow is insignificant. As a consequence, stellate ganglion or other nerve blocks do not increase the cerebral blood flow.[337] This fact is at variance with the clinical observation that a stellate ganglion block can sometimes be useful in a patient who is having a transient ischemic attack, particularly from unilateral carotid disease. It should be remembered that introducing needles into the stellate ganglion area causes pain. In turn, the pain may cause a rise in blood pressure that will increase the blood flow to an ischemic area.

Operation on Vessel

Resection of an occlusive or stenotic lesion from an artery is a proved means of increasing blood flow to the brain. After resection of an atherosclerotic plaque in the cervical portions in the carotid arteries there may be enormous increases in flow through the vessel. Boysen and co-workers reported a series of 17 patients in whom internal carotid artery flow and regional blood flow were measured simultaneously. Internal carotid flow after resection increased as much as from 0 to 500 ml per minute with a mean increase of carotid flow of 59 per cent in all 17 patients. In some patients the mean regional cerebral blood flow was unchanged despite significant increases in flow through the vessel from which the atherosclerotic plaque was removed.[29] The study demonstrates that whether the regional cerebral blood flow will be altered depends upon a number of factors such as the degree of stenosis of the cervical vessel, the adequacy of the intracranial collateral circulation, particularly through the circle of Willis, the presence of intracranial plaques that impede blood flow, and the condition of the microcirculation with regard to microemboli and sludging of the blood. The condition of the arteriole in microcirculation after a period of total occlusion of a carotid vessel is particularly important. After a few hours of occlusion of a cervical vessel, the changes that occur in this level of the circulatory system usually make operative resection of the cervical lesion a useless surgical exercise.[387]

If resection of a sclerotic plaque is to be performed, various techniques are available to test the tolerance to clamping of the carotid artery that is necessary for a brief time even if a bypass shunt is used. The purpose of all the techniques is to inform the surgeon when the cerebral oxygenation has fallen below a critical level. Lyons and associates advocated maintaining ipsilateral jugular venous oxygen saturations above 60 per cent.[230] Some authors have found electroencephalographic monitoring to be unsatisfactory because of the difficulty in interpreting the results and the fact that the study is influenced by the depth of anesthesia and the Pa_{CO_2} level.[44,127] Other authors have found the electroencephalogram to be quite helpful and advocate its routine use.[376] Regional cerebral blood flow studies are not readily available to all clinicians, and the information given by the technique is not available early enough after carotid clamping to give ideal guidance to the surgeon. It is, however, useful in helping to indicate the patient who is having a critical decrease in regional cerebral blood flow and in whom this would be expected to aggravate his neurological deficit postoperatively.[168,400] For instance, Jennett states that he has consistently found that if the regional cerebral blood flow is reduced by more than 25 per cent in the frontotemporal region during internal carotid clamping, then some degree of hemiparesis always ensues either immediately or at some period after the operation.[169,170] This complication was not seen in cases that had a lesser reduction of flow in the frontotemporal region.[169,170] Cerebral angiograms are a readily available means of investigating the circulation. Unfortunately, however, the presence of cross-filling of the intracranial vessels is of little predictive value in forecasting the capacity of the patient to tolerate a unilateral carotid ligation.[167]

Resection of an atherosclerotic plaque of a cervical vessel carries the risk of conversion of a partial stenosis to a complete occlusion owing to postoperative clotting at the operative site. Also, resection of the innervation of the carotid sinus may cause labile hypertension.[224,398] The occurrence of postoperative hypertension may be correlated with a higher incidence of postoperative neurological deterioration, and efforts to control the blood pressure with antihypertensive therapy have not given clearly beneficial results.

Techniques for intracranial resection of stenotic and occlusive lesions are being developed; however, they are still in the experimental phase.

Arterial anastomoses of extracranial to intracranial vessels have been developed in recent decades. The one most frequently used is the superficial temporal to middle cerebral artery anastomosis. Flowmeter observations taken soon after the anastomosis reveal flows ranging from 12 to 60 ml per minute.[42,313] Angiographic studies show that the anastomosis opens up during the weeks after it is made, and undoubtedly the flow figures become much higher. Vessels other than the superficial temporal artery have been used for anastomosis to the intracranial vessels. They include the occipital artery to the middle cerebral artery and the occipital artery to the posterior inferior cerebral artery.[191,372] A detailed discussion of these procedures is given in Chapter 44.

Elevation of Blood Pressure

As is well known by clinicians, lower blood pressures can be tolerated when the entire arterial system is intact and changes in cerebral vascular resistance can partially ameliorate the effects. When the system is compromised, the flow in the collateral system begins to have marked changes at about 80 to 90 mm of mercury arterial pressure.[78,87] Thus, the flow through an ischemic area or a collateral artery is unusually dependent on blood pressure.[381]

When an area of brain is ischemic, the autoregulation phenomenon is abolished and the flow is pressure dependent. Increasing the perfusion pressure causes a straight line increase in blood flow until adequate perfusion of the tissues is obtained.[195] When adequate tissue perfusion is obtained, the autoregulation phenomenon returns. As a result, increased perfusion pressure is the most reliable means of increasing flow through an ischemic area.[195,421] This is true regardless of whether the flow is inadequate because of a partial lesion in the main feeding vessel or because there is an occlusion and the flow has to come through collateral channels.[77]

After a severe ischemic episode, the integrity of the capillary wall may be impaired. As a result, increased blood pressure may increase the outflow of fluids into the tissues and cause edema. Also, if the ischemia has led to a frank infarction of the tissue, an increased perfusion pressure may rupture a necrotic vessel wall and convert a dry infarction to a hemorrhagic one.[416] The clinician has to consider the probability of benefit or harm as the blood pressure is elevated. This judgment can only be made with a full knowledge of the pathological process, how it has evolved to the present, and a fortunate guess as to its future course.

REFERENCES

1. Abreu, B. E., Liddle, G. W., Burks, A. L., Simon, A., Sutherland, V., and Gordan, G. S.: Effects of amphetamine, dihydroergotamine, and methadon on human cerebral blood flow and oxygen uptake. Fed. Amer. Soc. Exp. Biol., Proc., 7:201, 1948.
2. Aizawa, T., Tazaki, Y., and Gotoh, F.: Cerebral circulation in cerebrovascular disease. World Neurol., 2:635–645, 1961.
3. Alexander, S. C., and Lassen, N. A.: Cerebral circulatory response to acute brain disease: Implications for anesthestic practice. Anesthesiology, 32:60–68, 1970.
4. Alexander, S. C., James, F. M., Colton, E. T., Gleaton, H. R., and Wollman, H.: Effects of cyclopropane anesthesia on cerebral blood flow and carbohydrate metabolism of man. Anesthesiology, 29:170–171, 1968.
5. Allen, G. D., and Morris, L. E.: Central nervous system effects of hyperventilation during anaesthesia. Brit. J. Anaesth., 34:296–305, 1962.
6. Allen, G. S., Henderson, L. M., Chou, S. N., and French, L. A.: Cerebral arterial spasm. Part 1: In vitro contractile activity of vasoactive agents on canine basilar and middle cerebral arteries. J. Neurosurg., 40:433–441, 1974.
7. Alpers, B. J., and Berry, R. G.: Circle of Willis in cerebral vascular disorders. The anatomical structure. Arch. Neurol., 8:398–402, 1963.

8. Alpers, B. J., Berry, R. G., and Paddision, R. M.: Anatomical studies of the circle of Willis in normal brain. Arch. Neurol. Psychiat., *81*:409–418, 1959.

9. Altschule, M. D.: The significance of changes in the lung volume and its subdivisions during and after abdominal operations. Anesthesiology, *4*:385–391, 1943.

10. Antonini, F. M., Bertini, G., Fumagalli, C., Fieschi, C., Battistini, N., Violante, F., and Nori, A.: Effects of intravenous infusion of glycerol on regional cerebral blood flow in cerebral infarction. Gerontology, *23*:376–380, 1977.

11. Arutiunov, A. I., Baron, M. A., and Majorova, N. A.: Experimental and clinical study of the development of spasm of the cerebral arteries related to subarachnoid hemorrhage. J. Neurosurg., *32*:617–625, 1970.

12. Ausman, J. L., Van Nimwegen, D., and Owens, G.: Electron microscope evidence of potential blood flow from vein to capillary bed in brain. New York J. Med., *64*:2917–2919, 1964.

13. Bainton, C. R., and Mitchell, R. A.: Posthyperventilation apnea in awake man. J. Appl. Physiol., *21*:411–415, 1966.

14. Baldy-Moulinier, M., and Frèrebeau, P.: Cerebral blood flow in cases of coma following severe head injury. *In* Brock, M., Fieschi, C., Ingvar, D. H., Lassen, N. A., and Schurmann, K., eds.: Cerebral Blood Flow. Berlin, Springer-Verlag, 1969, pp. 216–218.

15. Barnes, B. D., Rosenblum, M. L., Pitts, L. H., Winestock, D. P., Parker, H., and Nohr, M. L.: Carotid-cavernous fistula: Demonstration of asymptomatic vascular "steal." J. Neurosurg., *49*:49–55, 1978.

16. Bassett, R. C., List, C. F., and Lemmen, L. F.: Surgical treatment of intracranial aneurysm. Surg. Gynec. Obstet., *95*:701–708, 1952.

17. Battacharji, S. K., Hutchinson, E. C., and McCall, A. J.: The circle of Willis—the incidence of developmental abnormalities in normal and infarcted brains. Brain, *90*:747–758, 1967.

18. Battey, L. L., Heyman, A., and Patterson, Jr., J. L.: Effects of ethyl alcohol on cerebral blood flow and metabolism. J.A.M.A., *152*:6–10, 1953.

19. Battey, L. L., Patterson, J. L., and Heyman, A.: Effects of methyl and ethyl alcohol on cerebral blood flow and oxygen consumption. Amer. J. Med., *13*:105, 1952.

20. Bayliss, N. M.: On the local reactions of the arterial wall to changes of internal pressure. J. Physiol. *28*:220–231, 1902.

21. Bentsen, N., Larsen, B., and Lassen, N. A.: Chronically impaired autoregulation of cerebral blood flow in long-term diabetes. Stroke, *6*:497–502, 1975.

22. Berglund, M., and Ingvar, D. H.: Cerebral blood flow and its regional distribution in alcoholism and in Korsakoff's psychosis. J. Stud. Alcohol, *37*:586–597, 1976.

23. Berglund, M., Nielsen, S., and Risberg, J.: Regional cerebral blood flow in a case of bromide psychosis. Arch. Psychiat. Nervenkr., *223*:197–201, 1977.

24. Betz, E.: Adaptation of regional cerebral blood flow in animals exposed to chronic alterations of PO_2 and PCO_2. Acta Neurol. Scand., *41*(Suppl. 14):121–128, 1965.

25. Bevegård, B. S., and Shepherd, J. T.: Regulation of the circulation during exercise in man. Physiol. Rev., *47*:178–213, 1967.

26. Boldrey, E., Maass, L., and Miller, E. R.: The role of atlantoid compression in the etiology of internal carotid thrombosis. J. Neurosurg., *13*:127–139, 1956.

27. Boschenstein, F. K., Reilly, J. A., Yahr, M. D.: and Correll, J. W.: Effect of low molecular weight dextran on cortical blood flow. *14*:288–293, 1966.

28. Boysen, G.: Cerebral blood flow measurement as a safeguard during carotid endarterectomy. Stroke, *2*:1–10, 1971.

29. Boysen, G., Ladegaard-Pedersen, H. J., Valentin, N., and Engell, H. C.: Cerebral blood flow and internal carotid artery flow during carotid surgery. Stroke, *1*:253–260, 1970.

30. Boysen, G., Engell, H. C., Pistolese, G. R., Fiorani, P., Agnoli, A., and Lassen, N. A.: On the critical level of cerebral blood flow in man with particular reference to carotid surgery. Circulation, *49*:1023–1025, 1974.

31. Brawley, B. W.: The pathophysiology of intracerebral steal following carbon dioxide inhalation, an experimental study. Scand. J. Clin. Lab. Invest., *22*(Suppl. 102):sect. 13:B, 1968.

32. Brawley, B. W., Strandness, D. E., and Kelly, W. A.: The biphasic response of cerebral vasospasm in experimental subarachnoid hemorrhage. J. Neurosurg., *28*:1–8, 1968.

33. Brodersen, P., and Gjerris, F.: Regional cerebral blood flow in patients with chronic subdural hematomas. Acta Neurol. Scand., *51*:233–239, 1975.

34. Brown, F. D., Hanlon, K, Crockard, H. A., and Mullan, S.: Effect of sodium nitroprusside on cerebral blood flow in conscious human beings. Surg. Neurol. *7*:67–70, 1977.

35. Brown, G. W., and Brown, M. L.: Cardiovascular responses to experimental cerebral concussion in the rhesus monkey. Arch. Neurol Psychiat., *71*:707–713, 1954.

36. Bruce, D. A., and Langfitt, T. W.: The prognostic value of ICP, CPP, CBF, and $CMRO_2$ in head injury. *In* McLaurin, R. L., ed.: Head Injuries. Second Chicago Symposium on Neural Trauma. 1975. New York, Grune & Stratton, 1976, pp. 23–25.

37. Buyniski, J. P., and Rapela, C. E.: Cerebral and renal vascular smooth muscle responses to adenosine. Amer. J. Physiol. *217*:1660–1664, 1969.

38. Caplan, L. R., and Sergay, S.: Positional cerebral ischaemia. J. Neurol. Neurosurg. Psychiat., *39*:385–391, 1976.

39. Carey, J. P., Stemmer, E. A., List, J. W., Chiu, S. C., Heber, R., and Connolly, J. E.: The hazards of using vasoactive drugs to augment peripheral and cerebral blood flow. Amer. Surg., *35*:12–22, 1969.

40. Carter, L. P., Morgan, M., and Urrea, D.: Psychological improvement following arteriovenous malformation excision. J. Neurosurg., *42*:452–456, 1975.

41. Case, E. H., and Stiles, J. A.: The effect of vari-

ous surgical positions on vital capacity. Anesthesiology, 7:29–31. 1946.

42. Chater, N.: Surgical results and measurements of intraoperative flow in microneurosurgical anastomoses. In Austin, G. M., ed.: Microneurosurgical Anastomoses for Cranial Ischemia. Springfield, Ill., Charles C Thomas, 1976, pp. 295– 304.

43. Chorobski, J., and Penfield, W.: Cerebral vasodilator nerves and their pathway from the medulla oblongata. Arch. Neurol. Psychiat., 28:1257–1289, 1932.

44. Clowes, G. H. A., Jr., Kretchmer, H. E.: McBurney, R. W., and Simeone, F. A.: The electroencephalogram in the evaluation of the effects of anesthetic agents and carbon dioxide accumulation during surgery. Ann. Surg., 138:558–569, 1953.

45. Cohen, P. J., Alexander, S. C., Smith, T. C., Reivich, M., and Wollman, H.: Effects of hypoxia and normocarbia on cerebral blood flow and metabolism in conscious man. J. Appl. Physiol., 23:183–189, 1967.

46. Cohen, P. J., Wollman, H., Alexander, S. C., Chase, P. E., and Behar, M. G.: Cerebral carbohydrate metabolism in man during halothane anesthesia: Effects of Pa_{CO_2} on some aspects of carbohydrate utilization. Anesthesiology, 25:185–191, 1964.

47. Connolly, R. C.: Cerebral ischaemia in spontaneous subarachnoid haemorrhage. Ann. Roy. Coll. Surg. Eng., 30:102–116, 1962.

48. Cooper, E. S., West, J. W., Jaffe, M. E., Goldberg, H. I., Kawamura, J., and McHenry, L. C.: The relation between cardiac function and cerebral blood flow in stroke patients. 1. Effect of CO_2 inhalation. Stroke, 1:330–347, 1970.

49. Cow, D.: Some reactions of surviving arteries. J. Physiol. (London), 42:125–143, 1911.

50. Crockard, H. A., Brown, F. D., and Mullen, J. F. (1976). Effects of trimethaphan and sodium nitroprusside on cerebral blood flow in rhesus monkeys. Acta Neurochir. (Wien), 35:85–89, 1976.

51. Crockard, H. A., Coppel, D. L., and Morrow, W. F. K.: Evaluation of hyperventilation in treatment of head injuries. Brit. Med. J., 4:634–640, 1973.

52. Cronqvist, S., and Agee, F.: Regional cerebral blood flow in intracranial tumors. Acta Radiol., 7:393–404, 1968.

53. Cronqvist, S., and Laroche, F.: Transitory hyperaemia in focal cerebral vascular lesions studied by angiography and regional cerebral blood flow measurements. Brit. J. Radiol., 40:270–274, 1967.

54. Cronqvist, S., Ingvar, D. H., and Lassen, N. A.: Quantitative measurements of regional cerebral blood flow related to neuroradiological findings. Acta Radiol. [Diagn.] (Stockholm), 5:760–766, 1966.

55. Cullen, C. F., and Swank, R. L.: Intravascular aggregation and adhesiveness of blood elements associated with alimentary lipemia and injections of large molecular substances. Circulation, 9:335–346, 1954.

56. Cullen, D. J., Cotev, S., Severinghaus, J. W., and Eger, E. I.: The effects of hypoxia and isovolemic anemia on the halothane requirement (MAC) of dogs. II. The effects of acute hypoxia on halothane requirement and cerebral-surface PO_2, PCO_2, pH, and HCO_3^-. Anesthesiology, 32:35–45, 1970.

57. Cushing, H.: Concerning a definite regulatory mechanism of the vaso-motor centre which controls blood pressure during cerebral compression. Bull. Johns Hopk. Hosp., 12:290–296, 1901.

58. Derrick, J. R., Kirksey, T. D., Estess, M., and Williams, D.: Kinking of the carotid arteries. Clinical considerations. Am. Surg., 32:503–506, 1966.

59. Desai, B., and Toole, J. F.: Kinks, coils, and carotids: A review. Stroke, 6:649–653, 1975.

60. Dintenfass, L.: Blood Microrheology—Viscosity Factors in Blood Flow, Ischemia and Thrombosis. New York, Appleton-Century-Crofts, 1971.

61. Dorland's Illustrated Medical Dictionary, 25th Ed. Philadelphia, W. B. Saunders Co., 1974.

62. Dugdale, M., Nofzinger, J. D., and Murphey, F.: Some effects of low molecular weight dextran on coagulation. Thromb. Diath. Haemorrh., 15:118–130, 1966.

63. Dumke, P. R., and Schmidt, C. F.: Quantitative measurements of cerebral blood flow in the macacque monkey. Amer. J. Physiol. 138:421–431, 1942–43.

64. Duret, H.: Recherches anatomiques sur la circulation de l'encéphale. Arch. de Physiol. Norm. ct Pathol., 2nd series. 1:60–91, 1874.

65. Echlin, F. A.: Current concepts in the etiology and treatment of vasospasm. Clin. Neurosurg., 15:133–160, 1968.

66. Eckenhoff, J. E., Enderby, G. E., Larson, A., Davies, R., and Judevine, D. E.: Human cerebral circulation during deliberate hypotension and head-up tilt. J. Appl. Physiol., 18:1130–1138, 1963.

67. Ehrenreich, D. L., Burns, R. A., Alman, R. W., and Fazekas, J. F.: Influence of acetazolamide on cerebral blood flow. Arch. Neurol. (Chicago), 5:227–232, 1961.

68. Eichhorn, O., and Schlict, L.: The importance of hydraulic principles in the regulation of cerebral blood flow. In Meyer, J. S., Lechner, H., and Eichhorn, O., eds.: Research on the Cerebral Circulation. Springfield, Ill., Charles C Thomas, 1969, pp. 332–346.

69. Ekberg, R., Cronqvist, S., and Ingvar, D. H.,: Regional cerebral blood flow in cerebrovascular disease. Acta Neurol. Scand., 14:164–168, 1965.

70. Ekstrom-Jodal, B., von Essen, C., and Haggendal, E.: Effects of noradrenaline on the cerebral blood flow in the dog. Acta Neurol. Scand., 50:11–26, 1974.

71. Ekstrom-Jodal, B., von Essen, C., and Haggendal, E., and Roos, B.-E.: Effects of L-dopa and L-tryptophan on the cerebral blood flow in the dog. Acta Neurol. Scand., 50:3–10, 1974.

72. Ellis, E. F., Nies, A. S., and Oates, J. A.: Cerebral arterial smooth muscle contraction by thromboxane A_2. Stroke, 8:480–483, 1977.

73. Ellis, E. F., Oelz, O., Roberts, L. J., II, Payne, N. A., Sweetman, B. J., Nies, A. S., and Oates, J. A.: Coronary arterial smooth muscle contraction by a substance released from platelets: Evidence that it is thromboxane A_2. Science, 193:1135–1137, 1976.

74. Endo, H., Larsen, B., and Lassen, N. A.: Regional cerebral blood flow alterations remote from the site of intracranial tumors. J. Neurosurg., *46*:271–281, 1977.

75. Engel, G. L.: Fainting, Physiological and Psychological Considerations. Springfield, Ill., Charles C Thomas, 1950.

76. Ernsting, J.: The effect of brief profound hypoxia upon the arterial and venous oxygen tensions in man. J. Physiol., *169*:292–311, 1963.

77. Farhat, S. M., and Schneider, R. C.: Observation on the effect of systemic blood pressure on intracranial circulation in patients with cerebral vascular insufficiency. J. Neurosurg. 27:441–445, 1967.

78. Fazekas, J. F., Kleh, J., and Parrish, A. E.: The influence of shock on cerebral hemodynamics and metabolism. Amer. J. Med. Sci., *229*:41–45, 1955.

79. Fazio, C.: The importance of the "intracerebral steal" in the pathogenesis of focal brain ischemia, *In* Meyer, J. S.: Reivich, M., Lechner, H., and Eichhorn, O., eds.: Research on the Cerebral Circulation. Springfield, Ill., Charles C Thomas, 1970, pp. 57–59.

80. Feindel, W., and Perot, P.: Red cerebral veins. J. Neurosurg., *22*:315–325, 1965.

81. Ferguson, R. W., Richardson, D. W., and Patterson, J. L., Jr.: Effects of mephentermine on cerebral circulation and metabolism. Fed. Proc. Amer. Soc. Exp. Biol., *15*:63, 1956.

82. Ferris, E. B., Capps, R. B., and Weiss, S.: Carotid sinus syncope and its bearing on the mechanism of the unconscious state and convulsions. A study of 32 additional cases. Medicine, *14*:337–456, 1935.

83. Fetterman, G. H., and Moran, T. J.: Anomalies of the circle of Willis in relation to cerebral softening. Arch. Path. (Chicago), *32*:251–257, 1941.

84. Fieschi, C., Agnoli, A., Battistini, N., Bozzao, L.: Regional cerebral blood flow in patients with brain infarcts. Arch. Neurol. (Chicago), *15*:653–663, 1966.

85. Fieschi, C., Agnoli, A., Battistini, N., and Bozzao, L.: Relationships between cerebral transit time and non-diffusible indicators and cerebral blood flow, a comparative study with krypton-85 and radioalbumin. Experientia. *22*:189–190, 1966.

86. Fink, B. R.: Influence of cerebral activity in wakefulness on regulation of breathing. J. Appl. Physiol., *16*:15–20, 1961.

87. Finnerty, F. A., Jr., Witkin, L., and Fazekas, J. F.: Cerebral hemodynamics during cerebral ischemia induced by acute hypotension. J. Clin. Invest., *33*:1227–1232, 1954.

88. Fisher, C. M.: The circle of Willis: Anatomical variations. Vasc. Dis., *2*:99–105, 1965.

89. Fitch, W.: Sodium nitroprusside and the cerebral circulation. Editorial. Brit. J. Anaesth., *49*: 399–400, 1977.

90. Fog, M.: Cerebral circulation: The reaction of pial arteries to fall in blood pressure. Arch. Neurol. Psychiat. *37*:351–364, 1937.

91. Fog, M.: Cerebral circulation: Reaction of pial arteries to epinephrine by direct application and by intravenous injection. Arch. Neurol. Psychiat., *41*:109–118, 1939.

92. Forbes, H. S., Finley, K. H., and Nason, G. I.: Cerebral circulation. Arch. Neurol. Psychiat., *30*:957–979, 1933.

93. Fraser, R. A. R., Stein, B. M., Barrett, R. E., and Pool, J. L.: Noradrenergic mediation of experimental cerebrovascular spasm. Stroke. *1*:356–362, 1970.

94. Fulton, J. F.: Observations upon the vascularity of the human occipital lobe during visual acuity. Brain, *51*:310–320, 1928.

95. Geiger, A., and Magnes, J.: The isolation of the cerebral circulation and the perfusion of the brain in the living cat. Amer. J. Physiol., *149*:517–537, 1947.

96. Géraud, J., Bès, A., Rascol, A., Delpla, M., and Marc-Vergnes, J. P.: Application de la méthode au krypton 85. Pharmacologie de la circulation cérébrale. Presse Méd., *73*:1577–1582, 1965.

97. Gibbs, F. A., Maxwell, H., and Gibbs, E. L.: Volume flow of blood through the human brain. Arch. Neurol. Psychiat., *57*:137–144, 1947.

98. Gillilan, L. A.: Significant superficial anastomoses in the arterial blood supply to the human brain. J. Comp. Neurol., *112*:55–74, 1959.

99. Gilroy, J., Barnhart, M. I., and Meyer, J. S.: Treatment of acute stroke with dextran 40. J.A.M.A., *210*:293–298, 1969.

100. Gordon, E., and Rossanda, M.: The importance of the cerebrospinal fluid acid base status in the treatment of unconscious patients with brain lesions. Scand. J. Clin. Lab. Invest., *22*(suppl. 102):sect. 9:C, 1968.

101. Gotoh, F., Tazaki, Y., and Meyer, J. S.: Transport of gases through brain and their extravascular vasomotor action. Exp. Neurol., *4*:48–58, 1961.

102. Gottstein, U.: Pharmacological studies of total cerebral blood flow in man with comments on the possibility of improving regional cerebral blood flow by drugs. Acta Neurol. Scand., suppl. *14*:136–141, 1965.

103. Gottstein, U., and Held, K: The effect of hemodilution caused by low molecular weight dextran on human cerebral blood flow and metabolism. *In* Brock, M., Fieschi, C., Ingvar, D. H., Lassen, N. A., and Schurmann, K., eds.: Cerebral Blood Flow. Berlin, Springer-Verlag, 1969, pp. 104–105.

104. Gottstein, U., and Paulson, O.B.: The effect of intracarotid aminophylline infusion on the cerebral circulation. Stroke *3*:560–565, 1972.

105. Gottstein, U., Held, K., Sebening, H., and Steiner, K.: Is decrease of cerebral blood flow after intravenous injections of theophylline due to direct vasoconstrictive action of the drug? Europ. Neurol., *6*:153–157, 1971–1972.

106. Green, H. D., Rapela, C. E., and Conrad, M. C.: Resistance (conductance) and capacitance phenomena in terminal vascular beds. Autoregulatory control of resistance vessels. *In* Hamilton, W. F., and Dow, P., eds.: Handbook of Physiology. Washington, D.C., Amer. Physiol. Soc., 1963, Sect. 2, vol. 2, pp. 942–948.

107. Greenfield, J. C., Jr., and Tindall, G. T.: Effect of acute increase in intracranial pressure on blood flow in the internal carotid artery of man. J. Clin. Invest., *44*:1343–1351, 1965.

108. Greenfield, J. C., Jr., and Tindall, G. T.: Studies of the effects of vasopressor drugs on internal carotid artery blood flow in man. *In* Bain, W. H., and Harper, A. M., eds.: Flow Through Organs and Tissues; Proceedings of an International Conference, Glasgow, 1967. Baltimore, Md., Williams & Wilkins Co., 1967, pp. 336–348.

109. Grenell, R. G.: Central nervous system resistance: I. The effects of temporary arrest of cerebral circulation for periods of two to ten minutes. J. Neuropath. Exp. Neurol., *5*:131–154, 1946.

110. Grubb, R. L., Jr., Raichle, M. E., Eichling, J. O., and Gado, M. H.: Effects of subarachnoid hemorrhage on cerebral blood volume, blood flow, and oxygen utilization in humans. J. Neurosurg., *46*:446–453, 1977.

111. Grubb, R. L., Raichle, M. E., Gado, M. H., Eichling, J. O., and Hughes, C. P.: Cerebral blood flow, oxygen utilization and blood volume in dementia. Neurology (Minneap.), *27*:905–910, 1977.

112. Guntheroth, W. G., Abel, F. L., and Mullins, G. L.: The effect of Trendelenburg's position on blood pressure and carotid flow. Surg. Gynec. Obstet., *119*:345–348, 1964.

113. Guyton, A.: Textbook of Medical Physiology. 5th Ed. Philadelphia, W. B. Saunders Co., 1976.

114. Hachinski, V. C., Iliff, L. D., Zilhka, E., DuBoulay, G. H., McAllister, V. L., Marshall, J., Russell, R. W. R., and Symon, L.: Cerebral blood flow in dementia. Arch. Neurol. (Chicago), *32*:632–637, 1975.

115. Hafkenschiel, J. H., and Friedland, C. K.: The effects of 1-hydrazinophthalzine on cerebral blood flow, vascular resistance, oxygen uptake and jugular oxygen tension in hypertensive subjects. J. Clin. Invest., *32*:655–660, 1953.

116. Hagberg, B., and Ingvar, D. H.: Cognitive reduction in presenile dementia related to regional abnormalities of the cerebral blood flow. Brit. J. Psychiat., *128*:209–22, 1976.

117. Haggendal, E.: Effects of some vasoactive drugs on the vessels of cerebral grey matter in the dog. Acta Physiol. Scand., suppl. *258*:55–79, 1965.

118. Haggendal, E., Nilsson, N. J., and Norback, B.: Effect of blood corpuscle concentration on cerebral blood flow. Acta Chir. Scand., suppl., *364*:3–12, 1966.

119. Haggendal, E., Ingvar, D. H., Lassen, N. A., Nilsson, N. J., Norlen, G., Wickbom, I., and Zwentnow, N.: Pre- and postoperative measurements of regional cerebral blood flow in three cases of intracranial arteriovenous aneurysms, J. Neurosurg., *22*:1–6, 1965.

120. Hamer, J., Hoyer, S., Stoeckel, H., Alberti, E., and Weinhardt, F.: Cerebral blood flow and cerebral metabolism in acute increase of intracranial pressure. Acta Neurochir. (Wien), *28*:95–110, 1973.

121. Hankinson, H. L., Smith, A. L., Nielsen, S. L., and Hoff, J. T.: Effect of thiopental on focal cerebral ischemia in dogs. Surg. Forum, *25*:445–447, 1974.

122. Hardesty, W. H., Roberts, B., Toole, J. F., and Royster, H. P.: Studies of carotid artery blood flow in man. New Eng. J. Med., *263*:944–946, 1960.

123. Hardesty, W. H., Roberts, B., Toole, J. F., and Royster, H. P.: Studies on carotid artery flow. Surgery., *49*:251–256, 1961.

124. Hardesty, W. H., Whitacre, B. W., Toole, J. F., and Royster, H. P.: Studies on vertebral artery blood flow. Surg. Forum, *13*:482–483, 1962.

125. Harper, A. M.: The inter-relationship between aP_{CO_2} and blood pressure in the regulation of blood flow through the cerebral cortex. Acta Neurol. Scand., *41*:suppl. 14:94–103, 1965.

126. Harper, A. M., and Glass, H. I.: Effect of alterations in arterial carbon dioxide tension of the blood flow through the cerebral cortex at normal and low arterial blood pressures. J. Neurol. Neurosurg. Psychiat., *28*:449–452, 1965.

127. Harris, E. J., Brown, W. H., Pavy, R. N., Anderson, W. W., and Stone, D. W.: Continuous electroencephalographic monitoring during carotid artery endarterectomy. Surgery, *62*:441–447, 1967.

128. Harrison, J. H., and Davalos, P. A.: Cerebral ischemia. Surgical procedure in cases due to tortuosity and buckling of the cervical vessels. Arch. Surg. (Chicago), *84*:103–112, 1962.

129. Hasegawa, T., Ravens, J. R., and Toole, J. F.: Precapillary arteriovenous anastomoses. Arch. Neurol. (Chicago), *16*:217–224, 1967.

130. Hashim, S. A., and Clancy, R. E.: Dietary fats and blood coagulation. New Eng, J. Med., *259*:1115–1123, 1958.

131. Hedlund, S.: Hemodynamic aspects of cerebral circulation. *In* Engel, A., and Larsson, T., eds.: Stroke—Thule International Symposium. Stockholm, Nordiska Bokhandelns Forlag, 1967, pp. 125–144.

132. Hedlund, S., Köhler, V., Nylin, G., Olsson, R., Regnström, O., Rothström, E., and Aström, K. E.: Cerebral blood circulation in dementia. Acta Psychiat. Neurol. Scand., *40*:77–106, 1964.

133. Heilbrun, M. P., and Olesen, J.: Regional cerebral blood flow studies in subarachnoid hemorrhage. *In* Cerebral Blood Flow and Intracranial Pressure. Proc. 5th Int. Symp., Roma-Siena, part II, Europ. Neurol., *8*:1–7, 1972.

134. Hekmatpanah, J.: Cerebral circulation and perfusion in experimental increased intracranial pressure. J. Neurosurg., *32*:21–29, 1970.

135. Hellinger, F. R., Bloor, B. M., and McCutchen, J. J.: Total cerebral blood flow and oxygen consumption using the dye-dilution method. J. Neurosurg., *19*:964–970, 1964.

136. Heros, R. C., Zervas, N. T., and Negoro, M.: Cerebral vasospasm. Surg. Neurol., *5*:354–362, 1976.

137. Heubner, J. O. L.: Die Luetische Erkrankung der Hirnarterien. Leipzig. Vogel, 1874, pp. 238–428.

138. Heyman, A., Patterson, J. L., Jr., and Duke, T. W.: Cerebral circulation and metabolism in sickle cell and other chronic anemias, with observations on the effects of oxygen inhalation. J. Clin. Invest., *31*:824–828, 1952.

139. Hill, L.: The Physiology and Pathology of the Cerebral Circulation. An Experimental Research. London, J. & A. Churchill, 1896, p. 5.

140. Himwich, W. A., Homburger, E., Maresca, R., and Himwich, H. E.: Brain metabolism in man: Unanesthetized and in pentothal narcosis. Amer. J. Psychiat., *103*:689–696, 1946.

141. Hirsch, H., and Schneider, M.: Durchblutung und Sauerstoffaufnahme des Gehirns. *In* Tönnis, O. H., ed: Handbuch der Neurochirurgie. Vol. 1, section 2. Berlin, Springer-Verlag, 1968, pp. 434–552.

142. Hirsch, H., Koch, D., Krenkel, W., and Schneider, M.: Die Erholungslatenz des Warmblütergehirns bei Ischämie und die Bedeutung des Restkreislaufs. Pfluegers. Arch., *261*:392–401, 1955.

143. Høedt-Rasmussen, K.: Regional cerebral blood flow. Acta Neurol. Scand., *43*:suppl. 27:8–81, 1967.

144. Høedt-Rasmussen, K., and Skinhøj, E.: Transneural depression of the cerebral hemispheric metabolism in man. Acta Neurol. Scand., *40*:41–46, 1964.

145. Høedt-Rasmussen, K., and Skinhøj, E., Paulson, O., Ewald, J., Bjerrum, J. K., Fahrenkrug, A., and Lassen, N. A.: Regional cerebral blood flow in acute apoplexy. The "luxury perfusion syndrome" of brain tissue. Arch. Neurol. (Chicago), *17*:271–281, 1967.

146. Hoff, J. T., Smith, A. L., Hankinson, H. L., and Nielsen, S. L.: Barbiturate protection from cerebral infarction in primates. Stroke, *6*:28–33, 1975.

147. Hohberger, C. P., Yamamoto, Y. L., Thompson, C. J., and Feindel, W.: On-line computer measurement of microregional cerebral blood flow by Xenon-133 clearance. Int. J. Nucl. Med. Biol., *2*:153–158, 1975.

148. Hossmann, K.-A., and Kleihues, P.: Reversibility of ischemic brain damage. Arch. Neurol. (Chicago), *29*:375–384, 1973.

149. Hougaard, K., Oikawa, T., Sveinsdottir, E., Skinhøj, E., Ingvar, D. H., and Lassen, N. A.: Regional cerebral blood flow in focal cortical epilepsy. Arch. Neurol. (Chicago), *33*:527–535, 1976.

150. Hulme, A., and Cooper, R.: Cerebral blood flow during sleep in patients with raised intracranial pressure. Progr. Brain Res., *30*:77–81, 1968.

151. Hutchinson, E. C., and Yates, P. O.: Caroticovertebral stenosis. Lancet.*1*:2–8, 1957.

152. Hwang, N. H. C., and Normann, N. A.: Methods for measurement of cerebral blood flow in man. *In* Cardiovascular Flow Dynamics and Measurements. Baltimore, University Park Press, 1977, pp. 217–243.

153. Ingenito, A. J., Barrett, J. P., and Procita, L.: An analysis of the effects of nicotine on the cerebral circulation of an isolated, perfused, in situ cat brain preparation. Stroke, *2*:67–75, 1971.

154. Ingvar, D. H.: The pathophysiology of the stroke related to findings in EEG and to measurements of regional cerebral blood flow. *In* Engel, A., and Larsson, T., eds.: Stroke—Thule International Symposium, Stockholm, Nordiska Bokhandelns Forlag, 1967, p. 105.

155. Ingvar, D. H., and Schwartz, M. S.: Blood flow patterns induced in the dominant hemisphere by speech and reading. Brain, *97*:273–288, 1974.

156. Ingvar, D. H., and Soderberg, U.: Cerebral vaso-

motor tone and EEG during injections of Umbradil. Acta Radiol., *47*:185–191, 1957.

157. Ingvar, D. H., Lubbers, D. W., and Siesjo, B.: Measurement of oxygen tension on the surface of the cerebral cortex of the cat during hyperoxia and hypoxia. Acta Physiol. Scand., *48*:373–381, 1960.

158. Ingvar, D. H., Rosen, I., and Elmqvist, D.: Effects of somatosensory stimulation upon rCBF. *In* Harper, M. B., et al., eds.: Proceedings of the Seventh International Symposium on Cerebral Blood Flow and Metabolism. Edinburgh, London and New York, Churchill-Livingstone, 1975, pp. 14–29.

159. Ingvar, D. H., Haggendal, E., Nilsson, N. J., Sourander, P., Wickbom, I., and Lassen, N. A.: Cerebral circulation and metabolism in a comatose patient. Arch. Neurol. (Chicago), *11*:13–21, 1964.

160. Ingvar, D., Obrist, W., Chivian, E., Cronquist, S., Risberg, J., Gustafson, L., Hägerdal, M., and Wittbom-Cigen, G.: General and regional abnormalities of cerebral blood flow in senile and presenile dementia. Scand. J. Clin. Lab. Invest., *102*:12:B, 1968.

161. Ishii, R.: Regional cerebral blood flow in patients with ruptured intracranial aneurysms. J. Neurosurg., *50*:587–594, 1979.

162. Ishikawa, S., Handa, J., Meyer, J. S., and Huber, P.: Haemodynamics of the circle of Willis and the leptomeningeal anastomoses: An electromagnetic flow meter study of intracranial arterial occlusion in the monkey. J. Neurol. Neurosurg. Psychiat., *28*:124–136, 1965.

163. Ivankovich, A. D., Miletich, D. J., Albrecht, R. F., and Zahed, B.: Sodium nitroprusside and cerebral blood flow in the anesthetised and unanesthetised goat. Anesthesiology, *44*:21–26, 1976.

164. Jackson, B. B.: The external carotid as a brain collateral. Amer. J. Surg., *113*:375–378, 1967.

165. Jacobson, I., Harper, A. M., and McDowall, D. G.: The effects of O_2 at 1 and 2 atmospheres on the blood flow and oxygen uptake of the cerebral cortex. Surg. Gynec. Obstet., *119*:737–742, 1964.

166. James, I. M.: Changes in cerebral blood flow and in systemic arterial pressure following spontaneous subarachnoid haemorrhage. Clin. Sci., *35*:11–22, 1968.

167. Jawad, K., Miller, J. D., Fitch, W., and Barker, J.: Predicting cerebral ischemia after carotid ligation. J. Neurol. Neurosurg. Psychiat., *38*:825–826, 1975.

168. Jawad, K., Miller, J. D., Wyper, D. J., and Rowan, J. O.: Measurement of CBF and carotid artery pressure compared with cerebral angiography in assessing collateral blood supply after carotid ligation. J. Neurosurg., *46*:185–196, 1977.

169. Jennett, W. B.: Experimental studies on the cerebral circulation: Clinical aspects. Proc. Roy. Soc. Med., *61*:606–610, 1968.

170. Jennett, W. B., Harper, A. M., and Gillespie, F. C.: Measurement of regional cerebral bloodflow during carotid ligation. Lancet, *2*:1162–1163, 1966.

171. Jennett, W. B., Barker, J., Fitch, W., and

McDowall, D. G.: Effect of anesthesia on intracranial pressure in patients with space-occupying lesions. Lancet, *1*:61–68, 1969.

172. Johnston, I. H., and Harper, A. M.: The effect of mannitol on cerebral blood flow. An experimental study. J. Neurosurg., *38*:461–471, 1973.

173. Johnston, I. H., Johnston, J. A., and Jennett, B.: Intracranial pressure changes following head injury. Lancet, *2*:433–436, 1970.

174. Johnston, I. H., Rowan, J. O., Park, D. M., and Rennie, M. J.: Raised intracranial pressure and cerebral blood flow. 5. Effects of episodic intracranial pressure waves in primates. J. Neurol., Neurosurg., Psychiat., *38*:1076–1082, 1975.

175. Kabat, H., Dennis, C., and Baker, A. B.: Recovery of function following arrest of the brain circulation. Amer. J. Physiol., *132*:737–747, 1941.

176. Kagstrom, E., Lindgren, P., and Tornell, G.: Changes in cerebral circulation during carotid angiography with sodium acetrizoate (Triurol) and sodium diatrizoate (Hypaque). An experimental study. Acta Radiol., *50*:151–159, 1958.

177. Kanai, N., Hayakawa, T., and Mogami, H.: Blood flow changes in carotid and vertebral arteries by hyperbaric oxygenation. Neurology (Minneap.), *23*:159–163, 1973.

178. Kaplan, H. A.: Collateral circulation of the brain. Neurology (Minneap.), *11*:pt. 2:9–15, 1961.

179. Kapp, J., Mahaley, M. S., Jr., and Odom, G. L.: Cerebral arterial spasm: Part 2: Experimental evaluation of mechanical and humoral factors in pathogenesis. J. Neurosurg., *29*:339–349, 1968.

180. Karlsberg, P., Elliott, H. W., and Adams, J. E.: Effect of various pharmacologic agents on cerebral arteries. Neurology (Minneap.), *13*:722–778, 1963.

181. Kavee, D. J., Lichtenstein, E., and Laufman, H.: Collateral arterial flow under normotensive and hypotensive conditions: Effect of autotransfusion, normal saline solution infusion, and dextran 40 infusion. Arch. Surg. (Chicago), *95*:395–401, 1967.

182. Kellie, G.: Some reflections on the pathology of the brain, Edinb. Med. Chir. Soc. Trans., *1*: 84–169, 1824.

183. Kelly, P. J., Gorten, R. J., Grossman, R. G., and Eisenberg, H. M.: Cerebral perfusion, vascular spasm, and outcome in patients with ruptured intracranial aneurysms. J. Neurosurg., *47*:44–49, 1977.

184. Kety, S. S.: Circulation and metabolism of the human brain in health and disease. Amer. J. Med., *8*:205–217, 1950.

185. Kety, S. S., and Schmidt, C. F.: The determination of cerebral blood flow in man by the use of nitrous oxide in low concentrations. Amer. J. Physiol., *143*:53–66, 1945.

186. Kety, S. S., and Schmidt, C. F.: The effects of active and passive hyperventilation on cerebral blood flow, cerebral oxygen consumption, cardiac output, and blood pressure of normal young men. J. Clin. Invest., *25*:107–119, 1946.

187. Kety, S. S., and Schmidt, C. F.: The nitrous oxide method for the quantitative determination of the cerebral blood flow in man: Theory,

procedure and normal values. J. Clin. Invest., *27*:476–483, 1948.

188. Kety, S. S., and Schmidt, C. F.: The effects of altered arterial tensions of carbon dioxide and oxygen on cerebral blood flow and cerebral oxygen consumption of normal young men. J. Clin. Invest., *27*:484–492, 1948.

189. Kety, S. S., Shenkin, H. A., and Schmidt, C. F.: The effects of increased intracranial pressure on cerebral circulatory functions in man. J. Clin. Invest., *27*:493–499, 1948.

190. Kety, S. S., Woodford, R. B., Harmel, M. H., Freyhan, F. A., Appel, K. E., and Schmidt, C. F.: Cerebral blood flow and metabolism in schizophrenia: The effects of barbiturate seminarcosis, insulin coma and electro-shock. Amer. J. Psychiat., *104*:765–770, 1948.

191. Khodadad, G., Singh, R. S., and Olinger, C. P.: Possible prevention of brain stem stroke by microvascular anastomosis in the vertebrobasilar system. Stroke, *8*:316–321, 1977.

192. Kindt, G., and Youmans, J.: Experimental studies of the effect of carbon dioxide on cerebral blood flow during carotid insufficiency. Scand. J. Clin. Lab. Invest., *22*:suppl. 102:16:H, 13:F, 1969.

193. Kindt, G., and Youmans, J. R.: The site of action of carbon dioxide on cerebral circulation. Surg. Forum, *20*:419–421, 1969.

194. Kindt, G. W., and Youmans, J. R.: The effect of stricture length on critical arterial stenosis. Surg. Gynec. Obstet., *128*:729–734, 1969.

195. Kindt, G. W., Youmans, J. R., and Albrand, O. W.: Factors influencing the autoregulation of the cerebral blood flow during hypotension and hypertension. J. Neurosurg., *26*:299–305, 1967.

196. Kindt, G. W., Hudson, J. S., Gosh, H. H., and Gabrielsen, T. O.: Relief of arterial spasm associated with cerebral aneurysms. Europ. Neurol., *8*:38–42, 1972.

197. King, B. D., Sokoloff, L., and Wechsler, R. L.: The effects of 1-epinephrine and 1-norepinephrine upon cerebral circulation and metabolism in man. J. Clin. Invest., *31*:273–279, 1952.

198. Kirgis, H. D., Fisher, W. L., Llewellyn, R. C., and Peebles, E. M.: Aneurysms of the anterior communicating artery and gross anomalies of the circle of Willis, J. Neurosurg., *25*:73–78, 1966.

199. Kolata, G. B.: Thromboxanes: The power behind the prostaglandins? Science, *190*:770–771, 1975.

200. Kong, Y., Lunzer, S., Heyman, A., Thompson, H. K., and Saltzman, H. A.: Effects of acetazolamide on cerebral blood flow of dogs during hyperbaric oxygenation. Amer. Heart J., *78*:229–237, 1969.

201. Kuhn, R. A.: The speed of cerebral circulation. New Eng. J. Med., *267*:689–695, 1962.

202. Ladurner, G., Zilkha, E., Iliff, L. D., Du Boulap, G. H., and Marshall, J.: Measurement of regional cerebral blood volume by computerized axial tomography. J. Neurol. Neurosurg. Psychiat. *39*:152–158, 1976.

203. Lambertsen, C. J., Kough, R. H., Cooper, D. Y., Emmel, G. L., Loeschke, H. H., and Schmidt, C. F.: Oxygen toxicity: Effects in man of oxygen inhalation at 1 and 3.5 atmospheres upon

blood gas transport, cerebral circulation, and cerebral metabolism. J. Appl. Physiol., 5:471–486, 1953.

204. Lambertsen, C. J., Owen, S. G., Wendel, H., Stroud, M. W., Lurie, A. A., Lochner, W., and Clark, G. F.: Respiratory and cerebral circulatory control during exercise at .21 and 2.0 atmospheres inspired pO_2. J. Appl. Physiol., 14:966–982, 1959.

205. Lambertsen, C. J., Semple, S. J. G., Smyth, M. G., and Gelfand, R.: H^+ and PCO_2 as chemical factors in respiratory and cerebral circulatory control. J. Appl. Physiol., 16:473–484, 1961.

206. Langfitt, T. W.: Increased intracranial pressure. Clin. Neurosurg. 16:436–471, 1969.

207. Langfitt, T. W., and Kassell, N. F.: Non-filling of cerebral vessels during angiography: Correlation with intracranial pressure. Acta Neurochir. (Wien), 14:96–104, 1966.

208. Langfitt, T. W., Weinstein, J. D., and Kassell, N. F.: Cerebral vasomotor paralysis produced by intracranial hypertension. Neurology (Minneap.), 15:622–641, 1965.

209. Langfitt, T. W., Marshall, W. J. S., Kassell, N. F., et al.: The pathophysiology of brain swelling produced by mechanical trauma and hypertension. Scand. J. Lab. Clin. Invest., 22:suppl. 102:14:B, 1968.

210. Langfitt, T. W., Weinstein, J. D., Kassell, N. F., and Shapiro, H. M.: Cerebrovascular dilatation and compression in intracranial hypertension. In Brock, M., Fieschi, C., Ingvar, D. H., Lassen, N. A., and Schurmann, K., eds.: Cerebral Blood Flow. Berlin, Springer-Verlag, 1969, pp. 177–178.

211. Lantz, B. M. T., Foerster, J. M., Link, D. P., and Holcroft, J. W.: Angiographic determination of splanchnic blood flow. Acta Radiol. [Diagn. (Stockholm),] 21:3–10, 1980.

212. Larson, C. P., Jr.: Anesthesia and control of the cerebral circulation. In Wylie, E. J., and Ehrenfeld, W. K., eds: Extracranial Occlusive Cerebrovascular Disease. Diagnosis and Management. Philadelphia, W. B. Saunders Co., 1970, pp. 152–183.

213. Lassen, N. A.: Cerebral blood flow and oxygen consumption in man. Physiol. Rev., 39:183–238, 1959.

214. Lassen, N. A.: The luxury-perfusion syndrome and its possible relation to acute metabolic acidosis localized within the brain. Lancet, 2:1113–1115, 1966.

215. Lassen, N. A.: Brain extracellular pH: The main factor controlling cerebral blood flow. Scand. J. Clin. Lab. Invest., 22:247–251, 1968.

216. Lassen, N. A., and Ingvar, D. H.: Regional cerebral blood flow in apoplexy: Studies of its pathophysiology, using 8 to 16 external detectors with the xenon 133 method. In Meyer, J. S., Lechner, H., and Eichhorn, O., eds.: Research on the Cerebral Circulation, Int'l. Salzburg Conference, Springfield, Ill., Charles C Thomas, 1969. pp. 96–102.

217. Lassen, N. A., and Ingvar, D. H.: Radioisotopic assessment of regional cerebral blood flow. Progr. Nucl. Med., 1:376–409, 1972.

218. Lassen, N. A., and Lane, M. H.: Validity of internal jugular blood for study of cerebral blood flow and metabolism. J. Appl. Physiol., 16:313–320, 1961.

219. Lassen, N. A., and Munck, O.: The cerebral blood flow in man determined by the use of radioactive krypton. Acta Physiol. Scand., 33:30–49, 1955.

220. Lassen, N. A., and Skinhøj, E.: Regional cerebral blood flow measurements disclosing abnormally perfused tissue components and "intracerebral steal" in cases of apoplexy and brain tumors. In Meyer, J. S., Reivich, M., Lechner, H., and Eichhorn, O. eds.: Research on the Cerebral Circulation, Springfield, Ill., Charles C Thomas, 1970, pp. 76–79.

221. Lavy, S., Melamed, E., and Portnoy, Z.: The effect of cerebral infarction on the regional cerebral blood flow of the contralateral hemisphere. Stroke, 6:160–163, 1975.

222. Lavy, S., Melamed, E., Portnoy, Z., and Carmon, A.: Interictal regional cerebral blood flow in patients with partial seizures. Neurology (Minneap.), 26:418–422, 1976.

223. Lehrer, G. M.: Arteriographic demonstration of collateral circulation in cerebrovascular disease. Neurology (Minneap.), 8:27–32, 1958.

224. Lehv, M. S., Salzman, E. W., and Silen, W.: Hypertension complicating carotid endarterectomy. Stroke, 1:307–313, 1970.

225. Lennox, W. G., Gibbs, F. A., and Gibbs, E. L.: Relationship of unconsciousness to cerebral blood flow and to anoxemia. Arch. Neurol. Psychiat., 34:1001–1013, 1935.

226. LePere, R. H., and Hardy, R. C.: Surgical improvement of collateral circulation to the brain. Texas Med., 62:55–58, 1966.

227. Lewis, B. M., Sokoloff, L., Wechsler, R. L., Wentz, W. B., and Kety, S. S.: A method for the continuous measurement of cerebral blood flow in man by means of radioactive krypton (Kr^{79}). J. Clin. Invest., 39:707–716, 1960.

228. Lewis, H. P., Ramirez, R., and McLaurin, R. L.: Intracranial blood volume after head injury. Surg. Forum, 19:433–435, 1968.

229. Liebow, A. A: Situations which lead to changes in vascular patterns. In Hamilton, W. F., and Dow, P., eds.: Handbook of Physiology, Washington, D.C., Amer. Physiol. Soc., 1963, Sect. 2, vol. 2, pp. 1251–1276.

230. Lyons, C., Clark, L. C., McDowell, H., and McArthur, K.: Cerebral venous oxygen content during carotid thrombintimectomy. Ann. Surg., 160:561–567, 1964.

231. Machleder, H. I., and Barker, W. F.: External carotid artery shunting during carotid endarterectomy. Arch. Surg. (Chicago), 108:785–788, 1974.

232. MacKenzie, E. T., McCulloch, J., and Harper, A. M.: Influence of endogenous norepinephrine on cerebral blood flow and metabolism. Amer. J. Physiol., 231:489–494, 1976.

233. Macpherson, P., and Graham, D. I.; Arterial spasm and slowing of the cerebral circulation in the ischaemia of head injury. J. Neurol. Neurosurg. Psychiat. 36:1069–1972, 1973.

234. Magaard, F., and Ryttman, A.: Regional cerebral blood flow and vertebral angiography at rest and in connection with arm work in patients with the "subclavian steal phenomenon."

Scand. J. Thorac. Cardiovasc. Surg., *10*:96–111, 1976.

235. Maggio, E.: Microhemocirculation; Observable Variables and Their Biologic Control. Springfield, Ill., Charles C Thomas, 1965, p. 194.

236. Magnussen, I., and Høedt-Rasmussen, K.: The effect of intraarterial administered aminophylline on cerebral hemodynamics in man. Acta Neurol. Scand., *55*:131–136, 1977.

237. Mangold, R., Sokoloff, L., Conner, E., Kleinerman, J., Therman, P. G., and Kety, S. S.: The effects of sleep on the cerebral circulation and metabolism of normal young men. J. Clin. Invest., *34*:1092–1100. 1955.

238. Mann, F. C., Herrick, J. F., Essex, H. E., and Baldes, E. J.: The effect on the blood flow of decreasing the lumen of a blood vessel. Surgery, *4*:249–252, 1938.

239. Marwardt, F.: Influence of drugs and enzymes on platelet 5-hydroxytryptamine. Ann. Med. Exp. Biol. Fenn., *46*:407–415, 1968.

240. Matakas, F., Leipert, M., and Franke, J.: Cerebral blood flow during increased subarachnoid pressure: The influence of systemic arterial pressure. Acta Neurochir. (Wien), *25*:19–36, 1971.

241. Mathew, N. T., Meyer, J. S., and Ott, E. O.: Increased cerebral blood volume in benign intracranial hypertension. Neurology (Minneap.), *25*:646–649, 1975.

242. Matsuda, M., Meyer, J. S., Deshmukh, V. D., and Tagashira, Y.: Effect of acetylcholine on cerebral circulation. J. Neurosurg., *45*:423–431, 1976.

243. Matsuda, M., Yoneda, S., Handa, H., and Gotoh, H.: Cerebral hemodynamic changes during plateau waves in brain-tumor patients. J. Neurosurg., *50*:483–488, 1979.

244. McDowall, D. G.: The effects of general anaesthetics on cerebral bloodflow and cerebral metabolism. Brit. J. Anaesth., *37*:236–245, 1965.

245. McDowall, D. G., Harper, A. M., and Jacobson. I.: Cerebral blood flow during halothane anesthesia. Brit. J. Anaesth., *35*:394–402, 1963.

246. McKissock, W., and Walsh, L.: Subarachnoid haemorrhage due to intracranial aneurysms. Brit. Med, J., *2*:559–565, 1956.

247. McNauthton, F. L.: The innervation of the intracranial blood vessels and dural sinuses. Res. Publ. Ass. Nerv. Ment. Dis., *18*:178–200. 1938.

248. Meffert, W., and Liebow, A. A.: Hormonal control of collateral circulation. Circ. Res., *18*:228–233, 1966.

249. Meier, P., and Zierler, K. L.: On the theory of the indicator-dilution method for measurement of blood flow and volume. J. Appl. Physiol., *6*:731–744, 1954.

250. Meyer, J. S., and Denny-Brown, D.: Studies of cerebral circulation in brain injury. II. Cerebral concussion. EEG Clin. Neurophysiol., *7*:529–544, 1955.

251. Meyer, J. S., and Denny-Brown, D.: The cerebral collateral circulation. Factors influencing collateral blood flow. Neurology (Minneap.), *7*:447–458, 1957.

252. Meyer, J. S., and Waltz, A. G.: Effects of changes in composition of plasma and blood flow. 1. Lipids and lipid fractions. Neurology (Minneap.), *9*:728–740, 1959.

253. Meyer, J. S., Fukuuchi, Y., Kanda, T., and Shimazu, K.: Interactions between cerebral metabolism and blood flow. *In* Russell, R. W. R., ed.: Brain and Blood Flow. London, Pitman Co., Ltd., 1971, pp. 156–164.

254. Meyer, J. S. Handa, J., Huber, P., and Yoshida, K.: Effect of hypotension on internal and external carotid blood flow. J. Neurosurg., *23*:191–198, 1965.

255. Meyer, J. S., Lavy, S., Ishikawa, S., and Symon, L.: Effects of drugs and brain metabolism on internal carotid arterial flow. An electromagnetic flowmeter study in the monkey. Amer. J. Med. Electronics. *3*:169–180, 1964.

256. Meyer, J. S., Tetsuaki, T., Sakamoto, K., and Kondo, A.: Central neurogenic control of cerebral blood flow. Neurology (Minneap.) *21*:247–262, 1971.

257. Meyer, J. S., Fukuuchi, Y., Shimazu, K., Ohuchi, T., and Ericsson, A. D.: Abnormal hemispheric blood flow and metabolism in cerebrovascular disease. II. Therapeutic trials with 5% CO_2 inhalation, hyperventilation and intravenous infusion of THAM and mannitol. Stroke, *3*:157–167, 1972.

258. Meyer, J. S., Shinohara, Y., Tadashi, K., Fukuuchi, Y., Kok, N. K., and Ericsson, A. D.: Abnormal hemispheric blood flow and metabolism despite normal angiograms in patients with stroke. Stroke, *1*:219–223, 1970.

259. Meyer, J. S., Shimazu, K., Fukuuchi, Y., Ohuchi, T., Okamoto, S., Koto, A., and Ericsson, A. D.: Impaired neurogenic cerebrovascular control and dysautoregulation after stroke. Stroke, *4*:169–186, 1973.

260. Miller, J. D.: The effect of space-occupying lesions on cerebral circulation. Int. Anesth. Clin., *7*:617–638, 1969.

261. Miller, J. D.: The effects of hyperbaric oxygen at 2 and 3 atmospheres absolute and intravenous mannitol on experimentally increased intracranial pressure. Europ. Neurol., *10*:1–11, 1973.

262. Miller, J. D., Stanek, A., and Langfitt, T. W.: Concepts of cerebral perfusion pressure and vascular compression during intracranial hypertension. Progr. Brain Res., *35*:411–432, 1971.

263. Miller, R. H., MacCarty, C. S., Kerr, F. W. L., Onofrio, B. M., Sundt, T. M., Jr., Laws, E. R., Jr., and Piepgras, D. G.: On the analysis of subarachnoid hemorrhage data. Arch. Neurol. (Chicago), *33*:309, 1976.

264. Millikan, C. H.: Cerebral vasospasm and ruptured intracranial aneurysm. Arch. Neurol. (Chicago), *32*:433–449, 1975.

265. Mitchell, O. C., de la Torre, E., Alexander, E., Jr., and Davis, C.: The nonfilling phenomenon during angiography in acute intracranial hypertension. J. Neurosurg., *19*:766–774, 1962.

266. Miyazaki, M.: Circulatory effect of cigarette smoking, with special reference to the effect on cerebral hemodynamics. Jap. Cir. J., *33*:907–912, 1969.

267. Monro, A.: Observations on the structure and function of the nervous system. Edinburgh, printed for William Creech, 1783.

268. Mount, L. A., and Taveras, J. M.: Arteriographic demonstration of the collateral circulation of the cerebral hemispheres. Arch. Neurol. Psychiat., *78*:235–253, 1957.

269. Mount, L. A., and Taveras, J. M.: Further observations of the significance of the collateral circulation of the brain as demonstrated arteriographically. Amer. Neurol. Ass. Trans., 85:109–113, 1960.

270. Moyer, J. H., and Morris, G.: Cerebral hemodynamics during controlled hypotension induced by the continuous infusion of ganglionic blocking agents (hexamethonium, Pendiomide and Arfonad). J. Clin. Invest., 33:1081–1088, 1954.

271. Moyer, J. H., Morris, G., and Snyder, H.: A comparison of the cerebral hemodynamic response to Aramine and norepinephrine in the normotensive and hypotensive subject. Circulation, 10:265–270, 1954.

272. Moyer, J. H., Snyder, H., and Miller, S. I.: Cerebral hemodynamic response to blood pressure reduction with phenoxybenzamine (Dibenzyline-688A). Amer. J. Med. Sci., 228:563–567, 1954.

273. Moyer, J. H., Pontius, R., Morris, G., and Hershberger, R.: Effect of morphine and n-allylnormorphine on cerebral hemodynamics and oxygen metabolism. Circulation, 15:379–384, 1957.

274. Muscholl, E., and Vogt, M.: The action of reserpine on the peripheral sympathetic system. J. Physiol. (London), 141:132–155, 1958.

275. Nagao, S., Okumura, S., and Nishimoto, A.: Effects of hyperbaric oxygenation on cerebral vasomotor tone in acute intracranial hypertension: an experimental study. Resuscitation, 4:51–59, 1975.

276. Nakano, J., Chang, A. C. K., and Fisher, R. G.: Effects of prostaglandins E_1, E_2, A_1, A_2, and F_2 on canine carotid arterial blood flow, cerebrospinal fluid pressure, and intraocular pressure. J. Neurosurg 38:32–39, 1973.

277. Neely, W. A., and Youmans, J. R.: Anoxia of canine brain without damage. J.A.M.A., 183:1085–1987, 1963.

278. Neuwirth, E.: Neurologic complications of osteoarthritis of the cervical spine. New York J. Med., 54:2583–2590, 1954.

279. Nierling, D. A., Wollschlaeger, P. B., and Wollschlaeger, G.: Ascending pharyngeal-vertebral anastomosis. Amer. J. Roentgen., 98:599–601, 1966.

280. Nilsson, B. W.: Cerebral blood flow in patients with subarachnoid haemorrhage studied with an intravenous isotope technique. Its clinical significance in the timing of surgery of cerebral arterial aneurysm. Acta Neurochir. (Wien), 37:33–48, 1977.

281. Norris, J. W., Hachinski, V. C., and Cooper, P. W.: Cerebral blood flow changes in cluster headache. Acta Neurol. Scand., 54:371–374, 1976.

282. Norwood, C. W., Poole, G. J., and Moody, D.: Treatment of experimental delayed cerebral arterial spasm with a beta$_2$-adrenergic stimulator and a phosphodiesterase inhibitor. J. Neurosurg., 45:491–497, 1976.

283. Novack, P., Shenkin, H. A., Bortin, L., Goluboff, B., and Soffe, A. M.: The effects of carbon dioxide inhalation upon the cerebral blood flow and cerebral oxygen consumption in vascular disease. J. Clin. Invest., 32:696–702, 1953.

284. Nylin, G., Hedlund, S., and Regnström, O.: Cerebral circulation studied with labelled red cells in healthy males. Acta Radiol., 55:281–304, 1961.

285. O'Brien, J. R.: Fat ingestion, blood coagulation and atherosclerosis. Amer. J. Med. Sci., 234:373–390. 1957.

286. O'Brien, M. D., and Veall, N.: Effect of cyclandelate on cerebral cortex perfusion-rates in cerebrovascular disease. Lancet, 2:729–730, 1966.

287. Obrist, W. D., Thompson, H. K., Jr., King, C. H., and Wang, H. S.: Determination of regional cerebral blood flow by inhalation of xenon[133]. Circ. Res., 20:124–135, 1967.

288. Oeconomos, D., Kosmaoglou, B., and Prossalentis, A.: rCBF studies in patients with arteriovenous malformations of the brain. In Brock, M., Fiesche, C., Ingvar, D. H., Lassen, N. A., and Schurmann, K., eds.: Cerebral Blood Flow. Berlin, Springer-Verlag, 1969, pp. 146–148.

289. Oeconomos, D., Kosmaoglou, B., and Prossalentis, A.: rCBF studies in intracranial tumors. In Brock, M., Fieschi, C., Ingvar, D. H., Lassen, N. A., and Schurmann, K., eds.: Cerebral Blood Flow, Berlin, Springer-Verlag, 1969, pp.172–175.

290. Oldendorf, W. H., and Kitano, M.: Radioisotope measurement of brain blood turnover as a clinical index of brain circulation. J. Nucl. Med., 8:570–587, 1967.

291. Osaka, K.: Prolonged vasospasm produced by the breakdown products of erythrocytes. J. Neurosurg., 47:403–411, 1977.

292. Ott, E. O., Lechner, H., and Aranibar, A.: High blood viscosity syndrome in cerebral infarction. Stroke, 5:330–333, 1974.

293. Ott, E. O., Mathew, N. T., and Meyer, J. S.: Redistribution of regional cerebral blood flow after glycerol infusion in acute cerebral infarction. Neurology (Minneap.), 24:1117–1126, 1974.

294. Overgaard, J., and Tweed, W. A.: Cerebral circulation after head injury. Part 1: Cerebral blood flow and its regulation after closed head injury with emphasis on clinical correlations. J. Neurosurg., 41:531–541, 1974.

295. Owens, G.: Evaluation of cerebral venous hypertension as therapy for cerebral infarction. Surg. Forum, 10:764–767, 1960.

296. Owens, G., and Ashby, R.: Intermittent jugular vein compression. Arch. Surg. (Chicago), 81:715–717, 1960.

297. Owens, G., and Stepanian, G.: Experimental evidence of potential blood flow from vein to capillary bed in brain. Neurology (Minneap.), 13:251–254, 1963.

298. Padget, D. H.: Development of cranial arteries in human embryo. Contrib. Embryol., 32:205–262, 1948.

299. Parrish, C. M., and Byrne, Jr., J. P.: Surgical correction of carotid artery obstruction in children. Surgery, 70:962–968, 1971.

300. Patterson, J. L., Jr., and Warren, J. V.: Mechanisms of adjustment in the cerebral circulation upon assumption of the upright position. J. Clin. Invest., 31:653, 1952.

301. Patterson, J. L., Jr., Heyman, A., Battery, L. L., and Ferguson, R. W.: Threshold of response of

the cerebral vessels of man to increase in blood carbon dioxide. J. Clin. Invest., *34*:1857–1864, 1955.

302. Paulson, O. B.: Regional cerebral blood flow in apoplexy due to occlusion of the middle cerebral artery. Neurology (Minneap.) *20*:63–77, 1970.

303. Paulson, O. B.: Restoration of autoregulation by hypocapnia. *In* Russell, R. W. R., ed.: Brain and Blood Flow. London, Pitman Co., Ltd., 1971, pp. 313–321.

304. Pierce, E. C., Jr., Lambertsen, C. J., Deutsch, S., Chase, P. E., Linde, H. W., Dripps, R. D., and Price, H. L.: Cerebral circulation and metabolism during thiopental anesthesia and hyperventilation in man. J. Clin. Invest., *41*:1664–1671, 1962.

305. Piraux, A., Jacquy, J., Lhoas, J. P., Wilmotte, J., and Noel, G.: Regional cerebral blood flow variations in mental alertness. Neuropsychobiology, *1*:335–343, 1975.

306. Pitts, F. W.: Variations of collateral circulation in internal carotid occlusion. Comparison of clinical and x-ray findings. Neurology (Minneap.). *12*:467–471, 1962.

307. Pletscher, A.: Metabolism, transfer and storage of 5-hydroxytryptamine in blood platelets. Brit. J. Pharmacol., *32*:1–16, 1968.

308. Quattlebaum, J. K., Wade, J. S., and Whiddon, C. M.: Stroke associated with elongation and kinking of the carotid artery: Long-term follow-up. Ann. Surg., *177*:572–579, 1973.

309. Raichle, M. E., and Plum, F.: Hyperventilation and cerebral blood flow. Stroke, *3*:566–575, 1972.

310. Regli, F., Yamaguchi, T., and Waltz, A. G.: Effects of inhalation of oxygen on blood flow and microvasculature of ischemic and nonischemic cerebral cortex. Stroke, *1*:314–319, 1970.

311. Regli, F., Yamaguchi, T., and Waltz, A. G.: Cerebral circulation; effects of vasodilating drugs on blood flow and the microvasculature of ischemic and nonischemic cerebral cortex. Arch. Neurol. (Chicago), *24*:467–474, 1971.

312. Reichelt, K. L.: The chemical basis for the intolerance of the brain to anoxia. Acta Anaesth. Scand. (suppl.), *29*:35–46, 1968.

313. Reichman, O. H.: Arteriographic flow patterns following sta-cortical MCA anastomosis. *In* Austin, G. M., ed.: Microneurosurgical Anastomoses for Cranial Ischemia. Springfield, Ill., Charles C Thomas, 1976, pp. 339–358.

314. Reinhold, H., de Rood, M., Capon, A., Mouawad, E., Fruhling, J., and Verbist, A.: Cerebral blood flow under enflurane anesthesia. Acta Anaesth. Belg., *27*:suppl.:250–258, 1976.

315. Reinmuth. O. M., Scheinberg, P., and Bourne, B.: Total cerebral blood flow and metabolism. Arch. Neurol. (Chicago), *12*:49–66, 1965.

316. Reiss, J., and Rosomoff, H. L.: Parenteral isoxsuprine and nylidrin. Arch. Neurol. (Chicago), *19*:213–217, 1968.

317. Reivich, M.: Regulation of the cerebral circulation. Clin. Neurosurg., *16*:378–418, 1968.

318. Reivich, M., Holling, H. E., Roberts, B., and Toole, J. F.: Reversal of blood flow through the vertebral artery and its effect on cerebral circulation. New Eng. J. Med., *265*:878–885, 1961.

319. Reivich, M., Dickson, J., Clark, J., Hedden, M., and Lambersten, C. J.: Role of hypoxia in cerebral circulatory and metabolic changes during hypocarbia in man: Studies in hyperbaric milieu. Scand. J. Clin. Lab. Invest., suppl. 102, IV:B, 1968.

320. Rob, C.: Surgical treatment of stenosis and thrombosis of the internal carotid vertebral and common carotid arteries. Proc. Roy. Soc. Med., *52*:549–552, 1959.

321. Roberts, B., Hardesty, W. H., Holling, H. E., Reivich, M., and Toole, J. F.: Studies on extracranial cerebral blood flow. Surgery, *56*:826–833, 1964.

322. Roe, B. B., Hepps, S. A., and Swenson, E. A.: Hemodilution with and without low-mole dextran: Laboratory studies and clinical experience. Circulation, *28*:792, 1963.

323. Roland, P. E., Larsen, Bo.: Focal increase of cerebral blood flow during stereognostic testing in man. Arch. Neurol. *33*:551–558, 1976.

324. Rosegay, H., and Welch, K.: Peripheral collateral circulation between cerebral arteries. J. Neurosurg., *11*:363–377, 1954.

325. Rosenberg, M. Z., and Liebow, A. A.: Effects of age, growth hormone, cortisone, and other factors on collateral circulation. Arch. Path. (Chicago), *57*:89–105, 1954.

326. Rosoff, C. B., Salzman, E. W., Gurewich, V., and Schroeder, H. K.: Reduction of platelet serotonin and the response to pulmonary emboli. Surgery, *70*:12–19, 1971.

327. Rowbotham, G. F., and Little, E.: A new concept of the circulation and the circulations of the brain. Brit. J. Surg., *52*:539–542, 1965.

328. Rowed, D. W., Stark, V. J., Hoffer, P. B., and Mullan, S.: Cerebral arteriovenous shunts reexamined. Stroke, *3*:592–600, 1972.

329. Roy, C. S., and Sherrington, C. S.: On the regulation of the blood-supply of the brain. J. Physiol. (London), *11*:85–108, 1889.

330. Sagawa, K.: Analysis of the CNS ischemic feedback regulation of the circulation. *In* Reeve, E. B., and Guyton, A. C., eds.: Physical Bases of Circulatory Transport. Philadelphia, W. B. Saunders Co., 1967, pp. 129–139.

331. Sagawa, K., and Guyton, A. C.: Pressure-flow relationships in isolated canine cerebral circulation. Amer. J. Physiol., *200*:711–714, 1961.

332. Sakai, F., and Meyer, J. S.: Regional cerebral hemodynamics during migraine and cluster headaches measured by the ^{133}Xe inhalation method. Headache, *18*:122–132, 1978.

333. Saphir, O.: Anomalies of the circle of Willis with resulting encephalomalacia and cerebral hemorrhage. Amer. J. Path., *11*:775–788, 1935.

334. Sarkari, N. B. S., Holmes, J. M., and Bickerstaff, E. R.: Neurological manifestations associated with internal carotid loops and kinks in children. J. Neurol. Neurosurg. Psychiat., *33*:194–200, 1970.

335. Schatz, I. J., Podolsky, S., and Frame, B.: Idiopathic orthostatic hypotension. J.A.M.A., *186*:537–540, 1963.

336. Schechter, M. M.: The occipital-vertebral anastomosis. J. Neurosurg., *21*:758–762, 1964.

337. Scheinberg, P.: Cerebral blood flow in vascular disease of the brain. Amer. J. Med., *8*:139–147, 1950.

338. Scheinberg, P., Jayne, H. W., Blackburn, I.,

Wich, M., and Belle, M. J.: Effects of intravenous papaverine and procaine on cerebral blood flow and metabolism. Amer. J. Med. *13*:106, 1952.

339. Scheinberg, P., Meyer, J. S., Reivich, M., Sundt, T. M., Jr., and Waltz, A. G.: XIII. Cerebral circulation and metabolism in stroke. Cerebral circulation and metabolism in stroke study group. Stroke, *7*:213–234, 1976.

340. Schieve, J. F., and Wilson, W. P.: The influence of age, anesthesia and cerebral arteriosclerosis on cerebral vascular activity to CO_2. Amer. J. Med., *15*:171–174, 1953.

341. Schieve, J. F., and Wilson, W. P.: The changes in cerebral vascular resistance of man in experimental alkalosis and acidosis. J. Clin. Invest., *32*:33–38, 1953.

342. Schieve, J. F., Scheinberg, P., and Wilson, W. P.: The effect of adrenocorticotrophic hormone (acth) on cerebral blood flow and metabolism. J. Clin. Invest., *30*:1527–1529, 1951.

343. Schmidt, C. F.: The influence of cerebral blood-flow on respiration. J. Physiol., *84*:202–259, 1928.

344. Schmidt, C. F., and Hendrix, J. P.: The action of chemical substances on cerebral blood vessels. Res. Publ. Ass. Nerv. Ment. Dis., *8*:229–276, 1938.

345. Schmidt, C. F., Kety, S. S., and Pennes, H. H.: The gaseous metabolism of the brain of the monkey. Amer. J. Physiol., *143*:33–52, 1945.

346. Schurr, P. H., and Wickbom, I.: Rapid serial angiography: Further experience. J. Neurol. Neurosurg. Psychiat., *15*:110–118, 1952.

347. Schutta, H. S., Kassell, N. F., and Langfitt, T. W.: Brain swelling produced by injury and aggravated by arterial hypertension. Brain, *91*:281–294, 1968.

348. Sechzer, P. H., Egbert, L. D., Linde, H. W., Cooper, D. Y., Dripps, R. D., and Price, H. L.: Effect of CO_2 inhalation on arterial pressure, ECG and plasma catecholamines and 17-OH corticosteroids in normal man. J. Appl. Physiol., *15*:454–458, 1960.

349. Seegers, W. H., Levine, W. G., and Johnson, S. A.: Inhibition of prothrombin activation with dextran. J. Appl. Physiol., *7*:617–620, 1955.

350. Severinghaus, J. W.: Role of cerebrospinal fluid pH in normalization of cerebral blood flow in chronic hypocapnia. Acta Neurol. Scand., *41*:suppl.14:116–120, 1965.

351. Shalit, M. N.: Effect of intracarotid artery administration of mannitol on cerebral blood flow and intracranial pressure in experimental brain edema. Israel J. Med. Sci., *10*: 577–580, 1974.

352. Shalit, M. N., Shimojyo, S., and Reinmuth, O. M.: Carbon dioxide and cerebral circulatory control: I. The extravascular effect. Arch. Neurol. (Chicago), *17*:298–303, 1967.

353. Shalit, M. N., Reinmuth, O. M., Shimojyo, S., and Scheinberg, P.: Carbon dioxide and cerebral circulatory control: III. The effects of brain stem lesions. Arch. Neurol. (Chicago), *17*:342–353, 1967.

354. Shapiro, C. M., and Rosendorff, C.: Local hypothalamic blood flow during sleep. Electroenceph. Clin. Neurophysiol. *39*:365–369, 1975.

355. Shapiro, H. M., Lafferty, M. D., Keyhah, M. M., Behar, M. G., Van Horn, K.: Barbiturates and intracranial hypertension. McLaurin, R.

L., ed.: Head Injuries. New York, Grune & Stratton, Inc., 1976.

356. Shellshear, J. L.: Arterial supply of cerebral cortex in chimpanzee (Anthropopithecus troglodytes). J. Anat., *65*:45–87, 1930.

357. Shenkin, H. A.: Effects of various drugs upon cerebral circulation and metabolism of man. J. Appl. Physiol., *3*:465–471, 1951.

358. Shenkin, H. A., Harmel, M. H., and Kety, S. S.: Dynamic anatomy of the cerebral circulation. Arch. Neurol. Psychiat., *60*:240–252, 1948.

359. Shenkin, H. A., Scheuerman, W. G., Spitz, E. B., and Groff, R. A.: Effect of change of position upon cerebral circulation of man. J. Appl. Physiol., *2*:317–326, 1949.

360. Simard, D., and Paulson, O. B.: Cerebral vasomotor paralysis during migraine attack. Arch. Neurol. (Chicago), *29*:207–209, 1973.

361. Simard, D. D., Olesen, J., Paulson, O. B., Lassen, N. A., and Skinhøj, E.: Regional cerebral blood flow and its regulation in dementia. Brain, *94*:273–288, 1971.

362. Skinhøj, E.: Determination of regional cerebral bloodflow in man. In Caveness, W. F., and Walker, A. E., eds.: Head Injury. Philadelphia, J. B. Lippincott Co., 1966, pp. 431–438.

363. Skinhøj, E., and Paulson, O. B.: Carbon dioxide and cerebral circulatory control. Arch. Neurol. (Chicago), *20*:249–252, 1969.

364. Skinhøj, E., and Paulson, O. B.: The mechanism of action of aminophylline upon cerebral vascular disorders. Acta Neurol. Scand., *46*:129–140, 1970.

365. Skinhøj, E., and Paulson, O. B.: Changes in focal cerebral blood flow within the internal carotid system during migraine attack. Acta Neurol. Scand., *46*:suppl. 43:254–255, 1970.

366. Skinhøj, E., Olesen, J., and Paulson, O. B.: Influence of smoking and nicotine on cerebral blood flow and metabolic rate of oxygen in man. J. Appl. Physiol., *35*:820–822, 1973.

367. Smith, A. L., Neigh, J. L., Hoffman, J. C., and Wollman, H.: Effect of blood pressure alterations on CBF during general anesthesia in man. In Brock, M., Fieschi, C., Ingvar, D. H., Lassen, N. A., and Schurmann, K., eds.: Cerebral Blood Flow. Berlin, Springer-Verlag. 1969, pp. 239–241.

368. Smith, G. W., and Sabiston, D. C.: A study of collateral circulation in vascular beds. Arch. Surg. (Chicago), *83*:702–706, 1961.

369. Soderberg, U.: Metabolic aspects of cerebral stroke. In Engel, A., and Larrson, T., eds.: Stroke—Thule International Symposium. Stockholm, Nordiska Bokhandelns Forlag. 1967, pp. 169–190.

370. Sokoloff, L.: Cerebral circulatory and metabolic changes associated with aging. In Milikan, C. H., ed.: Cerebrovascular Disease. Baltimore, Williams & Wilkins Co., 1966, pp. 237–251.

371. Soloway, M., Nadel, W., Albin, M. S., and White, R. J.: The effect of hyperventilation on subsequent cerebral infarction. Anesthesiology, *29*:975–980, 1968.

372. Spetzler, R., and Chater, N.: Occipital artery–middle cerebral artery anastomosis for cerebral artery occlusive disease. Surg. Neurol., *2*:235–238, 1974.

373. Steiner, S. H., Hsu, K., Oliner, L., and Behnke, R. H.: The measurement of cerebral blood

flow by external isotope counting. J. Clin. Invest., *41*:2221–2232, 1962.

374. Sukoff, M. H., Hollin, S. A., and Jacobson, J. H.: The protective effect of hyperbaric oxygenation in experimentally produced cerebral edema and compression. Surgery, *62*:40–46, 1967.

375. Sullivan, S. F., and Patterson, R. W.: Posthyperventilation hypoxia: Theoretical considerations in man. Anesthesiology, *29*:981–986, 1968.

376. Sundt, T. M., Jr., Sharbrough, F. W., Trautmann, J. C., and Gronert, G. A.: Monitoring techniques for carotid endarterectomy. Clin. Neurosurg., *22*:199–213, 1975.

377. Swank, R. L.: Changes in blood produced by fat meal and by intravenous heparin. Amer. J. Physiol., *164*:798–811, 1951.

378. Symon, L.: An experimental study of traumatic cerebral vascular spasm. J. Neurol. Neurosurg. Psychiat., *30*:497–505, 1967.

379. Symon, L.: Experimental features and therapeutic implications of "intracerebral steal". *In* Meyer, J. S., Reivich, M., Lechner, H., and Eichhorn, O., eds.: Research on the Cerebral Circulation. Springfield, Ill., Charles C Thomas, 1970, pp. 80–85.

380. Symon, L.: Vasospasm in aneurysm. *In* Moossey, J., ed.: Cerebral Vascular Disease. New York, Grune & Stratton, 1971, pp. 232–250.

381. Symon, L., Ishikawa, S., and Meyer, J. S.: Cerebral arterial pressure changes and development of leptomeningeal collateral circulation. Neurology (Minneap.), *13*:237–250, 1963.

382. Symon, L., Ishikawa, S., Lavy, S., and Meyer, J. S.: Quantitative measurement of cephalic blood flow in the monkey. A study of vascular occlusion in the neck using electromagnetic flowmeters. J. Neurosurg., *20*:199–218, 1963.

383. Szikals, J. J., and Spencer, R. P.: Transient abnormality on radionuclide cerebral dynamic study during a migraine attack. Headache, *14*:146–147, 1975.

384. Tada, K., Nukada, T., Yoneda, S., Kuriyama, Y., and Abe, H.: Assessment of the capacity of cerebral collateral circulation using ultrasonic Doppler technique. J. Neurol. Neurosurg. Psychiat., *38*:1068–1075, 1975.

385. Takeshita, H., Okuda, Y., and Sari, A.: The effects of ketamine on cerebral circulation and metabolism in man. Anesthesiology *36*:69–75, 1972.

386. Thomas, D. J., Marshall, J., Russell, R. W. R., Wetherley-Mein, G., du Boulay, G. H., Pearson, T. C., Symon, L., and Zilkha, E.: Cerebral blood-flow in polycythaemia. Lancet, July 23, 1977.

387. Thompson, J. E., Austin, D. J., and Patman, R. D.: Endarterectomy of the totally occluded carotid artery for stroke. Arch. Surg. (Chicago), *95*:791–801, 1967.

388. Tindall, G. T., Greenfield, J. C., Jr., Dillingham, W., and Lee, J. F.: Effect of 50 per cent sodium diatrizoate (Hypaque) on blood flow in the internal carotid artery of man. Amer. Heart J., *69*:215–219, 1965.

389. Tindall, G. T., Odom, G. L., Dillon, M. L., Cupp, H. B., Jr., Mahaley, M. S., Jr., and Greenfield, J. C., Jr.: Direction of blood flow in the internal and external carotid arteries following occlusion of the ipsilateral common carotid artery. J. Neurosurg., *20*:985–994, 1963.

390. Toole, J. F., and Tucker, S. H.: Influence of head position upon cerebral circulation. Arch. Neurol. (Chicago), *2*:616–623, 1960.

391. Torvik, A., and Skullerud, K.: How often are brain infarcts caused by hypotensive episodes? Stroke, *7*:255–257, 1976.

392. Townsend, R. E., Prinz, P. N., and Obrist, W. D.: Human cerebral blood flow during sleep and waking. J. Appl. Physiol., *35*:620–625, 1973.

393. Turner, J. M., Powell, D., Gibson, R. M., and McDowall, D. G.: Intracranial pressure changes in neurosurgical patients during hypotension induced with sodium nitroprusside or trimetaphan. Brit. J. Anaesth., *49*:419–425, 1977.

394. Ulano, H. B., Ascanio, G., Rice, V., O'Hern, R., Houmas, E., and Oppenheimer, M. J.: Effects of angiographic contrast media and hypertonic saline solutions on cerebral venous outflow in autoregulating brains. Invest. Radiol., *5*:518–533, 1970.

395. Vander Eecken, H. M., and Adams, R. D.: The anatomy and functional significance of the meningeal arterial anastomosis of the human brain. J. Neuropath. Exp. Neurol., *12*:132–157, 1953.

396. von Essen, C.: Effects of dopamine on the cerebral blood flow in the dog. Acta Neurol. Scand., *50*:39–52, 1974.

397. Voris, H. C.: Complications of ligations of the internal carotid artery. J. Neurosurg., *8*:119–131, 1951.

398. Wade, J. G., Larson, C. P., Hickey, R. H., and Ehrenfeld, W. K.: Effect of carotid endarterectomy on carotid chemoreceptor and baroreceptor function. Surg. Forum, *19*:144–145, 1968.

399. Waltz, A. G., and Sundt, T. M.: The microvasculature and microcirculation of the cerebral cortex after arterial occlusion. Brain, *90*:681–696, 1967.

400. Waltz, A. G., Sundt, T. M., Jr., and Michenfelder, J. D.: Cerebral blood flow during carotid endarterectomy. Circulation, *45*:1091–1096, 1972.

401. Wasserman, A. J., and Patterson, J. L. Jr.: The cerebral vascular response to reduction in arterial carbon dioxide tension. J. Clin. Invest., *40*:1297–1303, 1961.

402. Weil, M. H., and Whigham, H.: Head-down (Trendelenburg) position for treatment of irreversible hemorrhagic shock. Ann. Surg., *162*:905–909, 1965.

403. Welch, K. M. A., Hashi, K., and Meyer, J. S.: Cerebrovascular response to intracarotid injection of serotonin before and after middle cerebral artery occlusion. J. Neurol. Neurosurg. Psychiat., *36*:724–735, 1973.

404. Welch, K., Stephens, J., Huber, W., and Ingersoll, C.: The collateral circulation following middle cerebral branch occlusion. J. Neurosurg., *12*:361–368, 1955.

405. Wells, R. E., Jr.: Rheology of the blood in the microvasculature. New Eng. J. Med., *270*:832–839, 1964.

406. White, R. P., Hagen, A. A., Morgan, H., Dawson, W. N., and Robertson, J. T.: Experimental study on the genesis of cerebral vasospasm. Stroke, 6:52–57, 1975.

407. Wilkins, R. H., and Odom, G. L.: Intracranial arterial spasm associated with craniocerebral trauma. J. Neurosurg., 32:626–633, 1970.

408. Wilson, G., Riggs, H. E., and Rupp, C.: The pathologic anatomy of ruptured cerebral aneurysms. J. Neurosurg., 11:128–134, 1954.

409. Winsor, T., Hyman, C., and Knapp, F. M.: The cerebral peripheral circulatory action of nylidrin hydrochloride. Amer. J. Med. Sci., 239:594–600, 1960.

410. Wise, B. L., and Palubinskas, A. J.: Persistent trigeminal artery (carotid-basilar anastomosis). J. Neurosurg., 21:199–206, 1964.

411. Wolff, H. G., and Lennox, W. G.: Cerebral circulation: The effect on pial vessels of variations in the oxygen and carbon dioxide content of the blood. Arch. Neurol. Psychiat., 23:1097–1120, 1930.

412. Wollman, H., Alexander, S. C., and Cohen, P. J.: Cerebral circulation and metabolism in anesthetized man. In Harmel, M. H., ed: Clinical Anesthesia, Philadelphia, F. A. Davis Co., 1967, Vol. 3, pp. 1–15.

413. Wollman, H., Smith, A. L., and Alexander, S. C.: Effects of general anesthetics in man on the ratio of cerebral blood flow to cerebral oxygen consumption. In Brock, M., Fieschi, C., Ingvar, D. H., Lassen, N. A., and Schurmann, K., eds.: Cerebral Blood Flow. Berlin, Springer-Verlag, 1969, pp. 242–243.

414. Wollman, H., Alexander, S. C., Cohen, P. J., Stephen, G. W., and Zeiger, L. S.: Two-compartment analysis of the blood flow in the human brain. Acta Neurol. Scand., 41:suppl.14:49–82, 1965.

415. Wollman, S. B., and Orkin, L. R.: Postoperative human reaction time and hypocarbia during anesthesia. Brit. J. Anaesth., 40:920–925, 1968.

416. Wylie, E. J., Hein, M. F., and Adams, J. E.: Intracranial hemorrhage following surgical revascularization for treatment of acute strokes. J. Neurosurg., 21:212–215, 1964.

417. Yamamoto, Y. L., Feindel, W., Wolfe, L. S., Katoh, H., and Hodge, C. P.: Effects of prostaglandins on cerebral blood flow. Europ. Neurol., 6:144–152, 1971–1972.

418. Yamamoto, Y. L., Feindel, W., Wolfe, L. S., Katoh, H., and Hodge, C. P.: Experimental vasoconstriction of cerebral arteries by prostaglandins. J. Neurosurg., 37:385–397, 1972.

419. Youmans, J. R., and Kindt, G. W.: Effect of collateral artery impairment on blood flow through a constricted carotid artery. Circulation, 36:suppl.2:276, 1967.

420. Youmans, J. R., and Kindt, G. W.: Influence of multiple vessel impairment on carotid blood flow in the monkey. J. Neurosurg., 29:135–138, 1968.

421. Youmans, J. R., and Kindt, G. W.: Efficacy of carbon dioxide in treatment of cerebral ischemia. Surg. Forum, 19:425–426, 1968.

422. Youmans, J. R., and Scarcella, G.: Extracranial collateral cerebral circulation. Neurology (Minneap.), 11:166–169, 1961.

423. Youmans, J. R., Kindt, G. W., and Mitchell, O. C.: Extended studies of direction of flow and pressure in the internal carotid artery following common carotid artery ligation. J. Neurosurg., 27:250–254, 1967.

424. Zervas, N. T., Candia, M., Candia, G., Kido, D., Pessin, M. S., Rosoff, C. B., and Bacon, V.: Reduced incidence of cerebral ischemia following rupture of intracranial aneurysms. Surg. Neurol., 11:339–344, 1979.

425. Zucker, M. B., and Borrelli, J.: Quantity, assay and release of serotonin in human platelets. J. Appl. Physiol., 7:425–431, 1955.

426. Zwetnow, N. N.: Effects of increased cerebrospinal fluid pressure on the blood flow and on the energy metablism of the brain. Acta Physiol. Scand., 339:suppl.339:1–31, 1970.

24

INCREASED INTRACRANIAL PRESSURE AND THE CEREBRAL CIRCULATION

Brain swelling has plagued the neurosurgeon since the beginning of neurosurgery. It occurs in patients with head injuries, thrombotic and hemorrhagic strokes, brain tumors, and in fact, any space-occupying intracranial lesion, and is the most common cause of death in neurosurgical patients. Intracranial mass lesions and the brain swelling that accompanies them raise intracranial pressure, and for a long time it was assumed that death from a mass effect within the intracranial space was largely due to intracranial hypertension. For that reason, methods to reduce intracranial pressure, originally in the form of hypertonic solutions that dehydrate the brain, were added to the therapeutic armamentarium of the neurosurgeon.

Despite the association of brain swelling with intracranial hypertension and the common occurrence of the neurological signs of transtentorial herniation, until recent times there was little direct information on the incidence, magnitude, and clinical significance of increased intracranial pressure in patients with intracranial disease. The reason was that pressure was rarely measured directly from within the intracranial space. Instead, the measurements were made from the lumbar subarachnoid space; they were recorded infrequently and for brief periods of time, and under only those circumstances in which pressure measurements were most needed. Lumbar puncture was often contraindicated because of the possibility of inducing transtentorial or foramen magnum herniation.

The earliest continuous recordings of intracranial pressure on a strip chart recorder were performed by Guillaume and Janney; and in 1960, Lundberg published the first report of continuous recording of intracranial pressure in a large series of patients.[133,236] In the early 1960's, the author and his colleagues studied the effect of a variety of experimental intracranial lesions on intracranial pressure, cerebral blood flow, and vital signs: and these experimental observations helped explain a number of the clinical phenomena described by Lundberg.* It was not until the early 1970s, however, that large series of patients were reported, and therefore, only recently has it been possible to assess the incidence and significance of intracranial hypertension in patients with various intracranial disorders and the effects of increased intracranial pressure on the cerebral circulation and brain metabolism.

ANATOMY AND PHYSIOLOGY

The Craniospinal Space and Its Contents

The intracranial space is bounded by a thick layer of bone penetrated by several foramina. It is divided into two large compartments by the tentorium, and the compartments communicate through the tentorial incisura. Since the thick bone of the calvarium is essentially nondistensible, the volume of the intracranial space is virtually constant irrespective of the pressure gen-

---

* See references 210–213, 215, 216, 236, 420, 421, 423.

erated within it. The tentorium can be displaced upward or downward somewhat, resulting in reciprocal changes in volume in the supratentorial space and posterior fossa, but not in total intracranial volume. The intracranial space is filled to capacity with fluid and solid material, and its contents are nearly noncompressible. These facts, a rigid sphere filled to capacity with noncompressible contents, represent the basis of the Monro-Kellie doctrine.

Alexander Monro the younger was the son of the man who described the connection between the lateral and third ventricles. He was one of the most celebrated physiologists of his day and, in 1783, published his epochal "Observations on the Structure and Function of the Nervous System."[280] Among these was the concept that the intracranial space contains only two compartments that can change in volume, brain matter and intravascular blood. Since neither can be compressed, and the skull cannot be stretched, it follows that the volume of blood within the intracranial space must at all times be constant. Forty years later Kellie made several observations that appeared to support Monro's hypothesis.[193] Blood was still present in the brains of animals that died by exsanguination; the amount of blood in cerebral veins was not affected by changes in posture; cerebral congestion was not present in those who died by hanging, as would be expected if intracranial blood volume could be increased.

Despite the contribution of his father to our knowledge of the anatomy of the ventricular system, neither Monro, nor Kellie after him, apparently was aware of the cerebrospinal fluid. Burrows, in 1846, repeated some of the earlier experiments of Kellie in the light of observations on the cerebrospinal fluid system published by Magendie.[44] Burrows concluded that the blood volume of the brain does in fact change under a variety of circumstances and this change is accompanied by a reciprocal change in volume of one of the other intracranial compartments, either the brain or cerebrospinal fluid. This modification of the Monro-Kellie doctrine was generally accepted and was introduced into neurosurgery by Cushing.[70-73] Many of the critical experiments required to test the hypothesis were performed by Weed and his colleagues, as summarized by Weed in 1929.[417]

They found that the intravenous administration of hypertonic solutions in experimental animals resulted in a negative intracranial pressure and postulated that a pressure less than that of atmosphere could not develop in the intracranial space if the volume of the latter were not at all times constant. This was verified by demonstrating that a negative pressure, recorded in the spinal subarachnoid space, did not develop when the skull was open. Instead, the hypertonic solution caused shrinkage of the total volume of intracranial contents. Weed also made the important observation that the Monro-Kellie doctrine does not hold in infants because the skull is not yet rigid. The enlarged ventricles of hydrocephalus are accommodated primarily by expansion of the skull and only secondarily, if at all, by a reduction in total brain volume. In infants, hypertonic solutions cause not only dehydration of the brain but diminution in the size of the fontanelles and a reduction in total intracranial volume.

These and other observations on the Monro-Kellie doctrine can be summarized by stating that the craniospinal intradural space is *nearly* constant in volume and that its contents are *nearly* noncompressible. These qualifications, however, are very important and account for many of the clinically significant aspects of intracranial dynamics. Thus, the spinal dura is not in contact with the wall of the vertebral canal as it is in the intracranial space, permitting some changes in total volume at the expense of the blood volume in the spinal extradural veins. Since the dura can be stretched very little, these changes in volume are quite small. Furthermore, every substance can be either stretched or compressed if the applied force is great enough, and in physical terms these properties of the material are expressed in terms of elasticity.

Normal Intracranial Pressure

A consideration of the factors responsible for normal intracranial pressure can begin with examination of a few simple models. Figure 24–1 *A* illustrates a model of a patient in the lateral decubitus position with a needle in the spinal subarachnoid space. The plane of the needle passes

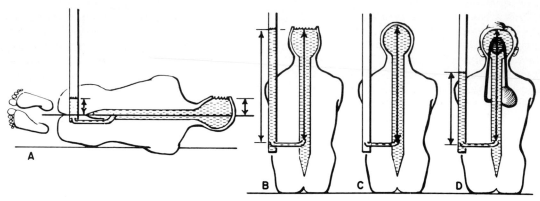

Figure 24-1 Models of craniospinal pressure. See text for explanation.

through the midsagittal plane of the skull. If the uppermost portion of the skull is open, forming a bowl, the pressure measured in the spinal canal is the distance between the midsagittal plane and the lateral wall of the skull. Thus, the pressure would be approximately 70 mm of water in this static open system. Water seeks its own level in a U-tube with both ends open to the atmosphere. When the model is tilted from the horizontal to the vertical position fluid rises in the manometer attached to the lumbar needle until it equals the fluid level in the skull (Fig. 24–1 B). On the other hand, if the skull were a completely closed, rigid container filled to capacity, no fluid would flow into the manometer when the model was tilted into the vertical position (Fig. 24–1 C). The reason is that the fluid in the needle in the spinal canal, but not the fluid in the head, is exposed to the atmosphere. If one places one end of a rubber tube into an automobile gas tank and the other end into a pail, gasoline does not flow from the tank. But if the car is raised approximately 34 feet, the pressure in the gas tank exceeds normal atmospheric pressure, and gasoline flows into the pail. An easier way to achieve the same result is to reduce atmospheric pressure at the end of the tube by applying suction. Figure 24–1 D illustrates a normal patient in the sitting position. Spinal fluid in an open manometer attached to the lumbar puncture needle rises to about the level of the cervicothoracic junction. Thus, actual spinal fluid pressure in the sitting position is less than it would be if the intracranial space were an open system and greater than if it were a completely closed system.

Weed and his colleagues investigated these phenomena extensively in experimental animals and attributed the pressure changes that occur in tilting from the horizontal to the head-down and tail-down positions to the elasticity of the craniospinal contents.[417–419] Pollock and Boshes, in an excellent application of physical principles to biological research, concluded that, on the contrary, the skull is an imperfectly closed container because a portion of atmospheric pressure is applied to the intracranial space through the blood vessels (Fig. 24–1 D).[316] Patients with large skull defects have higher than normal pressure in the sitting position because the system is further exposed to the atmosphere.

Another matter having to do with the mechanics of pressure measurements is the relationship of "absolute" to "relative" intracranial or spinal fluid pressure. In order to measure pressure in an open manometer, fluid must be dislocated into the manometer, thereby reducing the volume of fluid in the craniospinal intradural space; also the higher the pressure, the more fluid is required to measure it. This is often termed the relative pressure and is less than absolute pressure. Absolute pressure can be measured if the method does not permit escape of fluid. Originally this was performed with a "bubble manometer." A bubble of air is introduced at the hub of the needle and rises in the manometer during measurement of relative pressure. The manometer is then elevated until the dislocated fluid flows back into the spinal canal, and the bubble again rests at the bottom of the manometer. The problem of distinguishing between relative and absolute pressures is of less concern today with the wide use of pressure transducers. A transducer is attached to the hub of the needle at the time of insertion so that no fluid is lost, except that which may leak around the shaft of the needle. The volume of fluid displaced then is only that contained within the needle plus the minute quantity required to displace the diaphragm of the transducer.

In more recent studies of the effects of tilting the body from the lateral decubitus to the head-up position, Magnaes has called attention to two important points on the spine, the level of zero cerebrospinal fluid pressure (ZPS) and the hydrostatic indifferent point (HIP) (Fig. 24–2). Since in the sitting position the pressure in the lower part of the body is higher than the pressure in the upper part, there must be a point along the spine where cerebrospinal fluid pressure is zero. There must also be another point where the fluid pressure is the same in

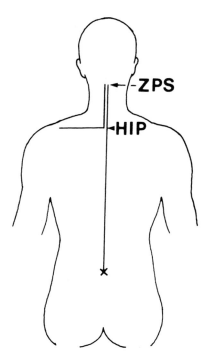

Figure 24–2 Drawing shows that the distance between level of zero cerebrospinal fluid pressure and hydrostatic indifferent point corresponds to the cerebrospinal fluid pressure in the lateral position(in millimeters of water). ZPS, level of zero cerebrospinal fluid pressure while in the sitting position. HIP, hydrostatic indifferent point for lateral and sitting positions. (From Magnaes, B.: Body position and cerebrospinal fluid pressure. Part 2: Clinical studies on orthostatic pressure and the hydrostatic indifferent point. J. Neurosurg., 44:698–705, 1976. Reprinted by permission.)

the lateral and sitting positions, and this is termed the hydrostatic indifferent point. The indifferent point is caudal to the zero point by a distance equal to the cerebrospinal fluid pressure measured in the lateral decubitus position.[240] Magnaes measured these points in a number of clinical situations. For example, in patients with skull defects, the zero and indifferent points were shifted cranially, while after cranioplasty, they were located within levels found in the control group.[241]

Of even greater interest were the transient alterations in lumbar cerebrospinal fluid pressure recorded in normal patients and in patients with intracranial disease in shifting from the lateral to the sitting position. In the normal patient, a primary rise in pressure of several hundred millimeters of water occurs as soon as the patient sits up, and is followed by a secondary transient increase in pressure that Magnaes attributes to increased cerebral blood volume as a manifestation of cerebral autoregulation.[240] In other words, when the patient sits up, the blood pressure in the cerebral arteries decreases transiently, and the cerebral resistance vessels dilate as a manifestation of autoregulation. Then as arterial pressure is restored to normal, the arteries constrict again, accounting for the transience of the pressure rise (Fig. 24–3). In patients with various types of intracranial disease, the secondary rise in cerebrospinal fluid pressure remained for much longer periods of time, and sometimes a sustained and progressive increase in pressure occurred. These constituted pressure waves, or the plateau waves of Lundberg.[236] The important point to be gained from these observations is that intracranial pressure is a dynamic phenomenon affected by a number of physiological variables within the intracranial space.

Normal intracranial pressure is a pulsatile pressure. The pulsations are mainly due to respirations and the cardiac pulse. For a long time the opinion was held that the cardiac pulse could be attributed entirely to the choroid plexus. There is good evidence, however, that the cerebral and spinal arteries also contribute to the pulsations.[29,85] Normally, the amplitude of the cardiac pulse is approximately 15 mm of water, and the combined cardiac and respiratory variation is about 45 mm of water.[29] As intracra-

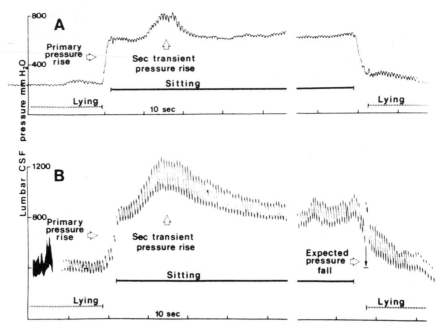

Figure 24–3 Tracings showing typical pattern of lumbar cerebrospinal fluid pressure during rapid tilting in a hydrocephalic patient, *A*, and a patient with subarachnoid hemorrhage, *B*. Sitting up: Rapid primary rise in hydrostatic pressure and secondary transient rise in filling pressure. Variation in amplitude of transient wave and phase of falling pressure. Lying down. The immediate drop in pressure was as expected in *A*, and less than expected in *B*. (From Magnaes, B.: Body position and cerebrospinal fluid pressure. Part 1: Clinical studies on the effect of rapid postural changes. J. Neurosurg., *44*:687–697, 1976. Reprinted by permission.)

nial pressure increases, the pulse pressure increases.

Since the intracranial cardiac pulsation has a complex wave form, another issue has been the intracranial vascular origins of the various components of the wave form. There is experimental evidence that under normal circumstances the pulsations are mainly arterial in origin.[140] There is a venous superimposition on the descending portion of the pulse curve, however. As intracranial pressure increases, not only does the amplitude of the pulse increase, but the venous component disappears, leaving an entirely arterial pulse. In contrast, during cardiac insufficiency and increased cerebral venous pressure, the cerebrospinal fluid pulse curve is venous in shape, with particular prominence of the wave whose origin is attributed to the right atrium.

Methods of Measurement

The first spinal tap appears to have been performed by Corning for the purpose of anesthetizing the spinal cord.[164] The first treatise on lumbar puncture was published by Quincke, who introduced the practice of measuring pressure with a fine glass pipet.[318] He described the normal pressure as 90 to 100 mm of water. In later years Jackson described spinal fluid pressure measurements with a mercury manometer in a variety of pathological conditions,[164] and the significance of examination of the spinal fluid in the diagnosis of intracranial tumors was thoroughly evaluated by Ayer.[9] The procedure was not used extensively, however, until it began to be applied in the management of head injuries. Sharpe published a monograph on brain injuries in which he stated that his principal criterion for operation was increased spinal fluid pressure.[375] Numerous reports of spinal fluid pressure measurements in head injury patients followed, and there was much disagreement on the indications for and danger of lumbar puncture and the reliability of the procedure in accurately measuring intracranial tension. Most authors did agree that a pressure in excess of 200 mm of water was definitely abnormal.

The two principal objections to lumbar puncture in the diagnosis of intracranial hypertension have been the danger of inducing acute brain stem compression, either at the tentorial incisura or the foramen magnum, and the contention that spinal fluid pressure is not an accurate reflection of intracranial pressure. The former concern has led to the admonition that a spinal tap should not be performed when there is clinical evidence of increased intracranial pressure, particularly in the presence of papilledema or signs of a tentorial pressure cone. Certainly the latter sign remains a contraindication to spinal tap under all except the most unusual circumstances. The value of analysis of the cerebrospinal fluid in patients with papilledema must be weighed against the dangers of the procedure. Lumbar puncture is not an innocuous procedure in patients with intracranial hypertension, but in experienced hands the danger appears to be minimal except in those patients who have a shift of the midline structure or those who already have signs of herniation or brain stem compression. The second reservation concerning lumbar puncture, that the spinal fluid pressure need not accurately reflect the intracranial pressure, is considered later.

Ventricular puncture for relief of increased intracranial pressure is one of the oldest practices in neurosurgery. Ventricular fluid pressure measurements during the procedure were described by a number of investigators, and occasionally ventricular and lumbar subarachnoid pressures were measured simultaneously. Prolonged pressure measurements were performed infrequently, however, because water and mercury manometers were cumbersome for this purpose and because of the risk of intracranial infection. Lundberg reviewed the early history of direct intracranial pressure mensuration in his monograph, "Continuous recording and control of ventricular fluid pressure in neurosurgical practice," a major milestone in the story of intracranial hypertension.[236]

Lundberg used a polyethylene cannula and stylet mounted on a stopcock. The cannula was inserted into the frontal horn of the right lateral ventricle through a burr hole. A rubber stopper through which the cannula was inserted was seated in the burr hole to prevent leakage of cerebrospinal fluid and to reduce the risk of infection. In 130 patients there were no hematomas that could be ascribed to the procedure. There were two cases each of extradural and intradural infections.[236] Intracranial pressure can also be measured from a catheter in the subdural space, but the tip of the catheter tends to become obstructed at high levels of intracranial pressure and the method does not permit removal of cerebrospinal fluid for examination or rapid reduction of pressure.[208]

In recent years there has been much interest in solid-state transducers that are not dependent for their function on contact with intracranial fluid and do not require penetration of the brain. The ideal transducer must meet many demands, and the goal has been to develop transducers for different purposes rather than one all-purpose device. The requirements range from long-term measurement of intracranial pressure in hydrocephalic infants to a quick method of recording intracranial pressure in patients with severe head injuries. The pressure changes in hydrocephalus are subtle, and the intracranial pulse pressure may be as important as the mean pressure in determining the ventricular size. The device should be implantable within the intracranial space for periods of months or longer, should operate efficiently at low pressures, and should have minimal baseline drift. A transducer for measuring intracranial pressure in patients with severe head injuries or other major cerebral insults should be adaptable to use in the emergency ward or intensive care unit. It should be small enough to pass through a twist drill hole in the skull, thus avoiding an open procedure in the operating room, and be rugged enough to withstand repeated use by personnel who have limited experience with the instrument.

In the 1960's, a number of devices were developed for measuring pressure from the extradural space. Since the extradural space does not contain fluid and, therefore, a hydraulic couple from the extradural space to an external transducer is not possible, it was necessary to develop a sensor that would accurately reflect changes in force applied to it from within the intradural space. Various types of fluid-filled bags were developed, which to some degree provided the basis for a hydraulic couple.[292] A number of devices were then developed in which the sensing elements themselves were encapsulated and placed within the extradural space. The earliest of these were small discs containing the arms of a Wheatstone bridge.[59,167] Several modifications of this basic concept, using a strain gauge and piezoelectric elements, have been introduced over the years.[79,80,121,291]

A number of investigators have aimed toward the ideal transducer, one that would be fully implantable within the extradural space and would record pressure accurately for an indefinite period of time. The earliest fully implantable device was developed by Collins and modified by Atkinson and co-workers to accomplish radiotelemetric measurements of intraventricular pressure.[6,64] Subsequently, a more sophisticated induction-powered oscillator transducer was described.[354] In these various induction devices, pressure is recorded by placing antenna coils over the scalp above the transducer. A modification of this concept uses a fully implanted differential intracranial pressure sensor with the advantage of zero point calibration. Pressure is applied to the scalp over the sensor until a balance of pressures is achieved; the applied pressure then equals the intracranial pressure.[436]

None of the solid-state or implantable transducers has yet attracted enough interest to be used widely. Instead, there is still considerable reliance on both intraventricular and subarachnoid or subdural measurements. Over the years there appears to have been general agreement that measurements of pressure from the intraventricular space are probably the most accurate of all. The tip of the cannula does occasionally become obstructed by the choroid plexus or the ependyma, but this is uncommon, and flushing with a milliliter or two of saline usually will clear the obstruction. There is, however, a significant risk of infection, and it is necessary to violate the brain in order to insert the cannula.[168] In patients with small or shifted ventricles, finding the ventricle can be difficult, but this problem has been ameliorated by CT scanning prior to insertion of the cannula.

The technique that now appears to be used as commonly as, and perhaps even more commonly than, intraventricular measurements is the subarachnoid screw or bolt first described by Vries and associates.[414] A twist drill hole ¼ inch in diameter is made through the skull, generally in the same location used to insert the intraventricular cannula, namely, at the level of the coronal suture and about 2 cm lateral to the midline over the nondominant hemisphere. The dura is then pricked through the twist drill hole until a small amount of cerebrospinal fluid is obtained, and the screw is inserted with a special hexagonal screwdriver. Tubing is attached to the screw and thence to an external transducer at the patient's bedside. The device has been modified to include a Millipore filter for protection against contamination of the intracranial space, and has also been modified for children.[169,170] A further modification of the device has also been described.[261]

The subarachnoid bolt appears to work quite well. In the beginning, there was concern that in the face of severe brain swelling, brain tissue might herniate into the internal orifice of the bolt, obstructing it and damping the recording. This appears to occur uncommonly, and as in the case of obstruction of an intraventricular cannula, the device can be cleared by injection of a small quantity of saline. The introduction of another subdural pressure-measuring device, a cup catheter, may reduce even further the incidence of damping.[427] The incidence of infection is low. Bruce and co-workers have recorded intracranial pressure with the pediatric version of the Richmond bolt for periods up to two weeks in children with severe head injuries without identified intracranial infection.[37]

Despite these many advances, to date an ideal device has not been developed. The most accurate measurements require hydrostatic coupling from the ventricular, subarachnoid, or subdural space to an external measuring device. Despite reports of an encouragingly low incidence of infection, this inside-outside connection must, in fact, increase the risk of infection more than an extradural placement of the measuring instrument and, especially, a fully implantable device. Although several of the latter methods have worked well in animals and in initial studies in patients, they have not been widely used. Probably there are a number of reasons. The more complex instruments, especially those that permit measurements by telemetry, are expensive, more difficult to calibrate than bolts and catheters, and more easily damaged, especially in the common situation in which the device is being used by many persons. Some of the most interesting methods have been described only recently, however, and may become acceptable with wider use.

Intracranial Volume-Pressure Relationship

Reciprocal changes among compartments occur during physiological alterations in the intracranial contents. Hypercapnia increases intracranial blood volume to values at least twice the control volume and is accompanied by an increase in intracranial pressure.[426] The rise in intracranial pressure appears to be damped, however, by expression of cerebrospinal fluid as the vasodilatation and increase in cerebral blood volume occur. When the fluid has already been displaced by prior brain swelling or a mass lesion, hypercapnia produces a much greater rise in intracranial pressure.[212] Presumably the increase in cerebral blood volume is the same, but the increase in intracranial pressure is greater, because less cerebrospinal fluid is available to be displaced.

During gradual expansion of a mass lesion, the volume displaced may be cerebrospinal fluid, intravascular blood, or brain tissue water. Long-term compression of the brain can produce atrophy and perhaps some reduction in the mineral content of the brain, but changes in brain solids must be very small in terms of total volume. Rosomoff estimated the cerebrospinal fluid volume in the dog to be approximately 9 per cent of total intracranial volume.[341] If all of this fluid were displaceable, the intracranial space could accommodate a mass 9 per cent of the total intracranial volume without an increase in intracranial tension. Measurements of cerebral blood volume vary considerably according to the technique used, and the methods have been reviewed recently by Sklar and associates.[387] Most investigators have found an average cerebral blood volume of about 2 per cent in postmortem determinations in animals. The animals were sacrificed by quick freezing the head, or attempts were made to prevent drainage of blood from the head at sacrifice. In vivo measurements of cerebral blood volume in man have yielded values as high as 7 per cent.[293] If the latter value is correct, there is in fact considerable blood within the intracranial space that could be expressed during expansion of a mass lesion. Reduction in total brain water as a means of compensation for an expanding mass has not been adequately investigated. Since the subarachnoid space over the cerebral hemispheres is obliterated and the ventricles are narrowed by expansion of a mass or by brain swelling, it appears that cerebrospinal fluid is the principal spatial buffer, although reduction in blood volume may be an important factor under some circumstances.

Another important factor is the time required for spatial compensation to take place. If, for example, cerebrospinal fluid could not be rapidly displaced, rapid expansion of even the smallest mass would produce an increase in intracranial pressure incompatible with life; that is, the intracranial space would behave as a completely closed container. Ryder and co-workers injected fluid into the lumbar subarachnoid space and then immediately withdrew fluid in sufficient amount to return the pressure to the baseline. Invariably the amount of fluid withdrawn was less than that injected, indicating that some of the fluid had rapidly escaped from the intradural space.[353] Foldes and Arrowwood infused the spinal subarachnoid space with saline and found that pressure remained constant at elevated levels during continuous infusion. Equilibrium was reached with an infusion rate of 4 drops per minute at 265 mm of cerebrospinal fluid, and with 16 drops per minute equilibrium pressure was 395 mm of cerebrospinal fluid.[105] Their observations suggest that as much as 1 ml of cerebrospinal fluid per minute can be expressed from the intradural space in the presence of elevated pressure. Thus, a large hematoma could be accommodated within a few hours without a dangerous rise in intracranial pressure. The complex anatomy of the cerebrospinal fluid spaces does not permit such a simple analogy, but the fact remains that the fluid can be driven out of the intracranial space rapidly, and were this not so, even the smallest extradural hematoma would cause swift death from intracranial hypertension.

In initial descriptions of the volume and pressure relationships within the intracranial space during expansion of a mass lesion, intracranial pressure was measured from one or more catheters in the subarachnoid space of the Rhesus monkey during gradual expansion of an extradural balloon.[212] When the balloon was expanded with water at a rate of approximately 1 ml per hour, by means of a slow-rate infusion pump, it appeared that there was no increase in intracranial pressure during infusion of the first few milliliters of water (Fig. 24–4). The data were interpreted to show that the volume added to the balloon was matched rather precisely by a decrease in volume of one or more of the intracranial compartments so that pressure remained constant. With further expansion of the balloon, the intracranial pressure began to rise, and at a volume of approximately 6 ml in the monkey, it began to rise very rapidly, nearly vertical to the horizontal axis. The flat portion of the curve was termed the period of spatial compensation, and the vertical portion, the period of spatial decompensation. According to the hypothesis, the rapid rise in pressure supervened when the amount of displaceable volume within the intracranial space had been reduced to the point that the volume added to the balloon exceeded the volume of fluid displaced, resulting in an increase in the net intracranial volume and, therefore, intracranial pressure.

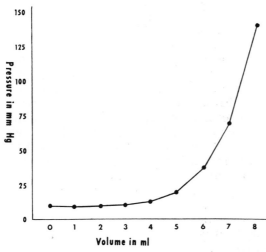

Figure 24–4 Volume-pressure graph. Volume is given in milliliters (abscissa), and pressure in millimeters of mercury (ordinate) in this and all subsequent illustrations. (From Langfitt, T. W., Weinstein, J. D., and Kassell, N. F., in Caveness, W. F., and Walker, A. E., eds.: Head Injury: Conference Proceedings. Philadelphia, J. B. Lippincott Co., 1966. Reprinted by permission.)

Those early experiments also demonstrated a shift of the vertical portion of the curve from right to left with either more rapid inflation of the balloon or the creation of pathological change that would decrease the amount of displaceable fluid before the balloon was expanded (Fig. 24–5). The marked leftward displacement of the vertical part of the curve was first noticed in a monkey that had had a period of accidental anoxia during preparation. As the balloon was expanded, the period of spatial compensation was very brief, presumably owing to brain swelling produced by the hypoxia.

The two groups of investigators who have contributed the most to our further understanding of the volume and pressure relationships within the intracranial space are Miller and Marmarou and their colleagues. The basic shape of the volume/pressure curve in the monkey was confirmed in children with hydrocephalus and in patients with raised intracranial pressure from a variety of other causes, including tumor, head injury, and cerebrovascular disease.[272,274,380]

The relationship of volume to pressure can be defined in terms of the compliance or elastance of the intracranial space.[230-233] Compliance is the amount of "give" that is available within the intracranial space; elastance is the inverse of compliance, in effect, the resistance offered to expansion of the mass or expansion of the brain itself. Compliance is expressed as dV/dP. A high degree of compliance, that is, much give within the intracranial space, would be reflected by a large change in volume producing a small change in pressure. The expression then would have a large number. Elastance, the inverse of compliance, can be expressed as dP/dV. This number is large when a small change in volume produces a large change in pressure. This is the situation on the vertical portion of the volume/pressure curve, where it can be said that the compliance of the intracranial space is low and the elastance is high.

Miller and Garibi introduced the volume/pressure response (VPR) to test the elastance of the intracranial space. In patients with a variety of disorders in whom ventricular pressure was measured continuously, 1 ml of saline was injected through the intraventricular cannula in one second, and the immediate change in intraventricu-

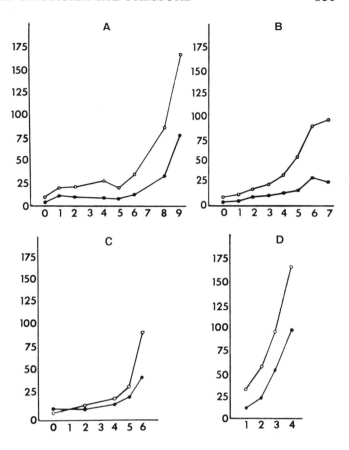

Figure 24–5 Intracranial volume-pressure curves in 4 animals (A, B, C, and D). Intracranial pressure (in millimeters of mercury) is shown on ordinate and intracranial balloon volume (in milliliters of water) on abscissa. Closed circles represent final pressure following each increment of water added to balloon, and open circles, at each point, the peak pressure produced by rapid injection of 0.5 ml of saline into cerebral subarachnoid space. Interval between balloon injections about 30 minutes; each 0.5 ml of saline injection made 10 minutes before subsequent balloon injection. Balloon injection time 50 seconds. Volume of deflated balloon about 1.5 ml in each experiment. (From Langfitt, T. W., Weinstein, J. D., and Kassell, N. F.: Cerebral vasomotor paralysis produced by intracranial hypertension. Neurology (Minneap.), *15*:622–641, 1965. Reprinted by permission.)

lar pressure was termed the volume/pressure response.[272] They found that the response was increased in parallel with intracranial pressure in experimental animals and in patients with intracranial disorders.[223,224,274] Only in patients with enlarged ventricles was this relationship less clear.[271] In view of the predictable relationship between the volume/pressure response and intracranial pressure in nearly all circumstances, it is surprising that both mannitol and steroids reduced the response much more than the intracranial pressure itself.[223,224]

The principal contribution of Marmarou and his colleagues to this field of research has been the development of mathematical models of the cerebrospinal fluid system. They identified four variables—the intracranial compliance, dural sinus pressure, resistance to absorption, and cerebrospinal fluid formation—and postulated that the interaction of these four variables would determine intracranial pressure and the characteristics of the volume/pressure response. The model and its experimental

verification are described in detail in a recent publication.[243] In brief, the volume/pressure relationship is defined as a nonlinear, exponential curve. The slope of the curve is a measure of the compliance of the system. Furthermore, compliance is not uniform throughout the full range of recorded pressures. According to the model, a sustained elevation of pressure can develop with an increase in cerebrospinal fluid formation, an increase in the resistance to the outflow of the fluid, or an increase in the venous pressure within the dural sinuses. The investigators concluded that increases in dural sinus pressure had a far greater effect on intracranial pressure than did either an increase in the rate of cerebrospinal fluid formation or an increase in outflow resistance.

Marmarou and colleagues also introduced the term "pressure/volume index" (PVI) as an alternative or a supplementary term to the volume/pressure response. The pressure/volume index is defined as the volume in milliliters necessary to raise intracranial pressure to a level 10 times the opening pressure. The concept has been applied in animals, but clearly has limited usefulness in patients, in whom every effort must be made not to raise intracranial pressure to dangerous levels during the course of testing intracranial compliance or elastance. Sullivan and associates have also studied the index in experimental animals. During expansion of an epidural balloon, they observed a progressive increase in the pressure/volume index and in elastance, and then, at high levels of intracranial pressure when the animals' pupils had become dilated, a marked decrease in cerebrospinal fluid elastance occurred.[397]

Throughout the recent history of these studies of intracranial compliance and elastance, distinctions have been made between the compliance of the cerebrospinal fluid system and the elasticity of the brain itself. In order to address this rather complicated issue, assume for the moment that the brain is a rigid body surrounded by dis-

placeable fluid, and the brain and fluid are incorporated within the essentially nondistensible cranium. If one now expands the mass, which must conform to the subarachnoid space, since the brain in this model is rigid and not displaceable, the intracranial volume/pressure curve is determined by cerebrospinal fluid compliance, which is a function of the volume of the fluid's formation, outflow resistance at the arachnoid granulation, and dural sinus pressures. In the actual situation, however, the brain is displaceable and moldable, and therefore it contributes to the total intracranial compliance and elastance. There is also displaceable intravascular blood both within the brain and in the veins that lie in the subdural and subarachnoid spaces.

Schettini and Walsh have developed a pressure-displacement transducer for studying the properties of brain tissue in vivo. In the transducer, a small pressure-sensing element is mounted at the end of a

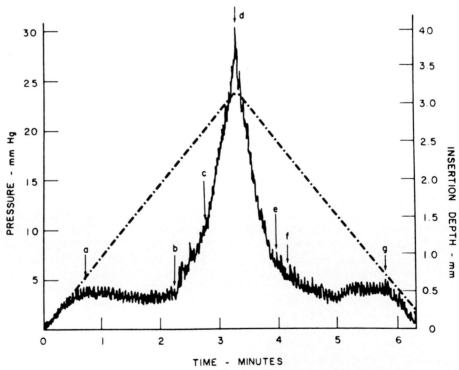

Figure 24–6 Pressure test recording. The solid line is the pressure response (in millimeters of mercury); the broken line is the insertion depth (in millimeters). Zero point represents initial dural contact of the piston. Point a, firm contact with the dura; a to b, the transducer measures pressure in the subarachnoid space as the piston advances slowly. Point b, contact with the subpial region b to d, the piston advances against the brain. From d to g, the piston was withdrawn at the same rate as it was inserted. (From Schettini, A., and Walsh, E. K.: Experimental identification of the subarachnoid and subpial compartments by intracranial pressure measurements. J. Neurosurg., *40*:609–616, 1974. Reprinted by permission.)

cylindrical piston that is coupled to a finely-threaded plunger. A rotational potentiometer is geared to the plunger, and as the potentiometer moves, the piston is advanced into or withdrawn from the intracranial space. In Figure 24–6, on the left-hand side of the illustration, the 0 pressure point represents contact of the piston with the dura. At point a, the piston is in firm contact with the dura, and as the piston continues to advance slowly from points a to b, the transducer measures pressure in the subarachnoid space. At point b, the subpial region is contacted, and from b to d, the piston advances against the brain. From d to g, the piston is withdrawn at the same rate as it was inserted. The difference in the shape of the two portions of the curve appears to be due at least in part to hysteresis, meaning that the compression and relaxation features of the cerebral tissue are different. The investigators made special note of the change in the slope of the compression portion of the curve marked by the letter c. They hypothesized that the slope from b to c represented the transition from the subarachnoid space through the pia into the subpial region, which is heavily vascularized, and the segment from c to d represented advancement of the piston through less vascular brain substance.[358,359,416] The method permits measurement of the depth of the subarachnoid space, which in turn provides an estimate of the amount of brain swelling, and it also measures the stiffness or the elastance of the brain determined by its resistance to compression.

Thus, in examining the relationships between volume and pressure within the intracranial space, it is necessary to distinguish between the compliance of the cerebrospinal fluid system and the elastance of the brain. The time element is important in making this distinction. For example, Sklar and Elashvili have questioned whether the volume/pressure response is serving one of its main functions, which is to determine "where the patient is on the pressure/volume curve."[386] Since 1 ml of fluid is injected within one second in order to measure the response, it would appear to provide a better estimate of brain elastance than of the compliance of the cerebrospinal fluid system, which provides information on the amount of available space for expansion within the intracranial cavity. In animal studies in which the volume and pressure relationship is defined by continuous infusion of fluid either into the subarachnoid space or into a balloon or with the injection of small aliquots of fluid, pressure is described as a semilogarithmic function of intracranial volume changes. These experiments do not, however, provide information on the relative contributions of brain elastance and cerebrospinal fluid system compliance to the volume/pressure curve in a given animal or patient. For example, it is not clear that such an exponential, semilogarithmic relationship necessarily exists in a patient with a long-standing intracranial mass lesion. If in fact a volume of cerebrospinal fluid or cerebral venous blood equal to the mass could be expressed during very slow expansion of the mass, the initial portion of the volume/pressure curve in this patient would, indeed, be flat. Furthermore, the stiffness or the elastance of the brain might have little or no influence on the pressure recorded from the lumbar subarachnoid space or a lateral ventricle as long as there was no change in intracranial volume.

These are important matters for further investigation, because there is still relatively little information on the pathophysiological basis of the reductions in intracranial pressure produced by a variety of therapeutic modalities. For example, hypertonic mannitol reduces brain fluid volume and thereby alters the elastance properties of the brain. Since there is evidence that the mannitol can greatly increase cerebral blood flow without a reduction in intracranial pressure, an increase in blood volume in addition to the decrease in tissue water volume would also contribute to changes in brain elastance.[41] Although not all of these issues have been resolved, the contributions of several investigators to a better understanding of the volume and pressure relationships within the intracranial space constitute one of the most important advances in the study of intracranial pressure in recent years.

Transmission of Intracranial Pressure

The term intracranial pressure is meaningful only if one can assume that pressure is everywhere equal. The pressure in brain adjacent to an expanding mass might be elevated at a time when intraventricular pressure is normal. If so, one must speak of intracranial *pressures,* and in this case the important measurement in terms of function is in the compressed brain. Lumbar subarachnoid pressure is usually equated with intracranial pressure, but if for any reason there is failure of communication of pressure from the intracranial space to the spinal canal the spinal fluid pressure will be misleading.

Methods for recording intracranial and intraspinal pressures were developed in the latter part of the nineteenth century, and some investigators noted that increased pressure was not transmitted consistently from the intracranial to the intraspinal space. Hill maintained that rapid injections of fluid into the supratentorial subarachnoid space caused displacement of the cerebral hemispheres and the cerebellum with obstruction at both the tentorial incisura and foramen magnum.[156] Cushing stated that severe effects of compression could occur locally with little or no transmission to remote areas of the brain.[71] On the other hand, Eyster argued that displacement of the brain could not occur because of the incompressible fluid in the spinal canal, which he believed had no means of escape.[92] In the experiments of Kahn and Meyers, an increase in pressure in the supratentorial space was not always fully communicated to the posterior fossa, but the difference in pressure was quite small.[190,269]

In simultaneous measurements of intracranial and spinal fluid pressures in patients with pathological intracranial conditions, Hodgson reported some difference between the two pressures in the majority of patients with posterior fossa mass lesions, but failure of communication of pressure was rare with supratentorial lesions.[157] Smyth and Henderson found a lower lumbar pressure in 8 of 33 patients with intracranial space-occupying lesions, most of which were tumors, but the maximum difference in pressure was 100 mm of water.[392] These observations contrast with the high incidence of transtentorial herniation caused by supratentorial mass lesions. At autopsy, Finney and Walker found transtentorial herniation in 55.4 per cent of an unselected series

of brain tumors, including an incidence of 88 per cent in glioblastomas of the cerebral hemispheres. In 23 per cent of supratentorial tumors, herniations at both the tentorial incisura and foramen magnum were present.[99] Many herniations, however, may not completely obstruct the basal cisterns. Kaufmann and Clark found lumbar subarachnoid pressure to be significantly less than intraventricular pressure in the majority of a series of patients with severe head injury.[192]

Observations in animals have demonstrated that obstruction to communication of pressure at both the incisura and the foramen magnum occurs uniformly during the expansion of mass lesions, but the issue of pressure transmission within the supratentorial space has not been completely resolved.[213,423] Pressure in an extradural mass may be manyfold the pressure recorded in the remainder of the intracranial space, because the dura is highly elastic and is often firmly attached to the inner table of the skull.

In the monkey, continued expansion of a supratentorial balloon invariably leads to obstruction at the tentorial incisura, and when obstruction is complete, elevating the intracranial pressure above the systolic blood pressure has no effect on the spinal fluid pressure.[213] In contrast, when the supratentorial pressure is raised to high levels by infusion of saline into the cerebrospinal fluid spaces, there is full communication of pressure throughout the craniospinal axis. These experiments demonstrate that the basal cisterns at the incisura must be blocked by brain tissue for a difference in pressure to occur and that this can be produced consistently by a mass lesion but not by infusion of the cerebrospinal fluid spaces. Injection of fluid into the spinal subarachnoid space or cisterna magna will reduce the block at the incisura created by a supratentorial mass, but the block redevelops immediately as long as the mass remains. Following evacuation of the mass, infusion of the cisterna magna with saline opens the tentorial cisterns and free communication of pressure throughout the craniospinal axis is re-established.

Herniation of brain through the tentorial incisura causes displacement and local compression of the brain stem and the familiar neurological signs of a tentorial pressure cone. If the pressure in the posterior fossa is normal, because of the obstruction at the incisura, the pons and medulla might be spared from the intracranial hypertension. In fact, increased supratentorial pressure is freely communicated through the brain stem to the medulla at a time when pressure in the cerebellopontine angle is normal by virtue of the incisural obstruction.[423]

The brain, particularly the cortical surface with its dense network of blood vessels, has important elastic properties that resist displacement and deformation. Thus, it would appear that in the course of expansion of a subdural hematoma, for example, the pressure within the deep gray matter and white matter might be different from the pressure in the subdural space and on the surface of the brain because of the elasticity of the intervening tissue.

The major problem in attempting to determine whether pressure gradients exist across the brain in various pathological circumstances has been the inability to measure tissue pressure accurately. Since the brain tissue itself does not contain fluid-filled spaces that are large enough to accommodate a pressure-measuring device, it has been necessary to create such a cavity in order to measure tissue pressure. In early experiments, tissue pressure was measured from several small intracerebral balloons during the expansion of another balloon, either in the subdural space or within the brain parenchyma.[423] When the pressure in the injection balloon was rapidly increased to 100 mm of mercury, the maximum difference in pressure measured across the brain was 35 mm of mercury, but this difference in pressure was rapidly dissipated. In subsequent experiments in the monkey, in which a transparent calvarium was used, expansion of a subdural or epidural mass produced focal compression of surface vessels at a time when surface vessels over the same hemisphere remote from the mass were normal.[422] Although pressures were not measured in these experiments, they lend support to the concept that differences in pressure do develop across the supratentorial compartment.

Brock and co-workers introduced the "wick method" for measuring brain tissue pressure.[32] A thin polyethylene catheter provided with a wick of long-stranded cotton wool that prevents obliteration of the tip of the catheter is inserted into the brain tissue, and the external end of the catheter is attached to a transducer. In experimental animals, simultaneous measurements of brain tissue pressure from several sites, by this method, and intraventricular pressure demonstrated the pressures to be equal and to rise and fall equally with infusion of fluid into the cerebrospinal fluid spaces.[315] Subsequently, Clark and associates found the catheter method to be unsatisfactory, presumably because of loss of fluid into the tissue. They used catheter transducers mounted on the distal end of a No. 5 French catheter and found that the method was accurate for monitoring rapid phasic changes but had serious limitations in measuring relatively small changes in intracranial pressure over time.[55] Finally, a number of investigators have implanted pressure-measuring devices of various kinds over the surface of the brain, in either the subdural or epidural spaces, in order to determine whether pressure gradients exist across the brain during the creation of experimental intracranial disorders.

The issue has not been resolved. Symon and colleagues, and Johnston and Rowan used either a subdural or extradural balloon to raise intracranial pressure while recording from multiple sites.[188,403] The former authors found significant differences in pressures between the region of the balloon and other regions in the supratentorial compartment, whereas the latter authors found no significant differences. It is of interest that in neither study was there a reduction in regional cerebral blood flow adjacent to or remote from the balloon. Undoubtedly this is a reflexion of well-preserved autoregulation throughout the brain. Clark's group did not find a pressure gradient across the brain in animals with experimental cerebral infarctions.[55] Reulen and Kreysch, however, found a pressure difference as large as 15 mm of mercury in animals with cold-induced cerebral edema. The difference in pressure appeared to develop as the spreading edema front within the white matter reached the catheters.[334] There have been few studies in man. Crockard and associates did find a sustained difference in pressures between the anterior and posterior portions of an obstructed lateral ventricle in a patient with a thalamic tumor.[69]

Although all the data do not quite fit the following conclusion, perhaps a consensus could be obtained that large pressure gradients do develop across the supratentorial space and the brain substance during rapid expansion of either an extracerebral or intracerebral mass lesion, and the pressure gradients then decline rather rapidly when the mass ceases to expand. Presumably, the dissipation of the gradients is due to "plastic creep" of the brain away from the mass.[423] During slower expansion of a mass, gradients either do not exist or are very small because the creep of the brain is continuous, and if plastic creep exceeds the elastic properties of the brain, as it were, pressure gradients do not develop. Spreading edema probably is quite different from expansion of a localized mass, and pressure gradients in this circumstance may be produced by the resistance of the tissue to the stretching effect of the advancing fluid front.[335]

PATHOLOGY OF RAISED INTRACRANIAL PRESSURE

Relationship Between Intracranial Hypertension and Disturbed Brain Function

A diffuse increase in intracranial pressure may have no detectable effect on brain function until mean intracranial pressure approaches the mean systemic arterial pressure. Figure 24–7 illustrates the intracranial and systemic arterial pressures mea-sured respectively from an intraventricular cannula and a catheter in the radial artery in a patient with obstructive hydrocephalus secondary to a cerebellar hemangioblastoma. The intraventricular cannula had been inserted in order to drain the ventricles slowly in preparation for removal of the tumor. At the time of this recording, which extended over several hours, the mean intracranial pressure approached the mean systemic arterial pressure on several occasions; for brief periods the cerebral perfusion pressure was as low as 6 to 10 mm of mercury. Throughout this time, the patient was alert and well-oriented. If intracranial pressure is such an important variable in assessing pathological conditions of the brain, how could the brain function normally in this patient at a time when the perfusion pressure across it had been virtually abolished?

There is ample evidence that the cause of the intracranial hypertension is as important as the level of intracranial pressure in determining brain function. The author has observed a number of patients with obstructive hydrocephalus or pseudotumor cerebri who have shown little or no ill effect from extraordinarily high intracranial pressure. The reason appears to be that the brain itself was essentially normal in these patients before the onset of their disease. Thus, cerebral autoregulation is intact, meaning that the perfusion pressure across the brain can be reduced to very low levels without causing a critical reduction in cerebral blood flow.

The situation is quite different in patients

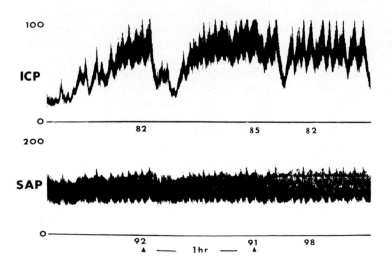

Figure 24–7 Intracranial pressure (ICP) recorded from a lateral ventricle and systemic arterial pressure (SAP) from the radial artery during spontaneous pressure waves. Intracranial pressure and corresponding systemic arterial pressure are indicated at peaks of pressure waves. (From Miller, J. D., Stanek, A., and Langfitt, T. W.: Concepts of cerebral perfusion pressure and vascular compression during intracranial hypertension. Progr. Brain Res., 35:411–432, 1971. Reprinted by permission.)

with parenchymal lesions of the brain such as certain tumors, hematomas, and contusions. These mass lesions cause a shift of brain structures and disturb autoregulation adjacent to the lesion. Furthermore, pressure in the brain tissue adjacent to the mass may be higher than intracranial pressure measured from a cerebrospinal fluid space. When a diffuse rise in intracranial pressure, produced by the volume effect of the mass, edema, or vascular dilatation from hypercarbia, is superimposed on the regional abnormality, function of the brain adjacent to the mass may be compromised at relatively low levels of intracranial pressure. Presumably this is due to compromised regional cerebral blood flow. The patient then develops focal neurological signs at intracranial pressures as low as 15 to 25 mm of mercury, and those signs are reversed when pressure is reduced to normal. This situation is in striking contrast to the patient with an essentially normal brain who remains neurologically normal with intracranial pressure that approaches the systemic arterial pressure.

It appears that increased intracranial pressure per se disturbs brain function by only two mechanisms: (1) a decrease in cerebral blood flow below the critical level required to provide the brain with an adequate amount of oxygen, and (2) transtentorial or foramen magnum herniation resulting in selective compression and ischemia in the brain stem at a time when the blood flow through the cerebral hemispheres is still adequate for tissue oxygenation. In other words, a critically located temporal lobe mass may produce uncal herniation and compression of the brain stem without a rise in intracranial pressure sufficient to reduce blood flow in the cerebral hemispheres.

Effect on Vital Signs of Increased Intracranial Pressure

Early clinical investigations of increased intracranial pressure suggested that changes in blood pressure, heart rate, and respiration might serve as an accurate index of the onset and degree of intracranial hypertension. Kocher defined four stages of cerebral compression and intracranial hypertension, based on changes in the vital signs and level of consciousness.[203] His observations did not receive wide attention, however, until the experiments of Cushing demonstrated that "an increase of intracranial tension occasions a rise of blood pressure which tends to find a level slightly above that of the pressure exerted above the medulla." The increase in arterial pressure did not occur until the intracranial pressure approached or equalled the mean arterial pressure, and thereafter the two pressures rose together.[70-72] Cushing also emphasized the importance of bradycardia and respiratory irregularities, but it is clear from his writings that he considered arterial hypertension the most diagnostic of the changes in vital signs. Cushing's observations were confirmed by many writers in the early part of the century, and Janeway stated that the highest blood pressures ever recorded were in patients with severe increased intracranial pressure.[173] The Cushing criteria were used particularly in the management of patients with head injuries, but several authors expressed the opinion that blood pressure was of little value in the management of head injuries.[164,327,376] Browder and Meyers recorded blood pressure and spinal fluid pressure intermittently in patients following head injury and found that blood pressure may be high without increased intracranial pressure, intracranial pressure may be elevated without a change in blood pressure, and blood pressure may increase as intracranial pressure is falling.[35] They concluded that changes in the arterial pressure were of no value in the diagnosis of cerebral compression and increased intracranial pressure. Evans and associates increased intracranial pressure to values in excess of 1000 mm of water by lumbar injections without necessarily altering the blood pressure.[91,351]

Many of the clinical studies were limited by a failure to demonstrate that patients who did not have increased arterial pressure did in fact have increased intracranial pressure. Kjallquist and co-workers were the first to record intraventricular fluid pressure (VFP) and arterial pressure continuously in brain tumor patients preoperatively.[197] They related spontaneous fluctuations in intracranial pressure, previously described in detail by Lundberg, to the arterial pressure.[236] Blood pressure did not increase with ventricular fluid pressure as high as 70 mm of mercury. In the first description of continuous recording of intracranial and blood pressures in postcraniotomy patients, the relationship was found to be unpredictable. In some patients intracranial pressure rose to the level of the mean arterial pressure without provoking a pressor response, whereas in others marked sustained increases in blood pressure occurred with intracranial pressure waves of relatively low magnitude.[208]

Expansion of a supratentorial mass in experimental animals almost always causes an arterial pressor response. The response persists following removal of the cerebral hemispheres and progressive maceration of the brain stem to a level at the superior border of the inferior olive, but with further destruction of the medulla it disappears.[108] Therefore, the vasopressor response to cerebral compression appears to arise in the medulla. It is accompanied by marked peripheral vasoconstriction that appears to be neurogenic in origin and it is abolished by sympathectomy.[36,93,110] Several mechanisms have been proposed to explain the vasopressor response. Cushing, following upon the earlier hypothesis of Kocher, believed that an increase in arterial pressure did not occur until the rise in intracranial pressure was sufficient to cause ischemia of the medullary vasomotor center. This conclusion was based primarily on the observation that arterial hypertension did not occur until intracranial pressure approached the level of the blood pressure, at which time it was assumed blood flow throughout the brain must be nearly abolished. Dickinson and McCubbin, however, found the vasopressor threshold in unanesthetized dogs to be far below the diastolic blood pressure.[77] There is experimental evidence that brain ischemia, produced by lowering the arterial pressure to the isolated dog head or by carotid and vertebral occlusion, does cause a marked rise in arterial pressure, but this vasopressor response need not be elicited by the same mechanism operative in intracranial hypertension.[355,401] Rodbard and Stone postulated a baroceptor mechanism responsible for the vasopressor response. They described a threefold cardiovascular response in the dog. Immediately after the onset of acute compression, blood pressure rises sharply, presumably owing to a direct neurogenic effect on peripheral arterioles.

A secondary rise, coming on several seconds after the onset of compression, was attributed to the release of pressor substances into the blood. A final increase in blood pressure was attributed to an increase in circulating blood volume. They postulated the existence of an intracranial receptor that is sensitive to differences in pressure between the intravascular space and the cerebrospinal fluid. Thus, a rise in intracranial pressure would be interpreted by the receptor as a fall in intravascular pressure, and peripheral vasoconstriction would be elicited.[339] Additional evidence in favor of the proposal by Rodbard and Stone is the demonstration by Weinstein and co-workers that during failure of the vasopressor mechanism a response still could be elicited by increasing intracranial pressure to several times the systolic arterial pressure, far beyond the level required for total cerebral ischemia.[421]

An additional contribution was the demonstration of the relationship of the vasopressor threshold to brain stem displacement or compression. Meyers noted that an increase in arterial pressure could be elicited more readily by injecting fluid into the ventricles than into the lumbar subarachnoid space and that the rapid ventricular injections were accompanied by the establishment of a difference in pressure between the ventricle and the cisterna magna.[269] This is best explained by a downward displacement or kinking of the brain stem. Thompson and Malina introduced the term "dynamic axial brain stem distortion" to explain the cardiorespiratory changes produced by increased intracranial pressure.[407] They demonstrated that the arterial pressor response, bradycardia, and respiratory irregularities occurred at a lower threshold with expansion of a supratentorial balloon than did elevation of intracranial pressure with lumbar fluid injections. Weinstein and associates quantified the vasopressor response in monkeys by alternating injections into a supratentorial extradural balloon and the lumbar subarachnoid space. They found that a vasopressor response could be elicited by a balloon injection to an intracranial pressure 50 mm of mercury below the mean arterial pressure at a time when it was necessary to raise the intracranial pressure to within 5 mm of mercury of the mean arterial pressure by lumbar injection in order to obtain the same increase in blood pressure.[421] Thus, patterns of brain stem distortion and displacement appear to be important in determining the nature and degree of the cardiorespiratory changes produced by an expanding mass. This mechanism cannot account for the vasopressor response produced by diffuse cerebral ischemia, however, nor for the fact that compression of the isolated spinal cord also causes a rise in arterial pressure.[421] The latter finding indicates that the medulla need not mediate the vasopressor response.

The changes in heart rate produced by intracranial hypertension have received less attention than the arterial pressor response, although it is well accepted that severe bradycardia may be the principal alteration in vital signs in acutely expanding lesions such as extradural hematoma. The bradycardia produced by intracranial hypertension in experimental animals is unaffected by denervation of the carotid sinuses, is abolished by section of the vagi, and is independent of the rise in blood pressure.[71,86]

The occurrence of respiratory irregularities with increased intracranial pressure was recognized in the earliest clinical reports. Respiratory and vasomotor collapse were the principal criteria of the end-stage of cerebral decompensation in Kocher's schema. Periodic respiration of the Cheyne-Stokes type was recognized in the nineteenth century in patients with primary cerebral disease. Jackson postulated that Cheyne-Stokes respiration is due to an interference in the neural connections between the respiratory center and higher levels.[165] Damage to the higher centers releases the respiratory mechanism in the medulla from a supranuclear control, and the periodic respiration is a manifestation of some inherent automatism within the medulla. A thorough study of levels of respiratory control was carried out by Hoff and Breckenridge, who described respiratory disorders in dogs and cats decerebrated at various levels between the hypothalamus and the medulla. Midpontine decerebration resulted in slow respirations that were succeeded by "ataxic" respirations when the level of section reached the pontomedullary level.[158] Ataxic breathing is grossly irregular and inefficient, usually leading to early death of the animal. The concept that periodic respiration is a release phenomenon caused by damage to supramedullary mechanisms is also supported by clinical studies.

Plum and associates were the first investigators to evaluate respiratory disorders systematically in patients with diencephalic and brain stem damage. They analyzed 52 cases with cerebral infarction, hemorrhage, trauma, or neoplasm. Level of consciousness, the status of the motor system, and numerous brain stem reflexes were analyzed in an attempt to establish the level of impairment within the brain stem or diencephalon. In the "diencephalic stage," a few patients respired normally, but the majority had Cheyne-Stokes respiration. As evidence of involvement of the midbrain and upper pons developed, periodic respiration was succeeded by sustained hyperventilation. When the level of dysfunction reached the upper medulla, respirations reverted to a nearly normal pattern, although somewhat more rapid and shallow, and in the final stage of medullary involvement breathing became ataxic.[262,311,312] Clinical ataxic breathing consists of intermittent, irregularly spaced pauses, deep sighs or gasps, and prolonged periods of apnea.

In recent years, several investigators have studied the sequence of changes in vital signs during gradual elevation of intracranial pressure, mostly by using extradural balloons. As the balloon is expanded in cats, dogs, and baboons, a decrease in heart rate occurs very early.[100,154] There are also a slight decrease in systemic arterial pressure and significant increases in arrhythmia.[100] The respiratory rate tends to decrease, but there is little or no change in the pulse pressure within the intracranial space.[100,154] Continuing the expansion of the balloon induces a Cushing response. The circumstances in which the systemic arterial pressor response occurs seem to vary considerably. Fitch and colleagues related the onset of the Cushing response to the supratentorial perfusion pressure and, as had Weinstein and co-workers in relating it to the pressure gradient between the supratentorial and the infratentorial spaces, found that the supratentorial perfusion pressure varies from 8 to 50 mm of mercury at the onset of the Cushing response. They also found considerable variability in the amplitude of the pressure gradient across the tentorium. Immediately before the onset of the increase in systemic arterial pressure, the gradient averaged 36 mm of mercury, and at the peak of the hypertensive response, it averaged 46 mm of mercury.[103,421] Hekmatpanah expressed the threshold of the Cushing response in terms of intracranial pressure rather than cerebral perfusion pressure and found the threshold to be about 50 mm of mercury.[154]

As the systemic arterial pressure rises, the heart rate, which decreases slowly during the early phase of the expansion of the balloon, begins to increase.[103,154] Events now occur rapidly with continued inflation of the balloon, terminating in severe bradycardia, pupillary dilatation, and cardiovascular collapse.

Because the animals did not survive long after the onset of the Cushing response, Fitch and his colleagues considered the onset of arterial hypertension as an essentially agonal event.[103] The author prefers the term "ominous" to "agonal," because the latter word suggests that the animal, and by inference a patient, is beyond recovery when the blood pressure rises in response to intracranial hypertension. Clinicians who are experienced in measuring intracranial pressure frequently observe increases in systemic arterial pressure with rises in intracranial pressure in patients who usually deteriorate neurologically during the course of these events but promptly improve when the intracranial pressure is lowered with appropriate therapy. Thus, the Cushing response is a dangerous but frequently reversible sign of raised intracranial pressure.

Generally respirations slow throughout expansions of the mass. Shortly following the onset of the Cushing response, respirations become short and shallow, associated with periods of apnea.[154] The ipsilateral pupil generally dilates at the time of the Cushing response, and when the arterial pressor response is fully developed and respirations are irregular, both pupils are dilated.

There are still a number of uncertainties about the origins of the Cushing response. Traditionally, it has been attributed to an increase in systemic vascular resistance produced by either ischemia of or pressure on the brain stem. Hoff and Reis identified regions in the brain stem and spinal cord that appear to be selectively sensitive to increases in focal pressure. They postulated that in addition to pressure-sensitive pressor centers in the brain stem, ischemia of the cerebral hemispheres could also elicit the Cushing response.[159,160] According to this explanation, the cerebral ischemia results in removal of supratentorial inhibition of brain stem vasopressor centers, resulting in the release of sympathomimetic influences, which in turn cause an increase in peripheral vasoconstriction. Although increased peripheral vascular resistance appears to be the major contributor to the Cushing response, increased cardiac output is also a factor.[124]

Fitch and co-workers analyzed the sequence of changes in the diagnostic signs of raised intracranial pressure in their balloon expansion experiments in the dog and baboon. The most common sequence of events was bradycardia, arrhythmia, pupillary constriction, unilateral pupillary dilatation, an increase in pulse pressure, and finally, an increase in the mean arterial pressure.[103]

Pulmonary Edema With Increased Intracranial Pressure

It has long been recognized that pulmonary edema occurs following severe head injuries and spinal cord injuries. There has, however, been difficulty in distinguishing pulmonary edema produced by brain injury and increased intracranial pressure from the pulmonary edema that is often seen in association with severe lung disease of other causes. Moutier noted pulmonary edema with various types of injuries to the central nervous system, especially gunshot wounds of the head.[285] Weisman found edema and congestion of the lungs in approximately 10 per cent of a group of patients who died from intracranial hemorrhage, mostly of traumatic origin.[424] Recent interest in the subject was stimulated particularly by the observations of Ducker. He described 11 patients with intracranial hypertension who died from pulmonary edema. None of them had received excess parenteral fluids, and all but two had normal central venous pressure. The only abnormality in the lungs at postmortem examination was diffuse noncellular edema.[81] On the basis of studies of experimental increased intracranial pressure in animals,

Ducker and Simmons concluded that the pulmonary vascular system shares in the systemic vascular responses to intracranial hypertension and that the edema is due primarily to increased pulmonary and venous pressures.[82,83]

Graf and Rossi retrospectively examined the records of 2100 patients with serious head injuries and 132 patients with cervical spine or spinal cord injuries seen at the University of Iowa over a five-year period. The incidence of pulmonary edema was quite low. The diagnosis was made clinically in 5 of the patients with head injuries, and in an additional 14 patients at postmortem examination. In 17 of the 19 patients, however, there were other pulmonary conditions such as aspiration pneumonitis and atelectasis that could have contributed to the formation of pulmonary edema. Pulmonary edema was seen infrequently in the patients with spine and spinal cord injuries who survived, but was present in three of nine patients who died. As in the head injury cases, there were other factors that could have contributed to the pulmonary edema in all three patients.[126] The distinction between pulmonary edema of central nervous system origin and edema as a complication of other pulmonary disease is made all the more difficult by the observations of Martin and co-workers that 89 of 100 patients who died of combat wounds incurred in Vietnam had various combinations of pulmonary edema, congestion, and alveolar hemorrhage.[251]

Despite these reservations, there can be little doubt that pulmonary edema secondary to raised intracranial pressure and independent of primary pulmonary disease, in fact, does occur. The most interesting case encountered by the author was a 15-year-old girl who was admitted for emergency treatment a few minutes after suffering a gunshot wound that had produced massive brain damage. The child was deeply comatose, but hyperventilating and normoxic. She was intubated and ventilated with an Ambu bag while preparations were being made to insert an intraventricular cannula to record intracranial pressure. Quite suddenly airway resistance to squeezing the bag increased, and frothy fluid began to pour from the endotracheal tube. The patient was then given a large intravenous bolus of 25 per cent mannitol. Over a period of 20 minutes more than a liter of fluid was aspirated from the lungs. The edema then ceased as swiftly as it had begun. The cessation of the edema coincided with a fall in systolic arterial pressure from 200 to approximately 140 mm of mercury. There seems little doubt the pulmonary edema was produced by the intracranial and arterial hypertension, which were relieved by the hypertonic mannitol. Although this type of occurrence would appear to be quite rare, the association of events observed in this patient would seem to leave little doubt about the cause of the pulmonary edema.

Two principal theories have been advanced to explain the pulmonary edema that occurs in association with increased intracranial pressure. According to the first theory, the intracranial hypertension generates increased sympathetic outflow to the pulmonary vessels, resulting in an edema that is primarily neurogenic in origin. Several studies were performed in the 1950's that suggested the existence of an "edemogenic center," and the hypothalamus, in particular, was implicated.[116,242] More recent studies have suggested that if there is such a sympathetic vasomotor center, it is more likely to be in the medulla or cervical spinal cord.[50]

A second theory has received more support from both clinical and animal observations than the concept of neurogenic constriction of pulmonary vessels. There is general agreement that increased hydrostatic pressure in the microvasculature of the lungs leads to transudation of fluid from the capillary bed into the alveoli.[301] Such increase in pressure in the pulmonary microvasculature can be produced by elevation of left atrial pressure, and there is experimental evidence that when left atrial pressure exceeds a value of 20 to 25 mm of mercury, pulmonary edema begins.[135] When systemic arterial hypertension produces such a large load on the left side of the heart that the ventricle begins to fail, left atrial pressure rises. On the basis of these facts, Luisada and Ducker and co-workers postulated the following sequence of events: an increase in intracranial pressure produces peripheral vasoconstriction that leads to systolic overload of the left ventricle with a shift of blood volume toward the right side of the heart and lungs; the resultant diastolic overload and inadequate relaxation of the left ventricle results in increases in left atrial pressure, pulmonary vein pressure, and ultimately capillary pressure with transudation of fluid. If the process continues, the left ventricle fails completely, and the subject passes into shock and dies.[84,235]

A number of studies in experimental animals have been directed toward determining the levels of intracranial pressure at which changes in systemic arterial oxygen tension occur. Valtonen was unable to produce arterial hypoxemia in rabbits in which intracranial pressure was elevated by a number of methods, including freezing lesions and massive vascular oil embolism.[410] Jennett and Hoff raised intracranial pressure by lumbar subarachnoid or intraventricular infusions to quite high levels and produced only moderate degrees of arterial hypoxemia.[181] Moody and associates produced severe hypoxemia in dogs in which intracranial pressure was elevated to very high levels by expansion of an extradural balloon. The hypoxemia occurred only in association with severe abnormalities of respiratory rate and rhythm, however.[283] Berman and co-workers performed similar studies in dogs. The decreases in arterial oxygen tension observed in their experiments occurred in the absence of gross or microscopic pathological change in the lungs. Thus, they postulated that the hypoxemia was due to pulmonary arteriovenous shunting and not to pulmonary edema.[21] Finally, the experiments of Maxwell and Goodwin have provided the most compelling evidence that pulmonary shunting is a direct function of the degree and duration of increased intracranial pressure.[257] In none of these various studies, however, were the investigators able to adduce convincing evidence in favor of either one of the two theories on the origin of pulmonary edema cited earlier.

Intracranial Pressure and Cerebral Blood Flow

The cerebral circulation is influenced by several anatomical and physiological features that are peculiar to the brain. It is the only major organ encased in a rigid container, and it is surrounded by the cerebrospinal fluid buffer that can expand and contract with changes in volume of the cerebrovascular bed. The organization of the vascular bed into arteries, capillaries, and veins is much the same as in other organs, but the collateral arterial and venous circulation is unusually rich.

The cerebrovascular mean pressure falls from approximately 90 mm of mercury in the carotid and vertebral arteries to 3 mm of mercury in the jugular and vertebral veins in normotensive subjects in the horizontal position. The largest fall in pressure per unit length of vessel is across the arterioles, but the loss of pressure across the arteries is also large. Small artery mean pressure in the dog averages 63 mm of mercury with a mean aortic pressure of 137 mm of mercury.[379] Shapiro and associates and Stromberg and Fox have viewed the cerebral circulation as comprising three segments in a series—the large arteries, the pial vessels, and the intracerebral vessels. By measuring the pressure drop across these segments, they showed that the total vascular resistance between the aorta and the cerebral veins was in the proportion 39 to 21 to 40. Thus, the resistance offered by the large arteries and the intracerebral vessels is the same.[374,396]

Autoregulation

The normal control of the cerebral circulation is complex, and the origins of the changes in the diameter of the cerebral vessels that occur in response to specific stimuli such as changes in systemic arterial pressure, hypoxia, and hypercarbia are largely unknown. These factors are discussed in this chapter and in Chapter 23. Whatever the mechanisms responsible for the regulation of cerebral blood flow, the purposes are clear—to provide enough oxygen and glucose to the brain so that it can carry out its metabolic processes.

When the systemic arterial pressure falls, or when there is an occlusion, complete or partial, of a major cerebral artery, the cerebral resistance vessels dilate in an attempt to maintain normal blood flow in the face of the decrease in perfusion pressure. When the systemic arterial pressure increases, cerebral vessels constrict in order to keep blood flow constant. This phenomenon is termed autoregulation and is sometimes referred to as pressure autoregulation in order to distinguish it from the changes in cerebral blood flow produced by changes in cerebral metabolism, which is called metabolic autoregulation.

If the systemic arterial pressure is lowered or raised quickly, cerebral blood flow decreases or increases passively with the change in arterial pressure. Blood flow then returns to the control value within a few seconds when autoregulation is intact. When autoregulation is impaired but still present, the adjustment of blood flow is slower and less complete, and when autoregulation is absent, blood flow passively follows changes in systemic arterial pressure. Thus, autoregulation is a quantitative, measureable variable in the control of the cerebral circulation and not an all-or-none phenomenon.

The lower limit of autoregulation to changes in mean systemic arterial pressure is approximately 50 mm of mercury, and the upper limit is about 160 mm of mercury. This means that as the arterial pressure is decreased, the resistance vessels dilate until they are maximally dilated in response to the decreased perfusion pressure. Below a mean pressure of 50 mm of mercury, blood flow declines steeply with further decrease in pressure. When arterial pressure is increased, the vessels constrict until the mean arterial pressure exceeds 160 mm of mercury, at which point the pressure head breaks through the vasoconstriction, causing passive dilatation and an increase in cerebral blood flow. Vital dyes usually enter the brain parenchyma at the moment of breakthrough, manifesting disruption of the blood-brain barrier.[87] Presumably this is a pressure phenomenon within capillaries and small veins—the barrier leaks because of sudden distention of vessels within the microcirculation. If autoregulation is impaired by hypoxia, hypercarbia, or minimal blunt trauma to the exposed surface of the brain, and the blood pressure is then raised quickly, not only is there extravasation of protein-bound dyes into the brain but the brain swells suddenly and often massively.*

The term "autoregulation" implies that the mechanism is intrinsic to the vascular bed of the brain and suggests a smooth muscle reflex somewhere within the system

of resistance vessels. Bayliss first proposed the myogenic theory in 1902 to explain the regulation of the circulation in muscle and other organs and tissues, and the theory was extensively explored in hind limb preparations by Folkow.[14,107] It is important to note, however, that autoregulation of cerebral vessels was not clearly proved until the early 1960's.[141] According to the myogenic hypothesis, the resistance vessels have a high degree of resting vasoconstrictor tone due mainly to smooth muscle contraction of the walls. An increase in intraluminal pressure stimulates a further increase in tone by stretching the muscle and causing a reactive shortening of radial fibers and a reduction in vascular diameter. A decrease in intraluminal pressure has the opposite effect. The effective pressure is not intraluminal pressure per se but the difference between intravascular and extravascular pressure, which is defined as transmural pressure. In recent years there has been surprisingly little evidence either in favor of or opposed to the myogenic theory of cerebral autoregulation. There has, however, been great interest in other mechanisms that influence cerebrovascular tone.

There is ample sympathetic innervation of the cerebral vessels, but there has been much dispute about the function of these sympathetic nerve terminals in the normal control of the cerebral circulation and in disease states. If sympathetic fibers are destroyed, blood flow during arterial hypotension is higher than in the hypotensive intact animal.[101] Stimulation of sympathetic nerves when the arterial pressure is elevated raises the upper limit of autoregulation.[24] The implication of these studies is that normally the sympathetics, not only the intrinsic smooth muscle tone of cerebral vessels, contribute to resting vasoconstriction. A vasodilator pathway to the brain was first described many years ago, and a number of vasodilator pathways have been postulated from more recent physiological studies.[51,210,239,323] The contribution of these postulated central neurogenic pathways to normal pressure autoregulation is unknown. Perhaps autoregulation is essentially myogenic in origin, but the myogenic response is modified in a complex fashion by the interplay of vasoconstrictor and vasodilator impulses.

There is conflicting evidence on the role

---

* See references: hypoxia, 3; hypercarbia, 138; blunt trauma, 332; and 250.

of baroreceptors in the control of the cerebral circulation. There is evidence that stimulation of the baroreceptors has no effect on cerebral blood flow, but there is other evidence that denervation of the carotid baroreceptors shifts the flow-pressure curve, and in the baboon the flow-pressure curve was found to be linear after baroreceptor denervation.[152,317,323]

An interesting development in recent years has been the hypothesis that different segments of the cerebrovascular bed respond differently to various types of stimuli. Several investigators have presented evidence that nerve stimulation affects primarily the large vessels, which includes the large cerebral arteries about the base of the brain and the pial arteries.[24,142] These observations have led to the hypothesis that the intracerebral vessels (from the small arteries down to the arterioles) are mainly controlled by smooth muscle reflexes—that is, true autoregulation. If this were the case, constriction of large arteries by sympathetic stimulation would result in reflex dilatation of intracerebral vessels and blood flow would remain constant. If myogenic autoregulation were defective, however, the sympathetic system would become a much more important regulator of the cerebral circulation.

Hypoxia and Hypercarbia

Systemic hypoxemia causes dilatation of cerebral vessels and an increase in cerebral blood flow. The purpose of the vascular dilatation, of course, is to increase the blood flow through the brain at a time when the volume of oxygen per unit volume of blood has been reduced. As long as the increase in blood flow can compensate for the reduction in the oxygen content of the blood, the oxygen needs of the brain are met, and the brain continues to metabolize normally. When the partial pressure of oxygen in the arterial blood (Pa_{O_2}) decreases to approximately 20 mm of mercury, the stimulus to vasodilatation has become maximal, and a further reduction of oxygen tension leads to anaerobic glycolysis and a decrease in oxidative phosphorylation, the cardinal signs of hypoxic metabolic derangement.[384]

The origin of the stimulus to cerebral vasodilatation produced by hypoxia is largely unknown. There have been several studies that suggest that the chemoreceptors in the aortic and carotid areas reflexly dilate the cerebral vessels in response to a hypoxic stimulus. Stimulus of the carotid body chemoreceptors with blood of altered composition increases regional cerebral blood flow measured by the [133]xenon method.[317] When the microsphere method is used, however, stimulation of the chemoreceptors has no effect on cerebral blood flow, and denervation of the chemoreceptors does not alter the cerebrovascular response to hypoxia.[12,153] Evidence that stimulation of the locus ceruleus can produce dilatation of the microvasculature raises the possibility that hypoxia has a selective effect on vasodilatory centers within the brain stem.[320]

The most common explanation for hypoxic vasodilatation has been chemical regulation through alterations in the composition of the extracellular space. According to this hypothesis, even a slight reduction in tissue oxygen tension induces lactic acidosis, which produces the dilatation. Although acidosis may contribute, it cannot be the primary cause of the vasodilatation, because lactic acid does not appear until many seconds after cerebral blood flow has increased.[27]

The most potent stimulus to cerebral vasodilatation is an increase in the partial pressure of carbon dioxide (Pa_{CO_2}) in the arterial blood. Teleologically, the reason for the vasodilatation is to prevent the fall in extracellular pH, which would be inevitable if cerebral blood flow did not increase. Since a change in carbon dioxide tension is also detected by the peripheral arterial chemoreceptors, a reflex pathway similar to that proposed for hypoxia might exist for hypercarbia. In support of this hypothesis: cortical blood flow increases when the chemoreceptors are stimulated with blood containing an elevated level of carbon dioxide; that response is abolished by section of the sinus nerves; the increase in cerebral blood flow produced by an increase in Pa_{CO_2} is reduced after section of fibers from vasosensory receptors; and lesions in the tegmental reticular formation reduce or abolish the cerebrovascular response to changes in Pa_{CO_2}.[171,172,319] Both carbon dioxide and the hydrogen ion act directly upon vascular smooth muscle.[369,415] Thus, as in hypoxia, the cerebrovascular response to hypercarbia may be largely locally mediated through vascular smooth muscle or through neurogenic vasodilator pathways or perhaps through a combination of the two mechanisms.

Metabolic Autoregulation

There is tight coupling between the demands of cerebral tissue for oxygen and glucose and the volume of blood flowing through that tissue. As metabolism increases, during seizures, for example, local flow at the site of the seizure focus increases, and when metabolism decreases, as in hypothermia, blood flow also decreases.[267] This association is termed metabolic autoregulation because the cerebrovascular bed is regulated to meet the needs of the tissue for metabolites. Perhaps the word "regulation" should be substituted for "autoregulation," because the latter term suggests that the cerebral vessels regulate themselves to effect the appropriate changes. In a pure sense, the term "autoregulation" should not be used if the stimulus to dilatation or constriction emanates from outside the vessel wall. It may, however, be too entrenched in the vocabulary of cerebrovascular physiology to warrant an attempt to make this distinction. Although there has been strong circumstantial evidence for very close regulation of local cerebral blood flow by changes in metabolic rate, it was not until the development of the [14]carbon deoxyglucose method for measuring glucose uptake in autoradiographs of the brain and subsequently the simultaneous measurements of glucose metabolism and local blood flow in the same regions by the [14]carbon iodoantipyrine method that this relationship was proved.[393]

There is general agreement that one or more chemical substances are responsible for the tight coupling between metabolism and flow. As in the case of the hypoxic stimulus to vasodilatation, extracellular lactic acidosis, or more specifically, the hydrogen ion, has been held to be that substance. According to the hypothesis, increased metabolism results in accumulation of hydrogen ions in the extracellular space, which produce vasodilatation; then when metabolism decreases to the prior level, the hydrogen ions are washed away and the cerebral vessels constrict to their former diameter. Recent studies using pH microelectrodes do not support the theory. In a variety of circumstances in which local flow increases greatly (bicuculline seizure, acute hypoxia, hypoglycemia) there was very little change in the pH of extracellular fluid in the cerebral cortex. Increased depolarization of neurons leads to the accumulation of larger quantities of potassium in the extracellular space, and therefore, potassium is another agent that has been postulated to be responsible for autoregulation. As in the case of the hydrogen ion, considerable changes in blood flow can occur in response to alterations in metabolism without a change in extracellular potassium.[5] The agent that has received the most attention recently is adenosine, a potent cerebral vasodilator.[349] As is true of all putative vasodilating agents, however, it will be necessary to demonstrate that adenosine in the fluid bathing the parenchymal vessels increases immediately as metabolism increases, that the concentrations of adenosine are sufficient to account for the increase in blood flow observed, and that the disappearance of adenosine correlates well with the decrease in blood flow as metabolism wanes.

Studies of regional cerebral blood flow and metabolism in patients with head injuries have demonstrated marked dissociations or unlinkage of the flow from metabolism.[41,295] Since the origin of metabolic autoregulation is so poorly understood, one can only guess at the cause of the dissociation. Perhaps it is due to the accumulation of a vasodilating agent within the brain in response to the insult, or to pathological stimulation of vasodilating centers, or to a diminution in vasoconstrictor tone mediated through sympathetic or directly ascending brain stem pathways.

Response to Increased Intracranial Pressure

If the stimulus to autoregulation of cerebral vessels produced by changes in systemic arterial pressure is a change in the transmural pressure across the vasoactive vessels, then it follows that an alteration in transmural pressure produced by raising intracranial pressure, rather than by lowering the intraluminal pressure, might have the

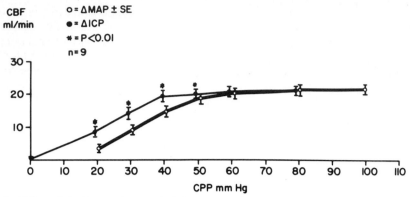

Figure 24–8 Effect of altering cerebral perfusion pressure (CPP) by decreasing arterial pressure (open circles) and by increasing intracranial pressure (closed circles) in dogs with intact autoregulation. Significance of variation between changes assessed by paired t-test. (From Miller, J. D., Stanek, A., and Langfitt, T. W.: Concepts of cerebral perfusion pressure and vascular compression during intracranial hypertension. Progr. Brain Res., *35*:411–432, 1971. Reprinted by permission.)

same effect. In early reports of the effects of increased intracranial pressure on cerebral blood flow, cerebral perfusion pressure was defined as the difference between mean aterial pressure and the mean intracranial pressure.[184,437] When intracranial pressure was increased in experimental animals, blood flow was found to adjust in much the same fashion as when systemic arterial pressure was decreased. Miller and co-workers have compared autoregulation in response to decreased systemic arterial pressure and increased intracranial pressure in the same animal. Not only was the cerebral circulation found to adjust to increased intracranial pressure, it did so to

levels of cerebral perfusion pressure that were significantly lower than in the circumstances of decreased arterial pressure (Fig. 24–8). In animals subjected to a period of intentional cerebral hypoxia, autoregulation became defective, but even then, the impaired autoregulation was better in response to increased intracranial pressure than to decreased arterial pressure (Fig. 24–9).[276]

From these and similar studies, there have arisen two views of the dynamics of the cerebral circulation, one describing autoregulation in response to increased intracranial pressure in terms of changes in cerebral perfusion pressure and the other

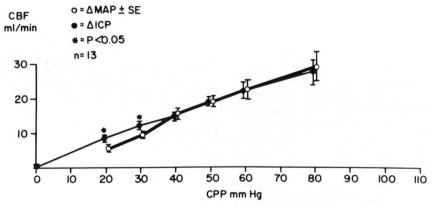

Figure 24–9 Effect of altering cerebral perfusion pressure (CPP) by decreasing arterial pressure (open circles) and increasing intracranial pressure (closed circles) in dogs with defective autoregulation. Significance of variation between changes assessed by paired t-test. Note that scatter of flow values above perfusion pressure of 50 mm of mercury is increased, indicated by increasing value for standard error of the mean. (From Miller, J. D., Stanek, A., and Langfitt, T. W.: Concepts of cerebral perfusion pressure and vascular compression during intracranial hypertension. Progr. Brain Res., *35*:411–432, 1971. Reprinted by permission.)

describing those changes in terms of resistance. Poiseuille's equation governing the laminar flow of Newtonian fluids through small-caliber rigid tubes is written:

$$Q = \frac{R^4 (P_1 - P_2)}{8 \, \eta \, 1}$$

where R = tube radius

P$_1$ − P$_2$ = perfusion pressure
η = viscosity of fluid
1 = length of tube

Although blood is a non-Newtonian fluid, and the cerebral vessels are anything but rigid, Poiseuille's equation is useful in attempting to distinguish changes in perfusion pressure from changes in resistance as the cause of a change in cerebral blood flow. Simplifying the equation:

Cerebral blood flow (CBF)

$$= \frac{\text{Carotid artery pressure} - \text{jugular vein pressure}}{\text{Cerebrovascular resistance (CVR)}}$$

where CVR = R arteries + R arterioles + R capillaries + R veins + R dural sinuses

The relationship of cerebral venous pressure to intracranial cerebrospinal fluid pressure has been controversial. In the past, it has been stated that the two pressures are always equal; that they are nearly always the same, but that either pressure may exceed the other; and that the sagittal sinus pressure is always greater than the cerebrospinal fluid pressure.[15,78,109,156] Cerebrospinal fluid pressure in man was found to always exceed jugular vein pressure.[286] It has been difficult to reconcile the observation that sagittal sinus or jugular vein pressure is higher than cerebrospinal fluid pressure with concepts of the bulk flow of fluid into the sinuses through valves. The pressure gradient should always be from cerebrospinal fluid to blood. Detailed measurements by Shulman and Verdier in dogs have demonstrated that sagittal sinus pressure is 60 per cent of torcular pressure and 30 per cent of cerebrospinal fluid pressure.[382] Pressures in the cerebral veins and sagittal sinus are about 14 and 7 mm of mercury respectively. Most important is the evidence that as intracranial pressure rises, cerebral venous pressure rises in concert, and the two pressures are equal or nearly so even to extremely high levels of intracranial pressure. Thus, when intracranial pressure is elevated, that value may be substituted for jugular venous pressure so that:

Cerebral blood flow (CBF)

$$= \frac{\text{carotid artery pressure} - \text{intracranial pressure}}{\text{CVR}}$$

The issue then is the sequence of events that maintains constant cerebral blood flow during a rise in intracranial pressure and that results in a decrease in cerebral blood flow when the capacity of autoregulation is exceeded. According to the perfusion pressure hypothesis, the decrease in transmural pressure produced by the increased extravascular pressure stimulates the resistance vessels to dilate to maintain blood flow in the face of a decrease in cerebral perfusion pressure. The venous system plays little, if any, role in this hypothesis. The alternative hypothesis places emphasis on compression of the venous system, produced by the rising intracranial pressure, rather than on changes in perfusion pressure. According to this theory, the perfusion is and remains the difference between carotid artery and jugular vein pressures; therefore, it does not change significantly with increased intracranial pressure. All of the alterations occur in cerebrovascular resistance. Again, the resistance vessels dilate because of the decrease in transmural pressure, and cerebral blood flow remains constant because compression of the cerebral veins precisely matches the dilatation of arteries and arterioles. The evidence for and against these two views has been summarized by Miller and colleagues.[276]

There have been numerous measurements of intracranial pressure, cerebral venous pressure, and sagittal sinus pressure in an attempt to determine whether compression of the cerebral venous system occurs during intracranial hypertension, and if so, at what levels of intracranial pressure the venous compression begins. Wright noted that bridging cerebral veins, observed through a cranial window, remained patent until rising intracranial pressure exceeded the blood pressure. When the collapse occurred, blood was forced proximally, indicating that the outflow resistance exceeded the resistance in the proximal vascular bed. He suggested that the intracranial hypertension caused constriction of the cerebral veins at their junction with the dural sinuses.[433] This explanation has received support from other investigators.[129,151,382] In experiments in which values were derived for the resistances in the venous and prevenous beds, during rising intracranial pressure the prevenous resistance decreased as the venous resistance rose.[382] When pressures were measured at various points along the dural sinuses from the anterior sagittal sinus to the jugular vein in Rhesus monkeys, the changes in pressures that occurred with increases and decreases in intracranial pressure indicated that both the sinuses and the cerebral veins were compressed by the intracranial hypertension.[215] There is also morphological evidence in animals and physiological evidence in man that supports venous sinus compression.[252,375] When cerebral blood flow begins to diminish, the increased venous resistance has overridden the effect of arterial dilatation.[234]

Recently, evidence has been presented that the site of venous compression is immediately proximal to the junction of the lateral lacunae and the superior sagittal sinus, and since the pressure drop across this region increases with even a minimal rise in intracranial pressure, the authors of that study concluded that venous compression is initiated as soon as intracranial pressure starts to increase.[288] These observations are important because prior evidence had suggested that venous compression becomes significant only after intracranial pressure is moderately elevated, or in the view of some investigators, markedly elevated. This has made the theory of venous compression difficult to accept. If venous compression begins immediately, however, the resistance theory of cerebral autoregulation receives more support and the definition of cerebral perfusion pressure as the difference between the arterial and jugular vein pressures, not the difference between the arterial and intracranial pressures, is more acceptable.

In early studies of the effect of increased intracranial pressure on cerebral blood flow, a simultaneous increase in blood flow and intracranial pressure, so that cerebral perfusion pressure remained constant, resulted in a relatively small but progressive increase in blood flow.[211] Subsequent studies have confirmed these observations and

have demonstrated further that the increase in flow in these circumstances is a function of the cause of the intracranial hypertension.[255,368] Blood flow increased in an animal model in which intracranial pressure and arterial pressure were raised by gradual inflation of an extradural balloon, but there was no increase in blood flow with rising arterial pressure and intracranial pressure when the latter was elevated by brain swelling.[368] These observations lend further support to the venous compression hypothesis. Presumably, in the balloon model the increase in the arterial pressure is capable of progressively overcoming increased venous resistance so as to increase cerebral blood flow in the face of a constant perfusion pressure. When the brain is damaged so as to produce brain swelling, however, the increase in arterial pressure probably induces further transudation of fluid from the microcirculation into the brain, resulting in compression of the microvasculature and a further increase in resistance. The transmission of the rising arterial pressure head into the microcirculation occurs because in the process of adjusting to the intracranial hypertension, the resistance vessels have become maximally dilated. There is recent evidence, in fact, that at the limits of autoregulation in response to intracranial hypertension, a sudden and unexplained additional decrease in resistance occurs.[402]

When intracranial pressure equals the systemic arterial pressure, cerebral blood flow ceases. Again, one could argue that cerebral circulation is arrested because the perfusion pressure across the brain has been abolished, or on the contrary, one could maintain that the perfusion pressure is still the difference between the arterial pressure and the jugular vein pressure, and therefore normal, and the arrest of blood flow is due to collapse of one or more portions of the cerebrovascular bed. There is considerable evidence in favor of the latter explanation. At extremely high levels of intracranial pressure produced by brain swelling, not only most cerebral veins but also the dural sinuses collapse.[375] Observations through a glass window demonstrate slowing of the cerebral circulation as intracranial tension increases, and as intracranial pressure approaches the blood pressure, arrest of the circulation occurs in more and more capillaries, then in larger and larger veins. Pallor spreads through the cortex as the vessels collapse, and those vessels that are still patent contain sludged red cells and emboli. When intracranial pressure is reduced, circulation is restored to some vessels but not to all of them, and the amount of restoration of blood flow is a function of the duration of the cerebral circulatory arrest.[155]

Collapse of the intracranial circulation, including the large arteries at the base of the brain, has been observed in a patient when intracranial pressure equaled the systemic arterial pressure. The patient had severe brain swelling from a gunshot wound. Cerebral blood flow was measured with the [133]xenon intracarotid injection technique, and there was no clearance of isotope from the brain, demonstrating cessation of the cerebral circulation. Mean intracranial pressure equaled the mean systemic arterial pressure at the time. Since there was some concern about the reliability of the intracranial pressure recording, an angiogram was performed. The contrast medium was arrested in the internal carotid artery just above the anterior clinoid process. A second, more forceful injection of contrast agent was then made into the internal carotid artery, resulting in filling of the proximal portions of markedly attenuated anterior and middle cerebral arteries. In subsequent films, the agent was seen to "back out" from the intracranial arteries, proving that they had been collapsed and were only temporarily opened by the injection.[41]

Response to a Mass Lesion

One of the most widely used models for the study of experimental increased intracranial pressure in animals has been expansion of an extracerebral balloon. It has the advantage of simplicity, reproducibility, and reasonable simulation of a clinical condition. In contrast to the intracranial hypertension produced by infusion of fluid into the cerebrospinal fluid spaces or diffuse brain swelling, the balloon not only increases intracranial pressure diffusely, but also produces compression and distortion of the brain. In particular, blood flow might be expected to decrease disproportionately at the site of balloon compression in comparison with the remainder of the brain.

A widely used model for the production of cerebral edema through the application of a cold plate or probe to the brain surface has also been used recently to study both the effect of a mass lesion on regional cerebral blood flow and the effect of spreading edema on regional flows remote from the lesion.[200] This model differs from the balloon model in that severe brain damage is produced at the site of the lesion, and the resultant edema spreads through the white matter in a reasonably predictable time course.

During gradual expansion of an extracerebral balloon, global blood flow, measured by the torcular venous outflow technique, did not fall until the cerebral perfusion pressure had been decreased to approximately 40 mm of mercury, about the same limit of autoregulatory capacity observed in similar animal experiments in which intracranial pressure was increased by cerebrospinal fluid infusion.[276,277] Slow expansion of the balloon to quite high levels of intracranial pressure also fails to reduce regional blood flow adjacent to the balloon, demonstrating good autoregulation in the resistance vessels in response not only to diffuse intracranial hypertension but also to focal compression.[188,403] There is conflicting evidence, however. Deep structures of the brain, in which blood flow was measured by the hydrogen clearance technique, did not adjust well to expansion of an extracerebral balloon.[390,391] The rate of expansion of the balloon is as important as the volume of the balloon and the level of intracranial pressure in determining the effect on cerebral blood flow, particularly regional flow beneath and adjacent to the mass. When a balloon is expanded very rapidly, brain immediately adjacent to it is rendered ischemic, and the volume of brain made ischemic can be expanded by increasing either the rate or volume of the injection.[423] At the completion of a rapid injection, the brain moves away from the balloon, and this plastic creep of the brain can be measured by recording the movement of a readily identifiable structure, such as the superior colliculus in sagittal sections of the cat brain. As the brain stem moves caudally, the volume of ischemic brain adjacent to the balloon decreases, presumably because of a progressive reduction in tissue pressure and reperfusion of the brain. Perhaps these observations help explain differences in experimental results. If the rate of expansion of the balloon is slow enough to permit brain to creep away from the balloon, thereby relieving tissue pressure, the vessels are able to adjust adequately, and blood flow is maintained. With more rapid expansion of the balloon, the brain does not have time to adjust, and tissue pressure exceeds the autoregulatory capacity of the vessels.

The results with cold lesions of the brain are quite different from those observed with expansion of an intracranial balloon. Regional blood flow was decreased adjacent to the lesion in short-term studies in which regional cerebral blood flow was measured from both hemispheres of the monkey following the placement of an occipital cold lesion, and the reduction in flow occurred long before edema had spread into the region from which the decreased flow was measured.[39] Of particular interest was the observation that the only other region of the brain that exhibited decreased flow was the homologous area of the contralateral hemisphere. Frei and associates postulated that the decrease in blood flow adjacent to the lesion was due to either increased tissue pressure produced by the lesion or a reduction in metabolism. They also postulated that reduction in transcallosal neuronal activity produced by an ipsilateral decrease in metabolism might explain the reduction in flow in the contralateral hemisphere. With spread of edema through the hemisphere, there is evidence substantiating a progressive increase in tissue pressure and reduction in regional flows.[111]

Brain Swelling From Intracranial Hypertension (Cerebral Vasomotor Paralysis)

The intracranial space contains three fluid compartments, cerebrospinal fluid, brain fluid, and intravascular blood. When intracranial pressure is increased by either cerebrospinal fluid infusion or expansion of an intracranial balloon, the vasodilatation that maintains cerebral blood flow must produce an increase in cerebral blood volume. This increase in volume must also contribute to the rise in intracranial pressure. In other words, a price is paid for autoregulation in the form of a higher intracranial pressure than is the case when autoregulation is impaired.

In experiments with monkeys conducted several years ago, the author and his colleagues observed progressive swelling of the brain when the intracranial balloon was expanded and deflated several times during the course of the experiment.[212] The changes in several variables including cerebral blood flow suggested that the brain swelling was due, in large part, to increased cerebral blood volume. In subsequent experiments, cerebral blood volume was measured by using [51]chromium-tagged red blood cells in animals in which brain swelling was produced by balloon expansion and deflation, blunt head injury, and cerebral ischemia.[216] Blood volume was increased in all three experimental designs, often markedly so, but in the balloon compression and head injury models, there was some extravascular blood. Although the concept of a progressive increase in blood volume with various forms of intracranial hypertension had been disputed, the results have been confirmed in experiments in which blood volume was measured by using the [15]oxygen method.[13,234]

When the brain swelling is severe, intracranial pressure approaches the systemic pressure and the cerebral vessels no longer respond to changes in carbon dioxide tension.[212] Although pressure autoregulation was not tested in these early studies, because at the time the experiments were performed autoregulation of the cerebral circulation had not been identified, there is good reason to believe that it also was absent at a time when the blood vessels did not respond to hypercarbia. The term "vasomotor paralysis" was coined to describe this phenomenon, and subsequent experience encourages this distinction between cerebral vasodilatation per se and cerebral vasodilatation that does not respond to an increase in systemic arterial pressure or hypocarbia.

Shortly after the term "vasomotor paralysis" was introduced, Lassen independently described the condition termed "luxury perfusion."[219] Luxury perfusion is focal or regional vasodilatation seen most commonly in the brain surrounding an area of ischemia. Presumably it is due to the diffusion into the surrouding normal brain of a vasodilating metabolite from the site of injury that dilates the normal vessels within that brain. Since the vasodilatation that led ultimately to vasomotor paralysis in the balloon compression experiments in monkeys also followed periods of cerebral ischemia produced by the intracranial hypertension, the etiology of vasomotor paralysis is probably the same as that of luxury perfusion. The term "luxury perfusion," however, refers to the fact that the amount of blood flowing through the tissue is in excess of metabolic needs and does not imply a particular state of responsiveness of the vessels. This is the difference, then, between luxury perfusion and vasomotor paralysis. In both conditions, the blood vessels are dilated, but in the first instance, they may respond well to hypocarbia, whereas in the second instance, the vessels are, by definition, paralyzed to all forms of stimulation.

Pressure Waves

In the past it was customary to consider intracranial pressure as a rather steady phenomenon, but in clinical practice lumbar subarachnoid pressure was measured infrequently and for brief periods of time. Cerebrospinal fluid in a manometer pulsates synchronously with the heart rate, and superimposed respiratory oscillations are also present. When intracranial pressure is elevated both oscillations increase in amplitude. In addition, low-amplitude four– to eight–per second waves were described by Lundberg in patients with intracranial hypertension.[236] These waves are synchronous with similar oscillations of blood pressure often referred to as Traube-Herring-Mayer waves. The latter were first described by several investigators in the nineteenth century in animals with experimental intracranial hypertension. They also occur in normal patients and seem to be of little clinical significance.

Over the years spontaneous fluctuations in cerebrospinal fluid pressure of greater magnitude have been described in occasional patients with intracranial lesions. Guillaume and Janny studied these pressure phenomena in some detail and commented particularly on large paroxysmal waves that developed for no apparent reason and were sometimes seen in association with flushing of the face.[133] They attributed them to disturbances in vasomotor control of the cerebral circulation. Lundberg recorded intraventricular pressure on a strip chart recorder for periods of days to weeks. Three types of pressure waves (A, B, and C) were described in his patients. Only the A waves were found to be of clinical significance and were observed in 21 of 48 patients. The A waves were divided into two types: rhythmic fluctuations in pressure occurring in 15- to 30-minute intervals, and "plateau waves" that persisted for longer periods of time. The rhythmic two– to four–per hour waves began spontaneously from a base of mild to moderately elevated intracranial tension, rose to values of 60 to 100 mm of mercury, and then subsided. Plateau waves were often in excess of 100 mm of mercury. Evacuation of ventricular fluid was always accompanied by a prompt fall in pressure.[236]

The ease of inducing pressure waves by hypoxia and hypercapnia, their response to hyperventilation, and their enhancement by an arterial pressor response favor alterations in cerebral blood volume as the most likely cause. An increase in cerebral blood flow is accompanied by a rise in intracranial pressure, and the effect on intracranial pressure is greater if the initial pressure is elevated.[211,352] Intracranial pressure rises during sleep, and in patients with space-occupying intracranial lesions, the pressure may increase to alarming levels.[66]

The intracranial hypertension is due to increased cerebral blood flow and blood volume either from respiratory depression and hypercapnia or from increased cerebral metabolism, as in rapid eye movement sleep. The increase in regional cerebral blood flow produced by increased metabolic activity has been demonstrated to be accompanied by augmentation of regional cerebral blood volume, and Risberg and associates clearly demonstrated increased cerebral blood volume during plateau waves in one patient with intracranial hypertension of unknown origin and in a second patient with an unverified cerebral glioma.[337] Halothane anesthesia increases cerebral blood flow and produces a moderate rise in intracranial pressure.[260] In brain tumor patients, however, intracranial pressure may rise to dangerously high levels.[182] Thus, hypoxia and hypercapnia dilate cerebral vessels and in normal man and animals cause a small increase in intracranial pressure. On the vertical portion of the volume-pressure graph, however, when most of the displaceable cerebrospinal fluid has been eliminated from the intracranial space, a small increase in blood volume produces an enormous rise in pressure. Therefore, mild respiratory insufficiency that may have no effect on brain function in normal patients can cause severe intracranial hypertension and a critical reduction in cerebral blood flow in patients with brain swelling or a space-occupying mass.

Cerebral Ischemia with Intracranial Hypertension

In a previous section of this chapter, the statement was made that increased intracranial pressure appears to produce brain damage by only two methods. The first method is a diffuse rise in intracranial pressure sufficient to critically reduce blood flow throughout the brain, and the second method is expansion of an intracranial mass lesion to the point that herniation of brain substance through the tentorial incisura or the foramen magnum causes compression and focal ischemia within the brain stem. An issue, then, is the means of identifying these two forms of brain damage and their incidence in patients with intracranial hypertension.

When intracranial pressure is elevated above the systemic arterial pressure so as to produce cerebral circulatory arrest in experimental animals, brain metabolism is disturbed immediately. There is an increase in anaerobic glycolysis with the accumulation of lactate, followed by a decrease in phosphocreatine and adenosine triphosphate.[229,249] After 15 minutes of ischemia, there is histological evidence of ischemic cell changes, primarily in the striatum, hippocampus, and thalamus, with relative sparing of the neocortex. When cerebral perfusion pressure is reduced but not abolished by raising intracranial pressure to within approximately 20 mm of mercury of the systolic arterial pressure, the oxygen supply to the brain is not adequate, and metabolism fails in much the same fashion as in complete ischemia. Morphological evidence of ischemic brain damage was not present in these animals, however.[248] Since intracranial pressure was elevated by infusion of cerebrospinal fluid into the lumbar subarachnoid space in these animal experiments, there were no shifts or herniations of the brain. Thus, the location of the histological changes can be attributed to the effects of reduced cerebral blood flow produced by diffuse intracranial hypertension.

The principal clinical contributions to this subject have been made by Adams and Graham from postmortem examinations of patients who died from severe head injuries.[1,2,127] In their initial studies, they examined the distribution and severity of hypoxic changes in fatal head injuries. Subsequently, they correlated these observations with known levels of intracranial pressure recorded prior to death. Herniation of brain through the tentorial incisura entrapping and compressing branches of the posterior cerebral artery against the edge of the tentorium is a well-known phenomenon. Often the result is infarction of portions of the occipital lobe including the calcarine cortex, and this was the most common finding in that material. In surviving patients, the lesion is diagnosed by a homonymous hemianopia. In patients who have experienced a period of shock and subsequently die, it is common to find ischemic changes in the boundary zones between the three major arterial territories of the brain. These are often referred to as watershed zones where a critical reduction in tissue perfusion occurs first. Boundary zone regions were seen in patients with severe head injuries and intracranial hypertension, but it was difficult to know whether the lesions were due to the increased intracranial pressure or to arterial hypotension, or to a combination of the two conditions.

In their most recent observations, Adams and Graham have identified regions of the brain that appear to be selectively vulnerable to raised intracranial pressure. The most common finding in patients with proved intracranial hypertension was pressure necrosis in one or both parahippocampal gyri.[2]

CLINICAL DIAGNOSIS

Signs and Symptoms of Increased Intracranial Pressure

Few of the signs and symptoms ordinarily attributed to intracranial hypertension are actually due to the increased pressure.

Intracranial pressure may reach high levels in pseudotumor cerebri, yet the patient shows little evidence of it. Headache usually is not severe, certainly less so than in many patients with brain tumors and intracranial hypertension. Vomiting is uncommon, and the patient is alert and feels well. But papilledema may be severe enough to threaten the patient's vision. The benign course of pseudotumor is due to the fact that the brain swells diffusely, intracranial pressure is equal throughout the craniospinal axis, and the brain is displaced little if at all. Sixth nerve palsies occur and are attributed to stretching of the nerve by caudal displacement (axial distortion) of the brain stem, but sixth nerve palsy is not common.

The headache associated with changes in intracranial pressure was described in detail by Wolff. The pain-sensitive structures within the intracranial space are the middle meningeal artery and its branches, the large arteries at the base of the brain, the sinuses and bridging veins, and the dura at the base of the cranial fossae. Headache was regularly induced in subjects in the erect position by withdrawal of cerebrospinal fluid. The headache was nearly always frontal or at the vertex. It developed at approximately the same reduction in pressure among all subjects and disappeared promptly when the pressure was returned to normal by injection of saline into the subarachnoid space.[431]

Wolff elevated intracranial pressure to values as high as 850 mm of cerebrospinal fluid for one to two minutes by intrathecal injections of saline. Headache was never recorded.[431] Similar observations were made by Ryder and co-workers in subjects whose intracranial pressure was elevated to values of 500 to 1000 mm of cerebrospinal fluid by inflation of a cuff around the neck or by the Valsalva maneuver.[344,351] Nine per cent of patients with elevated pressure developed headache, but a skull defect was present in most of them, and the pain was localized to the region of the defect.[351] Since intracranial pressure was elevated by artificial means in these patients for short periods of time, it could be argued that the procedures did not simulate clinical intracranial hypertension. The pressure waves described by Lundberg occurred spontaneously. Pressure waves to 60 to 70 mm of mercury occurred in his patients without headache or other symptoms of increased intracranial pressure.[236]

Thus, increased intracranial pressure even to very high levels is a rare cause of headache. This is explained by the postulated cause of headache with decreased intracranial pressure, or more properly with a decrease in cerebrospinal fluid volume. The brain rests on a cushion of fluid. When the volume of fluid is reduced, the brain sinks with the patient in the erect position or shifts to the dependent side when the patient is horizontal. At the same time cerebral vessels, particularly the veins, dilate to compensate for the reduction in cerebrospinal fluid volume. The combination of venous dilatation and traction on the bridging cerebral veins and stretching of the arteries at the base causes headache. When intracranial pressure is increased diffusely, displacement of and traction on blood vessels are minimal, insufficient to stimulate pain receptors, and headache does not occur. It follows that traction on blood vessels or compression and invasion of the pain-sensitive dura at the base of the cranium, not increased intracranial pressure, is the cause of headache in patients with space-occupying lesions.

The headache associated with increased intracranial pressure often is severe on awakening in the morning and is relieved by vomiting. Intracranial pressure increases during sleep and can reach dangerously high levels in patients with space-occupying lesions.[66] The most likely explanation is that there is brain swelling from vascular dilatation and perhaps edema that is secondary to carbon dioxide retention. Lundberg noted that pressure waves were terminated by vomiting when the vomiting was accompanied by hyperventilation.[236] Following on this argument, the headache is due not to the increased pressure but to increased traction or displacement of blood vessels produced by the brain swelling.

The cause of nausea and vomiting in patients with increased intracranial pressure is poorly understood. Vomiting that occurs without nausea suggests intracranial disease, particularly when it is precipitate. Since vomiting was not observed in the patients of Wolff and Ryder and associates with artificially induced increased intracranial pressure, it may also be more a function of displacement of intracranial structures than of pressure.

Papilledema is the only reliable clinical sign of increased intracranial pressure. The other neurological signs attributed to or associated with intracranial hypertension, such as sixth nerve palsy and the signs of tentorial or foramen magnum herniation, are due to displacement of brain tissue. The mechanisms of herniation are complex, and an increase in pressure, albeit small, may be necessary as the driving force behind the herniation. This raises again the issue of tissue pressure and intracranial pressure. If pressure or force in the medial temporal lobe adjacent to a tumor in the temporal fossa is increased, without elevated pressure in the rest of the intracranial cavity, herniation can occur without raised "intracranial pressure." In practice most patients with tentorial pressure cones do have a diffuse rise in intracranial tension.

Half of brain tumor patients have papilledema at the time the diagnosis is made. Some authors have attributed the absence of papilledema in the other half to anatomical variations of the optic nerve, sheath space, or papilla that preclude the development of papilledema. Local anomalies may account for the occasional finding of unilateral papilledema in a patient with a posterior fossa lesion, but most patients with brain tumor and no papilledema probably do not have increased intracranial pressure sufficient to cause it.

Tentorial Pressure Cone

In early studies of brain swelling and increased intracranial pressure, emphasis was placed on direct involvement of the medulla as the principal cause of coma and alterations in the vital signs. This was attributed in large part to medullary compression from herniation of the cerebellar tonsils into the foramen magnum. In recent times emphasis has shifted to transtentorial herniation as the principal cause of brain stem dysfunction with supratentorial mass lesions and cerebral swelling. Since the earliest days of neurology, clinicians have been puzzled by a number of false localizing signs in patients with expanding supratentorial lesions. Collier found sixth and third nerve palsies to be the most common neu-

rological signs that could not be attributed directly to the lesion.[63] Knapp described paresis of the ipsilateral oculomotor nerve as the most frequent sign of a temporal lobe tumor; occasionally both nerves or the contralateral one only were involved.[202]

Transtentorial herniation was first described by Meyer in autopsy specimens.[266] The significance of herniation in clinical terms was emphasized by the demonstration of grooving and an occasional partial transection of the contralateral cerebral peduncle by the edge of the tentorium.[195] Hasenjäger and Spatz brought attention to the marked displacement of both the diencephalon and midbrain that accompanies tentorial pressure cones, but lateral rather than caudal displacement was described.[145] Jefferson placed emphasis on transtentorial herniation as the cause of many signs and symptoms previously attributed to foramen magnum herniation, and his general discussion provided the first wide introduction of the problem to neurosurgeons.[180]

Many of the signs and symptoms often ascribed to transtentorial herniation and brain stem compression may be indistinguishable from those caused by the primary lesion. It is generally accepted that the most convincing evidence of herniation is a dilated pupil or other signs of third nerve dysfunction. Sunderland and Hughes considered this the surest indicator of the onset and degree of herniation.[398] Large tentorial pressure cones have, however, been demonstrated in patients who did not exhibit evidence of oculomotor abnormalities.[99,286] The third nerve palsy has been variously attributed to direct pressure by herniated tissue, midbrain ischemia, compression by the petroclinoid ligament, and compression or distortion of the nerve as it enters the cavernous sinus.[186,222,310,330] The most frequently quoted explanation is that the nerve is kinked across a displaced posterior cerebral artery or trapped between the posterior cerebral and superior cerebellar arteries.[399]

Transient obscurations of vision, appearing as hemianopic defects or intermittent total blindness, also are caused by transtentorial herniation. Ethelberg and Jensen attributed the symptoms to intermittent obstruction of one or both posterior cerebral arteries,[90] and Lindenberg described the posterior cerebral artery as the most frequently compressed large vessel in patients with severe brain swelling.[227] Visual symptoms also have been attributed to displacement or compression of the optic tracts in association with herniation.[47]

Contralateral weakness is such a common accompaniment of supratentorial mass lesions that it is usually difficult to assess the contribution of transtentorial herniation to the patient's neurological signs. The observations of Kernohan and Woltman show clearly the pathological changes that can occur in the cerebral peduncles, but the "Kernohan notch" appears to be a rather rare finding.[195] Nevertheless, Cabieses and Jeri contended that 50 per cent of patients with transtentorial herniation have contralateral motor signs on the basis of ipsilateral involvement of the brain stem by the herniation.[45]

Transection of the upper midbrain is the classic means of producing decerebration in experimental animals, and severe midbrain ischemia produced by transtentorial herniation might be expected to produce a high incidence of preterminal decerebration in patients. In fact, it has been described infrequently or incompletely, and in the retrospective series of brain tumor patients reported by Finney and Walker decerebration was present in only 9 per cent.[99] General experience, however, suggests that the incidence is much higher. Ingvar and Lundberg have described intermittent decerebration in brain tumor patients at the peak of intracranial pressure waves. Loss of consciousness and tonic extension of all four limbs occurred frequently, followed by complete recovery when intracranial pressure had returned to normal. Clonic convulsive movements were also observed in the presence of a remarkably normal electroencephalogram, and the authors identified the attacks with the "cerebellar fits" considered in detail by Penfield and Jasper.[163,309] Opisthotonus also was observed occasionally. The frequent occurrence of decerebrate phenomena in the material of Ingvar and Lundberg, both among patients and repeatedly in the same patient, emphasizes again the importance of brain stem dysfunction in the symptomatology of raised intracranial pressure.

The production of irreversible coma by brain stem injury has been clearly demonstrated in both experimental animals and man, and a decreasing level of consciousness would be expected to constitute one of the cardinal signs of brain stem dysfunction produced by transtentorial herniation. Munro and Sisson stated that nearly all patients with transtentorial herniations show progressive coma.[286]

Most authors who have written on the subject agree that the clinical diagnosis of transtentorial herniation is difficult in most cases, and the question arises whether the herniation is primarily responsible for the signs and symptoms of brain stem dysfunction.[99] In experimental animals, expansion of a supratentorial mass sufficient to cause transtentorial herniation always produced caudal displacement and distortion of the brain stem, and this direct effect on the brain stem might be sufficient to explain the clinical signs without need to invoke compression by herniated tissue.[407,423] Scheinker emphasized downward displacement of the midbrain through the incisura, as opposed to herniation, and Howell demonstrated that longitudinal buckling of the brain stem may occur without temporal lobe herniation.[161,357] Hassler examined the vertebral-basilar circulation by postmortem angiography in patients who had died from supratentorial mass lesions. In all patients there was severe caudal displacement and distortion of the brain stem and stretching of the paramedian branches of the basilar artery.[148]

A third mechanism requiring consideration is the one originally proposed by Cushing to explain the effect of a mass lesion on remote regions of the brain.[70] He postulated, as had Kocher, that dysfunction in the brain surrounding the lesion is due to capillary stasis and ischemia that gradually spreads to involve adjacent brain. McNealy and Plum believed that this or a similar mechanism is the most likely explanation for the orderly spread of brain stem dysfunction from above downward in their patients. Transtentorial herniation and caudal displacement of the brain stem were believed to play a minor role.[262]

Thus, several different mechanisms might account for the clinical signs and symptoms ordinarily attributed to transtentorial herniation alone, and identification of the significance of each factor is difficult because they appear to develop concurrently. Animal experiments have been helpful, but most have been short-term studies in anesthetized animals, conditions far removed from the clinical problem.

INCIDENCE AND SIGNIFICANCE IN CLINICAL DISORDERS

Head Injury

The incidence and significance of intracranial hypertension in head injury has been a controversial issue. Dandy, among others, believed that brain swelling and increased intracranial pressure were the rule and were the most common causes of death in patients with head injuries.[75] In contrast, Browder and Meyers, who measured the lumbar subarachnoid pressure in the same patient several times, observed marked intracranial hypertension infrequently. Furthermore, many patients who died did not have increased intracranial pressure at any time during the course of their illness.[35] Although these contradictory observations were made in the 1930's, and intracranial pressure has been measured directly and continuously in a large number of patients with head injuries in recent years, there is still some disagreement among investigators on the frequency of intracranial hypertension and its contribution to morbidity and death.

In the first report on continuous measurement of intracranial pressure in a large number of patients, Lundberg described various types of pressure waves, which are associated with his name, in patients with brain tumors.[236] Subsequently, Lundberg and his colleagues published the first observations of the course of intracranial pressure in patients with head injuries based on continuous ventricular recordings. Although only four cases were presented, they cover reasonably well the gamut of changes in intracranial pressure in head injury published since that time. The first patient had a contusion of the left frontal lobe that was not large, and intracranial pressure was only moderately elevated. The second patient had a contusion of the right temporal lobe with marked swelling and high intracranial pressure on admission. While the patient was being prepared for operation, a classical plateau wave developed

rapidly, intracranial pressure increased to 115 mm of mercury, and respirations ceased. The intracranial pressure responded immediately to hyperventilation and hypertonic urea.[238] All investigators who have had extensive experience with recording of intracranial pressure in patients with head injury have observed fatal or potentially fatal pressure waves, but the frequency of their occurrence has not been established. Another of Lundberg's patients had a normal carotid arteriogram except for some swelling of one hemisphere and had persistently normal intracranial pressure. Nevertheless, he had severe brain stem dysfunction during the acute phase of his illness and made a poor recovery.[238] This is now recognized to be the picture of diffuse impact injury in which intracranial pressure is usually normal or only slightly elevated but the outcome is almost always poor.

The first large series of patients in whom clinical outcome was related to the level of intracranial pressure on admission was reported by Vapalahti. The series contained 51 patients, all of whom were comatose at the time of admission to the hospital. Pressure levels were divided into four groups: below 15, 15 to 30, 30 to 60, and over 60 mm of mercury. Among the 11 patients in the lowest intracranial pressure category, only one died, and that death was considered to be of extracerebral causes. Thus, the mortality rate for intracranial disease in this group of patients was zero. In contrast, among the 15 patients who had a pressure over 60 mm of mercury, 12 died, and in all cases, the death was due to uncontrollable intracranial hypertension.[411] Moody and Mullan also found a good correlation between intracranial pressure and survival.[281] At the same time, however, Johnston and co-workers emphasized what the series of patients reported by Vapalahti in fact showed, namely, that intracranial pressure is not necessarily elevated in head injury, and normal intracranial pressure is not necessarily a favorable prognostic sign.[189]

In order to assess the incidence and significance of intracranial hypertension in terms of outcome, the author tabulated the results from several series of patients with head injury.[207] Table 24-1 shows the incidence of normal intracranial pressure and of mild, moderate, and severe intracranial

TABLE 24–1   INTRACRANIAL PRESSURE IN HEAD INJURY

	INTRACRANIAL PRESSURE (n = 280)			
REFERENCE	*Normal* *(0 to 10 mm Hg)*	*Mild (10, 11* *to 29, 30 mm Hg)*	*Moderate (30, 31* *to 50, 60 mm Hg)*	*Severe* *(>50, 60 mm Hg)*
Becker et al.*	10	32	14	10
Rossanda et al.*	13	6	6	5
Troupp et al.†	16	23	14	21
Kelly et al.‡	11	12	9	9
(Data given as <30 and >30 mm Hg)				
Bruce et al.§	6	7	5	4
Cold et al.*	14	28	5	0
Totals	70	108	53	49
Per cent of total	25	39	19	17

* *In* Lundberg, N., et al., eds.: Intracranial Pressure II. Berlin, Springer-Verlag, 1975.

† *In* Brock, M., and Dietz, H., eds.: Intracranial Pressure: Experimental and Clinical Aspects. Berlin, Springer-Verlag, 1973.

‡ *In* Langfitt, T. W., et al.: Cerebral Circulation and Metabolism. Berlin, Springer-Verlag, 1975.

§ Regional cerebral blood flow, intracranial pressure and brain metabolism in comatose patients. J. Neurosurg., 38:131–144, 1973.

hypertension in 280 patients from six series reported in the literature. Since the levels of intracranial pressure are grouped differently among reports, it was necessary to use some editorial license in regrouping the patients. The data demonstrate that about one quarter of the patients had normal intracranial pressure and about one sixth of the patients had an intracranial pressure in excess of 50 or 60 mm of mercury. There was considerable variability among the series. In one large series, the distribution of patients with normal to mild and moderate to severe increases in intracranial pressure is nearly equal, whereas in another series of comparable size, only a few patients had a moderate increase and none had a large increase in intracranial pressure.[60,409] These are very important observations because they demonstrate that even in a relatively large series of patients, the experience can vary considerably. Table 24–2 illustrates

one explanation for this difference in the experience among head injury units. Among 88 patients in whom a distinction was made between those patients who had a traumatic mass lesion and those who did not, elevated intracranial pressure was the rule in the patients with space-occupying masses and occurred in only a small percentage of those patients who did not have a mass lesion.

Table 24–3 presents data on the relationship between intracranial pressure and survival and the quality of survival from reports with a total of 236 patients.[17,60,189,194,409] Again, the varied description of the neurological status of the patients permitted division into only three groups, "recovered," vegetative, and dead. The designation "recovered" includes patients with a neurological status ranging from normal to severely impaired. Two thirds of patients

TABLE 24–2   INTRACRANIAL PRESSURE AND MASS LESION

	INTRACRANIAL PRESSURE (mm Hg) (88 PATIENTS)			
	0 to 10	*11 to 29*	*30 to 50*	*50*
Mass	1	9	12	12
No mass	13	32	6	3
	0 to 29	*Per Cent*	*>29*	*Per Cent*
Mass	10	18	24	73
No mass	45	82	9	27

TABLE 24–3   INTRACRANIAL PRESSURE AND SURVIVAL

	INTRACRANIAL PRESSURE*			
	Normal to Mild		*Moderate to Severe* *(>30, 40 mm Hg)*	
	No. of *Patients*	*Per Cent*	*No. of* *Patients*	*Per Cent*
"Recovered"	89	66	39	38
Vegetative	20	15	12	12
Dead	25	19	51	50

* Data from one report <11 (Normal to mild) and >11 (Moderate to severe) mm Hg.

TABLE 24-4   INTRACRANIAL PRESSURE AND SURVIVAL

INTRACRANIAL PRESSURE (mm Hg)	NUMBER OF PATIENTS	
	Recovered	Vegetative or Dead
Normal	50	22
Increased (>11, 15, 20, 30)	78	86
Normal	50	22
Severe increase (>60)	2	19

with normal or mildly increased intracranial pressure recovered, whereas half the patients with moderate or severe intracranial hypertension died. The number of vegetative patients in both groups is small. Table 24-4 presents the same data in a different format. The purpose is to demonstrate that when the patients are divided into only two groups (normal and increased intracranial pressure), and into two categories of survival (recovered and vegetative or dead), the presence or absence of increased intracranial pressure has little influence on the clinical results. When the patients with normal and severe increased intracranial pressure are compared, however, it is clear that very few patients with head injury with an increase in intracranial pressure over 60 mm of mercury survive. Of equal importance is the observation that many patients with normal intracranial pressure vegetate or die. The latter observation helped clarify some disagreements that had existed to that time. The fact that many patients who die following head injury do not have intracranial hypertension does not mean that intracranial hypertension is unimportant in head injuries. In fact, severe intracranial hypertension carries with it a very poor prognosis. Nevertheless, approximately one third of the death and severe morbidity occurs in patients with little or no increased intracranial pressure.

There have been a number of other clinical reports that generally support these results. Papo and Caruselli found no correlation between intracranial pressure and outcome when intracranial pressure did not exceed 50 mm of mercury. In contrast, every patient in the series who had a sustained pressure of 50 mm of mercury or more died.[302] DeRougemont and associates preferred to use the ratio of the mean intracranial pressure to the mean arterial blood pressure, rather than intracranial pressure alone, to assess the relationship of intracranial hypertension to outcome. They termed the ratio the brain vasomotor tone index and postulated that the mortality rate would increase with a rise in the value of the index. None of the patients died of intracranial disease with an index less than 0.25, and no surviving patient had an index above 0.50. The patients who died from extracerebral causes had indices that were widespread between 0.10 and 0.50.[76] Collice and co-workers recorded a mortality rate of 65 per cent in patients with high intracranial pressure and only 19 per cent in patients with normal intracranial pressure.[62]

The largest series reported from one neurosurgical unit is the 160 patients described in the report by Miller and colleagues. Generally, the observations support those of other investigators. The upper limit of normal intracranial pressure usually has been declared to be either 15 or 20 mm of mercury. In this series, however, the upper limit was set at 10 mm of mercury. The patients were divided into those who had an intracranial mass lesion and those who did not have a mass lesion and were therefore characterized as having diffuse brain injury. Among the 62 patients with a mass lesion, only 2 had normal intracranial pressure, and among the 98 with diffuse brain injury, 26 per cent had unequivocally normal pressure. Somewhat surprising was the observation that there was no apparent relationship between neurological dysfunction and the levels of intracranial pressure on admission in those patients with mass lesions who required operations. In contrast, in the diffuse brain injury group there was an inverse relationship between intracranial pressure and neurological function. The outcome was unaffected by intracranial tensions less than 40 mm of mercury, but above that level, the mortality rate was 69 per cent compared with a rate of only 14 per cent in patients with normal pressure. Of the 48 patients who died, 22 died from an intracranial cause, in every case, uncontrollable intracranial hypertension.[278]

In summary, increased intracranial pressure is common in patients with head injury. It is higher in patients with a mass lesion requiring operative intervention than in those patients who do not have mass lesions. As long as the intracranial pressure is below 40 to 50 mm of mercury, it does not increase the mortality rate owing to the head injury, although there is good evidence that neurological function deteriorates in patients with diffuse brain injury, even at relatively low levels of intracranial hypertension. The death rate rises rapidly with intracranial pressures above 50 mm of mercury, and in some series, all the patients with marked intracranial hypertension died. As a corollary of this statement, nearly all patients who die from an intracranial cause following head injury do so from uncontrollable intracranial hypertension, which usually approaches or equals the systemic arterial pressure prior to death.

Marked intracranial hypertension represents the greatest challenge to therapy. At the present time there is little to offer patients with diffuse brain injury. In fact, nearly all therapy for patients with head injury is directed toward reducing intracranial pressure and therefore is applicable only to those with intracranial hypertension. Although even now there are some who question the value of continuous recording of intracranial pressure in head injury patients, the weight of evidence is in favor of recording intracranial pressure continuously in all patients who remain comatose for any period of time following their injury.[104] The rise in intracranial pressure can be diagnosed and treated early, and the important observations of Miller and his colleagues that neurological function deteriorates with even mild to moderate increases in intracranial pressure suggest that therapy should be applied at lower levels of intracranial pressure than has been the custom in most neurosurgical units.

Bruce and associates have made important observations about the pathophysiology of head injury in children that are particularly important in understanding the role of intracranial hypertension in the pediatric age group. In a large series of unconscious patients with head injury, approximately 40 per cent demonstrated smallness or absence of the ventricles and basal cisterns on CT scans. Subarachnoid hemorrhage was fairly common in association with this picture of diffuse brain swelling, but parenchymal hemorrhage and extracerebral collections of blood were rare. The authors postulated that the brain swelling is due primarily to cerebrovascular dilatation, not cerebral edema.[40,42] The facts that the density of the swollen brain is normal or increased, rather than decreased as would be expected with cerebral edema, and cerebral blood flow is increased throughout the swollen brain, rather than decreased as in adults, support the hypothesis.

In the first series of 53 children, intracranial pressure was measured continuously in 25 patients, and was found to be increased to 20 mm of mercury or more in 68 per cent. The outcome in this series was extremely good. Two patients died from systemic complications of the head injury, and one died from uncontrollable intracranial hypertension. Several other children, however, had very high intracranial pressures that were clearly responsible for neurological deterioration, and the children survived only because intracranial pressure could be controlled.[40]

A diffuse rise in intracranial pressure, without brain displacement or herniation, causes a decrease in cerebral blood flow when the limits of autoregulation have been exceeded. In normal animals, the lower limit of autoregulation to increased intracranial pressure is in the range of 30 to 40 mm of mercury. In recent years, there have been a number of investigations relating intracranial pressure, systemic arterial pressure, and cerebral blood flow in patients with head injury. In nearly all the studies, regional cerebral blood flow has been measured by the intracarotid [133]xenon technique developed by Lassen and Ingvar.[220] More recently, a noninvasive technique for measuring regional cerebral blood flow with [133]xenon has been developed by Obrist and co-workers.[294] Xenon is administered by inhalation or by intravenous injection as suggested by Austin and associates.[8] Measurements of cerebral blood flow have been made in the steady state and in response to changes in systemic arterial pressure and carbon dioxide tension in order to test cerebrovascular reactivity. In a few series of patients, the cerebral metabolic rate of oxygen utilization has also been measured. Cerebral metabolism of oxygen is calculated from the difference in oxygen content of arterial blood and of cerebral venous blood. The latter is obtained by inserting a catheter percutaneously into the jugular vein and threading it into the jugular bulb. At the time the cerebral blood flow study is performed, samples of arterial and jugular venous blood are obtained simultaneously, and the difference in oxygen content is measured. Then the cerebral metabolic rate of oxygen utilization (CMR_{O_2}) is calculated by multiplying the arteriovenous difference of oxygen content (AVD_{O_2}) times mean cerebral blood flow (mCBF) and dividing by 100.

$$CMR_{O_2} = \frac{AVD_{O_2} \times mCBF}{100}$$

The value for CMR_{O_2} is expressed as milliliters of oxygen utilized per 100 gm of brain per minute. Using the intracarotid ^{133}xenon technique, with which the normal value for CBF is approximately 50 ml per 100 gm per minute, the normal value for CMR_{O_2} is approximately 3.5 ml per 100 gm per minute.

There are potential errors of considerable magnitude in calculating oxygen utilization on the basis of the intracarotid ^{133}xenon technique. Although cerebral blood flow is measured from multiple regions in one hemisphere, much of the hemisphere is not included, and cerebral blood flow in the opposite hemisphere is excluded from the equation. Ordinarily blood is taken from the right jugular bulb to obtain blood flowing mainly from the sagittal sinus. Normally the contribution of blood flow from each hemisphere into the sagittal sinus should be about equal. Therefore, an average arteriovenous oxygen difference across the cerebral cortex of both hemispheres is multiplied by mean cerebral blood flow through a portion of only one of those hemispheres. The ^{133}xenon noninvasive technique is much superior for the calculation of metabolic rate, because values are averaged for the two hemispheres. An even better method is the original Kety-Schmidt technique for measuring global cerebral blood flow, using the nitrous oxide technique or modifications of that procedure, such as the argon method, which has been used to measure both cerebral blood flow and oxygen metabolism in patients with head injury.[146] With this method, there is greater certainty that blood is flowing through the same tissue from which oxygen is extracted.

In early reports of the study of the cerebral circulation and metabolism in patients with severe head injuries, emphasis was placed on levels of cerebral blood flow and metabolism in relation to the patient's neurological status and on the interrelationships between intracranial pressure and cerebral blood flow. In addition, cerebrovascular reactivity to changes in blood pressure and arterial carbon dioxide tension were studied in a number of patients. As a general rule, mean cerebral blood flow from the hemisphere studied was reduced and reached very low levels in patients in deep coma.[41,98,298] When the initial blood flows were averaged over a large series of patients, however, there was no statistically significant correlation between blood flow and neurological status. In the series reported by Bruce and associates mean cerebral blood flow ranged from zero (brain death) to 114 ml per 100 gm per minute. The overall mean value was 39 ml per 100 gm per minute. In contrast to the cerebral blood flow findings, the cerebral metabolic rate of oxygen utilization was always depressed. The highest value recorded was 2.85 ml per 100 gm per minute, but the value was in excess of 2.0 in only 5 of the 18 patients in whom metabolism was measured. The mean value for the group was 1.53 ml per 100 gm per minute.[41] Examination of the data from individual patients makes it clear that blood flow and metabolism were decreased proportionately in some patients, whereas in others metabolism was depressed much more than blood flow. Thus, blood flow had become dissociated or unlinked from metabolism. As noted previously, metabolic autoregulation is a normal property of the brain. When metabolism is either increased or decreased, blood flow follows metabolism, and the purpose is to provide the brain with the appropriate quantity of oxygen and glucose required to meet the metabolic demand. In clinical head injury, therefore, metabolic autoregulation often is defective.

Not only is blood flow dissociated from metabolism in unconscious patients with head injury, cerebral blood flow values often are normal or above normal. Hyperemia may be focal at the site of a contusion, where a cerebral angiogram will show evidence of the luxury perfusion syndrome, and focal hyperemia is common in the brain adjacent to a hematoma that has been evacuated.[217] Blood flow may, however, be uniformly increased throughout the cerebral hemisphere, and in studies using the noninvasive ^{133}xenon technique, blood flow was found to be increased throughout both hemispheres in some patients.[41,98,217]

Marked, diffuse hyperemia appears to be a response mainly of the young brain. In the series of Obrist and colleagues, a normal or supernormal value was observed in 7 of 20 patients. The mean age of this group was 19 compared with 41 for those patients with a mean cerebral blood flow value less than normal. When patients who had had a seizure not long before the blood flow study was performed or who were in peripheral shock at the time of admission to the hospital were excluded, the difference between the two groups was even more impressive.[295] Overgaard also divided his series of head injury patients according to the initial blood flow values. In the hyperemia group, the age range was 6 to 33 years, with an average age of 18 years. The average age of patients with severe depression of flow was 19 years, and among patients with values ranging from normal to about half normal, the average age was also 19 years.[297] In this series, therefore, hyperemia was not confined to the younger age group.

Table 24–5 provides the mean cerebral blood flow values from a total of 180 patients reported in the literature. The mean values range from 22 to 43 ml per 100 gm per minute. Table 24–6 provides the principal explanation for this marked variability among series. Fewer than 1 in 10 of the pa-

TABLE 24–5 MEAN CEREBRAL BLOOD FLOW IN PATIENTS WITH HEAD INJURY

REFERENCE	NUMBER OF PATIENTS	MEAN CEREBRAL BLOOD FLOW (ml/100 gm/min)
Hass et al.*	45	43.4
Enevoldsen et al.†	23	30
Overgaard and Tweed‡	43	26
Kelly et al.§	17	42.7
Baldy-Moulinier and Frerebeau‖	30	22.1
Bruce et al.¶	22	39.5
Total	180	

  * In Harper, A. M., et al., eds.: Blood Flow and Metabolism in the Brain. Edinburgh, Churchill Livingstone, 1975.
  † Dynamic changes in regional CBF, intraventricular pressure, CSF pH, and lactate levels during the acute phase of head injury. J. Neurosurg., 44:191–214, 1976.
  ‡ Cerebral circulation after head injury. Part I. J. Neurosurg., 41:531–541, 1974.
  § In Langfitt, T. W., et al., eds.: Cerebral Circulation and Metabolism. Berlin, Springer-Verlag, 1975.
  ‖ In Cerebral Blood Flow. Brock, M., et al., eds.: Berlin, Springer-Verlag, 1969.
  ¶ Regional cerebral blood flow, intracranial pressure and brain metabolism in comatose patients. J. Neurosurg., 38:131–144, 1973.

TABLE 24–6 HYPEREMIA IN HEAD INJURY

Enevoldsen et al.*
  (normal 50 ml/100 gm/min)
  2 of 23 patients > 50—mean 53 ml/100 gm/min
Overgaard and Tweed†
  (CBF initially normal—58.7 ml/100 gm/min)
  0 to 24 hours 2 of 15 > 58.7—mean 64 ml/100 gm/min
  1 to 7 days—10 of 20 > 58.7—mean 68 ml/100 gm/min
Bruce et al.‡
  (normal 50 ml/100 gm/min)
  Patients with no mass lesion
    4 of 12 > 50—mean 74.7 ml/100 gm/min
    8 of 12 < 50—mean 34.6 ml/100 gm/min

  * Dynamic changes in regional CBF, intraventricular pressure, CSF pH, and lactate levels during the acute phase of head injury. J. Neurosurg., 44:191–214, 1976.
  † Cerebral circulation after head injury. Part I. J. Neurosurg., 41:531–541, 1974.
  ‡ Regional cerebral blood flow, intracranial pressure and brain metabolism in comatose patients. J. Neurosurg., 38:131–144, 1973.

tients reported by Enevoldsen and co-workers had hyperemia, whereas two thirds of the patients reported by Bruce and his associates had supernormal blood flows, and in the series of Overgaard and Tweed, hyperemia was infrequent during the first day, then appeared in half the patients between the first and seventh days.[41,89,298]

There is surprisingly little information on the relationship between intracranial pressure and cerebral blood flow in patients with head injury. At levels of intracranial hypertension below 50 to 60 mm of mercury, that is, below those levels that significantly influence the mortality rate, there is no predictable relationship between intracranial pressure and blood flow.[41,89,98,364] As intracranial pressure continues to rise, however, blood flow invariably declines. When the intracranial pressure equals the systemic arterial pressure, cerebral blood flow ceases.[41,298] If the intracarotid [133]xenon technique is used, either the isotope fails to enter the brain or small amounts are detectable within the intracranial space, then fail to clear. With a noninvasive [133]xenon method, the clearance curve appears to be derived entirely from scalp.[295]

There is also little correlation between regional cerebral blood flow subjacent to a mass lesion and regional flow elsewhere in the same hemisphere. Similar observations have been made in experimental brain compression, and the data demonstrate that the cerebral vessels beneath an expanding mass, in both the experimental and clinical situations, can adjust quite well to the increase in pressure produced by the mass. When the mass is very large, however, marked focal or regional reductions in flow do occur. Figure 24–10 illustrates this situation in a patient with a very large intracerebral hematoma. Blood flow was markedly reduced throughout the hemisphere and had been virtually abolished over the posterior half of the brain overlying the hematoma. Following evacuation of most of the hematoma, blood flow tended to equalize throughout the hemisphere, and it increased with arterial hypertension, demonstrating defective autoregulation. Following the administration of hypertonic mannitol, cerebral blood flow approached

normal in three of the six regions, despite the fact that a significant mass effect remained within the hemisphere. Overgaard and Tweed diagnosed brain edema radiologically from cerebral angiograms and ventriculograms in a series of head injury patients. When the patients were divided into two groups, those with and those without edema, the mean intracranial pressure in the edema group was 27 mm of mercury compared with 14 mm of mercury in the patients without edema. There was, however, no difference between the two groups in hemispheric blood flow.[300] In contrast, Enevoldsen and Jensen did find differences between normal brain tissue, cortical contusion, and severely edematous brain when the clearance curves were submitted to

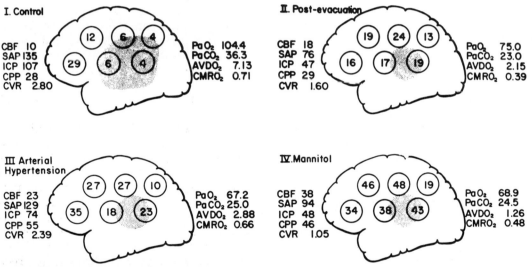

Figure 24–10 A patient with a large intracerebral hematoma in the left hemisphere, probably of traumatic origin. The controlled value of cerebral blood flow (CBF) determined by the intracarotid ^{133}xenon technique was 10 ml per 100 gm per minute compared with a normal value of 50 ml per 100 gm per minute. Cerebral blood flow was virtually abolished in brain tissue overlying the hematoma (stippled area). The systemic arterial pressure (SAP) was moderately elevated, and intracranial pressure was 107 mm of mercury, resulting in a perfusion pressure (CPP) of 28 mm of mercury and a calculated cerebrovascular resistance (CVR) of 2.80. The patient was well oxygenated and slightly hypocapnic on a ventilator. The arteriovenous difference of oxygen across the brain (AVDO$_2$) was 7.13, and the cerebral metabolic rate of oxygen utilization (CMRO$_2$) was 0.71 ml per 100 gm per minute compared with a normal value of 3.5 ml per 100 gm per minute. The hematoma, which had been identified by angiography only immediately prior to the control studies, was then evacuated through a burr hole, and repeat studies were performed (II Post-evacuation). Cerebral blood flow increased throughout the hemisphere except for the left frontal region, where it decreased, suggesting an intracerebral steal phenomenon. Intracranial pressure was greatly reduced, but oxygen utilization declined even further. This observation, plus the fact that the patient had been deeply comatose from the time of admission, indicated that survival was very unlikely. Because systemic arterial pressure had also dropped precipitously with the decline of intracranial pressure, so that perfusion pressure was still greatly reduced, systemic arterial pressure was then raised with angiotensin, resulting in a large increase in intracranial pressure (III, Arterial Hypertension). Although perfusion pressure improved considerably, there was only a modest increase in mean cerebral blood flow throughout the hemisphere. This is the phenomenon known as false autoregulation. Finally, 1 gm per kilogram of a 25 per cent solution of mannitol was administered intravenously, and the studies were repeated 30 minutes later. There was marked improvement in cerebral blood flow throughout the hemisphere, and intracranial pressure was again reduced. There was, however, no improvement in the rate of oxygen utilization, and a few hours after these studies were performed, the patient died.

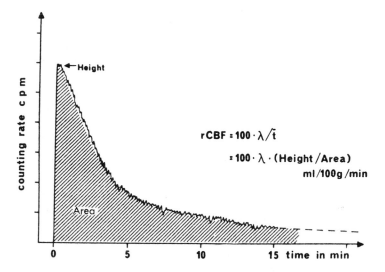

Figure 24–11 Clearance curve for [133]xenon injected via the internal carotid artery. Shaded area and height of curve are basis for height to area, or stochastic, method for calculation of mean cerebral blood flow (CBF) from a region. $\bar{t}$, Area/height per minute. (From Lassen, N. A., and Ingvar, D. H.: Radioisotopic assessment of regional cerebral blood flow. Progr. Nucl. Med., *1*:376–409, 1971. Reprinted by permission.

compartmental analysis instead of the height to area method for analyzing the curves that has been reported by most investigators.[88]

Figure 24–11 illustrates the height to area method of analysis, which gives a single mean value for the 15-minute clearance curve. Even casual inspection of the curve reveals an initial fast clearance followed by a slower clearance of the isotope. The method of bicompartmental analysis is illustrated in Figure 24–12. In normal brain the fast compartment is gray matter and the slow compartment is white matter. Unfortunately for analytic purposes, the blood flow compartments break down in patients with severe insults. As gray matter flow decreases, it becomes indistinguishable from that of white matter, and when cerebral

blood flow is markedly reduced, the clearance curve approaches a monoexponential function.[38] Despite these limitations, Enevoldsen and Jensen were able to identify three types of clearance curves in patients with severe head injuries. The curves from fairly normal brain tissue were typically biexponential. Clearance of the isotope from regions of severe cortical contusion showed a very fast third component, often referred to as a tissue peak, and in regions with marked edema, the clearance curve approached the monoexponential shape.[88]

The status of pressure autoregulation also varies greatly among head injury patients.[41,98,298] It may be either diffusely intact or diffusely defective in comatose patients. It may be intact in one hemisphere and defective throughout the opposite hem-

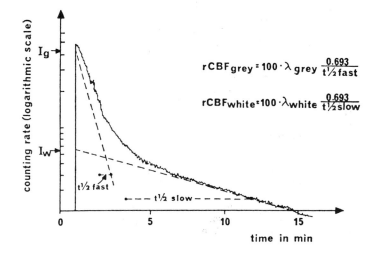

Figure 24–12 Bicompartmental or biexponential analysis of the [133]xenon clearance curve. Flows for gray and white matter are calculated from the steep and the flat dotted lines, respectively. (From Lassen, N. A., and Ingvar, D. H.: Radioisotopic assessment of regional cerebral blood flow. Progr. Nucl. Med., *1*:376–409, 1972. Reprinted by permission.)

isphere. As a general rule, it is defective adjacent to mass lesions, whether the resting blood flow has increased or decreased prior to the test of autoregulation. Figure 24–13 illustrates cerebral blood flow that was diffusely decreased throughout the hemisphere in a patient with a contused temporal lobe. Regional flow adjacent to the

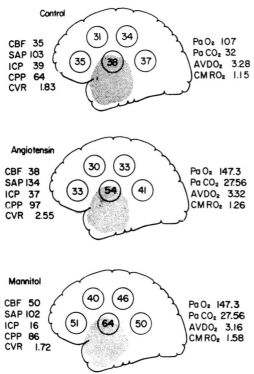

Control

CBF 35
SAP 103
ICP 39
CPP 64
CVR 1.83

31   34
35   38   37

Pa O₂ 107
Pa CO₂ 32
AVDO₂ 3.28
CM RO₂ 1.15

Angiotensin

CBF 38
SAP 134
ICP 37
CPP 97
CVR 2.55

30   33
33   54   41

Pa O₂ 147.3
Pa CO₂ 27.56
AVDO₂ 3.32
CM RO₂ 1.26

Mannitol

CBF 50
SAP 102
ICP 16
CPP 86
CVR 1.72

40   46
51   64   50

Pa O₂ 147.3
Pa CO₂ 27.56
AVDO₂ 3.16
CM RO₂ 1.58

Figure 24–13 A patient with head injury involving extensive contusion and edema of the left temporal lobe resulting in a large mass effect. Cerebral blood flow (CBF) was reduced throughout the hemisphere during the control period but no more so in brain overlying the contusion. Intracranial pressure (ICP) was moderately elevated, and the metabotic rate of oxygen utilization (CMRO₂) was reduced to about one third the normal value. Following administration of angiotensin, the systemic arterial pressure (SAP) increased by 31 mm of mercury, intracranial pressure remained the same, and mean cerebral blood flow for the hemisphere also remained the same. There was, however, a marked increase in cerebral blood flow adjacent to the contusion as a manifestation of defective autoregulation. The angiotensin was discontinued, and systemic arterial pressure returned to the control value. Hypertonic mannitol, 1 gm per kilogram of a 25 per cent solution, was administered intravenously, and the measurements were repeated 30 minutes later. Intracranial pressure was reduced to normal, and cerebral blood flow increased to the normal value. The greatest increase took place in brain overlying the contusion. There was only a marginal increase in oxygen utilization, and the patient subsequently died.

contusion was the same as elsewhere within that hemisphere. On elevation of the systemic arterial pressure with angiotensin, regional flow increased significantly only adjacent to the contusion, demonstrating focal defective autoregulation. Following administration of mannitol, blood flow increased throughout the hemisphere, more so adjacent to the mass lesion.

A number of observations, some of them at variance with each other, have been made on the responsiveness of the cerebral vessels to changes in arterial carbon dioxide levels in unconscious patients with head injury. According to some reports, cerebrovascular responsivity to hypocapnia and hypercapnia is as unpredictable as the status of autoregulation. Cold and associates found that hypocapnia tended to increase the homogeneity of regional flow patterns, mainly through a reduction in the number of focal hyperemic regions.[61] Fieschi and his colleagues found that carbon dioxide activity was abolished in nearly half their patients at the time of the initial cerebral blood flow study, then the responsivity gradually recovered with improvement in the patients' neurological status.[98] In all of seven patients who were in particularly deep coma following head injury, Gennarelli and co-workers found intact carbon dioxide reactivity. Cerebral blood flow failed to respond to changes in carbon dioxide only when the patients had acquired the clinical criteria of brain death.[118]

A final matter of interest in studies of the cerebral circulation in head injury is the prognostic value of cerebral blood flow and cerebral metabolism. There is general agreement that patients with markedly reduced cerebral blood flow do poorly, but the level below which death is a virtual certainty has not been established clearly. In Overgaard's series, all patients with a blood flow value of one third of normal or less either died or remained in a vegetative state.[297] A normal or hyperemic flow does not, however, necessarily indicate a favorable outcome. Obrist and co-workers found an excellent correlation between cerebral blood flow and the patient's neurological status when patients with hyperemia were excluded. The patients with hyperemia were adolescents and young adults and patients who had either had a seizure immediately prior to the study or were admitted in peripheral shock. In patients without hyperemia, cerebral blood flow increased toward normal in every patient who recovered and decreased in every patient who died. In patients with brain death, cerebral blood flow had ceased or virtually so, even when intracranial pressure was normal and the perfusion pressure across the brain was adequate.[295] This is an intriguing observation that has been made before.[299] Cessation of the cerebral circulation is easily explained when the intracranial pressure equals the blood pressure, thereby abolishing the cerebral perfusion pressure. But why does the cerebral circulation cease when the brain stops functioning but a normal perfusion pressure still exists across the cerebrovascular bed? Perhaps some metabolic activity is necessary to keep open the cerebrovascular bed; whatever the mechanism responsible for metabolic autoregulation, when the substance that links metabolism to flow is abolished, the vascular bed "snaps shut," arresting the circulation. This is not a very satisfactory answer because the cerebral resistance vessels are presumed to be dead also at this time, and therefore they should passively dilate to the pressure head that should still be present within the intracranial arteries. In other words, in a dead brain, the vessels should be paralyzed to changes in either blood pressure or metabolism and therefore should passively dilate, not constrict to the extent that cerebral blood flow is abolished as brain function ceases. Further insight into some of the remaining mysteries of cerebral blood flow and metabolism may lie within the explanation of this most intriguing phenomenon.

Brain Tumors

In contrast to the experience with head injury, reports on continuous recording of intracranial pressure in patients with intracranial tumors have been few. In Lundberg's original monograph, most of the 140 patients on whom those data were based were brain tumor patients awaiting operation. It was in these patients that pressure waves, particularly the dangerous plateau waves, were first demonstrated. Lundberg was able to show conclusively that intermittent headache, alterations in level of consciousness, and focal neurological signs that had been recognized in brain tumor patients for so long were due to fluctuations in intracranial pressure. Marked rhythmic fluctuations in pressure to levels as high as 80 mm of mercury often were not manifested clinically, however, either in the form of changes in the patient's neurological status or as alterations in vital signs. One of the most important observations made was the marked increase in intracranial pressure that occurred during sleep. The most dangerous condition was the plateau wave that did not terminate spontaneously or in response to involuntary hyperventilation, but continued to increase, resulting in coma, dilated fixed pupils, and respiratory arrest. Prompt withdrawal of fluid from the ventricular cannula, induced hyperventilation, or rapid intravenous administration of a hypertonic solution usually reduced intracranial pressure promptly, and if intracranial pressure had not been elevated to extremely high levels for too long, the patient recovered.[236]

In the first study of plateau waves in patients in whom the systemic arterial pressure was also recorded continuously, the prolonged or terminal plateau wave always produced a marked rise in systemic arterial pressure.[208] In fact, the authors believed that they were witnessing the same pressure phenomena that had been observed earlier in animal experiments in which an extracerebral balloon was slowly inflated.[212] It appeared that a plateau wave would terminate spontaneously unless an arterial pressor response was initiated. The rise in arterial pressure caused a slight further increase in intracranial blood volume, which raised the intracranial pressure, inducing a further increase in blood pressure. As the cycle was repeated, the two pressures rose together. Since the intracranial pressure rose more than the arterial pressure, however, cerebral perfusion pressure decreased progressively as the plateau wave continued to develop. In patients in whom it could not be controlled, the intracranial pressure ultimately reached the level of the mean arterial pressure, either in the form of a succession of higher and higher plateau waves or as a steady rise in intracranial tension. When mean intracranial pressure equalled the mean arterial pressure, contrast medium injected into the internal carotid artery failed to enter the intracranial space, demonstrating arrest of the cerebral circulation.[209] Then when the arterial pressure was varied by increasing or decreasing the rate of infusion of a vasopressor agent, intracranial pressure followed the arterial pressure passively. When fluid was removed quickly from the ventricular cannula, intracranial pressure fell to normal levels but rebounded within a few seconds to the level of the arterial pressure. The authors postulated that this represented the state of cerebral vasomotor paralysis described in their animal experiments. As fluid was removed from the ventricular system, paralyzed vessels dilated passively, increasing cerebral blood volume. The brain expanded quickly to fill in the space previously occupied by the ventricular fluid, and once again intracranial pressure equalled the systemic arterial pressure. Cerebral perfusion pressure had now been permanently abolished; it could not be restored either by increasing the arterial pressure or by decreasing intracranial pressure through a reduction in the volume of any of the intracranial compartments.[212]

Becker and co-workers recorded intracranial pressure preoperatively and postoperatively in 50 patients with supratentorial or infratentorial neoplasms. The measurements were most useful during the postoperative period. Characteristically (38 patients), intracranial pressure was normal or unrecordable in the intensive care unit immediately following the operation. It then increased to 10 to 15 mm of mercury toward the end of the first day and slowly declined thereafter. In the few patients with large infiltrating tumors in whom the internal decompression was limited, intracranial pressure was elevated as soon as it was recorded postoperatively, but declined with routine therapy. In only 4 of the 50 patients was intracranial hypertension a significant postoperative problem because of brain swelling, ventricular dilatation, or loculation of fluid in a tumor bed.[16]

Considering the wide use of intracranial pressure monitoring today and the fact that it is used routinely in the management of unconscious head injury patients in many neurosurgical units, the paucity of data in brain tumor patients suggests that most neurosurgeons have not found it to be a useful tool in the management of these problems. There is other evidence to support this assumption. Most benign tumors can be removed completely, and the postoperative brain swelling that plagued the neurosurgeon only a few years ago has now been largely eliminated by modern neuroanesthesia, steroids, a reduction in pulmonary complications, and perhaps most importantly, the application of microsurgical concepts, if not always micro-operative technique itself, in the removal of intracranial tumors. Most of these patients awaken immediately after operation and follow a benign postoperative course. If intracranial pressure does rise, the increase is insufficient to compromise brain function. There are a few circumstances, however, in which continuous recording of intracranial pressure may be useful in management of the brain tumor patient.

The first circumstance is one in which the patient has a glioma in or adjacent to vital regions of the brain and in a position where a lobectomy cannot be performed. The internal decompression is limited in volume, and the brain swells to fill in the cavity so that some protrusion through the craniotomy is present at the completion of the operation. Often the neurosurgeon elects to remove the craniotomy flap. This produces an external decompression, but vital regions may be damaged by herniation of brain through the craniotomy defect during the postoperative period. Continuous measurement of intracranial pressure is helpful when the craniotomy flap has been replaced, but probably is of limited value when the flap has been removed. In the latter situation, a large amount of herniation and brain destruction can occur with no more than a moderate rise in intracranial pressure because of plastic creep of brain through the opening. When the skull is closed, the same circumstances are present that existed preoperatively, and if the brain continues to swell following operation, vigorous therapy for the intracranial hypertension often is required in order to save the patient's life. This indication for recording intracranial pressure is encountered less frequently now than in the past because patients with deep, malignant gliomas are not subjected to operation as often as before, and many neurosurgeons make a special point of doing anterior frontal or temporal lobectomy whenever possible.

The second situation in which measurements of intracranial pressure can prove to be useful is in patients with inoperable tumors who are candidates for radiotherapy or chemotherapy. Ordinarily, the patient's neurological signs can be controlled with steroids, but if the tumor is quite large, or there are multiple metastases, other methods may be required to control intracranial pressure. If hypertonic mannitol, oral glycerol, or another dehydrating agent is to be used for a period of several days or longer, in the hope that the effect of therapy on the tumor will be rapid, continuous recording of intracranial pressure can be helpful in establishing the dose and frequency of administration of the agent. The technique is most useful when the tumor is producing obstructive hydrocephalus and the principal means of controlling intracranial pressure is intermittent drainage of ventricular fluid.

A common complication of a posterior fossa operation is obstructive hydrocephalus, either persistence of preoperative hydrocephalus or hydrocephalus as a complication of the procedure. Of all of the indications for measuring intracranial pressure in brain tumor patients, probably this is the most compelling one. Postoperative dilatation of the ventricular system can occur quickly and lead to rapid clinical deterioration of the patient. Plateau waves are more common in obstructive hydrocephalus than in any other single intracranial condition. Postoperative monitoring of ventricular fluid pressure will detect early evidence of obstruction, and fluid can be vented into a drainage system at any desired level of pressure. Periodically, the drainage system can be clamped off to test the cerebrospinal fluid circulation. In the past, the author postulated that normal circulation of cerebrospinal fluid could be stimulated by permitting intracranial pressure to rise to rather high levels for a short period of time as long as the patient's neurological status did not change. In fact, there has not been clear evidence that this has promoted "flushing" of the cerebrospinal fluid pathways. Also, the argument can be advanced that these patients should have permanent shunts installed as soon as it is clearly evident that the cerebrospinal fluid pathways are obstructed. The argument is that a shunt probably will be required ultimately, and if it is installed after even several days of continuous recording of intraventricular pressure, the risk of infection will be greater than if it is installed immediately. Empirical data to resolve the issue are not available. In the experience of the author, resolution of the hydrocephalus is common enough to warrant a few days of intraventricular recording and drainage.

Subarachnoid Hemorrhage

At the moment of hemorrhage from an intracranial aneurysm, intracranial pressure rises to very high levels in both experimental animals and man.[149,150,289] Studies in experimental animals also demonstrate the immediate onset of severe vasospasm.[385] The patient usually loses consciousness for a variable period of time. The mortality rate from aneurysm rupture is very high, and those patients who die usually do not recover consciousness between the ictus and their death. Irreversible brain damage and death have been attributed to the volume of hemorrhage within the intracranial space and within the brain, cerebral ischemia from prolonged vasospasm, cerebral ischemia from brain edema, and an undefined noxious effect of blood elements on brain cells. There is not nearly enough information from clinical observations to assess the relative contribution of these factors to the morbidity and mortality rates of subarachnoid hemorrhage, but continuous recording of intracranial pressure in patients following hemorrhage has helped to clarify the role of intracranial hypertension in the process.

Nornes and Magnaes were the first investigators to record intracranial pressure continuously in patients following aneurysm rupture; in several patients rerupture occurred during the course of the recording. They described two types of recurrent hemorrhage. In the first type, intracranial pressure increased suddenly to values in excess of 1000 mm of water, then immediately began to decline (Fig. 24–14 A). The patients usually lost consciousness and exhibited other neurological signs at the time of rupture. Intracranial pressure then declined toward normal values, in which event the patient recovered quickly; or, as illustrated in Figure 24–14 A, a secondary

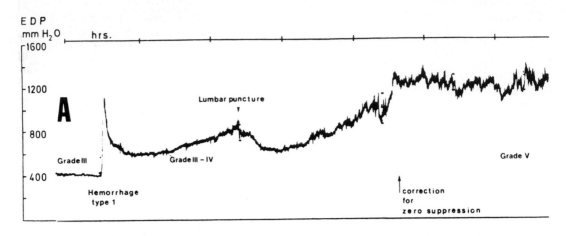

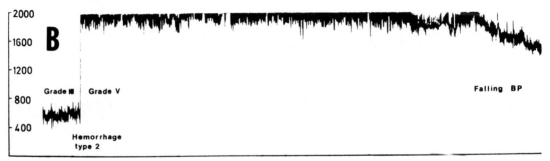

Figure 24–14 *A*. Subarachnoid hemorrhage type 1. Initial pressure peak and secondary increase in intracranial pressure due to edema. *B*. Subarachnoid hemorrhage type 2. Instant increase in pressure followed by a high pressure plateau. Terminal drop is due to falling blood pressure. Tracing partly off scale. EDP, extradural pressure. (From Nornes, H., and Magnaes, B.: Intracranial pressure in patients with ruptured saccular aneurysm. J. Neurosurg., *36:*537–547, 1972. Reprinted by permission.)

increase in pressure occurred and led to the death of the patient. At postmortem examination, there was severe brain swelling but only a small amount of blood within the intracranial space.[290]

A second type of subarachnoid hemorrhage was invariably fatal (Fig. 24–14 *B*). Pressure increased to the range of 2000 mm of water, which was to the level of or in excess of the diastolic arterial pressure, and remained there. The patient was immediately rendered deeply comatose, respirations ceased, and death occurred within minutes or hours. In contrast to the first type of hemorrhage, there were large volumes of blood within the intracranial space, and the intracranial hypertension was due mainly to the mass effect of the blood.[290]

Nornes and Magnaes described a third type of spontaneous change in intracranial pressure in patients following hemorrhage that they termed warning episodes. The increases in pressure occurred suddenly,

were quite transient, and produced little in the way of clinical signs or symptoms. In patients who underwent operation shortly after a warning episode, there was no evidence that the aneurysm had reruptured. Nevertheless, a full-fledged rupture was common in patients who had repeated warning episodes, and the episodes were never seen in intracranial pressure recordings of patients following aneurysm clipping.[290] The authors postulated that they are due to very slight amounts of bleeding that are not detectable at the time of operation or to vasomotor instability. Why the latter phenomenon would predispose the aneurysm to rerupture is difficult to explain.

Assuming that the principal force that leads to rupture or rerupture of an aneurysm is the transmural pressure across the weakest point in the wall of the aneurysm, increased intracranial pressure should protect against rupture. In fact, one might postulate that the optimal situation is one in which intracranial pressure is just below the threshold for compromise of brain function. Nornes described experiences that lend weight to this hypothesis. Three of his patients were subjected to "decompressive management." In one patient, lumbar cerebrospinal fluid was removed as soon as possible following the hemorrhage. Intracranial pressure fell immediately, only to increase to an even higher level moments later, strongly suggesting another hemorrhage from the aneurysm. A second patient was given a bolus of hypertonic mannitol, and intracranial pressure fell to below the pre-rebleed level, then increased in a succession of pressure peaks. At postmortem examination, extensive intracranial hemorrhage was found. A third case showed similar multiple pressure peaks following ventricular drainage immediately after rupture.[289]

Nornes summarized information from the literature on healing of the rent in the aneurysm. The wall contains collagen fibrils, which probably initiate platelet aggregation. The platelets accumulate to form a plug, and at the site of injury in other vessels, the plug can build up in the course of one or two minutes. For a time, however, some leakage may occur through the channels of the plug until all of the platelets have become tightly adherent. Fibrin is then deposited in the platelet mass, which now becomes a hemostatic clot. Over the next two weeks, normal fibrinolytic activity can lead to dissolution of the clot and rerupture. Assuming that this sequence of events in fact does occur at the site of aneurysm rupture, it is clear that a very high intracranial pressure, virtually eliminating transmural pressure, is beneficial for a few minutes following rupture of the aneurysm. Of course, it is equally clear that a critical reduction in cerebral perfusion pressure will produce irreversible ischemic brain damage in a very short period of time.

Cerebral blood flow is reduced in patients following subarachnoid hemorrhage.[130,289,305] This is not surprising. Cerebral metabolism is also reduced, and at least in adults, both metabolism and flow decrease with almost any form of diffuse cerebral insult.[130] Vasospasm is also present in many of these patients and could contribute to the decrease in blood flow.

Grubb and associates observed an increase in cerebral blood volume in patients who had a decrease in both cerebral blood flow and metabolism, and the increase in blood volume was greatest in those patients who also had vasospasm demonstrated by angiography.[130] They postulated that the increase in blood volume was probably due to an autoregulatory dilatation of the microcirculation in response to a decrease in perfusion pressure caused by the vasospasm.

In comparison with the data on head injury, there is little information on the relationship of intracranial pressure to outcome in patients following subarachnoid hemorrhage. The one study in which the patients' neurological status, according to the Hunt and Hess criteria, was compared with intracranial pressure showed a good correlation. The mean intracranial pressure levels ranged from 15 to 40 mm of mercury in grade III patients, from 30 to 75 mm of mercury in grade IV patients, and 75 mm of mercury or more in all grade V patients. All of the latter patients died of uncontrollable intracranial hypertension within a few days of the hemorrhage.[149]

On the basis of these observations, there appear to be several circumstances in which continuous recording of intracranial pressure is valuable in the management of patients with subarachnoid hemorrhage. The best guides to selecting patients for pressure recording are the neurological status and the CT scan, which is invaluable in establishing the location and extent of intracranial hemorrhage. The first circumstance in which recording of intracranial pressure should be considered is an intracerebral hematoma adjacent to the aneurysm. If the hematoma is large and the patient's condition is critical, there is no substitute for immediate evacuation of the hematoma with or without definitive treatment of the aneurysm. There are many patients, however, in whom the hematoma is sizeable but stable, the patient's neurological status is also stable, and one wishes to avoid the potential complications of an emergency operation on the brain freshly insulted by a subarachnoid hemorrhage. The author has found intracranial pressure to be elevated in many of these patients, and intracranial pressure waves are common. If the hematoma is not expanding, pressure can be controlled with the methods available, and the operation can be performed electively.

The second situation in which intracranial pressure, or more precisely, intraventricular pressure recordings, can be useful is hemorrhage of an aneurysm or arteriovenous malformation into the ventricle. Since rupture of an aneurysm into the ventricular system carries such a high mortality rate, even with the most vigorous therapy, the procedure appears to be most useful with rupture of a malformation. With the patient in the supine position, computed tomography demonstrates layering of blood and cerebrospinal fluid within the ventricles, and even when the hemorrhage has been extensive, usually there is room to insert a cannula into a pocket of cerebrospinal fluid in the anteriormost portion of the lateral ventricle. By the time the cannula has been inserted, blood within the ventricle is clotting, and it may be difficult to remove it. Freshly formed cerebrospinal fluid, however, can be removed, and within a short time, the clot begins to lyse. Then it can be removed slowly with suction and irrigation with very small quantities of saline. Irrigation is dangerous if there is little compliance within the intracranial space, and there is still not enough experience to judge the value of attempting to remove the clot compared with controlling intracranial pressure by other means and ignoring the clot. Bruce and co-workers have described their experience with this form of management in children with ruptured arteriovenous malformation.[37]

A third reason for recording intracranial pressure in patients with ruptured aneurysms is the oldest reason, but perhaps the least acceptable now. Klafta and Hamby reported improved results when operations on aneurysms were delayed until lumbar cerebrospinal fluid pressure had fallen to about 200 mm of water, even in those patients whose neurological status had been satisfactory for the procedure before that level of intracranial pressure was reached.[199] The observations of Nornes support this recommendation.[289] It is difficult to see how this could be an important factor in the results of aneurysm operations. The decline in pressure probably is the result of removal of blood from the intracranial space, improved cerebrospinal fluid circulation, decreased brain edema, or perhaps a combination of all three factors. Granted that the neurosurgeon wishes to operate under optimal circumstances, the results with aneurysm procedures in grade I patients in recent times has been so good, one questions whether waiting for intracranial pressure to decline a bit further would improve them. And there is always the risk of rerupture from waiting.

Brain Ischemia and Anoxia

Neurologists and neurosurgeons are often called upon to manage patients who have suffered a severe neurological deficit caused by hypoxia. The causes of the brain insult in these patients are numerous and include complications of anesthesia and cardiopulmonary operations, peripheral shock, respiratory obstruction, and various toxic and metabolic conditions. Emergency treatment is provided for the primary condition, when it is possible to do so, and the question then asked is how to treat the brain damage. It is common practice to manage the patient with steroids, and sometimes various other forms of therapy, which have as their major goal a reduction in brain volume and intracranial pressure. Within the present context, the two issues posed by hypoxic brain damage are the incidence of increased intracranial pressure and, if it is present, whether intracranial hypertension is contributing to the poor neurological state of the patient.

With these questions in mind, the author and his colleagues recorded intracranial pressure continuously in nine patients who were comatose following acute brain insults that ranged from cardiac arrest to a case of accidental anoxia in a patient with tetanus. Intracranial pressure was increased in all of the patients. Maximum intracranial tension ranged from 40 to 60 mm of mercury in patients who were comatose following open heart procedures and was as high as 60 mm of mercury in the patient with tetanus. Six of the nine patients demonstrated spontaneous pressure waves, in one patient to a value in excess of 90 mm of mercury. All the patients were treated vigorously to control intracranial pressure, and in none of them was the pressure uncontrollable. Nevertheless, eight of the nine patients died from extracranial complications of coma.[214]

The experience is not encouraging, nor should a different outcome be expected. If the patient remains comatose following an episode of cerebral hypoxia, vital regions of the brain are almost surely irreversibly damaged. The likelihood that moderate levels of sustained intracranial hypertension will materially affect the outcome of these patients would appear to be slight. Therefore, within the limits of our current understanding of the problem, continuous recording of intracranial pressure probably has little place in the management of these patients.

Normal-Pressure Hydrocephalus

The condition termed normal-pressure hydrocephalus has created as much controversy as any subject in neurosurgery. It came into being because of the suggestion by Hakim and Adams that many patients with dementia and enlarged ventricles in whom cerebral atrophy had been diagnosed might actually have hydrocephalus.[139] The challenge, then, was to establish a differential diagnosis between the two conditions on the assumption that the patients with normal-pressure hydrocephalus would respond to a shunt procedure. A thorough review of the problem is beyond the scope of this presentation. It is sufficient to say that a multitude of tests have been purported to be diagnostic, but it has been difficult to confirm observations among series of patients. The only means of establishing the accuracy of a test distinguishing between atrophy and hydrocephalus is to compare the results of that test with the clinical results of shunting in a series of patients. There is evidence that most of the criteria for distinguishing between normal-pressure hydrocephalus and Alzheimer's disease, which were in vogue in the early 1970's, do not correlate well with the results of shunting.[394]

Chawla and associates measured intracranial pressure continuously in patients with dementia and found that some of them had flat intracranial pressure recordings, whereas others showed various types of pressure waves. They concluded that the first group of patients probably had atrophy and the second group might have normal-pressure hydrocephalus. Among the first group, none improved with shunting, whereas all the patients who had had pressure waves preoperatively did show improvement.[49] Symon and co-workers made similar observations, but the results from shunting could be described as more suggestive than convincing.[400] Measurements of cerebral blood flow, either alone or in combination with continuous recording of intracranial pressure, have been suggested as another means of distinguishing between the two conditions. Grubb and co-workers divided 30 patients with dementia into one group with presumed normal-pressure hydrocephalus and another group with presumed cerebral atrophy on the basis of a variety of criteria. Cerebral blood flow, metabolism of oxygen, and intracranial pressure were then measured in all the patients. There was no difference between the two groups in any of the variables measured.[132]

In the series reported by Stein and Langfitt, patients with a likely cause for their ventricular enlargement and a relatively rapid development of symptoms responded well to shunting, whereas those with a more chronic history and no apparent cause responded poorly. The first group of patients were categorized as having "secondary hydrocephalus," and this appeared to be a more useful term than "normal-pressure hydrocephalus" in selecting patients to receive a shunt.[394] These patients are also more likely to have intermittent elevations of intracranial pressure. Continuous recording of pressure may prove to be most useful in patients who are suspected of having secondary hydrocephalus, but the other criteria used to distinguish between hydrocephalus and atrophy are equivocal.

Reye's Syndrome

Reye's syndrome is an acute encephalopathy associated with fatty changes in the viscera.[336] The diagnosis is strongly suggested by a cluster of clinical and biochemical findings, but a definitive diagnosis probably can be made only by liver biopsy.[115] The children with Reye's syndrome are comatose, and the mortality rate has been very high. The cause of death has been at issue. Since the changes in the viscera appear to be reversible in most cases, a number of clinicians have postulated that brain swelling and intracranial hypertension are the most common cause of death.

Kindt and colleagues observed increased intracranial pressure in every child with Reye's syndrome in whom intracranial pressure was measured continuously. The pressure was usually higher than 40 mm of mercury and was punctuated by pressure waves up to 90 mm of mercury. The intracranial hypertension was treated vigorously with all available methods, and eight of the children survived and were neurologically normal. The authors concluded that many of the children would have died without vigorous management of the brain swelling.[48,196] Similar observations were made by Berman and colleagues. The principal method of therapy in their 10 patients was exchange transfusion, however, and they found that intracranial pressure was reduced and remained much more controllable following the transfusions.[22] There is conflicting evidence that exchange transfusions may not be beneficial in control of intracranial pressure.[377] When all other methods fail, decompressive craniectomy may be beneficial.[7]

In contrast to anoxic encephalopathy, Reye's syndrome is an excellent example of the benefits to be derived from continuous monitoring of intracranial pressure to guide therapy.

Pseudotumor Cerebri

Pseudotumor cerebri, or benign intracranial hypertension, is diffuse brain swelling that is usually of undetermined etiology. It can be secondary to obstruction of a lateral or sigmoid sinus from chronic temporal bone infections, but cases of this origin are rare today. More commonly, it is seen in young women, and many of the patients are overweight. Thus, another suggested cause has been hormonal imbalance, particularly among the sex hormones.

The patients present with headache and papilledema and sometimes a sixth nerve palsy presumably due to downward displacement of the brain stem, which is the only localizing or lateralizing sign permissible within a diagnosis of pseudotumor. The diagnosis has always been one of exclusion. In the past, cerebral angiography and pneumoencephalography were required to rule

out another cause of the patient's signs and symptoms, but the diagnosis can now be made with a high degree of certainty with computed tomography. The ventricles are normal or reduced in size, and the basal cisterns, particularly the perimesencephalic cisterns, are reduced in volume or are obliterated. Intracranial pressure is always elevated, sometimes markedly so. In a series of 20 patients studied by Johnston and Paterson, the mean intracranial pressure was always in excess of 15 mm of mercury, and more importantly, all the patients exhibited pressure waves. In some patients, the pressure waves peaked as high as 80 mm of mercury.[187]

In the absence of a space-occupying lesion the intracranial hypertension of pseudotumor cerebri must be due to expansion of one or more of the three fluid compartments of the intracranial space: brain water, cerebral blood volume, or cerebrospinal fluid. Since the cerebrospinal fluid spaces in fact are reduced in volume, the increased pressure must be due to expansion of the brain in turn caused by either edema or cerebrovascular congestion. Traditionally, the brain swelling has been attributed to edema, and edema was said to be present in brain biopsies from patients in whom pseudotumor had been diagnosed.[356] Early suggestions that the swelling is due to an increase in cerebral blood volume received support from observations by Foley, who demonstrated an increase in cerebral blood flow in three patients.[106] Mathew and coworkers found a decrease in cerebral blood flow in two patients, but in contrast, cerebral blood volume was increased, and in fact was nearly double the control value.[256] Similar observations have been made by Raichle and colleagues. Blood volume was increased only about one third above normal in their patients, however, and the authors doubted that the volume effect could produce a sufficient increase in brain bulk to account for the levels of intracranial hypertension. They believed that edema must also be present and, on the basis of a number of experimental observations, postulated that the decrease in blood flow was a result of the edema.[321] Although their logic is persuasive, it is still important to note that an increase in cerebral blood volume has now been proved quite conclusively in pseudotumor patients, whereas an increase in the fluid content of the brain has not been clearly demonstrated. That a combination of problems in vascular control and fluid balance within the brain is caused by hormonal abnormalities remains an intriguing hypothesis to explain the etiology of pseudotumor in many patients.

The terms "pseudotumor cerebri" and "benign intracranial hypertension" often are used synonymously. There is the occasional case, however, in which the clinical course is not benign. Langfitt and Kassell observed a patient who clearly would have died without vigorous therapy for intracranial pressure that approached the level of the blood pressure and who, in fact, was left a neurological cripple despite vigorous therapy.[208]

TREATMENT

General Principles

Increased intracranial pressure disturbs brain function by a reduction in cerebral blood flow or by herniation of brain beneath the falx cerebri, through the tentorial incisura, through the foramen magnum, or through a traumatic or operative defect in the skull. The reduction in blood flow that occurs in the brain stem with transtentorial or foramen magnum herniation is most critical for survival of the patient. The goals of treatment, therefore, are to reduce intracranial pressure in order to increase cerebral blood flow above that critical level required for oxygenation of the brain and to relieve herniation.

Several general principles in the selection of the various methods available to treat intracranial hypertension can be stated. The first principle addresses the various causes of increased intracranial pressure. They are four in number. The first cause is a mass lesion such as a tumor or hematoma. The most effective means of lowering intracranial pressure in the face of a mass lesion is to remove all of the mass, or as much of it as can be removed safely. When the mass is in a vital region and direct attack carries a great risk for the patient, other methods of reducing intracranial pressure must be used. The second cause of intracranial hypertension is hydrocephalus. Treatment consists of removal of cerebrospinal fluid

from the intracranial space either by a permanent shunt or by intermittent drainage through a ventriculostomy. The third cause is edema, which is defined as an increase in the volume of fluid within brain tissue. Treatment consists of a reduction in brain fluid content. The fourth compartment within the intracranial space that can enlarge to raise pressure is the cerebrovascular bed. Cerebrovascular dilatation is now recognized to be the cause of intracranial hypertension in a number of conditions in which the cause was formerly believed to be edema.

In describing the four compartments within the intracranial space that can enlarge to produce intracranial hypertension, three of them normal compartments, it is important to note that increased intracranial pressure, irrespective of its cause, can be lowered by reducing the volume of any one of those compartments even when the volume of that compartment is normal. Although the volume of cerebrospinal fluid normally contained within the ventricles is quite small, removal of even a few milliliters of ventricular cerebrospinal fluid at the peak of a pressure wave can be lifesaving. Hypertonic solutions significantly reduce the fluid content of normal brain, and normal cerebral blood volume is decreased by hyperventilation. Thus, intracranial pressure can be reduced by attacking that compartment within the intracranial space that is responsible for the intracranial hypertension or by reducing the volume of a normal compartment. Since, with a defective blood-brain barrier, edematous tissue cannot be dehydrated effectively with hypertonic solutions and sometimes a dilated cerebrovascular bed will not respond to hyperventilation, it is necessary then to direct attention to those intracranial compartments that are responsive to therapy.

The second general principle in the treatment of increased intracranial pressure has to do with the speed of action of various agents in reducing intracranial tension. Of course, the treatment of increased pressure is most important when it is very high and life-threatening. The challenge then is to select that method that will reduce intracranial pressure as quickly as possible, irrespective of the etiology of the increased pressure. The quickest way is always removal of ventricular cerebrospinal fluid.

For this reason, many neurosurgeons still prefer an intraventricular cannula to other methods of measuring intracranial pressure in any patient who has enlarged ventricles and particularly in patients with obstructive hydrocephalus. When the cerebral vessels are normally responsive to changes in arterial carbon dioxide tension, hyperventilation reduces intracranial pressure almost as quickly and by as much as withdrawal of cerebrospinal fluid. An intravenous bolus of hypertonic mannitol usually will reduce intracranial pressure below critical levels within a few minutes. Barbiturates also appear to act quickly, but hypothermia takes longer to reduce intracranial tension. There are, however, fewer data on correlations of changes in intracranial pressure with hypothermia, barbiturates, and steroids than with the other methods of treatment.

The third principle relates to the convenience and the risk of administration of the various methods of treatment. Steroids are easiest to administer in contrast to a combination of hypothermia and barbiturates, which requires continuous attention by a team of professionals. Hyperventilation reduces intracranial pressure primarily by constricting cerebral vessels and reducing cerebral blood volume. But this therapeutic effect is achieved by reduction of cerebral blood flow, which can result in cerebral ischemia at severe levels of hypocapnia. The effectiveness of hypertonic solutions is a function of the increase in serum osmolarity, but excessive increases in serum osmolarity cause complications such as renal damage. In each instance, the risk of treatment must be weighed against the potential benefits in the individual patient. The ideal method is one that is easily administered, is always effective, and carries minimal risk. The information presented in the sections that follow demonstrates that the ideal method neither exists nor appears to be in the offing in the near future.

The fourth principle in the management of intracranial hypertension is a rather obvious one but one that still requires emphasis. Increased intracranial pressure cannot be treated properly without continuous recording of intracranial pressure. In the absence of a continuous assessment of intracranial tension, the only criterion available for establishing the effect of an agent is the clinical status of the patient.

Assume, for illustrative purposes, that in treating a comatose patient with an intravenous bolus of hypertonic mannitol, the patient's neurological status does not change. What are the potential explanations for the patient's failure to improve? Perhaps the patient did not have increased intracranial pressure in the first place. Second, intracranial pressure was increased, but the mannitol failed to reduce it. Third, intracranial pressure was increased prior to the therapy and was reduced to normal by it, but the pressure returned to hypertensive levels before the patient had a chance to improve neurologically. Finally, intracranial pressure was increased, and the mannitol therapy was effective in reducing it for a long period of time, but the brain had already been irreversibly damaged by the intracranial hypertension, and therefore, the patient failed to improve despite the reduction in pressure.

There is limited information on the value of the various methods of treatment of increased intracranial pressure because few investigators have chosen to evaluate or have had the luxury of using only one method of treatment at a time. When intracranial pressure approaches threatening levels, the objective is to reduce the pressure by any means available in order to save the patient's life. It is difficult to adhere to a clinical research protocol under these circumstances. In the sections on specific methods of treatment, emphasis is placed on those studies that have been most successful in testing the method in isolation in various clinical disorders. Analysis of the additive effects of two or more agents has not been sufficient to warrant more than passing comment.

Management of the Comatose Patient

In many ways the treatment of intracranial hypertension is indistinguishable from management of the comatose patient. In terms of brain function, the correction of shock and pulmonary insufficiency have as their principal goal the restoration of adequate oxygenation of the brain. Not only does the correction of pulmonary insufficiency improve the amount of oxygen carried in the blood, it also reduces intracranial pressure, thereby increasing the volume of blood flowing through the brain Many of the methods used to reduce intracranial pressure—hyperventilation, hypertonic solutions, hypothermia, barbiturates, steroids—are also used in the short-term management of coma. The prototype condition for discussion of the management of the unconscious patient is severe head injury. Head injury units throughout the world have continued to develop regimens for the treatment of traumatic coma, and probably it is accurate to state that no two units treat the patient in the same way. Because of the importance of head injury and because the management of the unconscious patient is always an appropriate introduction to the treatment of intracranial hypertension, a description of the protocol employed by the Head Injury Clinical Research Center at the University of Pennsylvania in the management of the comatose patient with head injury in the late 1970's follows.

On admission to the emergency ward, the unconscious patient with head injury is quickly evaluated by the personnel in the emergency ward, and a neurosurgical resident is called. The airway and the status of the systemic circulation are evaluated immediately. Peripheral shock is treated appropriately; the specific therapy is beyond the scope of this presentation. In each instance, an attempt is made to draw an arterial sample for blood gas determination before the airway is treated in order to determine whether the patient had systemic hypoxemia on admission. An intravenous line and a Foley catheter are inserted. A blood sample is sent for measurement of alcohol content if that appears to be indicated. Blood studies are performed for other central nervous system depressants only if a suspicion of drug intoxication is raised by peculiarities of the case.

Every patient who clearly has a severe head injury is intubated. This can be a difficult decision to make in borderline cases. For example, if the patient arrives in the emergency ward within a few minutes of the injury and the neurological examination suggests that he may begin to improve spontaneously before long, intubation is deferred. Intubation is performed by an anesthesiologist under optimal conditions. The deleterious increase in intracranial pressure that can be produced by a traumatic intubation may more than offset the benefits of the procedure. The patient is then transferred immediately to the radiology department for a CT scan and, if necessary, is paralyzed and mechanically ventilated in order to obtain the best possible scan. A lateral x-ray of the cervical spine and a chest x-ray are obtained along with anteroposterior and lateral x-rays of the skull.

In the emergency ward, the patient receives a loading dose of 20 mg of dexamethasone, followed by dexamethasone 0.1 to 0.2 mg per kilogram every six hours for the first day. Then the steroid is tapered gradually over the next week, depending on the clinical status of the patient. Most unconscious head injury patients hyperventilate spontaneously to a Pa_{CO_2} of less than 35 mm of mercury. During the initial phase of evaluation of the patient, the aim is to maintain Pa_{CO_2} between 30 and 35 mm of mercury. If, however, the patient is in extremis on admission with evidence of a space-occupying mass, vigorous hyperventilation is performed, and hypertonic mannitol is administered as an intravenous bolus of 1.5 to 2.0 gm per kilogram of a 25 per cent solution. A CT scan is obtained, and if a hematoma is demonstrated, the patient is taken immediately to the operating theater for evacuation of the hematoma. If vigorous therapy to reduce intracranial pressure is introduced immediately, even in the decerebrate patient with a dilated, fixed pupil, there is time for computed tomography in nearly every instance. The value of the scan in clearly identifying the intracranial lesion, compared to blind exploration of the intracranial space through a few burr holes, is incalculable.

Following evacuation of the hematoma, or if the patient does not require an operation, he is transferred to the neurosurgical intensive care unit for continued therapy. A subarachnoid bolt (the Richmond screw) is inserted in the operating room at the completion of the procedure or in the intensive care unit in patients who are not operated on. A catheter is inserted into a radial artery, and the intracranial pressure and systemic arterial pressure are displayed on an oscilloscope and on a strip chart recorder. Subsequent management is based on the responses of the patient's neurological status, intracranial pressure, and systemic arterial pressure to various modes of therapy. In addition, regional cerebral blood flow and the cerebral metabolic rate of oxygen utilization are measured in nearly every patient soon after admission to the intensive care unit. The results of these studies are also used to guide therapy. This is feasible because the noninvasive [133]xenon method is used. Since it is noninvasive, it can be repeated frequently throughout the course of management of the patient.

Increased intracranial pressure is defined as a sustained elevation in pressure above 15 to 20 mm of mercury or intermittent pressure waves, either B-waves or plateau waves. In the past, patients with mild to moderate levels of intracranial hypertension, that is, patients with pressures as high as 40 mm of mercury, often were not treated unless there was evidence of neurological deterioration. That policy has changed with the passage of time because of the belief that even moderate intracranial hypertension superimposed on a damaged brain can produce more damage that is not evident clinically.

The first step in the management of intracranial pressure that meets the criteria for treatment is to quiet the patient. Often sustained elevations of pressure, and especially pressure waves, are produced by straining or by involuntary movements such as decerebrate posturing. If the movements are mild, ordinarily they can be controlled with morphine, 2 to 4 mg every two to four hours. If morphine will not control the movements sufficiently to maintain intracranial pressure within normal limits, the patient is paralyzed and artifically ventilated.

The second method of management of intracranial hypertension in the intensive care unit is through the control of carbon dioxide tension. Pa_{CO_2} is reduced from 30 to 35 to 25 to 30 mm of mercury. It is lowered below 25 mm of mercury only when other methods of therapy have been attempted and have failed. Traditionally the next method of treatment, when intracranial hypertension still cannot be controlled, has been hypertonic mannitol. If the pressure is rising rapidly, the mannitol is given as a loading dose of 1.0 to 2.0 gm per kilogram of a 25 per cent solution as an intravenous bolus. Otherwise, the mannitol is given either in intermittent boluses or as an infusion of 0.05 to 0.15 gm per kilogram per hour. Serum osmolarity is measured at frequent intervals, and the maximum permissible osmolarity is 320 mOsm. Urine output is measured hourly, and 75 per cent of the output is replaced with half-normal saline and potassium supplement. Recently furosemide or ethacrynic acid has been tried as a substitute for hypertonic mannitol. The experience is too limited to compare these agents with mannitol.

It is important to recall that when the various methods for treating intracranial hypertension fail successively, the possibility of an expanding intracranial process must never be far from mind. Delayed intracerebral hemorrhage has been described, even in patients in whom there is no evidence at all of the hemorrhage at the time of the initial CT scan. If the initial scan was performed very quickly following the injury, the beginnings of an extracerebral collection of blood might have been missed. Acute hydrocephalus is uncommon in head injury but can occur when there has been extensive bleeding into the subarachnoid space.

When steroid therapy, muscular paralysis that prevents movement, hyperventilation, and hypertonic solutions fail to control intracranial pressure, barbiturate coma is induced. Pentobarbital is administered at a rate of 0.5 to 3 mg per kilogram per hour in order to achieve serum levels of 2.5 to 3.5 mg per 100 ml. The electroencephalogram is also helpful. The maintenance of a burst-suppression pattern is a substitute for more frequent measurements of serum barbiturate levels. When intracranial pressure still is uncontrollable with all of these methods of therapy, extensive, bilateral craniectomies are considered. If the problem is diffuse brain swelling and therefore the cerebral hemispheres and brain stem have been spared from hemorrhage or infarction, insofar as can be determined on repeat CT scans, the operation is performed. Since the procedure has had so little appeal to the neurosurgeon in the past, unfortunately it is often performed too late; the intracranial hypertension has already produced irreversible brain damage.

Measurements of regional cerebral blood flow and metabolism have been useful in patient management. Whether they will be useful enough to warrant routine application of these methods in the management of patients with head injury remains to be determined.

Anesthesia for Intracranial Procedures

During induction of anesthesia for intracranial operations, intracranial pressure can increase to dangerously high levels. This is particularly true if the patient has a mass lesion causing intracranial hypertension or if a mass lesion has resulted in a reduction in intracranial compliance, even though resting intracranial pressure may not be elevated. Straining results in an increase in cerebral blood volume, which can trigger a plateau wave, and the augmentation of blood volume required to produce the rise in intracranial pressure is quite small when the volume-pressure relationship is on the vertical portion of the curve illustrated in Figure 24–4.

Volatile anesthetic agents such as halothane, methoxyflurane, and trichloroethylene produce increases in cerebral blood flow, cerebral blood volume, and intracranial pressure that are dose dependent.[183,389] Initially, enflurane appeared to have an advantage over halothane, but there is evidence that enflurane can create the same problems.[370] Thus, it appears likely that any volatile agent will produce the same effect. The vasodilatory action of these agents, tending to increase intracranial pressure when compliance is reduced, can be countered by maneuvers to improve compliance at the time of induction, such as hyperventilation, barbiturates, and osmotic agents. The patient can be managed with an intracranial monitor in place, but the complications of using the volatile agents have not been common enough to warrant pressure monitoring prior to operation.

Ketamine can also produce marked rises in intracranial pressure.[372] A relaxant technique employing droperidol and fentanyl does not increase intracranial pressure, and may in fact reduce it, but systemic arterial pressure may decrease significantly with the two agents, resulting in a fall in cerebral perfusion pressure.[102] Another agent that is used frequently in intracranial procedures, mainly to lower blood pressure during aneurysm operations, is sodium nitroprusside. When sodium nitroprusside was given prior to opening the dura at the time of craniotomy, there was a significant increase in intracranial pressure and a decrease in systemic arterial pressure sufficient to produce a marked reduction in perfusion pressure.[67]

Hyperventilation

Changes in arterial carbon dioxide tension significantly affect intracranial pressure. Lundberg and co-workers were the first to demonstrate that hyperventilation consistently reduced intracranial pressure in brain tumor patients with intracranial hypertension.[237] Since then, the observation has been made repeatedly, and hyperventilation has come to be regarded as one of the most effective means of controlling intracranial tension. In addition, hyperventilation has been declared to improve the outcome in patients with severe brain insults, especially closed head injuries. Evidence that hyperventilation is beneficial in head injury patients, however, irrespective of whether or not intracranial pressure is increased, is not convincing to many observers.

Hyperventilation reduces intracranial tension by decreasing cerebral blood flow and cerebral blood volume. The relationship between cerebral blood flow and the carbon dioxide content of arterial blood has been well described in normal man and animals.[331] Cerebral blood flow changes approximately 2 per cent per millimeter of mercury change in Pa_{CO_2}. This is in part, if not entirely, a reflection of intracranial compliance. As the cerebral vessels dilate, cerebrospinal fluid can be displaced from the intracranial space into the spinal canal, thereby attenuating the response of intracranial pressure. As this buffering mechanism is reduced, the rate of the rise in intracranial pressure increases. Similarly, hypocapnia has been demonstrated to increase intracranial compliance proportionally to the reduction of intracranial pressure in patients with intracranial lesions. In baboons in which intracranial pressure was raised by expansion of an extradural balloon, however, hyperventilation decreased intracranial pressure without much change in the volume-pressure response, which was used to evaluate intracranial compliance.[348]

There is conflicting evidence that cerebral blood flow, and therefore blood volume, tend to return toward normal with prolonged hyperventilation to a constant arterial carbon dioxide level. Initially the evidence against normalization of blood flow was very strong.[23,314,367,432] The results of experiments in fully conscious, healthy men strongly suggest, however, that a factor other than the carbon dioxide content of arterial blood is responsible for controlling cerebrovascular resistance.[319]

The reduction in intracranial pressure produced by a decrease in cerebral blood volume is at the expense of a reduction in cerebral blood flow. Therefore, there is the potential of relieving the cerebral ischemia produced by intracranial hypertension only to replace it with cerebral ischemia produced by intense cerebral vasoconstriction. There is, in fact, evidence in both man and experimental animals that when Pa_{CO_2} is reduced below 20 mm of mercury, the amount of oxygen available to the brain is inadequate to maintain normal metabolism. The abnormal metabolism is manifested by alterations in the electroencephalogram and cerebrospinal fluid acidosis.[74] When hyperventilation is superimposed on the cerebral vasodilatation that is often the cause of or accompanies intracranial hypertension, however, Pa_{CO_2} may be reduced to values considerably below 20 mm of mercury without causing a critical reduction in blood flow. Furthermore, the decrease in cerebral blood flow may not be proportional to the constriction of the resistance vessels produced by the hypocapnia. As intracranial pressure rises, the cerebral resistance vessels dilate, increasing cerebral blood volume and tending to increase cerebral blood flow. The increase in blood volume tends to increase brain volume and raise intracranial pressure. At this time, cerebral blood flow becomes a function of both the cerebral resistance vessels, which are controlled by the manipulation of Pa_{CO_2}, and the venous outflow track, which is compressed by the increased intracranial pressure. If the cerebral resistance vessels are dilated by the autoregulatory response to intracranial hypertension, before hyperventilation is initiated, the vasoconstriction produced by the hypocapnia may be more than offset by the relief of venous compression produced by the decrease in intracranial pressure;

therefore, the net change in resistance across the cerebrovascular bed either may not change or may decrease. In this circumstance, hyperventilation may produce an *increase* in cerebral blood flow, even though the resistance vessels constrict normally to the decrease in arterial carbon dioxide tensions.

A second mechanism whereby changes in Pa_{CO_2} may affect brain function, independently of changes in intracranial pressure, is through alterations in regional cerebral blood flow. In regions of cerebral infarction, blood flow is usually reduced and may be completely eliminated in the infarcted area. Surrounding the infarction there is often an area of hyperemia, which has been termed luxury perfusion because the blood flow through the tissue is in excess of the metabolic need. Presumably the hyperemia is due to metabolic acidosis produced by the period of ischemia.[219] The dilated vessels may not respond to changes in the carbon dioxide level, which results in paradoxical changes in blood flow through the affected region. Thus, when Pa_{CO_2} is increased, dilating normal cerebral vessels, blood may be shunted away from the region of luxury perfusion.[31,307] This phenomenon has been termed the intracerebral steal. Conversely, when Pa_{CO_2} is reduced by hyperventilation, blood may be shunted from normal brain, where vasoconstriction takes place, into the affected region where the dilated vessels are paralyzed and cannot constrict in response to the hypocapnia.[307] On the basis of these observations, hyperventilation has been advocated in the treatment of acute stroke in order to improve blood flow to the damaged brain through the reverse steal phenomenon. Other mechanisms whereby hyperventilation might improve function in damaged brain are through the restoration of autoregulation and a reduction in brain tissue acidosis.[125,136,308]

Hyperventilation significantly reduces intracranial pressure in the majority of, but by no means all, patients with various forms of intracranial disease. It reduced intracranial tension in half of a series of deeply comatose patients who had suffered periods of severe cerebral anoxia.[214] Hyperventilation was also assessed in 50 trials in 34 patients who had various intracranial disorders. In two thirds of the trials, intracranial pressure was reduced by 10 to 80 per cent with a mean reduction of just less than 50 per cent. The time from initiation of hyperventilation to maximum reduction in pressure ranged from 2 to 30 minutes with a mean of 7.6 minutes. After cessation of hyperventilation, intracranial pressure returned to control values in less than five minutes in all cases. In 14 trials, the hyperventilation was maintained after it had been demonstrated to reduce intracranial pressure. In 9 of the 14 trials, the pressure returned to control values in 12 to 80 minutes, despite continued hyperventilation at the same rate and volume that reduced intracranial tension in the first place. In the remaining five trials, intracranial pressure was reduced for periods ranging from 2 to 30 hours.[168] These results demonstrate quite clearly that intracranial pressure does tend to return to hypertensive levels despite continued hyperventilation. Whether this phenomenon is due to normalization of cerebral blood flow and cerebral blood volume or some other factor has not been determined.

In this series of patients there was a significant difference in the response to hyperventilation according to the nature of the intracranial lesion. Among the 50 trials in the 34 patients, 22 trials were on individuals with intracranial tumor and brain swelling either due to systemic disease or of unknown origin. In only two of the 22 trials did the intracranial pressure fail to respond to the hyperventilation. In contrast, in 8 of 12 trials in patients with severe head injury or subarachnoid hemorrhage, intracranial pressure did not respond to the hyperventilation. These observations suggest that the brain was more severely damaged in the latter patients, and therefore, cerebrovascular reactivity was less. Similar observations have been made by Paul and co-workers. They categorized three types of patients with head injuries according to the response of intracranial pressure to hyperventilation. In the first type, patients who appeared to have brain stem injuries with preservation of the cerebral hemispheres, intracranial pressure decreased immediately and rapidly with hyperventilation. In the second type of patient, resting intracranial pressure was higher and was characterized by pressure waves. In these patients the response to hyperventilation was slower. The third type was characterized by complete vasomotor paralysis.[306]

Despite the clear evidence that hyperventilation does reduce intracranial pressure in most patients, there is still doubt that prolonged hyperventilation influences the outcome in patients with acute brain insults, particularly head injury and stroke. It is said to reduce morbidity and death among children with a variety of intracranial lesions and in patients with both closed and penetrating injuries of the head.[68,270] The strongest advocates of hyperventilation in the treatment of severe brain injuries have been Gordon and Rossanda and her colleagues.[125,345] Although they have presented evidence for a reduction in morbidity and death, it has been difficult to be sure of the results without a controlled study, which is so difficult to perform in patients with head injury.

A controlled clinical study was performed to determine whether prolonged hyperventilation influenced the outcome in stroke patients. Of 50 patients with severe stroke, 24 were subjected to hyperventilation to a Pa_{CO_2} of 25 mm of mercury, and 26 were hyperventilated, but carbon dioxide was added to the breathing mixture so that Pa_{CO_2} was maintained at the normocapnic level of 40 mm of mercury. These two groups of patients were then compared with a third group of 21 comparable stroke patients who were not treated with a ventilator. There was no difference in the clinical course or the mortality rate among the three groups, nor were there significant differences in the appearance of the brains at autopsy in those patients who failed to survive.[53] In a companion study, the cerebrospinal fluid lactate level was found to be elevated, and average intracranial pressure was on the borderline of normal in these stroke patients. There was, however, no correlation between the mortality rate and the cerebrospinal fluid lactate levels or intracranial pressure.[52]

Hyperbaric Oxygen

The critical reduction in cerebral blood flow produced by intracranial hypertension damages the brain because the supply of oxygen is insufficient to maintain normal metabolism. In contused and edematous brain, the microcirculation may be impaired with the same results, ischemic hypoxia. The methods of alleviating the problem are to increase cerebral blood flow or to increase the oxygen content per unit volume of blood flowing through the tissue. At a very high oxygen content in the inspired air, hemoglobin is nearly fully saturated, and therefore, increasing the partial pressure of oxygen beyond 1 atm cannot significantly increase the amount of oxygen carried by hemoglobin. Normally, some oxygen is dissolved in the plasma, but this amount is very small compared to the amount of oxygen carried by hemoglobin. When the partial pressure of oxygen is increased beyond 1 atm, the volume of dissolved oxygen rises. This is the rationale for the treatment of cerebral ischemia with hyperbaric oxygen. If the ischemia cannot be relieved or if blood flow is increased but is still inadequate, increasing the volume of dissolved oxygen in the blood might make the difference.

Hypoxia dilates and hyperoxia constricts cerebral vessels. Thus, the effects on the diameter of the cerebrovascular bed produced by changing the arterial oxygen tension are just the opposite of the changes produced by alterations in arterial carbon dioxide tension. Hyperoxia should lower intracranial pressure when it is increased by the same mechanism as hypocapnia, namely a reduction in cerebral blood volume. Miller and colleagues investigated the effect of hyperbaric oxygen on increased intracranial pressure produced by expansion of an extradural balloon and by a cold lesion of the cerebral cortex. In the balloon experiments, they found that intracranial pressure decreased by about one third of the control value with the application of hyperbaric oxygen, and the drop in intracranial tension occurred in the presence of a normal arterial carbon dioxide level. When vasomotor paralysis, manifested by failure of intracranial pressure to increase with hypercapnia, had been produced by continued expansion of the balloon, the response to hyperbaric oxygen was also lost. In both these experiments and in those with cold lesions, intracranial pressure tended to rebound above the pretreatment levels on discontinuation of hyperbaric oxygen therapy. Also, the rebound seemed to be greater the longer the period of treatment.[273,275]

The effect of hyperbaric oxygen on cerebral blood flow under normal conditions is not so clear. In studies performed by Lambertsen and associates, global cerebral blood flow was reduced by 25 per cent at 3.5 atm of hyperbaric oxygen in normal, awake man. The subjects hyperventilated somewhat, however, decreasing the carbon dioxide tension, and the investigators could not be sure how much of the decrease in blood flow was due to the hyperbaric oxygen and how much to the hypocapnia.[205] Subsequently, Jacobson and co-workers observed a mean reduction in cortical blood flow of 21 per cent in the presence of normocapnia.[166] Thus, the reduction in cerebral blood flow produced by hyperbaric oxygen almost surely is due to cerebral vasoconstriction. In the animal studies of Miller and co-workers, hyperbaric oxygen appeared to reduce cerebral blood flow, but the reduction was only about one third that produced by hyperventilation.[273] Artru and associates studied cerebral blood flow and the cerebral metabolic rates of oxygen, glucose, and lactate, as well as cerebrospinal fluid lactate, in a series of head injury patients. Both blood flow and the metabolic rate of oxygen utilization fell with hyperbaric oxygen therapy, and cerebrospinal fluid lactate concentration rose, suggesting increased, not decreased, cerebral ischemia.[4]

The effects of hyperbaric oxygen therapy on the morbidity and mortality rates of severe brain insults are uncertain. Mullan and colleagues studied the effects of isovolemic hemodilution and hyperbaric oxygen on the death rate produced by expanding an extradural balloon in dogs. Hemodilution reduced the mortality rate from a value of 95 per cent with no treatment to 50 per cent, and the combination of hemodilution and hyperbaric oxygen at 2 atm reduced it to 20 per cent.[264,284] Fasano and associates saw some improvement in comatose patients with head injury, and Mogami and co-workers stated that about one third of head injury patients treated with hyperbaric oxygen at 2 atm were greatly improved.[94,279] The problems in interpreting these data are no less than the problems encountered in evaluating the beneficial effects of hyperventilation, and in fact, any other form of therapy. The number of variables is so great and they are so difficult to control that there appears to be no substitute for a randomized trial.

Hypertonic Solutions

The anatomical blood-brain barrier consists of tight junctions between endothelial cells. The barrier prevents diffusion of water-soluble substances from the blood across the wall of the capillary into the extracellular space of the brain. Even atoms as small as sodium will not pass through the tight junction. Thus, all water-soluble materials that normally enter the brain must do so by active transport across the endothelial cell, and this requires the expenditure of energy. Lipid-soluble materials such as gases and a substance like antipyrine, which is used to measure cerebral blood flow, diffuse rapidly across the blood-brain barrier just as they diffuse across all cell membranes. When the concentration of a substance normally present in the blood, such as urea, is increased, that substance diffuses readily across open capillary junctions and there is no change in the fluid content of the organ or tissue into which it freely diffuses. This is not true in the brain. An increase in the blood concentration of a wide variety of substances decreases the fluid content of the brain because of the increase in osmotic pressure driving fluid from brain to blood.

These principles were first applied to the study of intracranial pressure by Weed and McKibben in 1919. They observed a marked fall in pressure in cats following the administration of hypertonic solutions of sodium chloride, sodium bicarbonate, sodium sulfate, and glucose. A decrease in brain volume was also observed in animals with the skull open. The high concentrations of sodium salts caused respiratory and cardiac disturbances, but hypertonic glucose appeared to be without untoward effect.[418] Hypertonic solutions were then used in the treatment of patients with severe head injury, and decreases in lumbar subarachnoid pressure were observed. Fifty per cent glucose was used most frequently in the initial studies. The decrease in intracranial pressure was brief, however, and rebound above the control pressure was described.[34,128] Several other complications of using hypertonic glucose were re-corded, including headache, backache, peripheral nerve pains, and transient fever.[254] Substances such as magnesium sulfate and sodium arabinate were also tried but were soon abandoned.[96,97,162]

The rebound in intracranial pressure was of particular concern to a number of investigators and was attributed to the rapid passage of glucose from the blood into the brain. According to the explanation, as the plasma concentration of glucose fell, the brain concentration exceeded the plasma concentration, resulting in rehydration of the brain and a rebound in intracranial pressure above the control value. Sucrose was then introduced as a material that does not diffuse into the brain or cerebrospinal fluid to a significant degree.[43] Despite encouraging results in animals, the use of the agent in clinical trials was deemed unsatisfactory.[30]

Urea

Not much was accomplished in the treatment of intracranial hypertension with hypertonic solutions until the introduction of urea by Javid in the 1950's.[174-176,178,179] In 1961, he summarized the results in 700 patients and described a marked, sustained fall in intracranial pressure in nearly all cases.[176] A number of vehicles were investigated, and 30 per cent urea in 10 per cent invert sugar at a dosage of 1 gm per kilogram of body weight appeared to give the best results. Several complications were described, however. Infiltration of the subcutaneous tissue during intravenous therapy could cause sloughing of the skin, and hemoglobinuria also was described frequently.[177] Abnormal prothrombin times were also described.[253] Although Javid and his colleagues did not observe rebound, it was described quite clearly in other clinical and animal studies.[206,263] The rebound was greater when the initial intracranial pressure was elevated.

The mode of action of urea in dehydrating the brain was studied extensively, and these studies have remained one of the most important contributions to our understanding of the basic mechanisms of hypertonic solutions. Javid and Anderson demonstrated that the reduction in intracranial pressure was not dependent upon diuresis. In fact, reduced pressure was better maintained in monkeys with bilateral nephrectomy than in controls.[178] Urea is a nonpolar, un-ionized, water-soluble material that rapidly penetrates most capillaries. In the steady state, cellular and extracellular concentrations of urea are the same in most tissue. Thus it has been used to measure total body water. If urea penetrated brain as freely as it does other organs and tissues, however, dehydration of nervous tissue would not occur, and the effect of hypertonic urea on intracranial pressure could not be explained by a difference in osmotic pressure between blood and brain. Kleeman and associates, using [14]carbon-labeled urea, found that the steady state concentration of the water of white matter was about equal to the concentration in plasma water, but gray matter contained a higher (ratio 1.18) and cerebrospinal fluid a lower (ratio 0.78) concentration of urea.[201] They suggested that some of the urea might be adsorbed on intracellular proteins in neurons but not in glial cells. The decreased concentration of urea, from gray matter to white matter to cerebrospinal fluid, could then be explained by the number of neurons in each compartment, from a large number in the gray matter to none, of course, in the fluid. This explanation also permits the assumption that there is equilibrium between free brain urea and cerebrospinal fluid, a necessary condition if the absence of a barrier between brain and cerebrospinal fluid is accepted. It also follows that the concentration of urea in cerebrospinal fluid and free urea in the brain are less than plasma, indicating a blood-brain barrier to urea.

A barrier to diffusion of urea from blood to brain, in fact, has been amply confirmed. [14]Carbon-labeled urea penetrates the brain far more slowly than it penetrates muscle and enters white matter more slowly than it enters gray matter.[119,201,262] Equilibration takes place in gray matter in less than 2 hours but not until 12 hours in white matter. The difference might be explained by the greater vascularity of gray matter, but it is likely that other factors contribute.[28] Reed and Woodbury studied the penetration of hypertonic urea (2 gm per kilogram) into the brain of rats and recorded brain urea concentration, brain water volume, and cerebrospinal fluid pressure at various times following administration of the agent. The kinetics of the uptake of urea by the brain indicated a two-compartment system with half times of 23 minutes and 2.5 hours. Both cerebrospinal fluid and brain water volume decreased rapidly following injection of urea. The surprising finding was that both pressure and water volume began to return toward normal at a time when a large urea osmotic gradient from brain to blood still existed. They postulated that both the fast and slow compartments of the brain were rapidly dehydrated by the initial high concentration of urea in the plasma. After equilibrium had been reached in the fast compartment, urea continued to enter the slow compartment, carrying water with it and accounting for the parallel rise in brain water and urea concentration over the next several hours. The rapid return of cerebrospinal fluid pressure toward normal was explained by some vasodilatation and particularly by increased production or decreased absorption of cerebrospinal fluid.[328] Subsequently it was demonstrated, in fact, that cerebrospinal fluid pressure returned to normal more slowly following administration of hypertonic urea when the rate of fluid formation was reduced with acetazolamide.[329] Probably this is also the explanation for the rebound in intracranial pressure above control levels. As the water content of the brain returns to normal, the brain expands into a space made smaller by the accumulation of cerebrospinal fluid and the dilatation of cerebral vessels.

Urea was the first agent used to determine whether the fluid content of edematous brain could be reduced. In theory, if the blood-brain barrier were intact in edematous brain at the time the agent was administered, the brain tissue containing edema fluid should be dehydrated as well as normal brain. On the other hand, if the blood-brain barrier were defective, urea should enter the brain quickly, equilibrium should be established between the vascular bed and the extracellular space, and little if any edema fluid would be removed. Levy and co-workers studied the effect of hypertonic urea on the water content of white matter made edematous by triethyltin intoxication.[226] The blood-brain barrier is intact in this type of experimental edema, and the edema appears to have little effect on cerebral blood flow or neurological function.[246] Hypertonic urea reduced both the sodium and the water content of the edematous white matter, but the response was delayed more than would be expected on the basis of hyperosmolarity alone. Pappius and Dayes studied the effect of hypertonic urea on brain made edematous by a freezing lesion compared with normal brain in the same preparation. Large amounts of water were removed from the normal brain, but the water content of edematous brain was unchanged.[303] Similar observations have been made by others.[58]

Mannitol

Hypertonic urea was largely abandoned in the 1960's. Probably the two most important reasons for doing so were the very high incidence of hemoglobinuria and sloughing of the skin, sometimes so severe as to require skin grafting, when the solution infiltrated the subcutaneous tissue. An even more compelling reason for discontinuing the use of urea was the introduction of mannitol. Mannitol is the alcohol of the 6-carbon sugar mannose. Its molecular configuration is similar to that of glucose, but it is not metabolized to any extent and, unlike urea, it appears to remain entirely in the extracellular compartment. Thus, mannitol is an excellent diuretic and was used in research in renal physiology for many years prior to its introduction into neurosurgery.[366] Wise and Chater demonstrated in dogs that in comparison with urea, mannitol decreased cerebrospinal fluid pressure as effectively, for longer periods of time, and with no rebound in intracranial pressure.[429] McQueen and Jeanes compared urea and mannitol in normal dogs and in dogs with intracranial hypertension produced by subarachnoid injections of blood. The decrease in pressure was about the same with equivalent amounts of the two agents, but the effect of mannitol lasted longer. Some rebound in pressure occurred with mannitol in the animals with intracranial hypertension, but it was minimal compared with the large rebound observed with urea.[263] In contrast to these observations, Beks and terWeeme found that increased intracranial pressure produced by cold lesions in cats was reduced more rapidly and more profoundly by urea than by mannitol, and the duration of action was about equal with the two agents.[18]

The first clinical results in a series of neurosurgical patients were reported in the early 1960's.[378,430] Since then clinical investigations of mannitol have been extensive. The issues that have been addressed in particular have been the rapidity of onset of the reduction in pressure, the maximum pressure response, and the duration of action; the optimal dosage related both to the amount of mannitol administered and to the resultant serum osmolarity; the complications of therapy; comparisons with other agents; and the effects of mannitol on the cerebral circulation and metabolism.

Gobiet used a standard dose of 1 gm per kilogram infused over a period of 15 minutes and found that the time from infusion to the maximum effect averaged 22 minutes, intracranial pressure was always reduced below 25 mm of mercury (when it was effective), and the average length of time for the pressure to again exceed 25 mm of mercury was 3.7 hours. In several deeply comatose patients, neither mannitol nor any other dehydrating agents in multiple doses reduced intracranial pressure.[120] James and co-workers made similar measurements. Hypertonic mannitol was administered as a bolus (0.18 to 2.5 gm per kilogram of a 25 per cent solution in 2 to 10 minutes) 73 times in 44 patients with a variety of intracranial lesions ranging from pseudotumor cerebri to severe head injury accompanied by deep coma. A reduction in intracranial pressure, defined as a decrease from control value of 10 per cent or more, occurred 67 times in a range of 10 to 98 per cent and a mean reduction of 52 per cent. The time from completion of the bolus injection to the maximum response was 20 to 360 minutes, with a mean of 88 minutes. The time from completion of the bolus injection to return of intracranial pressure to the control value ranged from 45 minutes to 11 hours with a mean of 210 minutes. Among the six administrations in which no response was obtained, three could not be evaluated properly because of the introduction of other variables; one patient subsequently responded to a larger dose, and one patient had already responded to five previous doses of mannitol, suggesting the possibility of tachyphylaxis to the agent.[168] Thus, in this study, hypertonic mannitol almost always reduced increased intracranial pressure irrespective of the intracranial disease. The amplitude and the length of the response varied greatly; as a rule, the higher the initial intracranial pressure, the shorter was the response to mannitol.

One of the problems in evaluating any agent that reduces intracranial pressure is defining the criterion for an effect. Should it be any detectable reduction in pressure, a defined reduction in terms of percentage of control value, or a reduction to the normal range? Should the agent be termed effective if the defined reduction in pressure occurs even transiently or should the pressure remain below the defined level for a specific period of time? Should pressure waves be averaged for a specified length of time? Szewczykowski and associates used a specially designed automatic digital recording system for intracranial pressure and a computer to analyze the results. They began their analysis with a pre-mannitol period divided into a subperiod of normal pressure and another subperiod in which intracranial pressure rose to approximately 40 mm of mercury, which was the criterion for the initiation of therapy. Mannitol was then infused for three hours at a dosage of 0.6 gm per kilogram. The mean pressure was determined for each one-hour period during the time of administration, and then for each of three hours following discontinuation of the infusion. Mannitol decreased intracranial pressure, but at this dosage level, the reduction in pressure was minimal in 2 of 10 cases, and not very great in any of the remainder.[404] The point is, however, that to date this study represents the most systematic effort to study the effect of any dehydrating agent on intracranial pressure.

The dose of mannitol used has varied widely. This has been because uniformity in defining a response to mannitol is lacking and serum osmolarities were not measured routinely until recent times. The studies by Marshall and associates indicate that the dose used in most neurosurgical units has been too large. The reduction in intracranial pressure produced by a dose of 0.25 gm per kilogram was equivalent to the response obtained with doses of 0.5 and 1.0 gm per kilogram in a series of patients with acute head injuries. Furthermore, detectable reductions in intracranial pressure occurred with increases in osmolarity of no more than 10 mOsm. The mean control serum osmolarity in the patients was approximately 280 mOsm. At the three dosage levels, 0.25, 0.5, and 1.0 gm per kilogram, serum osmolarity was 293, 294, and 304 mOsm respectively at a time when the maximum response to intracranial pressure had been achieved.[247] In desperation, much larger doses of mannitol have been given in an attempt to reduce otherwise uncontrollable intracranial hypertension. In 10 such patients who had severe head injuries and ultimately died from increased intracranial pressure, Becker and Vries administered mannitol until peak osmolarities varied from 374 to 475 mOsm. Among the 10 patients, 8 had systemic acidosis, and 3 of these developed frank renal failure.[16] It is no surprise that severe hyperosmolarity produced by mannitol causes renal damage. It is important that relatively small increases in serum osmolarity will reduce intracranial pressure in many patients, and values far in excess of the threshold osmolarity are needed to produce renal damage.

Leech and Miller have studied the effect of mannitol on both intracranial pressure and intracranial compliance in baboons in which intracranial pressure was elevated by inflation of an extradural balloon.[224] Patients also were studied.[271] The interesting observation in the animals was that mannitol improved compliance out of proportion to the reduction in intracranial pressure, and this contrasted with hypocapnia, in which ventricular fluid pressure and the volume-pressure response were reduced equally. The observations with mannitol were confirmed in a large series of patients in whom intraventricular pressure was monitored continuously. Whereas the maximum average reduction in intracranial pressure was about one third of the control value, the reduction in the volume-pressure response approached three fourths of the control value.

Much has been made of the possibility of rebound of intracranial pressure above the control value with all dehydrating agents. The information available can be summarized by stating that rebound with hypertonic mannitol is rare, and when it occurs, it is of doubtful clinical significance. Troupp and associates observed no rebound in patients with severe head injury.[408] James and co-workers observed rebound after only 3 of 73 administrations, and the maximum value was 20 mm of mercury above the control value.[168]

Glycerol

Glycerol has been introduced as a potential substitute for mannitol. In 1961, Virno and colleagues reported that either orally or intravenously administered glycerol was effective in reducing experimental cerebral edema in rabbits, and a few years later, Cantore and associates described marked reductions in cerebral edema and intracranial pressure with orally administered glycerol in patients.[46,413] Although hemoglobinuria was common, Sloviter had demonstrated that quite large quantities of glycerol dissolved in normal electrolyte solution could be administered intravenously to man without complications.[388] The obvious appeal of glycerol was the fact that it can be administered orally. This presented the opportunity of treating intracranial hypertension from malignant intracranial tumors and pseudotumor cerebri, for example, on an outpatient basis. Meyer and colleagues described beneficial effects in stroke patients.[268] Rebound of some significance has also been described.[134] Glycerol solutions at concentrations of 10 per cent are said to be effective, but the margin of safety may be small because 20 per cent can cause hemolysis and renal failure.

Cerebrovascular and Metabolic Responses to Hypertonic Agents

Some of the most intriguing responses to hypertonic agents have been their effects on cerebral blood flow and the cerebral metabolism of oxygen. Goluboff and co-workers observed that both urea and mannitol increased cerebral blood flow and cerebral oxygen consumption.[123] The decrease in cerebrospinal fluid pressure was small and inconstant, and therefore, they concluded that the decreased intracranial pressure produced by the agents could not be the sole explanation for the changes observed. They noted that Harper and Bell found no increase in cortical blood flow in normal dogs to which urea was administered and concluded that the changes observed in the patients probably represented the response of pathological brain tissue.[143] Ott and asso-

ciates found a redistribution of regional flow in stroke patients following glycerol therapy. Flow increased in ischemic regions and concomitantly decreased in adjacent hyperemic zones.[296] The most striking changes in cerebral blood flow that have been observed were reported by Bruce and colleagues in comatose patients following the administration of hypertonic mannitol. Mannitol increased blood flow in 11 of 14 patients, and in many patients the increase was independent of the level of intracranial pressure before or after mannitol administration. In patients with space-occupying masses and marked reductions in flow, hemisphere blood flow as much as doubled following mannitol, and even in patients with diffuse brain insults increases in blood flow of as much as 50 per cent were observed. The cerebral metabolism of oxygen also increased in 10 of 14 patients, but the significance of this observation was uncertain because the method used to measure the cerebral metabolic rate of oxygen utilization was less accurate than the method used to measure cerebral blood flow.[41]

The implications of these observations are very important. Traditionally, if a hypertonic agent has no effect on raised intracranial pressure, it is declared to be clinically ineffectual and is not administered again or is given in a larger dose. As noted earlier, the purpose of reducing raised intracranial pressure is to improve cerebral blood flow. If cerebral blood flow can be increased without a reduction in intracranial pressure, then it follows that changes in intracranial pressure are not an adequate guide to therapy in some patients. The cause of the increase in blood flow with little or no change in intracranial tension remains obscure. Bruce and co-workers postulated that blood flow might have been reduced in their patients, at least in part, by swelling of endothelial cells. The dehydration of the endothelial cells resulted in enlargement of the capillary bed and an increase in flow. Intracranial pressure decreased little, if at all, because the decrease in water content of the endothelial cells, and perhaps the perivascular glial cells, was matched by an increase in blood volume secondary to dilatation of the capillary bed. Since net intracranial volume did not change, neither did intracranial pressure.[41] This hypothesis receives some support from the fact that hypertonic mannitol administered to animals through the internal carotid artery transiently opens the blood-brain barrier. Rapoport and his colleagues postulated that the opening of the barrier was due to dehydration of endothelial cells causing separation of the tight junctions.[324,325]

The increases in metabolism observed with urea, mannitol, and glycerol are even more difficult to explain than the improvements in cerebral blood flow. Two explanations come to mind. If the brain was ischemic at the time the hypertonic agent was administered, and therefore, the metabolism of oxygen was reduced because of the ischemic condition of the tissue, improvement in blood flow would improve the delivery of oxygen to the tissue, metabolism would be restored toward normal, and the rate of oxygen utilization would increase. The difficulty with this explanation is that the metabolism increases when blood flow has been only moderately reduced, almost surely still above the threshold for ischemia. The alternative explanation is even less satisfactory because it postulates that the primary effect is on metabolism, and the increase in blood flow is secondary because of intact metabolic autoregulation.

Steroids

Steroids, particularly the glucocorticoid dexamethasone, have been used extensively in the treatment of a wide variety of pathological conditions affecting the nervous system. In fact, dexamethasone is one of the most widely used drugs in the treatment of organic diseases of the nervous system. Beneficial effects occur so quickly and are so dramatic in many conditions that there can be no question about the effectiveness of the agent. In many other clinical conditions the results are not so clear.

The first reports of the clinical effectiveness of steroids in the treatment of acute brain insults were of its use in stroke patients.[338,350] Kofman and associates described marked improvement in the neurological status of patients with cerebral metastases from carcinoma of the breast.[204] The reports of Galicich and co-workers, and Rasmussen and Gulati were principally responsible for the introduction of steroid therapy into neurosurgery. In the former

study, 14 patients with brain tumors and increased intracranial pressure were treated with dexamethasone. Thirteen of them showed definite clinical improvement, and in two cases, angiography during treatment showed a decrease in the size of the total mass.[114] Rasmussen and Gulati compared steroid-treated patients who underwent temporal lobectomy for epilepsy with a series of untreated patients. The incidence of hemiparesis, early seizures, and other signs ordinarily attributed to edema during the postoperative period was reduced in the treated patients.[326] In 1964, French and Galicich reviewed their experience with 300 neurosurgical patients treated with dexamethasone. They concluded that the treatment was effective in the postoperative management of a variety of intracranial disorders that frequently cause cerebral edema. The ordinary dose employed was 16 mg of dexamethasone a day in divided doses. There were a few complications. Several patients on long-term treatment developed water retention, but arterial hypertension was not observed, and serum electrolyte abnormalities were rare. Wound healing was delayed in a few patients, but factors other than the catabolic and antifibroblastic action of the glucocorticoid appeared to be the explanation. The incidence of wound infection was not increased. Gastrointestinal hemorrhage was seen in only four patients and was apparent in only one of them prior to death.[112] There is little additional information about the incidence and significance of the side effects of dexamethasone therapy since this landmark report.

Of all the intracranial conditions in which dexamethasone has been used, it has been most effective in the treatment of gliomas and metastatic tumors. In patients in whom intracranial pressure has been measured continuously, it has been reduced significantly with steroid therapy.[33,120,360] Following administration of the steroid, samples of brain tissue adjacent to tumors have been removed at the time of craniotomy, and significant reductions in the fluid content of both gray and white matter have been described.[360] Regional cerebral blood flow has been measured adjacent to the tumor and in normal brain within the same hemisphere. In general, there was a good correlation between clinical improvement, reduction in mass effect demonstrated by cerebral angiography, and an increase in regional flow adjacent to the tumor.[422] There is also evidence that cerebrovascular reactivity to changes in both arterial carbon dioxide tension and systemic arterial pressure is improved in peritumoral brain tissue by dexamethasone therapy.

The dose of dexamethasone employed has varied greatly among clinical studies, but in general, the dosage has gradually increased with the passage of time. The dose level of 16 mg per day in four divided doses, advocated by French and Galicich, was standard treatment for many years.[112] Then neurosurgeons began to increase the dosage in brain tumor patients who no longer responded to the original schedule.[333] There have been a number of interesting observations in these patients that have not been described thus far in the literature. Patients who require 16 mg per day during the postoperative period following partial removal of a malignant glioma may require no steroid therapy only a few weeks later. When the patient begins to deteriorate clinically, a daily dose of 16 mg or more may be required to return his neurological status to normal, but again, often it is possible to greatly reduce and even occasionally eliminate the steroid treatment over the next several weeks. In the later phases of the illness, the requirement for steroid therapy increases steadily, at which time the patient's clinical status can be titrated with the dexamethasone. The author has observed a case in which 100 mg per day improved the patient, whereas 80 mg per day was ineffectual. The striking benefits of steroid treatment in patients with malignant brain tumors have led to the advocacy of biopsy and high-dosage steroid therapy in patients with deep tumors, especially in the dominant hemisphere.[244] The average survival time in a series of patients treated in this manner was 29 weeks, not very different from other therapeutic regimens.

Dexamethasone has been said to be beneficial in the acute phase of stroke. In one of the few well-controlled studies of the effect of dexamethasone on mortality rates in both hemorrhagic and thrombotic stroke, however, Tellez and Bauer found no significant difference in outcome. The patients with intracerebral hemorrhage were divided into two groups, those who were severely disabled but responsive, and those who were in coma or deep stupor on admission. Patients from both groups were treated with either a placebo or dexamethasone. The dosage of dexamethasone was tapered after the first three days of a maximum dose of 18 mg per day. The total dosage over a ten-day period was 120 mg. The mortality rate was extremely high in all patients, and there was no difference between patients who received dexamethasone and those who received the placebo.[406] One wonders, however, whether any type of therapy would be beneficial in this type of patient, and the dose of dexamethasone was small compared with the very large doses that are being used at this time. In a companion study to the series of patients with intracerebral hemorrhage, another series of patients with acute cerebral infarction were studied. A clinical score was derived for each patient on admission, then the change in the scores was compared in patients who were treated with dexamethasone and in those who received a placebo. Excluding patients who were semicomatose, there was no significant difference between the two groups among those patients who were improved, unchanged, worse, or dead.[13]

Most neurosurgeons have been discouraged about the treatment of severe head injuries with steroids. It has been difficult to evaluate the effects of steroids, because in the most severely ill patients, other forms of therapy are invariably superimposed upon the steroid treatment. The only randomized double-blind study that has been reported was carried out by Faupel and colleagues. On admission, patients received either dexamethasone or a placebo. The dexamethasone-treated patients were in turn divided into two subgroups, one receiving an initial dose of 12 mg intravenously, followed by 4 mg every six hours for eight days, then a tapering dose. The second subgroup received an initial dose of 100 mg intravenously, 100 mg intramuscularly at six hours following admission, then a regimen identical to the first subgroup. A score sheet was used to evaluate the neurological status. At the end of the study, when the double-blind code was broken, 28 patients had received placebo, 32 the low-dosage dexamethasone, and 34 the high-dosage dexamethasone course of treatment. The mortality rates were 57 per cent in the placebo group, 30 per cent in the low-dosage dexamethasone group, and 18 per cent in the high-dosage dexamethasone group of patients.[95] In terms of the ultimate outcome, the number of patients who recovered totally or who were left with only moderate neurological deficit did not differ significantly between the placebo and dexamethasone groups. Thus, unfortunately, in this particular series, those patients who would have died without treatment did not recover; rather, they were left in a vegetative state or a stable state with severe neurological deficit. This series of patients has been presented in considerable detail because it does represent the first detailed evaluation of dexamethasone therapy in patients with head injury. It is to be hoped that a combination of dexamethasone and other forms of therapy will reduce the severe morbidity.

Steroids have been studied extensively in experimental models of acute brain insults. The two most common models employed have been various simulations of stroke and the simulation of a cerebral contusion with a freezing lesion of the cerebral cortex. The results in the stroke models have been inconclusive. The effect of steroids has been tested in various models of vascular occlusion, including ligation or clipping of large arteries, and microembolization. The therapy has been found to be effective in some models and ineffectual in others.* Steroids have been found to reduce the volume of edema produced by extracerebral compression with a balloon and triethyl tin intoxication, but had no effect on the water content of brain made edematous by a laser injury.†

The most dramatic effects have been in the white matter edema produced by a freezing lesion of the cortex.[25,258,304,347] When the steroid was administered following production of the lesion, there was little effect during the first 24 hours, then the reduction in the volume of edema was progressive.[304] Pretreatment with a steroid was more effective in preventing edema than was steroid therapy at any time after the lesion had been made.[258] The mechanism of action of steroids in improving brain function is poorly understood. First, a

distinction must be made between improvement in brain function, measured clinically by improvement in the patients' neurological status, and a reduction in the fluid content of the brain. The issue is whether and under what specific conditions brain edema is the cause of brain dysfunction or simply an epiphenomenon of the pathological condition. There is evidence that at least one form of massive edema of the white matter, namely, triethyltin intoxication, does not alter neurological status and decreases cerebral blood flow only as a dilutional effect of the edema.[246] Recent experiences with serial computed tomography in brain tumor patients have demonstrated that the patients' neurological status may improve greatly at the same time that the volume of peritumoral edema, estimated from the CT scan, has not changed or has even increased slightly.[265,361] The author believes that edema per se does not disturb brain function unless it produces a critical reduction in cerebral blood flow either by an increase of tissue pressure within edematous brain or by a diffuse rise in intracranial pressure.

Very little is known about the effect of steroids on neuronal and glial functions. It is often stated that steroids stabilize cell membranes, but this says very little. In studies of cold injuries in the rat, dexamethasone suppressed the activity of three lysosomal enzymes in the injured hemisphere. In the untreated rat, alkaline phosphatase increased significantly in the injured tissue, and dexamethasone eliminated this rise in activity following injury.[25] Most alkaline phosphatase in brain tissue resides in blood vessels. Since alkaline phosphatase activity has also been tied to the blood-brain barrier, the results suggest that a reduction in edema, which has been demonstrated in this model with dexamethasone, may be due to improvement in blood-brain barrier function. There is also evidence that dexamethasone reduces the production of cerebrospinal fluid, which would enhance whatever other effect the steroid has in reducing intracranial pressure.[425]

Hypothermia

In the past, hypothermia was used principally in the treatment of patients with severe craniocerebral trauma or anoxia and in intracranial and cardiovascular operations.

---

* See references: effective, 11, 144; ineffectual, 191, 228, 313, 383.

† See references: balloon compression, 434; triethyl tin, 405; laser injury, 19.

Despite encouraging reports of the effectiveness of hypothermia in reducing morbidity and mortality rates in head injury and in intracranial procedures, particularly for aneurysms, it fell into disfavor among most neurosurgeons. The principal reason appears to have been a lack of convincing evidence that hypothermia is, in fact, an effective treatment of brain injury, cerebral swelling, and increased intracranial pressure.

Sedzimir treated 30 consecutive patients with severe head injury with hypothermia. He found it difficult to interpret the contributions of hypothermia, but believed that it was probably beneficial. He emphasized, however, that tracheostomy was also performed in these patients and could well have accounted for the improved mortality rate, compared with another series of patients who received neither hypothermia nor tracheostomy.[365] Lazorthes and Campan were more enthusiastic about the beneficial effects of hypothermia in patients with severe head injuries and stated that the results in this series probably would have been even better if the patients had come to treatment earlier following the injury.[221] Lundberg and his colleagues observed a dramatic reduction in intracranial pressure, including cessation of pressure waves, with hypothermia in one patient with a head injury. Pressure was normal about two hours after cooling was begun.[238] Gravel and co-workers, and Williams and Spencer reported improvement in patients with cardiac arrest treated with hypothermia.[113,428]

The effect of hypothermia on intracranial pressure in five patients who were comatose following periods of severe cerebral hypoxia were highly variable. When the body temperature was reduced to a mean of 32.8° C, the mean fall in intracranial pressure among the patients was 45 per cent, with a maximum of 80 per cent.[214] It is interesting that the effects of hypothermia on intracranial hypertension were about the same in these patients as the effects of hypertonic mannitol. In a study by James and associates, alluded to in previous sections on therapy, hypothermia was induced in 40 patients with intracranial hypertension due to many causes. Hypothermia was induced by placing the patients between thermal blankets, with or without the addition of ice bags between the legs and beneath the arms. Mild hypothermia (32° to 36° C) decreased intracranial pressure by 10 per cent or more in 13 of 32 trials. There was no response in 13, and in 6 trials the results were indeterminate because of the introduction of other variables. The mean reduction in intracranial pressure in the 13 patients was 51 per cent, and the time from induction of hypothermia to the maximum response of intracranial pressure was 240 to 720 minutes with a mean of 516 minutes. Moderate hypothermia (27° to 31° C) was used in eight trials, in addition to the 32 trials of mild hypothermia. A reduction in intracranial pressure was obtained in four trials, in two trials there was no response, and two trials were indeterminate. The mean reduction in intracranial pressure was about the same as with mild hypothermia. In nearly every instance the decline in intracranial pressure followed the reduction in body temperature. Figure 24–15 illustrates the relationship of intracranial pressure to body temperature in one patient.[168]

In 1971, McDowall reported the results of a survey of neurosurgical anesthetists in Britain to determine the use of hypothermia in neurosurgical procedures at that time. He found that there were wide variations among centers. For example, London hospitals used virtually no hypothermia; it was used in about 15 per cent of major intracranial operations in some Midland centers; and in Liverpool, hypothermia was used in approximately 30 per cent of cases. Cooling was induced mainly with thermal blankets; shivering during recovery was treated with chlorpromazine and promazine; and serious cardiac arrhythmias were described as being extremely rare during the course of hypothermia.[259]

Many studies of experimental hypothermia have been carried out over the years. During a fall in body temperature from normal to 25° C, systemic arterial and venous pressures fall, cerebral blood flow declines, and cerebral metabolic rate for oxygen also decreases.[20,267,343,395] Cerebral glucose metabolism decreases in proportion to oxygen consumption.[20] Polarographic measurements of oxygen availability in the cortex show no change, again demonstrating the parallel response of cerebral flow and metabolism to the hypothermia.[267] Hagerdal and associates found that cerebral oxygen metabolism decreased linearly with temperature in the range of 37° to 22° C, decreasing about 5 per cent per degree cen-

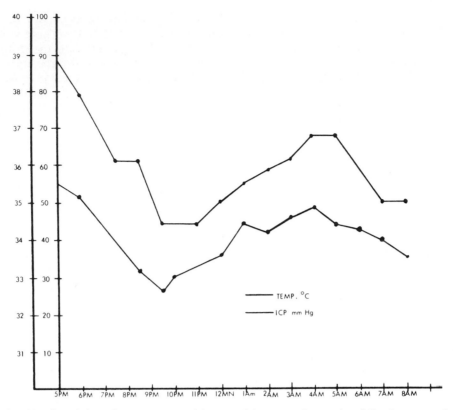

Figure 24–15 Correlation of temperature and intracranial pressure in a patient following removal of a large intracerebral hematoma. (From Langfitt, T. W., Kumar, V. S., James, H. E., and Miller, J. D.: Continuous recording of intracranial pressure in patients with hypoxic brain damage. *In* Brierley, J. B., and Meldrum, B. S., eds: Brain Hypoxia. Clinics in Developmental Medicine. Vol. 39–40. London, Spastics International Medical Publications, 1971. Reprinted by permission.)

tigrade. At the lowest temperature investigated, 22° C, both cerebral blood flow and metabolism were reduced to about 25 per cent of normal.[137] Meyer and Hunter have presented evidence that the neurons are affected in a descending manner, the cortex first, and the medullary centers and spinal cord only at deep levels of hypothermia.[267]

Under hypothermia the brain idles and should be able to function for longer periods of time with a reduction in available oxygen and metabolites. This is the basis for the use of hypothermia in intracranial and cardiovascular operations in which periods of systemic or local cerebral circulatory arrest may be necessary. The protective effect of hypothermia in this regard has been clearly demonstrated in experimental animals. Ganshirt and co-workers demonstrated that survival time after total cerebral ischemia was a function of the depth of hypothermia and was particularly significant below 30° C. Recovery time was also measured in their experiments and was found to increase rapidly below 30° C. They

concluded, therefore, that optimum protection of the brain was produced by temperatures between 27° and 30° C.[117] Hypothermia also reduced brain bulk and intracranial pressure in experimental animals. Lowering of the temperature in dogs to 25° C resulted in a reduction in brain volume of 4.1 per cent.[342] Lemmen and Davis measured lumbar cerebrospinal fluid pressure in patients during hypothermia induced in preparation for craniotomy. It fell in patients with little or no initial pressure elevation, but when intracranial hypertension was present, the pattern varied considerably, and in some patients there was no significant decrease in pressure.[225] In comparison with animal studies, however, the period of hypothermia was brief. Shulman and Rosomoff demonstrated that hypothermia at 25° C significantly reduces the mortality rate in dogs with brain swelling produced by cold lesions of the cerebral cortex.[381] These results were confirmed by Laskowski and associates. The amount of edema was less in the protected animals, blood-brain barrier permeability was less affected, and the enlargement and PAS-positive staining of glial cells was less pronounced than in the control animals.[218] Clasen and colleagues demonstrated a decrease in both hemorrhage and edema in the hemisphere damaged by a cold lesion with sustained systemic hypothermia and with interrupted hypothermia.[57] Rosomoff and co-workers emphasized a reduction in the inflammatory response in the hypothermic animals compared with controls.[344] Hypothermia has also been demonstrated to protect the blood-brain barrier against iodopyracet (Diodrast).[185]

The principal fear among those using hypothermia to treat patients with severe brain insults or as an adjunct to neurological operations has been that body temperature might be reduced to a level that causes cardiac arrhythmias or cardiac arrest. Since the threshold for cardiac arrhythmia occurs almost always at 26° to 27° C, careful maintenance of body temperature above that level has made cardiac problems very infrequent. Bloch has described other complications during rewarming following prolonged hypothermia. Central nervous system complications in patients who have been treated for cerebral astrocytoma included persistent drowsiness, seizures, and increased intracranial pressure. Rarely acute neurogenic pulmonary edema was also observed. The severity of the complications appeared to be related to both the duration of the hypothermia and the rate of return of body temperature to normal.[26]

The discrepancy between the experimental studies of hypothermia, which clearly show reduced cerebral metabolism and protection against mechanical and anoxic injury, and the clinical results have probably been due to the timing of the treatment and the nature of the lesions being treated. Hypothermia has been most effective in experimental animals when it has been administered prior to rather than after the creation of the injury. Clearly this is not possible in head injuries and stroke, for example. Where intracranial pressure is the problem, hypothermia is frequently effective in reducing intracranial pressure, often as effective as hypertonic solutions, but several hours may be required to reduce intracranial tension maximally. Since most investigations of hypothermia in the treatment of head injury were reported many years ago, a re-evaluation of the treatment would appear to be in order, particularly in light of a more complete understanding of intracranial and cerebral circulatory dynamics. In particular, a combination of hypothermia and barbiturate therapy might be more effective than either treatment alone.

Barbiturate Therapy

Barbiturate therapy has been introduced into the armamentarium of methods for treating intracranial hypertension only recently. It has been known for some time that barbiturates do protect the brain from anoxia, ischemia, and vasogenic cerebral edema.[56,122,435] In persistent hypertension that became resistant to treatment with diuretics, steroids, and hyperventilation, thiopental and pentobarbital were effective in reducing intracranial pressure. The decrease in pressure often was rapid, and abrupt increases in intracranial pressure could be aborted with barbiturate treatment.[373] Barbiturate therapy was clearly lifesaving in a child with a severe brain insult who had not responded to other methods of treatment.[245]

The use of barbiturates and of neuromuscular blocking agents to prevent movement in semicomatose patients has been resisted by neurosurgeons because the neurological examination is lost during the period of unresponsiveness. The risks of inducing deep coma or paralysis are greatly reduced, however, if not entirely eliminated, in patients who are ventilated and under careful respiratory control with frequent measurements of blood gases and in whom intracranial pressure is measured continuously. In fact, one can state that these forms of treatment should never be instituted unless intracranial pressure is recorded continuously. The complication of the intracranial insult that could further damage the brain, for example, a hematoma or cerebral edema, will invariably manifest themselves by an increase in intracranial pressure, which is about the only mechanism whereby these complications can produce further brain damage. In other words, if blood pressure and blood oxygenation are adequate, and if intracranial pressure remains within the normal range, one can be reasonably sure that significant complications within the intracranial space are not in process during the time when the patient is in deep coma or paralyzed.

Operative Decompression

Since the dawn of neurosurgery, internal and external cranial decompression have been used to combat brain swelling and intracranial pressure. Internal decompression, which is the resection of brain tissue, has been employed most frequently during craniotomy for brain tumors and in order to have access to lesions at the base of the brain. The surgeon may elect to do an anterior temporal lobectomy, for example, in a patient with a large deep glioma in the temporocentral region of the brain that cannot be removed completely, particularly when the brain is swollen. Experience has taught that the survival rate of patients with marked brain swelling at the time of closure of the craniotomy is poorer than that of patients with a slack brain, despite the many treatments to combat cerebral edema that are available. As a general statement, however, internal decompressions are performed less frequently now than used to be the case because of the availability of various agents to reduce brain swelling, and particularly because of the many advances in neurosurgical anesthesia.

External cranial decompression is used frequently in neurosurgical practice. Some neurosurgeons prefer to leave the dura open and do not wire down the bone flap in many of their craniotomy cases. Others, probably the majority, are guided by the circumstances in each patient. They do a reconstructive closure if the brain is slack, and they leave a large opening for decompression if it is swollen. If swelling is severe, the craniotomy can be enlarged.

From time to time, external decompression has been advocated for uncontrollable brain swelling, particularly in patients with severe craniocerebral trauma. Moody and co-workers studied the procedure experimentally. Marked increased intracranial pressure was produced by inflating an extracerebral balloon. The entire cranial vault except for the bone over the sagittal sinus was removed in half the animals. The survival rate was significantly higher among those animals than among the controls, but the quality of survival was poor. All animals remained comatose, and fungus cerebri developed routinely within 10 days following operation.[282] Clark and associates reported a discouraging experience in two patients with severe head injuries who had "circumferential craniotomy." They describe marked upward displacement of the brain stem in one of these patients.[54] Ransohoff and his colleagues compared a series of unconscious patients with head injury with acute subdural hematoma treated by extensive unilateral craniectomy with a previous series of patients in their own unit treated by multiple burr holes. The mortality rate appeared to be greatly reduced in the patients treated by decompressive craniectomy.[322] In a subsequent paper based on analysis of another 50 patients, however, the results were much more discouraging. Only 10 per cent of these patients survived, and only 4 per cent of the total survived with reasonably good neurological function.[65] Other authors have advocated bifrontal decompressive craniectomy in the treatment of patients with severe brain swelling secondary to head injury.[198,412]

The author has performed bilateral craniectomies in a few patients with massive brain swelling secondary to head injury. One 17-year-old boy had massive bilateral brain swelling without an extracerebral collection of blood or angiographic evidence of parenchymal brain injury. When the intracranial pressure rose to 80 mm of mercury despite vigorous medical therapy to control intracranial hypertension, bilateral decompressive craniectomies were performed. The patient had been comatose and decerebrate prior to the operation, but all brain stem reflexes were intact and he made a complete recovery. The other patients died or were left with severe neurological deficits. The conclusions from this experience were that the procedure is ineffectual in patients with diffuse impact injuries of the brain and in patients in whom the operation was performed as a desperation effort after the brain had already been irreversibly damaged by ischemia secondary to the intracranial hypertension. Finally, if the decompression is to be performed at all, it should be very extensive.

CONCLUSION

Increased intracranial pressure is common in neurosurgical patients. It is caused by a mass lesion, brain edema, cerebrovascular congestion of the brain, or hydrocephalus. The increased intracranial pressure damages the brain either by a reduction in cerebral blood flow focally or generally within the cerebral hemispheres or by inducing herniation and ischemia of the brain stem.

The only means of determining whether intracranial hypertension is present and contributing to the patient's neurological status is to record the pressure continuously directly from the intracranial space. Many methods are available. Although none is entirely accurate or risk-free, the two methods that have gained the greatest favor are an intraventricular cannula and a subarachnoid bolt.

The treatment of intracranial hypertension is based on the premise that reduction in the volume of any one of the normally present intracranial compartments—brain water, intravascular blood, cerebrospinal fluid—or reduction in the volume of a mass lesion will reduce pressure. If the compartment that is the target of the particular therapy is increased in volume, so much the better, but the objective is to reduce intracranial pressure with whatever method works. A better understanding of the pathophysiology of increased intracranial pressure has improved the rationale for specific treatments. Despite this improved knowledge, however, the selection of methods is still largely empirical. If the patient is carefully monitored and the various forms of therapy available are applied vigorously and intelligently, death from uncontrollable intracranial hypertension is now rather uncommon.

An unresolved problem is the contribution of intracranial hypertension to morbidity and death from specific disorders, particularly head injury, cerebrovascular accidents, systemic hypoxemia, encephalitis and encephalopathies, and a variety of systemic conditions that tend to cause brain swelling. When the intracranial pressure is increased in a patient who has been devastated neurologically, often the intracranial hypertension is an epiphenomenon of the brain insult and not the cause of the patient's neurological state. On the other hand, when the patient is relatively intact, intracranial pressure is rising, and the patient's neurological status begins to deteriorate with the rising pressure, the increased pressure is clearly life-threatening. This is the circumstance that makes the past two decades of research worthwhile. The

neurosurgeon is in control of the situation. He can observe the pressure continuously and correlate it with the neurological status of the patient. If one method of treatment does not work, he can add another, and still another, method. When the pressure rises out of control and the patient becomes comatose only to recover when another treatment regimen reduces the pressure to normal, the neurosurgeon is convinced that intracranial hypertension is an important problem in the practice of neurosurgery, and he derives immense satisfaction from a therapeutic triumph that is the equal of most in the operating theater.

REFERENCES

1. Adams, J. H.: Hypoxic brain damage. Brit. J. Anaesth., 47:121–129, 1975.
2. Adams, J. H., and Graham, D. I.: The relationship between ventricular fluid pressure and the neuropathology of raised intracranial pressure. Neuropath. Appl. Neurobiol., 2:323–332, 1976.
3. Alexander, S. C., and Lassen, N. A.: Cerebral circulatory response to acute brain disease. Anesthesiology, 32:60–68, 1970.
4. Artru, F., Philippon, B., Gau, F., Berger, M., and Deleuze, R.: Cerebral blood flow, cerebral metabolism and cerebrospinal fluid biochemistry in brain-injured patients after exposure to hyperbaric oxygen. Europ. Neurol., 14:351–364, 1976.
5. Astrup, J., Heuser, D., and Lassen, N. A.: Evidence against H+ and K+ as the main factors in the regulation of cerebral blood flow during epileptic discharges, acute hypoxemia, amphetamine intoxication, and hypoglycemia. A micro-electrode study. In Betz, E., ed.: Ionic Actions in Vascular Smooth Muscle. Berlin, Springer-Verlag, 1976.
6. Atkinson, J. R., Shurtleff, D. B., and Foltz, E. L.: Radiotelemetry for the measurement of intracranial pressure. J. Neurosurg., 27:428–432, 1967.
7. Ausman, J. I., Rogers, C., and Sharp, H. L.: Decompressive craniectomy for the encephalopathy of Reye's syndrome. Surg. Neurol., 6:97–99, 1976.
8. Austin, G., Horn, N., Rouhe, S., and Hayward, W.: Description and early results of an intravenous radioisotope technique for measuring regional cerebral blood flow in man. Europ. Neurol., 8:43–51, 1972.
9. Ayer, J. B.: Analysis of the lumbar cerebrospinal fluid in sixty-seven cases of tumors and cysts of the brain. Res. Publ. Ass. Res. Nerv. Ment. Dis., 8:189–199, 1927.
10. Baldy-Moulinier, M., and Frerebeau, P.: Cerebral blood flow in cases of coma following severe head injury. In Brock, M., Fieschi, C., Ingvar, D. H., Lassen, N. A., and Schurmann, K., eds.: Cerebral Blood Flow. Berlin, Springer-Verlag, 1969.

11. Bartko, D., Reulen, H. J., Hodgko, C. H. H., and Schurman, N. K.: Effect of dexamethasone on early edema following occlusion of the middle cerebral artery in cats. *In* Reulen, H. J., and Schurman, K., eds.: Steroids and Brain Edema. Berlin, Springer-Verlag, 1972.

12. Bates, P., and Sundt, T. M.: The relevance of peripheral baroreceptors and chemoreceptors to regulation of cerebral blood flow in the cat. Circ. Res., *38*:488–493, 1976.

13. Bauer, R. B., and Tellez, H.: Dexamethasone as treatment in cerebrovascular disease. 2. A controlled study in acute cerebral infarction. Stroke, *4*:547–555, 1973.

14. Bayliss, W. M.: On the local reactions of the arterial wall to changes of internal pressure. J. Physiol. (London), *28*:220–231, 1902.

15. Becht, F. C.: Studies on the cerebrospinal fluid. Amer. J. Physiol., *52*:1–125, 1920.

16. Becker, D. P. and Vries, J. K.: The alleviation of intracranial pressure by the chronic administration of osmotic agents. *In* Brock, M., and Dietz, H., eds.: Intracranial Pressure. Berlin, Springer-Verlag, 1972.

17. Becker, D. P., Vries, J. K., Young, H. F., and Ward, J. D.: Controlled cerebral perfusion pressure and ventilation in human mechanical brain injury. Prevention of progressive brain swelling. *In* Lundberg, N., Ponten, U., and Brock, M., eds.: Intracranial Pressure II. Berlin, Springer-Verlag, 1975.

18. Beks, J. W. F., and terWeeme, C. A.: The influence of urea and mannitol on increased intraventricular pressure in cold-induced cerebral oedema. Acta Neurochir., *16*:97–107, 1967.

19. Benson, V. M., McLaurin, R. L., and Foulkes, E. C.: Traumatic cerebral edema: An experimental model with evaluation of dexamethasone. Arch. Neurol. (Chicago), *23*:179–186, 1970.

20. Bering, E. A., Jr., Taren, J. A., McMurrey, J. D., and Bernhard, W. F.: Studies on hypothermia in monkeys. II. The effect of hypothermia on the general physiology and cerebral metabolism of monkeys in the hypothermic state. Surg. Gynec. Obstet., *102*:134–138, 1956.

21. Berman, I. R., Ducker, T. B., and Simmons, R. L.: The effects of increased intracranial pressure upon the oxygenation of blood in dogs. J. Neurosurg., *30*:532–536, 1969.

22. Berman, W., Pizzi, F., Schut, L., Raphaely, R., and Holtzapple, P.: The effect of exchange transfusion on intracranial pressure in patients with Reye's syndrome. J. Pediat., *87*:887–891, 1975.

23. Betz, E., Pickerodt, V., and Weidner, A.: Respiratory alkalosis: Effect on CBF, pO_2 and acid-base relation in cerebral cortex with a note on water content. Scand. J. Lab. Clin. Invest., *22*:suppl. 102:4:D, 1968.

24. Bill, A., and Linder, J.: Sympathetic control of cerebral blood flow in acute arterial hypertension. Acta. Physiol. Scand., *96*:114–121, 1976.

25. Bingham, W. G., Paul, S. E., and Sastry, K. S. S.: Effect of steroid on enzyme response to cold injury in rat brain. Neurology (Minneap.), *21*:111–121, 1971.

26. Bloch, M.: Cerebral effects of rewarming following prolonged hypothermia: Significance for the management of severe craniocerebral injury in acute pyrexia. Brain, *90*:769–784, 1967.

27. Borgstrom, L., Johansson, H., and Siesjo, B. K.: The relationship between arterial PCO_2 and cerebral blood flow in hypoxia. Acta Physiol. Scand., *93*:423–432, 1975.

28. Bradbury, M. W. B., and Coxon, R. V.: The penetration of urea into the central nervous system at high blood levels. J. Physiol. (London), *163*:423–435, 1962.

29. Bradley, K. C.: Cerebrospinal fluid pressure. J. Neurol. Neurosurg. Psychiat., *33*:387–397, 1970.

30. Bragdon, F. H.: Alterations observed in craniocerebral injuries following the use of dehydrating agents. Res. Publ. Ass. Res. Nerv. Ment. Dis., *24*:545–561, 1943.

31. Brawley, B. W., Strandness, D. E., and Kelly, W. A.: The physiologic response to therapy in experimental cerebral ischemia. Arch. Neurol. (Chicago), *17*:180–187, 1967.

32. Brock, M., Winkelmuller, W., Poll, W., Markakis, E., and Dietz, H.: Measurement of brain tissue pressure. Lancet, *2*:595–596, 1972.

33. Brock, M., Wiegand, H., Zillig, C., Zywietz, C., Mock, P., and Dietz, H.: The effect of dexamethasone on intracranial pressure in patients with supratentorial tumors. *In* Pappius, H. M., and Feindel, W., eds.: Dynamics of Brain Edema. Berlin, Springer-Verlag, 1976.

34. Browder, J.: Dangers in the use of hypertonic solutions in the treatment of brain injuries. Amer. J. Surg., *8*:1213–1217, 1930.

35. Browder, J., and Meyers, R.: Observations on behavior of the systemic blood pressure, pulse and spinal fluid pressure following craniocerebral injury. Amer. J. Surg., *31*:403–426, 1936.

36. Brown, F. K.: Cardiovascular effects of acutely raised intracranial pressure. Amer. J. Physiol., *185*:510–514, 1956.

37. Bruce, D. A., Goldberg, D., and Schut, L.: Intracranial pressure monitoring in critical care pediatrics. Intensive Care Med., *3*:184, 1977.

38. Bruce, D. A., Schutz, H., Vapalahti, M., and Langfitt, T. W.: Pitfalls in the interpretation of xenon CBF studies in head injured patients. *In* Langfitt, T. W., McHenry, L. C., Reivich, M., and Wollman, H., eds.: Cerebral Circulation and Metabolism. Berlin, Springer-Verlag, 1975.

39. Bruce, D. A., Vapalahti, M., Schutz, H., and Langfitt, T. W.: rCBF, $CMRO_2$ and intracranial pressure following a local cold injury of the cortex. *In* Brock, M., and Dietz, H., eds.: Intracranial Pressure I. Berlin, Springer-Verlag, 1972.

40. Bruce, D. A., Schut, L., Bruno, L. A., Wood, J. H., and Sutton, L. N.: Outcome following severe head injuries in children. J. Neurosurg., *48*:679–688, 1978.

41. Bruce, D. A., Langfitt, T. W., Miller, J. D., Schutz, H., Vapalahti, M. P., Stanek, A., and Goldberg, H. I.: Regional cerebral blood flow, intracranial pressure and brain metabolism in comatose patients. J. Neurosurg., *38*:131–144, 1973.

42. Bruce, D. A., Raphaely, R. C., Goldberg, A. I., Zimmerman, R. A., Bilaniuk, L. T., Schut, L., and Kuhl, D.: The pathophysiology, treatment and outcome following severe head injury in children. Child's Brain, in *5*:74–191, 1979.

43. Bullock, L. T., Gregersen, M. I., and Kinney, R.: The use of hypertonic sucrose solution intravenously to reduce cerebrospinal fluid pressure without a secondary rise. Amer. J. Physiol., *112*:82–96, 1935.

44. Burrows, G.: Disorders of the Cerebral Circulation. London, 1846.

45. Cabieses, F., and Jeri, R.: Transtentorial temporal lobe herniation. Acta Neurol. Lat. Amer., *1*:167–179, 1955.

46. Cantore, G. P., Guidetti, B., and Virno, M.: Oral glycerol for the reduction of intracranial pressure. J. Neurosurg., *21*:278–283, 1964.

47. Carrillo, R.: Hernias cisternales. Arch. Neurochir., *7*:498–590, 1950.

48. Chandler, W. F., and Kindt, G. W.: Monitoring and control of intracranial pressure in nontraumatic encephalopathies. Surg. Neurol., *5*:311–314, 1976.

49. Chawla, J. H., Hulme, A., and Cooper, R.: Intracranial pressure in patients with dementia and communicating hydrocephalus. J. Neurosurg., *40*:376–380, 1974.

50. Chen, H. I., Sun, S. C., and Chai, C. Y.: Pulmonary edema and hemorrhage resulting from brain compression. Amer. J. Physiol., *224*:223–229, 1973.

51. Chorobski, J., and Penfield, W.: Cerebral vasodilator nerves and their pathway from the medulla oblongata. Arch. Neurol. Psychiat., *28*:1257–1289, 1932.

52. Christensen, M. S., Brodersen, P., Olesen, J., and Paulson, O. B.: Cerebral apoplexy (stroke) treated with or without prolonged artificial hyperventilation: 2. Cerebrospinal fluid acid-base balance and intracranial pressures. Stroke, *4*:620–631, 1973.

53. Christensen, M. S., Paulson, O. B., Olesen, J., Alexander, S. C., Skinhoj, E., Dam, W. H., and Lassen, N. A.: Cerebral apoplexy (stroke) treated with or without prolonged artificial hyperventilation: 1. Cerebral circulation, clinical course and cause of death. Stroke, *4*:568–618, 1973.

54. Clark, K., Nash, T. M., and Hutchison, G. C.: The failure of circumferential craniotomy in acute traumatic cerebral swelling. J. Neurosurg., *29*:367–371, 1968.

55. Clark, R. M., Capra, N. F., and Halsey, J. H.: Method for measuring brain tissue pressure: Response to alteration in pCO_2, systemic blood pressure and middle cerebral artery occlusion. J. Neurosurg., *43*:1–8, 1975.

56. Clasen, R. A., Pandolfi, S., and Casey, D.: Furosemide and pentobarbital cryogenic cerebral injury and edema. Neurology (Minneap.), *24*:642–648, 1974.

57. Clasen, R. A., Pandolfi, S., and Hass, G. M.: Interrupted hypothermia in experimental cerebral edema. Neurology (Minneap.), *20*:279–282, 1970.

58. Clasen, R. A., Prouty, R. R., Bingham, W. G., Martin, F. A., and Hass, G. M.: Treatment of experimental cerebral edema with intravenous hypertonic glucose, albumin and dextran. Surg. Gynec. Obstet., *104*:591–606, 1957.

59. Coe, J. E., Nelson, W. J., Rudenberg, F. H., and Garza, R.: Technique for continuous intracranial pressure recording. Technical note. J. Neurosurg., *27*:370–375, 1967.

60. Cold, G. E., Enevoldsen, E., and Malmros, M.: The prognostic value of continuous intraventricular pressure recording in unconscious brain injury patients under controlled ventilation. *In* Lundberg, N., Ponten, U., and Brock, M., eds.: Intracranial Pressure II. Berlin, Springer-Verlag, 1975.

61. Cold, G. E., Jenson, F. T., and Malmros, R.: The effects of $PaCO_2$ reduction on regional cerebral blood flow in the acute phase of brain injury. Acta Anaesthes. Scand., *21*:359–367, 1977.

62. Collice, M., Rossanda, M., Beduschi, A., and Porta, M.: Management of head injury by means of ventricular fluid pressure monitoring. *In* Beks, J. W. F., Bosch, D. A., and Brock, M., eds.: Intracranial Pressure III. Berlin, Springer-Verlag, 1976.

63. Collier, J.: The false localizing signs of intracranial tumors. Brain, *27*:490–508, 1904.

64. Collins, C. C.: Miniature passive pressure transensor for implanting in the eye. IEEE Trans. Biomed. Engin., *14*:74–83, 1967.

65. Cooper, P. R., Rovit, R. L., and Ransohoff, J.: Hemicraniectomy in the treatment of acute subdural hematoma: A re-appraisal. Surg. Neurol., *5*:25–28, 1976.

66. Cooper, R., and Hulme, A.: Intracranial pressure and related phenomena during sleep. J. Neurol. Neurosurg. Psychiat., *29*:564–570, 1966.

67. Cottrell, J. E., Patel, K., Turndorf, H., and Ransohoff, J.: Intracranial pressure changes induced by sodium nitroprusside in patients with intracranial mass lesions. J. Neurosurg., *48*:329–331, 1978.

68. Crockard, H. A., Coppell, D. L., and Morrow, W. F. K.: Evaluation of hyperventilation in treatment of head injuries. Brit. Med. J., *4*:634–640, 1973.

69. Crockard, H. A., Hanlon, K., Ganc, E., and Duda, E. E.: Intracranial pressure gradients in a patient with a thalamic tumor. Surg. Neurol., *5*:151–155, 1976.

70. Cushing, H.: Concerning a definite regulatory mechanism of the vasomotor centre which controls blood pressure during cerebral compression. Bull. Johns Hopk. Hosp., *12*:290–292, 1901.

71. Cushing, H.: Some experimental and clinical observations concerning states of increased intracranial tension. Amer. J. Med. Sci., *124*:375–400, 1902.

72. Cushing, H.: The blood-pressure reaction of acute cerebral compression, illustrated by cases of intracranial hemorrhage. Amer. J. Med. Sci., *125*:1017–1045, 1903.

73. Cushing, H.: Studies in Intracranial Physiology and Surgery. London, Oxford University Press, 1925.

74. Czernicki, Z., Jurkiewicz, J., Kunicki, A.: Intracranial hypertension in head injury. Clinical significance and relation to respiration. *In* Lundberg, N., Ponten, U. and Brock, M., eds.: Intracranial Pressure II. Berlin, Springer-Verlag, 1975.

75. Dandy, W. E.: Diagnosis and treatment of injuries of the head. J.A.M.A., *101*:772–775, 1933.

76. deRougemont, J., Benabid, A. L., Chirossel, J. P., and Barge, M.: The brain vasomotor index

as prognosis leader in severe head injuries. *In* Beks, J. W. F., Bosch, D. A., and Brock, M., eds.: Intracranial Pressure III. Berlin, Springer-Verlag, 1976.

77. Dickinson, C. J., and McCubbin, J. W.: Pressor effect of increased cerebrospinal fluid pressure and vertebral artery occlusion with and without anesthesia. Circ. Res., *12*:190–202, 1963.

78. Dixon, W. E., and Halliburton, W. D.: The cerebro-spinal fluid. II. Cerebro-spinal pressure. J. Physiol. (London), *48*:128–153, 1914.

79. Dorsch, N. W. C., and Symon, L.: A practical technique for monitoring extradural pressure. J. Neurosurg., *42*:249–257, 1975.

80. Dorsch, N. W. C., Stephens, R. J., and Symon, L.: An intracranial pressure transducer, Biomed. Engin., *6*:452–457, 1971.

81. Ducker, T. B.: Increased intracranial pressure and pulmonary edema. Part 1: Clinical study of eleven cases. J. Neurosurg., *28*:112–117, 1968.

82. Ducker, T. B., and Simmons, R. L.: Increased intracranial pressure and pulmonary edema, Part 2: Hemodynamic response of dogs and monkeys to increased intracranial pressure. J. Neurosurg., *28*:118–123, 1968.

83. Ducker, T. B., and Simmons, R. L.: Increased intracranial pressure and pulmonary edema. Part 3: The effect of increased intracranial pressure on the cardio-vascular hemodynamics of chimpanzees. J. Neurosurg., *29*:475–483, 1968.

84. Ducker, T. B., Simmons, R. L., Anderson, R. W., and Kempe, L. G.: Hemodynamic cardiovascular response to raised intracranial pressure. Med. Ann. D.C., *37*:523–574, 1968.

85. Dunbar, H. S., Guthrie, T. C., and Karpell, B.: A study of the cerebrospinal fluid pulse wave. Arch. Neurol. (Chicago), *14*:624–639, 1966.

86. Edholm, O. G.: The relation of heart rate to intracranial pressure. J. Physiol. (London), *98*:442–445, 1940.

87. Ekstrom-Jodal, B., Haggendal, E., Johannson, B., Linder, L. E., and Nilsson, N. J.: Acute arterial hypertension and the blood-brain; an experimental study in dogs. *In* Langfitt, T. W., McHenry, L. C., Reivich, M., and Wollman, H., eds.: Cerebral Circulation and Metabolism. Berlin, Springer-Verlag, 1975.

88. Enevoldsen, E. M., and Jensen, F. T.: Compartmental analysis of regional cerebral blood flow in patients with acute severe head injury. J. Neurosurg., *47*:699–712, 1977.

89. Enevoldsen, E. M., Cold, G., Jensen, F. T., and Malmros, R.: Dynamic changes in regional CBF, intraventricular pressure, CSF pH, and lactate levels during the acute phase of head injury. J. Neurosurg., *44*:191–214, 1976.

90. Ethelberg, S., and Jensen, V. A.: Obscurations and further time-related paroxysmal disorders in intracranial tumors. Syndrome of initial herniation of parts of the brain through the tentorial incisure. Arch. Neurol. Psychiat., *68*:130–149, 1952.

91. Evans, J. P., Espey, F. F., Kristoff, F. V., Kimbell, F. D., and Ryder, H. W.: Experimental and clinical observations on rising intracranial pressure. Arch. Surg. (Chicago), *63*:107–114, 1951.

92. Eyster, J. A. E.: Clinical and experimental obser-

vations upon Cheyne-Stokes respiration. J. Exp. Med., *8*:565–613, 1906.

93. Eyster, J. A. E., Burrows, M. T., and Essick, C. R.: Studies on intracranial pressure. J. Exp. Med., *11*:489–514, 1909.

94. Fasano, V. A., Broggi, G., Urciuoli, R., DeNunno, T., and Lombard, G. F.: Clinical applications of hyperbaric oxygen and traumatic coma. *In* DeWets, A. C., ed.: Proceedings of the Third International Congress of Neurological Surgery. Excerpta Med., *110*: 502–505, 1966.

95. Faupel, G., Reulen, J., Muller, D., and Schurmann, K.: Double-blind study on the effects of steroids on severe closed head injury. *In* Pappius, H. M., and Fidel, W., eds.: Dynamics of Brain Edema. Berlin, Springer-Verlag, 1976.

96. Fay, T.: Comparative values of magnesium sulphate and sodium chloride for relief of intracranial tension. J.A.M.A., *82*:766–769, 1924.

97. Fay, T.: The control of intracranial pressure. J.A.M.A., *84*:1261, 1925.

98. Fieschi, C., Battistini, N., Beduschi, A., Boselli, L., and Rossanda, M.: Regional cerebral blood flow and intraventricular pressure in acute head injuries. J. Neurol. Neurosurg. Psychiat., *37*:1378–1388, 1974.

99. Finney, L. A., and Walker, A. E.: Transtentorial herniation. Springfield, Ill., Charles C Thomas, 1962.

100. Fitch, W., and McDowall, D. G.: Systemic vascular responses to increased intracranial pressure: 1. Effects of progressive epidural balloon expansion on intracranial pressure and systemic circulation. J. Neurol. Neurosurg. Psychiat., *40*:833–842, 1977.

101. Fitch, W., MacKenzie, E. T., and Harper, A. M.: Effects of decreasing arterial blood pressure on cerebral blood flow in the baboon. Circ. Res., *37*:550–557, 1975.

102. Fitch, W., Barker, J., Jennett, W. B., and McDowall, D. G.: The influence of neuroleptanalgesic drugs on cerebrospinal fluid pressure. Brit. J. Anaesth., *41*:800–806, 1969.

103. Fitch, W., McDowall, D. G., Keaney, M. P., and Pickerodt, V. W. A.: Systemic vascular responses to increased intracranial pressure: 2. The "Cushing" response in the presence of intracranial space-occupying lesions; systemic and cerebral haemodynamic studies in the dog and the baboon. J. Neurol. Neurosurg. Psychiat., *40*:843–852, 1977.

104. Fleischer, A. S., Payne, N. S., and Tindall, G. T.: Continuous monitoring of intracranial pressure in severe closed head injury without mass lesions. Surg. Neurol., *6*:31–34, 1976.

105. Foldes, F. F., and Arrowood, J. G.: Changes in cerebrospinal fluid pressure under the influence of continuous subarachnoidal infusion of normal saline. J. Clin. Invest., *27*:346–351, 1948.

106. Foley, J.: Benign forms of intracranial hypertension—"toxic" and "otitic" hydrocephalus. Brain, *78*:1–41, 1955.

107. Folkow, B.: Intravascular pressure as a factor regulating the tone of small vessels. Acta Physiol. Scand., *17*:289–310, 1948.

108. Forster, F. M.: The role of the brain stem in arterial hypertension subsequent to intracranial

hypertension. Amer. J. Physiol., *139*:347–350, 1943.

109. Frazier, C. H., and Peet, M. M.: The action of glandular extracts on the secretion of cerebrospinal fluid. Amer. J. Physiol., *36*:464–487, 1915.

110. Freeman, N. E., and Jeffers, W. A.: Effects of progressive sympathectomy on hypertension produced by increased intracranial pressure. Amer. J. Physiol., *128*:662–671, 1939–1940.

111. Frei, H. J., Poll, M., Reulen, H. J., Brock, M., and Schurmann, K.: Regional energy metabolism, tissue lactate content, and rCBF in cold injury oedema. *In* Russell, R., ed.: Brain and Blood Flow. London, Pitman Publishing Ltd., 1971.

112. French, L. A., and Galicich, J. H.: The use of steroids for control of cerebral edema. Clin. Neurosurg., *10*:212–223, 1964.

113. Gravel, J. A., Dechene, J. P., and Beaulieu, N.: L'hypothermie dans la prévention des lésions cérébrales consécutives à l'arrêt cardiaque. Laval Méd., *29*:48–60, 1960.

114. Galicich, J. H., French, L. A., and Melby, J. C.: Use of dexamethasone in treatment of cerebral edema associated with brain tumors. Lancet, *81*:46–53, 1961.

115. Gall, D. G., Cuty, E., McClung, H. J., and Greenberg, M. L.: Acute liver disease and encephalopathy mimicking Reye syndrome. J. Pediat., *87*:869–874, 1975.

116. Gamble, J. E., and Patton, H. D.: Pulmonary edema and hemorrhage from preoptic lesions in rats. Amer. J. Physiol., *172*:623–631, 1953.

117. Ganshirt, H., Hirsch, H., Krenkel, W., Schneider, M., and Zylka, W.: Über den Einfluss der Temperatursenkung auf die Erholungsfahigkeit des Warmblütergehirns. Arch. Exp. Path. Pharmak., *222*:431–449, 1954.

118. Gennarelli, T. A., Obrist, W. D., Langfitt, T. W., and Segawa, H.: Vascular and metabolic reactivity to changes in PCO_2 in head injured patients. *In* Bourke, R. S., ed.: Proceedings of the Third Chicago Symposium on Neural Trauma. New York, Raven Press, 1978.

119. Gilboe, D., Javid, M., and Frechette, P.: The fate and distribution of hypertonic urea solutions: A preliminary report. Surg. Forum, *11*:390–391, 1960.

120. Gobiet, W.: Monitoring of intracranial pressure in patients with severe head injury: A review of 100 cases. Acta Neurochir. (Wien), *20*:35–47, 1977.

121. Gobiet, W., Bock, W. J., Liesegant, J., and Grote, W.: Experience with an intracranial pressure transducer readjustable in vivo. Technical note. J. Neurosurg., *39*:272–276, 1974.

122. Goldstein, A., Jr., Wells, B. A., and Keats, A. S.: Increased tolerance to cerebral anoxia by pentobarbital. Arch. Int. Pharmacodyn. Ther., *161*:138–143, 1966.

123. Goluboff, B., Shenkin, H. A., and Haft, H.: The effects of mannitol and urea on cerebral hemodynamics and cerebrospinal fluid pressure. Neurology (Minneap.), *14*:891–898, 1964.

124. Gonzalez, N. C., Oberman, J., and Maxwell, J. A.: Circulatory effects of moderately and severely increased intracranial pressure in the dog. J. Neurosurg., *6*:721–726, 1972.

125. Gordon, E.: Post-traumatic and post-operative treatment of severe brain injuries with controlled hyperventilation. Acta Anaesth. Belg., *27*:suppl., 291–297, 1976.

126. Graf, C. J., and Rossi, N. P.: Pulmonary edema and the central nervous system. A clinicopathological study. Surg. Neurol., *4*:319–325, 1975.

127. Graham, D. I., and Adams, J. H.: Ischemic brain damage in fatal head injuries. *In* Brierley, J. B., and Meldrum, B. S., eds.: Brain Hypoxia. London, William Heinemann, Ltd., 1971.

128. Grant, F. C.: Value of hypertonic solutions in reducing intracranial pressures. Res. Publ. Ass. Res. Nerv. Ment. Dis., *8*:437, 1927.

129. Greenfield, J. C., and Tindall, G. T.: Effect of acute increase in intracranial pressure on blood flow in the internal carotid artery of man. J. Clin. Invest., *44*:1343–1351, 1965.

130. Grubb, R. L., Raichle, M. E., Eichling, J. O., and Gado, M. H.: The effects of subarachnoid hemorrhage upon regional cerebral blood volume, blood flow and oxygen utilization in man. *In* Harper, A. M., Jennett, B., Miller, D., and Rowan, J., eds.: Blood Flow and Metabolism in the Brain. Edinburgh, Churchill Livingstone, 1975.

131. Grubb, R. L., Raichle, M. E., Phelps, M. E., and Ratcheson, R. A.: Effects of increased intracranial pressure on cerebral blood volume, blood flow and oxygen utilization in monkeys. J. Neurosurg., *43*:385–398, 1975.

132. Grubb, R. L., Raichle, M. E., Gado, M. H., Eichling, J. O., and Hughes, C. P.: Cerebral blood flow, oxygen utilization, and blood volume in dementia. Neurology (Minneap.), *27*:905–910, 1977.

133. Guillaume, J., and Janny, P.: Manométrie intracranienne continue. Intérêt physiopatologique et clinique de la méthode. Press Méd., *59*:953–955, 1951.

134. Guisado, R., Tourtellotte, W. W., Arieff, A. I., Tomiyasu, U., Mishra, S. K., and Shotz, M. C.: Rebound phenomenon complicating cerebral dehydration with glycerol. J. Neurosurg., *42*:226–228, 1975.

135. Guyton, A. C., and Lindsey, A. W.: Effect of elevated left atrial pressure and decreased plasma protein concentration on the development of pulmonary edema. Circ. Res., *7*:649–657, 1959.

136. Hadjidimos, A., Steingass, U., Fischer, F., Reulen, H. J., and Schurmann, K.: The effect of dexamethasone on rCBF and cerebral vasomotor response in brain tumors. Europ. Neurol., *10*:25, 1973.

137. Hagerdal, M., Harp, J., Nilsson, L., and Siesjo, P. K.: The effect of induced hypothermia upon oxygen consumption in the rat brain. J. Neurochem., *24*:311–316, 1975.

138. Haggendal, E., and Johansson, B.: Effects of arterial carbon dioxide tension and oxygen saturation on cerebral blood flow and autoregulation in dogs. Acta Physiol. Scand., *66*:suppl. 258:27–53, 1965.

139. Hakim, S., and Adams, R. D.: The special clinical problem of symptomatic hydrocephalus with normal cerebrospinal fluid pressure. J. Neurol. Sci., *2*:307–327, 1965.

140. Hamer, J., Alberti, E., Hoyer, S., and Wiedemann, K.: Influence of systemic and cerebrovascular factors on the cerebrospinal fluid pulse waves. J. Neurosurg., 46:36–45, 1977.

141. Harper, A. M.: Autoregulation of cerebral blood flow, influence of the arterial blood pressure on the blood flow through the cerebral cortex. J. Neurol. Neurosurg. Psychiat., 29:398–403, 1966.

142. Harper, A. M., Deshmukh, V. D., Rowan, J. O., et al.: Influence of sympathetic nervous activity on cerebral blood flow. Arch. Neurol. (Chicago), 27:1–6, 1972.

143. Harper, M. A., and Bell, R. A.: The failure of intravenous urea to alter the blood flow to the cerebral cortex. J. Neurol. Neurosurg. Psychiat., 26:69–70, 1973.

144. Harrison, M. J. G., and Russel, R. W. R.: The effects of dexamethasone on experimental cerebral infarction in the gerbil. J. Neurol. Neurosurg. Psychiat., 35:520–521, 1972.

145. Hasenjäger, T., and Spatz, H.: Über örtliche Veränderungen der Konfiguration des Gehirns beim Hirndruck. Arch. Psychiat., 107:193–222, 1937.

146. Hass, W. K., Wald, A., Ransohoff, J., et al.: Argon and nitrous oxide cerebral blood flow simultaneously monitored by mass spectrometry in patients with head injury. Europ. Neurol., 8:164–168, 1972.

147. Hass, W. K., Kobayashi, M., Hochwald, G. M., Wald, A., Durogi, P., and Ransohoff, J.: Relationship of cerebral metabolic rate to brainstem injury. In Harper, A. M., Jennett, W. B., Miller, J. D., and Rowan, J. O., eds.: Blood Flow and Metabolism in the Brain. Edinburgh, Churchill Livingstone, 1976.

148. Hassler, O.: Arterial pattern of human brainstem. Normal appearance and deformation in expanding supratentorial conditions. Neurology (Minneap.), 17:368–375, 1967.

149. Hayashi, M., Marukawa, S., Fujii, H., Kitano, T., Kobayashi, H., and Yamamoto, S.: Intracranial hypertension in patients with ruptured intracranial aneurysm. J. Neurosurg., 46:584–590, 1977.

150. Haykawa, T., and Waltz, A. G.: Experimental subarachnoid hemorrhage from a middle cerebral artery. Stroke, 8:42–46, 1977.

151. Hedges, T. R., Weinstein, J. D., Kassell, N. F., and Stein, S.: Cerebrovascular responses to increased intracranial pressure. J. Neurosurg., 21:292–297, 1964.

152. Heistad, D. D., and Marcus, M. L.: Total and regional cerebral blood flow during stimulation of carotid baroreceptors. Stroke, 7:239–243, 1976.

153. Heistad, D. D., Marcus, M. L., Ehrhardt, J. C., et al.: Effect of stimulation carotid chemoreceptors on total and regional cerebral blood flow. Circ. Res., 38:20–25, 1976.

154. Hekmatpanah, J.: The sequence of alterations in the vital signs during acute experimental increased intracranial pressure. J. Neurosurg., 32:16–20, 1970.

155. Hekmatpanah, J.: Cerebral circulation and perfusion in experimental increased intracranial pressure. J. Neurosurg., 32:21–29, 1970.

156. Hill, L.: The physiology and pathology of the cerebral circulation: An experimental research. London, J. & A. Churchill Ltd., 1896.

157. Hodgson, J. S.: The relation between increased intracranial pressure and increased intraspinal pressure. Changes in the cerebrospinal fluid in increased intracranial pressure. Res. Publ. Ass. Res. Nerv. Ment. Dis., 8:182–188, 1927.

158. Hoff, H. E., and Breckenridge, C. G.: Intrinsic mechanisms in periodic breathing. Arch. Neurol. Psychiat., 72:11–42, 1954.

159. Hoff, J. T., and Reis, D. J.: The Cushing reflex. Localization of pressure-sensitive area in brainstem and spinal cord of cat. Neurology (Minneap.), 19:308, 1969.

160. Hoff, J. T., and Reis, D. J.: Localization of regions mediating the Cushing response in CNS of cats. Arch. Neurol. (Chicago), 23:228–240, 1970.

161. Howell, D. A.: Longitudinal brain stem compression with buckling. Arch. Neurol. Psychiat., 4:116–123, 1961.

162. Hughes, J., and LaPlace, L.: Effect of hypertonic solutions of sodium arabinate on cerebrospinal fluid pressure. J. Pharmacol. Exp. Ther., 38:363–383, 1930.

163. Ingvar, D. H., and Lundberg, N.: Paroxysmal symptoms in intracranial hypertension, studied with ventricular fluid pressure recording and electroencephalography. Brain, 84:446–459, 1961.

164. Jackson, H.: The management of acute cranial injuries by the early exact determination of intracranial pressure, and its relief by lumbar drainage. Surg. Gynec. Obstet., 34:494–508, 1922.

165. Jackson, J. H.: Neurological fragment. XV. Superior and subordinate centres of the lowest level. Lancet, 1:476–478, 1895.

166. Jacobson, I., Harper, A. M., and McDowall, D. G.: The effects of oxygen under pressure on cerebral blood flow and cerebral venous oxygen tension. Lancet, 2:549, 1963.

167. Jacobson, S. A., and Rothballer, A. B.: Prolonged measurement of experimental intracranial pressure using a subminiature absolute pressure transducer. J. Neurosurg., 26:603–608, 1967.

168. James, H. E., Langfitt, T. W., and Kumar, V. S.: Treatment of intracranial hypertension: Analysis of 105 consecutive continuous recordings of intracranial pressure. Acta Neurochir. (Wien), 36:189–200, 1977.

169. James, H. E., Bruno, L., Schut, L., and Shalna, E.: Intracranial subarachnoid pressure monitoring in children. Surg. Neurol., 3:313–315, 1975.

170. James, H. E., Bruno, L., Shapiro, H., Levitt, J. D., Adinas, S., Langfitt, T. W., and Shalna, E.: Methodology for intraventricular and subarachnoid continuous recording of intracranial pressure in clinical practice. Acta Neurochir. (Wien), 33:45–51, 1976.

171. James, I. M., and MacDonnell, L. A.: The role of baroreceptors and chemoreceptors in the regulation of the cerebral circulation. Clin. Sci. Mol. Med., 49:465–471, 1975.

172. James, I. M., Miller, R. A., and Purves, M. J.:

Observations on the extrinsic neural control of cerebral blood flow in the baboon. Circ. Res., 25:77–93, 1969.

173. Janeway, T. C.: The clinical study of blood pressure. New York, D. Appleton & Co., 1904.

174. Javid, M.: Urea—new use of an old agent. Reduction of intracranial and intraocular pressure. Surg. Clin. N. Amer., 38:907–928, 1958.

175. Javid, M.: A valuable new method for the reduction of intracranial and intraocular pressure by the use of urea. Trans. Amer. Neurol. Ass., pp. 113–116, 1958.

176. Javid, M.: Urea in intracranial surgery. A new method. J. Neurosurg., 18:51–57, 1961.

177. Javid, M., and Anderson, J.: Observations on the use of urea in rhesus monkeys. Surg. Forum, 9:686–690, 1958.

178. Javid, M., and Anderson, J.: The effect of urea on cerebrospinal fluid pressure in monkeys before and after bilateral nephrectomy. J. Lab. Clin. Med., 53:484–489, 1959.

179. Javid, M., and Settlage, P.: Effect of urea on cerebrospinal fluid pressure in human subjects. Preliminary report. J.A.M.A., 160:943–949, 1956.

180. Jefferson, G.: Tentorial pressure cone. Arch. Neurol. Psychiat., 40:857–876, 1938.

181. Jennett, S., and Hoff, J. T.: Arterial blood gases during raised intracranial pressure in anesthetized cats under controlled ventilation. J. Neurosurg., 48:390–401, 1978.

182. Jennett, W. B., McDowall, D. G., and Barker, J.: The effect of halothane on intracranial pressure in cerebral tumors. Report of two cases. J. Neurosurg., 26:270–274, 1967.

183. Jennett, W. B., Barker, J., Fitch, W., et al.: Effect of anesthesia on intracranial pressure in patients with space-occupying lesions. Lancet, 1:61–64, 1969.

184. Jennett, W. B., Harper, A. M., Miller, J. D., and Rowan, J. O.: Relation between cerebral blood flow and cerebral perfusion pressure. Brit. J. Surg., 57:390, 1970.

185. Jeppsson, P. G., and Nielsen, K.: The effect of hyperthermia on lesions of the blood-brain barrier produced by Umbradil. Excerpta Med., sec. 8:848–849, 1955.

186. Johnson, R. T., and Yates, P. O.: Tentorial herniation and midbrain deformity. A clinicopathological study. In Proceedings of the Second International Congress of Neuropathology. London, 1955, pp. 329–332.

187. Johnston, I. H., and Paterson, A.: Intracranial pressure monitoring in patients with benign intracranial hypertension. In Lundberg, N., Ponten, U., and Brock, M., eds.: Intracranial Pressure II. Berlin, Springer-Verlag, 1975.

188. Johnston, I. H., and Rowan, J. O.: Intracranial pressure gradients and cerebral blood flow. In Langfitt, T. W., McHenry, I. C., Reivich, M., and Wollman, H., eds.: Cerebral Circulation and Metabolism. Berlin, Springer-Verlag, 1975.

189. Johnston, I. H., Johnston, J. A., and Jennett, B.: Intracranial pressure changes following head injury. Lancet, 2:433–436, 1970.

190. Kahn, A. J.: Effects of variations in intracranial pressure. Arch. Neurol. Psychiat., 51:508–527, 1944.

191. Kahn, K., Pranzarone, G. F., and Newman, T.: Dexamethasone treatment of experimental cerebral infarction. Neurology (Minneap.), 22:406–407, 1972.

192. Kaufmann, G. E., and Clark, W. K.: Transmission of increased intracranial pressure across the tentorium in man. Surg. Forum, 20:437, 1969.

193. Kellie, G.: An account of the appearances observed in the dissection of two of three individuals presumed to have perished in the storm of the 3D, and whose bodies were discovered in the vicinity of Leith on the morning of the 4th, November 1821 with some reflections on the pathology of the brain. Trans. Med. Chir. Soc. Edinb., 1:84–169, 1824.

194. Kelly, P. J., Iwata, K., McGraw, C. P., and Tindall, G. T.: Intracranial pressure, cerebral blood flow and prognosis of patients with severe head injuries. In Langfitt, T. W., McHenry, L. C., Reivich, M., and Wollman, H., eds.: Cerebral Circulation and Metabolism. Berlin, Springer-Verlag, 1975.

195. Kernohan, J. W., and Woltman, H. E.: Incisura of the crus due to contralateral brain tumor. Arch. Neurol. Psychiat., 21:274–287, 1929.

196. Kindt, G. W., Walman, J., Kohl, S., Baublis, J., and Tucker, R.: Intracranial pressure in Reye's syndrome. J.A.M.A., 231:822, 1975.

197. Kjallquist, A., Lundberg, N., and Ponten, U.: Respiratory and cardiovascular changes during rapid spontaneous variations of ventricular fluid pressure in patients with intracranial hypertension. Acta Neurol. Scand., 40:291–317, 1964.

198. Kjellberg, R. N., and Prieto, A.: Bifrontal decompressive craniotomy for massive cerebral edema. J. Neurosurg., 34:488–493, 1971.

199. Klafta, L. A., and Hamby, W. B.: Significance of cerebrospinal fluid pressure in determining time for repair of intracranial aneurysms. J. Neurosurg., 31:217–219, 1969.

200. Klatzo, I., Wisniewski, H., Steinwall, O., and Steicher, E.: Dynamics of cold injury edema. In Klatzo, I., and Seitelberger, F., eds.: Brain Edema. New York, Springer-Verlag, 1967.

201. Kleeman, C. R., Davson, H., and Levin, E.: Urea transport in the central nervous system. Amer. J. Physiol., 203:739–747, 1962.

202. Knapp, A.: Die Tumoren des Schlaffenlappens. Z. Ges. Neurol. Psychiat., 42:226–289, 1918.

203. Kocher, T.: Hirnerschütterung, Hirndruck und chirurgische Eingriffe bei Hirnerkrankungen Nothnagel's specielle Pathologie und Therapie. Bid. ix, 3 Teil, 2 Abteilung, s 81, 1901.

204. Kofman, S., Garvin, J. S., Nagamani, D., and Taylor, S. G.: III. Treatment of cerebral metastases from breast carcinoma with prednisolone. J.A.M.A., 163:1473–1476, 1957.

205. Lambertsen, C. J., Kough, R. H., Cooper, D. Y., Emmell, G. L., Louschke, H. H., and Schmidt, C. F.: Oxygen toxicity: Effects in man of oxygen inhalation at 1 and 3.5 atmospheres upon blood gas transport, cerebral circulation and cerebral metabolism. J. Appl. Physiol., 5:471–486, 1953.

206. Langfitt, T. W.: Possible mechanisms of action of hypertonic urea in reducing intracranial pres-

sure. Neurology (Minneap.), *11*:196–209, 1961.

207. Langfitt, T. W.: The incidence and importance of intracranial hypertension in head injured patients. *In* Beks, J. W. F., Bosch, D. A., and Brock, M., eds.: Intracranial Pressure III. Berlin, Springer-Verlag, 1976.

208. Langfitt, T. W., and Kassell, N. F.: Acute brain swelling in neurosurgical patients. J. Neurosurg., *24*:975–983, 1966.

209. Langfitt, T. W., and Kassell, N. F.: Non-filling of cerebral vessels during angiography: Correlation with intracranial pressure. Acta Neurochir. (Wien), *14*:96–104, 1966.

210. Langfitt, T. W., and Kassell, N. F.: Cerebral vasodilatation produced by brainstem stimulation. Neurogenic control versus autoregulation. Amer. J. Physiol., *215*:90–97, 1968.

211. Langfitt, T. W., Kassell, N. F., and Weinstein, J. D.: Cerebral blood flow with intracranial hypertension. Neurology (Minneap.), *15*:761–773, 1965.

212. Langfitt, T. W., Weinstein, J. D., and Kassell, N. F.: Cerebral vasomotor paralysis produced by intracranial hypertension. Neurology (Minneap.), *15*:622–641, 1965.

213. Langfitt, T. W., Weinstein, J. D., Kassell, N. F., and Simeone, F. A.: Transmission of increased intracranial pressure. I. Within the craniospinal axis. J. Neurosurg., *21*:989–997, 1964.

214. Langfitt, T. W., Kumar, V. S., James, H. E., and Miller, J. D.: Continuous recording of intracranial pressure in patients with hypoxic brain damage. *In* Brierley, J. B., and Meldrum, B. S., eds.: Brain Hypoxia. Philadelphia, J. B. Lippincott Co., 1971.

215. Langfitt, T. W., Weinstein, J. D., Kassell, N. F., Gagliardi, L. J., and Shapiro, H. M.: Compression of cerebral vessels by intracranial hypertension. I. Dural sinus pressures. Acta Neurochir. (Wien), *15*:212–222, 1966.

216. Langfitt, T. W., Weinstein, J. D., Sklar, F. H., Zaren, H. A., and Kassell, N. F.: Contribution of intracranial blood volume to three forms of experimental brain swelling. Johns Hopkins Med. J., *122*:261–270, 1968.

217. Langfitt, T. W., Obrist, W. D., Gennarelli, T. A., O'Connor, M. J., and terWeeme, C. A.: Correlation of cerebral blood flow with outcome in head injured patients. Ann. Surg., *186*:411–414, 1977.

218. Laskowski, E. J., Klatzo, I., and Baldwin, M.: Experimental study of the effects of hypothermia on local brain injury. Neurology (Minneap.), *10*:499–505, 1960.

219. Lassen, N. A.: The luxury-perfusion syndrome and its possible relation to acute metabolic acidosis localized within the brain. Lancet, *2*:1113–1116, 1966.

220. Lassen, N. A., and Ingvar, D. H.: Regional cerebral flow measurement in man. Arch. Neurol. (Chicago), *9*:615, 1963.

221. Lazorthes, G., and Campan, L.: Hypothermia in the treatment of craniocerebral traumatism. J. Neurosurg., *15*:162–167, 1958.

222. Lazorthes, G., and Gaubert, J.: Les rapports du III de la clinoïde postérieure à sa pénétration dans le sinus caverneux. Bull. Ass. Anat., *40*:161–164, 1953.

223. Leech, P., and Miller, J. D.: Intracranial volume-pressure relationships during experimental brain compression in primates. 2. Effects of induced changes in arterial pressure. J. Neurol. Neurosurg. Psychiat., *37*:1099–1104, 1974.

224. Leech, P. J., and Miller, J. D.: Intracranial volume-pressure relationships during experimental brain compression of primates. 3. The effect of mannitol and hypocapnia. J. Neurol. Neurosurg. Psychiat., *37*:1105–1111, 1974.

225. Lemmen, L. J., and Davis, J. S.: Studies of cerebrospinal fluid pressure during hypothermia in intracranial surgery. Surg. Gynec. Obstet., *106*:555–558, 1958.

226. Levy, W. A., Taylor, J. M., Herzog, I., and Scheinberg, L. C.: The effect of hypertonic urea on cerebral edema in the rabbit induced by triethyl tin sulfate. Arch. Neurol. (Chicago), *13*:58–64, 1965.

227. Lindenberg, R.: Compression of brain arteries as pathogenetic factor for tissue necroses and their areas of predilection. J. Neuropath. Exp. Neurol., *14*:223–243, 1955.

228. Lippert, R. G., Svien, H. J., Grindlay, J. H., Goldstein, N. P., and Gastineau, C. F.: The effect of cortisone on experimental cerebral edema. J. Neurosurg., *17*:583–589, 1960.

229. Ljunggren, B., Granholm, L., Schutz, H., et al.: Energy state of the brain during and after compression ischemia. *In* Brock, M., and Dietz, H., eds.: Intracranial Pressure: Experimental and Clinical Aspects. Berlin, Springer-Verlag, 1972.

230. Lofgren, J.: Effects of variations in arterial pressure and arterial carbon dioxide tension on the cerebrospinal fluid pressure-volume relationship. Acta Neurol. Scand., *49*:586–598, 1973.

231. Lofgren, J., and Zwetnow, N. N.: Cranial and spinal components of the cerebrospinal fluid pressure-volume curve. Acta Neurol. Scand., *45*:575–585, 1973.

232. Lofgren, J., and Zwetnow, N. N.: Influence of a supratentorial expanding mass on intracranial pressure-volume relationship. Acta Neurol. Scand., *49*:599–612, 1973.

233. Lofgren, J., VonEssen, C., and Zwetnow, N. N.: The pressure-volume curve of the cerebrospinal fluid space in dogs. Acta Neurol. Scand., *49*:557–574, 1973.

234. Lowell, H. M., and Bloor, B. M.: The effect of increased intracranial pressure on cerebrovascular hemodynamics. J. Neurosurg., *34*:760–769, 1971.

235. Luisada, A. A.: Mechanism of neurogenic pulmonary edema. Amer. J. Cardiol., *20*:66–68, 1967.

236. Lundberg, N.: Continuous recording and control of ventricular fluid pressure in neurosurgical practice. Acta Psychiat. Scand., *36*:suppl. 149:1–193, 1960.

237. Lundberg, N., Kjallquist, A., and Bien, C.: Reduction of increased intracranial pressure by hyperventilation. Acta Psychiat. Scand., *34*:suppl. 139:1–64, 1959.

238. Lundberg, N., Troupp, H., and Lorin, H.: Continuous recording of the ventricular-fluid pressure in patients with severe acute traumatic brain injury. A preliminary report. J. Neurosurg., *22*:581–590, 1965.

239. MacKenzie, E. T., McGeorge, A. P., Graham, D. I., et al.: Breakthrough of cerebral autoregulations and the sympathetic nervous system. Acta Neurol. Scand., *56*:suppl. 64:48–49, 1977.

240. Magnaes, B.: Body position and cerebrospinal fluid pressure. Part 1: Clinical studies on the effect of rapid postural changes. J. Neurosurg., *44*:687–697, 1976.

241. Magnaes, B.: Body position and cerebrospinal fluid pressure. Part 2: Clinical studies on orthostatic pressure and the hydrostatic indifferent point. J. Neurosurg., *44*:698–705, 1976.

242. Maire, F. W., and Patton, H. D.: Neural structures evidence in the genesis of "preoptic pulmonary edema," gastric erosions and behavioral changes. Amer. J. Physiol., *184*:345–350, 1956.

243. Marmarou, A., Shulman, K., and Rosende, R. M.: A nonlinear analysis of the cerebrospinal fluid system and intracranial pressure dynamics. J. Neurosurg., *48*:332–344, 1978.

244. Marshall, L. F., and Langfitt, T. W.: Needle biopsy, high dose corticosteroids and radiotherapy in the treatment of malignant gliotumors. Conference on Modern Concepts in Brain Tumor Therapy. Laboratory and Clinical Investigation, National Cancer Institute, Monograph 46, 1977.

245. Marshall, L. F., Bruce, D. A., Bruno, L. A., and Schut, L.: Role of intracranial pressure monitoring and barbiturate therapy in malignant intracranial hypertension. J. Neurosurg., *47*:481–484, 1977.

246. Marshall, L. F., Bruce, D. A., Graham, D. I., and Langfitt, T. W.: Alterations in behavior, brain electrical activity, cerebral blood flow and intracranial pressure produced by triethyl tin sulfate induced cerebral edema. Stroke, *7*:21–25, 1976.

247. Marshall, L. F., Smith, R. W., Rauscher, L. A., and Shapiro, H. M.: Mannitol dose requirements in brain-injured patients. J. Neurosurg., *48*:169–172, 1978.

248. Marshall, L. F., Welsh, F., Durity, F., Lounsbury, R., Graham, D. I., and Langfitt, T. W.: Experimental cerebral oligemia and ischemia produced by intracranial hypertension. Part 2: Brain morphology. J. Neurosurg., *43*:318–322, 1975.

249. Marshall, L. F., Welsh, F., Durity, F., Lounsbury, R., Graham, D. I., and Langfitt, T. W.: Experimental cerebral oligemia and ischemia produced by intracranial hypertension. Part 3: Brain energy metabolism. J. Neurosurg., *43*:323–328, 1975.

250. Marshall, W. J. S., Jackson, J. L. F., and Langfitt, T. W.: Brain swelling caused by trauma and arterial hypertension. Arch. Neurol. (Chicago), *21*:545–553, 1969.

251. Martin, S. M., Simmons, R. L., and Heisterkamp, C. A.: Respiratory insufficiency in combat casualties. I. Pathologic changes in the lungs of patients dying of wounds. Ann. Surg., *170*:30–37, 1969.

252. Martins, A. N., Kobine, A. I., and Larsen, D. F.: Pressure in the sagittal sinus during intracranial hypertension in man. J. Neurosurg., *40*:603–608, 1974.

253. Mason, M. S., and Raaf, J.: Physiological alterations and clinical effects of urea-induced diuresis. J. Neurosurg., *18*:645–653, 1961.

254. Masserman, J. H.: Effects of intravenous administration of hypertonic solutions of dextrose. With special reference to the cerebrospinal fluid pressure. J.A.M.A., *102*:2084–2086, 1934.

255. Matakas, F., Eibs, G., and Cuypers, J.: Effect of systemic arterial blood pressure on cerebral blood flow in intracranial hypertension. J. Neurol. Neurosurg. Psychiat., *38*:1206–1210, 1975.

256. Mathew, N. T., Meyer, J. S., and Ott, E. O.: Increased cerebral blood volume in benign intracranial hypertension. Neurology (Minneap.), *25*:646–649, 1975.

257. Maxwell, J. A., and Goodwin, J. M.: Neurogenic pulmonary shunting. J. Trauma, *13*:368–373, 1973.

258. Maxwell, R. E., Long, D. M., and French, L. A.: The effects of glucosteroids on experimental cold-induced brain edema: Gross morphological alterations in vascular permeability changes. J. Neurosurg., *34*:477–487, 1971.

259. McDowall, D. G.: The current usage of hypothermia in British neurosurgery. Brit. J. Anaesth., *43*:1084–1087, 1971.

260. McDowall, D. G., Barker, J., and Jennett, W. B.: Cerebro-spinal fluid measurements during anaesthesia. Anaesthesia, *21*:189–201, 1966.

261. McGraw, C. P.: Continuous intracranial pressure monitoring: Review of techniques and presentation of method. Surg. Neurol., *6*:149–155, 1976.

262. McNealy, D. E., and Plum, F.: Brain stem dysfunction with supratentorial mass lesions. Arch. Neurol. Psychiat., *7*:10–32, 1962.

263. McQueen, J. D., and Jeanes, L. D.: Dehydration and rehydration of the brain with hypertonic urea and mannitol. J. Neurosurg., *21*:118–128, 1964.

264. Mead, C. O., Moody, R. A., Ruamsuke, S., and Mullan, S. F.: Effect of isovolemic hemodilution on cerebral blood flow following experimental head injury. J. Neurosurg., *32*:40–50, 1970.

265. Meinig, G., Aulich, A., Wende, S., and Reulen, H. J.: The effect of dexamethasone and diuretics on peritumor brain edema: Comparative study of tissue water content and CT dynamics of brain edema. *In* Pappius, H. M., and Feindel, W., eds.: Dynamics of Brain Edema. Berlin, Springer-Verlag, 1976.

266. Meyer, A.: Herniation of the brain. Arch. Neurol. Psychiat., *4*:387–400, 1920.

267. Meyer, J. S., and Hunter, J.: Effects of hypothermia on local blood flow and metabolism during cerebral ischemia and hypoxia. J. Neurosurg., *14*:210–227, 1957.

268. Meyer, J. S., Fukuuchi, Y., Shimazu, K., Ohuchi, T., and Ericsson, A. D.: Effect of intravenous infusion of glycerol on hemispheric blood flow and metabolism in patients with acute cerebral infarction. Stroke, *3*:168–180, 1972.

269. Meyers, R.: Systemic vascular and respiratory effects of experimentally induced alterations in intraventricular pressure. J. Neuropath. Exp. Neurol., *1*:241–264, 1942.

270. Mickell, J. J., Reigel, D. H., Cook, D. R., Binda, R. E., and Safar, P.: Intracranial pressure: Monitoring and normalization therapy in children. Pediatrics, 59:606–613, 1977.

271. Miller, J. D., and Leech, H. P.: Effects of mannitol and steroid therapy on intracranial volume-pressure relationship in patients. J. Neurosurg., 42:274–281, 1975.

272. Miller, J. D., and Garibi, J.: Intracranial volume-pressure relationships during continuous monitoring of ventricular fluid pressure. In Brock, M., and Dietz, H., eds.: Intracranial Pressure: Experimental and Clinical Aspects. Berlin, Springer-Verlag, 1972.

273. Miller, J. D., and Levingham, I. A.: Reduction of increased intracranial pressure: Comparison between hyperbaric oxygen and hyperventilation. Arch. Neurol. (Chicago), 24:210–216, 1971.

274. Miller, J. D., Garabi, J., and Pickard, J. D.: Induced changes of cerebrospinal fluid volume. Effects during continuous monitoring of ventricular fluid pressure. Arch. Neurol. (Chicago), 28:265–269, 1973.

275. Miller, J. D., Levingham, I. A., and Jennett, W. B.: Effects of hyperbaric oxygen on intracranial pressure and cerebral blood flow in experimental cerebral edema. J. Neurol. Neurosurg. Psychiat., 33:745–755, 1970.

276. Miller, J. D., Stanek, A., and Langfitt, T. W.: Concepts of cerebral perfusion pressure and vascular compression during intracranial hypertension. Progr. Brain Res., 35:411–432, 1971.

277. Miller, J. D., Stanek, A. E., and Langfitt, T. W.: Cerebral blood flow regulations during experimental brain compression. J. Neurosurg., 39:186–196, 1973.

278. Miller, J. D., Becker, D. P., Ward, J. D., Sullivan, H. G., Adams, W. E., and Rosner, M. J.: Significance of intracranial hypertension in severe head injury. J. Neurosurg., 47:503–516, 1977.

279. Mogami, H., Hayakawa, T., Kanai, N., Kuroda, R., Yamada, R., Ikeda, T., Katsurada, K., and Sugimoto, T.: Clinical application of hyperbaric oxygenation in the treatment of acute cerebral damage. J. Neurosurg., 31:636–643, 1969.

280. Monro, A.: Observations on the Structure and Function of the Nervous System. Edinburgh, Creech & Johnson, 1783.

281. Moody, R. A., and Mullan, S.: Head injury monitoring: A preliminary report. J. Trauma, 11:458–462, 1971.

282. Moody, R. A., Ruamsuke, S., and Mullan, S. F.: An evaluation of decompression in experimental head injury. J. Neurosurg., 29:586–590, 1968.

283. Moody, R. A., Ruamsuke, S., and Mullan, S.: Experimental effects of acutely increased intracranial pressure on respiration and blood gases. J. Neurosurg., 30:482–493, 1969.

284. Moody, R. A., Mead, C. O., Ruamsuke, S., and Mullan, S. F.: Therapeutic value of oxygen at normal and hyperbaric pressure in experimental head injury. J. Neurosurg., 32:51–54, 1970.

285. Moutier, F.: Hypertension et mort par oedème pulmonaire aigu chez les blessés crân-

ioencéphaliques (relation de ces faits aux recherches récentes sur les functions des capsules surrénales). Presse Méd., 26:108, 1918.

286. Munro, D., and Sisson, W. R., Jr.: Hernia through the incisura of the tentorium cerebelli in connection with craniocerebral trauma. New Eng. J. Med., 247:699–708, 1952.

287. Myerson, A., and Loman, J.: Internal jugular venous pressure and its relationship to cerebral spinal fluid pressure. J. Nerv. Ment. Dis., 74:192–194, 1931.

288. Nakagawa, Y., Mitsuo, T., and Yada, K.: Site and mechanism for compression of the venous system during experimental intracranial hypertension. J. Neurosurg., 41:427–434, 1974.

289. Nornes, H.: The role of intracranial pressure in the arrest of hemorrhage in patients with ruptured intracranial aneurysm. J. Neurosurg., 39:226–234, 1973.

290. Nornes, H., and Magnaes, B.: Intracranial pressure in patients with ruptured saccular aneurysm. J. Neurosurg., 36:537–547, 1972.

291. Nornes, H., and Serck-Hanssen, F.: Miniature transducer for intracranial pressure monitoring in man. Acta Neurol. Scand., 46:203–214, 1970.

292. Numoto, M., Wallman, J. K., and Donaghy, R. M. P.: Pressure indicating bag for monitoring intracranial pressure. Technical note. J. Neurosurg., 39:784–787, 1973.

293. Nylin, G., Hedlund, S., and Regnstrom, O.: Studies of the cerebral circulation with labeled erythrocytes in healthy man. Circ. Res., 9:664–674, 1961.

294. Obrist, W. D., Thompson, H. K., King, C. H., and Wang, H. S.: Determination of regional cerebral blood flow by inhalation of 133-Xenon. Circ. Res., 20:124–135, 1967.

295. Obrist, W. D., Langfitt, T. W., terWeeme, C. A., O'Connor, M. J., Gennarelli, T. W., Zimmerman, R. A., and Kuhl, D. E.: Non-invasive, long-term serial studies of rCBF in acute head injury. In Ingvar, D. H. and Lassen, N. A., ed.: Cerebral Function, Metabolism and Circulation. Copenhagen, Munksgaard, 1977.

296. Ott, E. O., Matthew, N. T., and Meyer, J. S.: Redistribution of regional cerebral blood flow after glycerol infusion in acute cerebral infarction. Neurology (Minneap.), 24:1117–1126, 1974.

297. Overgaard, J.: Reflections on prognostic determinants in acute severe head injury. In McLaurin, R. L., ed.: Head Injuries, Second Chicago Symposium on Neural Trauma. New York, Grune & Stratton Inc., 1976.

298. Overgaard, J., and Tweed, W. A.: Cerebral circulation after head injury. Part I: Cerebral blood flow and its regulation after closed head injury with emphasis on clinical correlations. J. Neurosurg., 41:531–541, 1974.

299. Overgaard, J., and Tweed, W. A.: rCBF in impending brain death. Acta Neurochir. (Wien), 31:167–175, 1975.

300. Overgaard, J., and Tweed, W. A.: Cerebral circulation after head injury. Part 2. The effects of traumatic brain edema. J. Neurosurg., 45:292–300, 1976.

301. Paine, R., Smith, J. R., Butcher, H. R., and Howard, F. A.: Heart failure and pulmonary

edema produced by certain neurologic stimuli. Circulation, 5:759–765, 1952.

302. Papo, I., and Caruselli, G.: Intracranial pressure monitoring in intensive care patients suffering from acute head injuries. *In* Beks, J. W. F., Bosch, D. A., and Brock, M., eds.: Intracranial Pressure III. Berlin, Springer-Verlag, 1976.

303. Pappius, H. M., and Dayes, L. A.: Hypertonic urea. Arch. Neurol. (Chicago), 13:395–402, 1965.

304. Pappius, H. M., and McCann, W. P.: Effects of steroids on cerebral edema in cats. Arch. Neurol. (Chicago), 20:207–216, 1969.

305. Parkes, J. D., and James, I. M.: Electroencephalographic and cerebral blood flow changes following spontaneous subarachnoid hemorrhage. Brain, 94:69–76, 1971.

306. Paul, R. L., Polanco, B., Turney, S. Z., McAslan, T. C., and Cowley, R. A.: Intracranial pressure responses to alterations in arterial carbon dioxide pressure in patients with head injuries. J. Neurosurg., 36:714–720, 1972.

307. Paulson, O. B.: Regional cerebral blood flow in apoplexy due to occlusion of the middle cerebral artery. Neurology (Minneap.), 20:63–77, 1970.

308. Paulson, O. B., Olesen, J., and Christensen, M. S.: Restoration of autoregulation and cerebral blood flow by hypocapnia. Neurology (Minneap.), 22:286–293, 1972.

309. Penfield, W., and Jasper, H.: Epilepsy and the functional anatomy of the human brain. Boston, Little, Brown & Co., 1954.

310. Penfield, W., and MacEachern, D.: Intracranial tumors. Oxford Medicine, Chap. VI, pp. 137–216, 1938.

311. Plum, F.: Neural mechanisms of abnormal respiration in humans. Arch. Neurol. (Chicago), 3:484–487, 1960.

312. Plum, F., and Swanson, A. G.: Central neurogenic hyperventilation in man. Arch. Neurol. Psychiat., 81:535–549, 1959.

313. Plum, F., Alvord, E. C., and Posner, J. B.: The effect of steroids on experimental cerebral infarction. Arch. Neurol. (Chicago), 9:571–573, 1963.

314. Plum, F., Posner, J. B., and Zee, D.: The relationship of cerebral blood flow to CO_2 tension in the blood and pH in the cerebrospinal fluid respectively. Scand. J. Lab. Clin. Invest., 22:suppl. 102:8:F, 1968.

315. Poll, W., Brock, M., Markakis, E., Winkelmuller, W., and Dietz, H.: Brain tissue pressure. *In* Brock, M., and Dietz, H., eds.: Intracranial Pressure: Experimental and Clinical Aspects. Berlin, Springer-Verlag, 1973.

316. Pollock, L. J., and Boshes, B.: Cerebrospinal fluid pressure. Arch. Neurol. Psychiat., 36:931–974, 1936.

317. Ponte, J., and Purves, M. J.: The role of the carotid body chemoreceptors and carotid sinus baroreceptors in the control of cerebral blood vessels. J. Physiol. (London), 237:315–340, 1974.

318. Quincke, H.: Ueber meningitis serosa und verwandte Zustande. Deutsch. Z. Nervenheilk., 9:149, 1897.

319. Raichle, M. E., and Plum, F.: Hyperventilation in cerebral blood flow. Stroke, 3:566–575, 1972.

320. Raichle, M. D., Hartmann, B. K., Eichling, J. O., et al.: Central noradrenergic regulation of cerebral blood flow and vascular permeability. Proc. Nat. Acad. Sci. U.S.A., 72:3726–3730, 1975.

321. Raichle, M. E., Grubb, R. L., Phelps, M. E., Gada, J. H., and Caronna, J. J.: Cerebral hemodynamics and metabolism in pseudotumor cerebri. Ann Neurol., 4:104–111, 1978.

322. Ransohoff, J., Benjamin, M. V., Gage, E. L., and Epstein, F.: Hemicraniectomy in the management of acute subdural hematoma. J. Neurosurg., 34:70–76, 1971.

323. Rapela, C. A., Green, H. D., and Denison, A. B.: Baroreceptor reflexes and autoregulation of cerebral blood flow in the dog. Circ. Res., 21:559–568, 1967.

324. Rapoport, S. I.: The effect of concentrated solutions on blood brain barrier. Amer. J. Physiol., 219:270–274, 1970.

325. Rapoport, S. I., Hori, M., and Klatzo, I.: Testing of a hypothesis for osmotic blood-brain barrier. Amer. J. Physiol., 223:323–331, 1972.

326. Rasmussen, T., and Gulati, D.: Cortisone in the treatment of postoperative cerebral edema. J. Neurosurg., 19:535–544, 1962.

327. Rawling, L. B.: Cerebral oedema (excess cerebrospinal fluid). Its causation and surgical treatment. Brit. Med. J., 1:499–502, 1918.

328. Reed, D. J., and Woodbury, D. M.: Effect of hypertonic urea on cerebrospinal fluid pressure and brain volume. J. Physiol. (London), 164:252–264, 1962.

329. Reed, D. J., and Woodbury, D. M.: Effect of urea and acetazolamide on brain volume and cerebrospinal fluid pressure. J. Physiol. (London), 164:265–273, 1962.

330. Reid, W. L.: Cerebral herniation through the incisura tentorii. Surgery, 8:756–770, 1940.

331. Reivich, M.: Arterial pCO_2 and cerebral hemodynamics. Amer. J. Physiol., 206:25–35, 1964.

332. Reivich, M., Marshall, W. J. S., and Kassell, N.: Loss of autoregulation produced by cerebral trauma. *In* Brock, M., Fieschi, E., Ingvar, D. H., Lassen, N. A., and Schurmann, K., eds.: Cerebral Blood Flow. Berlin, Springer-Verlag, 1969.

333. Renaudin, J., Fewer, D., Wilson, C. B., Boldren, E. B., Calogero, J., Enot, K. J.: Dose dependency of Decadron in patients with partially excised brain tumors. J. Neurosurg., 39:302–305, 1973.

334. Reulen, H. J., and Kreysch, H. G.: Measurement of brain tissue pressure in cold induced cerebral edema. Acta Neurochir. (Wien), 29:29–40, 1973.

335. Reulen, H. J., Graham, R., Spatz, M., and Klatzo, I.: Role of pressure gradients and bulk flow in dynamics of vasogenic brain edema. J. Neurosurg., 46:24–35, 1977.

336. Reye, R. D. K., Morgan, G., and Barol, J.: Encephalopathy and fatty degeneration of the viscera: A disease entity in childhood. Lancet, 2:749, 1963.

337. Risberg, J., Lundberg, N., and Ingvar, D. H.: Regional cerebral blood volume during acute transient rises of the intracranial pressure (pla-

teau waves). J. Neurosurg., *31*:303–310, 1969.

338. Roberts, H. J.: Supportive adrenocortical steroid therapy in acute and subacute cerebrovascular accidents, with particular reference to brainstem involvement. J. Amer. Geriat. Soc., 6:686–702, 1958.

339. Rodbard, S., and Stone, W.: Pressor mechanisms induced by intracranial compression. Circulation, *12*:883–889, 1955.

340. Rosner, M. J., and Becker, D. P.: ICP monitoring: Complications and associated factors. Clin. Neurosurg., *23*:494–519, 1975.

341. Rosomoff, H. L.: Method for simultaneous quantitative estimation of intracranial contents. J. Appl. Physiol., *16*:395–396, 1961.

342. Rosomoff, H. L., and Gilbert, R.: Brain volume and cerebrospinal fluid pressure during hypothermia. Amer. J. Physiol., *183*:19–22, 1955.

343. Rosomoff, H. L., and Holaday, D. A.: Cerebral blood flow and cerebral oxygen consumption during hypothermia. Amer. J. Physiol., *179*:85–88, 1954.

344. Rosomoff, H. L., Clasen, R. A., Hartstock, R., and Bebin, J.: Brain reaction to experimental injury after hypothermia. Arch. Neurol. (Chicago), *13*:337–345, 1965.

345. Rossanda, M., Selematia, Villa, C. and Beduschia: J. Neurol. Sci., *17*:265–270, 1973.

346. Rossanda, M., Collice, M., Porta, M., and Roselli, L.: Intracranial hypertension in head injury. Clinical significance and relation to respiration. *In* Lundberg, N., Ponten, U., and Brock, M., eds.: Intracranial Pressure II Berlin, Springer-Verlag, 1975.

347. Rovit, R. L., and Hagan, R.: Steroids and cerebral edema: The effects of glucocorticoids on abnormal capillary permeability following cerebral injury in cats. J. Neuropath. Exp. Neurol., *27*:277–299, 1968.

348. Rowed, D. W., Leech, P. J., Reilly, P. L., and Miller, J. D.: Hypocapnia and intracranial volume-pressure relationship. Arch. Neurol. (Chicago), *32*:369–373, 1975.

349. Rubio, R., Berne, R. M., Bockman, E. L., et al.: Relationship between adenosine concentration and oxygen supply in rat brain. Amer. J. Physiol., *228*:1896–1902, 1975.

350. Russek, H. I., Zohman, B. L., and Russek, A. S.: Cortisone in the immediate therapy of apoplectic stroke. J. Amer. Geriat. Soc., 2:216–228, 1954.

351. Ryder, H. W., Rosenauer, A., Penka, E. J., Espey, F. F., and Evans, J. P.: Failure of abnormal cerebrospinal fluid pressure to influence cerebral function. Arch. Neurol. Psychiat., *70*:563–586, 1953.

352. Ryder, H. W., Espey, F. F., Kimbell, F. D., Penka, E. J., Rosenauer, A., Podolsky, B., and Evans, J. P.: Influence of changes in cerebral blood flow on the cerebrospinal fluid pressure. Arch. Neurol. Psychiat., *68*:165–169, 1952.

353. Ryder, H. W., Espey, F. F., Kimbell, F. D., Penka, E. J., Rosenauer, A., Podolsky, B., and Evans, J. P.: The mechanism of the change in cerebrospinal fluid pressure following an induced change in the volume of the fluid space. J. Lab. Clin. Med., *41*:428–435, 1953.

354. Rylander, H. G., Taylor, H. L., Wissinger, J. P., and Story, J. L.: Chronic measurement of epidural pressure with an induction-powered oscillator transducer. J. Neurosurg., *44*:465–478, 1976.

355. Sagawa, K., Ross, J. M., and Guyton, A. C.: Quantitation of cerebral ischemic pressor response in dogs. Amer. J. Physiol., *200*:1164–1168, 1961.

356. Sahs, A. L., and Joynt, R. J.: Brain swelling of unknown cause. Neurology (Minneap.), 6:791–803, 1956.

357. Scheinker, I. M.: Transtentorial herniation of the brain stem. Characteristic clinico-pathological syndrome. Pathogenesis of hemorrhages in brain stem. Arch. Neurol. Psychiat., *53*:289–303, 1945.

358. Schettini, A., and Walsh, E. K.: Pressure relaxation of the intracranial system in vivo. Amer. J. Physiol., *225*:513–517, 1973.

359. Schettini, A., and Walsh, E. K.: Experimental identification of the subarachnoid and subpial compartments by intracranial pressure measurements. J. Neurosurg., *40*:609–616, 1974.

360. Schmiedek, P., Baethmann, A., Brendel, W., Schneider, E., Enzenbach, R., and Marguth, F.: Treatment of cerebral edema in man with spirolactone. *In* Brock, M., and Dietz, H., eds.: Intracranial Pressure: Experimental and Clinical Aspects. Berlin, Springer-Verlag, 1973.

361. Schmiedek, P., Guggemos, L., Baethmann, A., Lanksch, W., Kazner, E., Picha, P., Olteanu-Nerbe, V., Enzenbach, R., Brendel, W., and Marguth, F.: Re-evaluation of short-term steroid therapy for perifocal edema. *In* Pappius, H. M., and Feindel, W., eds.: Dynamics of Brain Edema. Berlin, Springer-Verlag, 1976.

362. Schoolar, J. C., Barlow, C. F., and Roth, L. J.: The penetration of carbon-14 urea into cerebrospinal fluid and various areas of the cat brain. J. Neuropath. Exp. Neurol., *19*:216–227, 1960.

363. Schut, L., and Bruce, D. A.: Case report: Giant aneurysms of middle cerebral artery in infants. Proceedings from the Scientific Session, 2nd International Society for Pediatric Neurosurgery, Jerusalem, September, 1978.

364. Schutz, H., and Taylor, F. A.: Intracranial pressure and cerebral blood flow monitoring in head injuries. Canad. Med. Ass. J., *116*:609–613, 1978.

365. Sedzimir, C. R.: Therapeutic hypothermia in cases of head injury. J. Neurosurg., *16*:407–414, 1959.

366. Selkurt, E. E.: The changes in renal clearance following complete ischemia of the kidney. Amer. J. Physiol., *144*:395–403, 1945.

367. Severinghaus, J. W., and Lassen, N.: Step hypocapnia to separate arterial from tissue pCO_2 in the regulation of cerebral blood flow. Circ. Res., *20*:272–278, 1967.

368. Shalit, M. N., and Cotev, S.: Interrelationship between blood pressure and regional cerebral blood flow in experimental intracranial hypertension. J. Neurosurg., *40*:594–602, 1974.

369. Shalit, M. N., Shimojyo, S., and Reinmuth, O. M.: Carbon dioxide and cerebral circulatory control. I. The extra-vascular effect. Arch. Neurol. (Chicago), *17*:298–303, 1967.

370. Shapiro, H. M., and Aidinis, S. J.: Neurosurgical anesthesia. Surg. Clin. N. Amer., 55:913–928, 1975.

371. Shapiro, H. M., Langfitt, T. W., and Weinstein, J. D.: Compression of cerebral vessels by intracranial hypertension. II. Morphological evidence for collapse of vessels. Acta Neurochir. (Wien), 12:223–233, 1966.

372. Shapiro, H. M., Wyte, S. R., and Harris, A. B.: Ketamine anesthesia in patients with intracranial pathology. Brit. J. Anaesth., 44:1200–1204, 1972.

373. Shapiro, H. M., Wyte, S. R., and Loeser, J.: Barbiturate-augmented hypothermia for reduction of persistent intracranial hypertension. J. Neurosurg., 40:90–100, 1974.

374. Shapiro, H. M., Stromberg, D. D., Lee, D. R., et al.: Dynamic pressures in the pial arterial microcirculation. Amer. J. Physiol., 221:279–283, 1971.

375. Sharpe, W.: The Diagnosis and Treatment of Brain Injuries. Philadelphia, J. B. Lippincott Co., 1920, pp. 108–137.

376. Sharpe, W.: Repeated lumbar punctures and spinal drainage: Diagnostic and therapeutic value in traumatic and allied lesions of the central nervous system. J.A.M.A., 104:959–965, 1935.

377. Shaywitz, B. A., Leventhal, H. J., Cramer, M. S., and Venes, J. L.: Prolonged continuous monitoring of intracranial pressure in severe Reye's syndrome. Pediatrics, 59:595–605, 1977.

378. Shenken, H. A., Goluboff, B., and Haft, H.: The use of mannitol for the reduction of intracranial pressure in intracranial surgery. J. Neurosurg., 19:897–901, 1962.

379. Shulman, K.: Small artery and vein pressures in the subarachnoid space of the dog. J. Surg. Res., 5:56–61, 1965.

380. Shulman, K., and Marmarou, K.: Pressure-volume considerations in infantile hydrocephalus. Develop. Med. Child Neurol., 13:suppl. 25:90–95, 1971.

381. Shulman, K., and Rosomoff, H. L.: Effect of hypothermia on mortality in experimental injury to the brain. Amer. J. Surg., 98:704–705, 1959.

382. Shulman, K., and Verdier, G. R.: Cerebral vascular resistance changes in response to cerebrospinal fluid pressure. Amer. J. Physiol., 213:1084–1088, 1967.

383. Siegel, B. A., Studer, R. K., and Potchen, E. J.: Steroid therapy of brain edema: Ineffectiveness in experimental cerebral microembolism. Arch. Neurol. (Chicago), 27:209–212, 1972.

384. Siesjo, B. K., and Plum, F.: The brain in normoxia and in hypoxia. Acta Anesthes. Scand., suppl., 45:81–101, 1972.

385. Simeone, F. A., Ryan, K. G., and Cotton, J. R.: Prolonged experimental cerebral vasospasm. J. Neurosurg., 29:357–366, 1968.

386. Sklar, F. H., and Elashvili, I.: The pressure-volume function of brain elasticity: Physiological considerations and clinical applications. J. Neurosurg., 47:670–679, 1977.

387. Sklar, F. H., Burke, E. F., Jr., and Langfitt, T. W.: Cerebral blood volume: Values obtained with ^{51}Cr-labeled red blood cells and RISA. J. Appl. Physiol., 24:79–82, 1968.

388. Sloviter, H. A.: Effects of intravenous administration of glycerol solutions to animals and man. J. Clin. Invest., 37:619–626, 1958.

389. Smith, A. L., and Wollman, H.: Cerebral blood flow and metabolism. Anesthesiology, 36:378–400, 1972.

390. Smith, D. R., Jacobson, J., Kobrine, A. I., and Rizzoli, H. V.: Regional cerebral blood flow with intracranial mass lesions. Part I. Local alterations in cerebral blood flow. Surg. Neurol., 7:233–237, 1977.

391. Smith, D. R., Jacobson, J., Kobrine, A. I., and Rizzoli, H. V.: Regional cerebral blood flow with intracranial mass lesions. Part II. Autoregulation in localized mass lesion. Surg. Neurol., 7:238–240, 1977.

392. Smyth, G. E., and Henderson, W. R.: Observations on the cerebrospinal fluid pressure on simultaneous ventricular and lumbar punctures. J. Neurol. Psychiat., 1:226–237, 1938.

393. Sokoloff, L.: Influence of functional activity on local cerebral glucose utilization. In Ingvar, D. A., and Lassen, N. A., eds.: Brain Work. The Coupling of Function, Metabolism and Blood Flow in the Brain. New York, Academic Press, 1975.

394. Stein, S., and Langfitt, T. W.: Normal pressure hydrocephalus. J. Neurosurg., 4:463–470, 1974.

395. Stern, W. E., and Good, R. G.: Studies of the effects of hypothermia upon cerebrospinal fluid oxygen tension and carotid blood flow. Surgery, 48:13–30, 1960.

396. Stromberg, D. D., and Fox, J. R.: Pressures in the pial arterial microcirculation of the cat during changes in systemic arterial blood pressure. Circ. Res., 31:229–239, 1972.

397. Sullivan, H. G., Miller, J. D., Becker, D. P., Flora, R. E., and Allen, G. A.: The physiological basis of intracranial pressure change with progressive epidural brain compression. J. Neurosurg., 47:532–550, 1977.

398. Sunderland, S.: The tentorial notch and complications produced by herniations of the brain through that aperture. Brit. J. Surg., 45:422–438, 1958.

399. Sunderland, S., and Hughes, E. S. R.: The pupilloconstrictor pathway and the nerves to the ocular muscles in man. Brain, 69:301–309, 1946.

400. Symon, L., and Dorsch, N. W. C.: Use of long-term intracranial pressure measurement to assess hydrocephalic patients prior to shunt surgery. J. Neurosurg., 42:258–273, 1975.

401. Symon, L., Ischikawa, S., and Meyer, J. S.: Cerebral arterial pressure changes and development of leptomeningeal collateral circulation. Neurology (Minneap.), 13:237–250, 1963.

402. Symon, L., Crockard, H. A., Juhasz, J., and Branston, N. M.: The effect of intracranial hypertension on cerebrovascular resistance. An experimental study. Acta Neurochir. (Wien), 35:221–232, 1976.

403. Symon, L., Pasztor, E., Dorsch, N. W. C., and Branston, N. M.: Differential pressures recorded in acute epidural expanding lesions, correlation with local cerebral blood flow by hydrogen clearance in baboons. In Langfitt, T.

W., McHenry, L. C., Reivich, M., and Wollman, H., eds.: Cerebral Circulation and Metabolism. Berlin, Springer-Verlag, 1975.

404. Szewczykowski, J., Sliwkaskunicki, A., Korsaksliwka, J., Dziduszkojdytko, P., and Augustyniak, B.: Computer-assisted analysis of intraventricular pressure after mannitol administration. J. Neurosurg., 43:136–141, 1975.

405. Taylor, J. M., Levy, W. A., Herzog, I., et al.: Prevention of experimental cerebral edema by corticosteroids. Neurology (Minneap.), 15:667–674, 1965.

406. Tellez, H., and Bauer, R. B.: Dexamethasone as treatment in cerebrovascular disease. I. A controlled study in intracerebral hemorrhage. Stroke, 4:541–546, 1973.

407. Thompson, R. K., and Malina, S.: Dynamic axial brain-stem distortion as a mechanism explaining the cardiorespiratory changes in increased intracranial pressure. J. Neurosurg., 16:664–675, 1959.

408. Troupp, H., Valtonen, S., and Vapalahti, M.: Intraventricular pressure after administration of dehydrating agents to severely brain-injured patients. Acta Neurochir. (Wien), 24:89–95, 1971.

409. Troupp, H., Kuurne, T., Kaste, M., Vapalahti, M., and Valtonen, S.: Intraventricular pressure after severe brain injuries: Prognostic value and correlation with blood pressure and jugular venous oxygen tension. In Brock, M., and Dietz, H., eds.: Intracranial Pressure. Berlin, Springer-Verlag, 1972.

410. Valtonen, S.: Arterial oxygen tension and high intracranial pressure. Acta Neurochir. (Wien), 31:161–165, 1975.

411. Vapalahti, M.: Intracranial pressure, acid-base status of blood and cerebrospinal fluid, and pulmonary function in the prognosis of severe brain injury. Thesis, Helsinki, 1970.

412. Venes, J. L., and Collins, W. F.: Bifrontal decompressive craniectomy in the management of head trauma. J. Neurosurg., 42:429–433, 1975.

413. Virno, M., Chiavarelli, S., and Cantore, G. P.: Azione del glicerolo sull'edema cerebrale nel conigilo dopo craniectomia. Gaz. Int. Med. Chir., 66:3509–3515, 1961.

414. Vries, J. K., Becker, D. P., and Young, H. F.: A subarachnoid screw for monitoring intracranial pressure. Technical note. J. Neurosurg., 39:416–419, 1973.

415. Wahl, M., Deetjen, P., and Thurau, K., et al.: Micropuncture evaluation of the importance of perivascular pH for the arteriolar diameter on the brain surface. Pfleuger. Arch. Ges. Physiol., 316:152–163, 1970.

416. Walsh, E. K., and Schettini, A.: A pressure-displacement transducer for measuring brain tissue properties in vivo. J. Appl. Physiol., 38:187–189, 1975.

417. Weed, L. H.: Some limitations of the Monro-Kellie hypothesis. Arch. Surg. (Chicago), 18:1049–1068, 1929.

418. Weed, L. H., and McKibben, P. S.: Pressure changes in cerebrospinal fluid following intravenous injection of solutions of various concentrations. Amer. J. Physiol., 48:512–530, 1919.

419. Weed, L. H., Flexner, L. B., and Clark, J. H.: The effect of dislocation of cerebrospinal fluid upon its pressure. Amer. J. Physiol., 100:246–261, 1932.

420. Weinstein, J. D., and Langfitt, T. W.: Responses of cortical vessels to brain compression: Observations through a transparent calvarium. Surg. Forum, 18:430–432, 1967.

421. Weinstein, J. D., Langfitt, T. W., and Kassell, N. F.: Vasopressor response to increased intracranial pressure. Neurology (Minneap.), 14:1118–1131, 1964.

422. Weinstein, J. D., Toy, F. J., Jaffe, M. E., and Goldberg, H. I.: The effect of dexamethasone on brain edema in patients with metastatic brain tumors. Neurology (Minneap.), 23:121–129, 1973.

423. Weinstein, J. D., Langfitt, T. W., Bruno, L. A., Zaren, H. A., and Jackson, J. L. F.: Experimental study of patterns of brain distortion and ischemia produced by an intracranial mass. J. Neurosurg., 28:513–521, 1968.

424. Weisman, S. J.: Edema and congestion of the lungs resulting from intracranial hemorrhage. Surgery, 6:722–729, 1939.

425. Weiss, M. H., and Nulsen, F. E.: The effective glucocorticoids on CSF flow in dogs. J. Neurosurg., 32:452–458, 1970.

426. White, J. C., Verlot, M., Selverstone, B., and Beecher, H. K.: Changes in brain volume during anesthesia. The effects of anoxia and hypercapnia. Arch. Surg. (Chicago), 44:1–21, 1942.

427. Wilkinson, H. A.: The intracranial pressure-monitoring cup catheter: Technical note. Neurosurgery, 1:139–141, 1977.

428. Williams, G. R., and Spencer, F. C.: The clinical use of hypothermia following cardiac arrest. Amer. J. Surg., 148:462–465, 1958.

429. Wise, B. L., and Chater, N.: Effect of mannitol on cerebrospinal fluid pressure. Arch. Neurol. (Chicago), 4:96–98, 1961.

430. Wise, B. L., and Chater, N.: The value of hypertonic mannitol solution in decreasing brain mass and lowering cerebrospinal-fluid pressure. J. Neurosurg., 19:1038–1043, 1962.

431. Wolff, H. G.: Headache and other head pain. New York, Oxford University Press, 1963.

432. Wollman, H., Smith, P. C., Stephen, G. W., et al.: Effects of extremes of respiratory and metabolic alkalosis on cerebral blood flow in man. J. Appl. Physiol., 24:60–65, 1968.

433. Wright, R. D.: Experimental observations on increased intracranial pressure. Aust. New Zeal. J. Surg., 7:215–235, 1938.

434. Yamaguchi, M., Chirakata, S., Taomoto, K., and Matsumoto, S.: Steroid treatment of brain edema. Surg. Neurol., 4:5–8, 1975.

435. Yatsu, F. M., Diamond, I., Graziano, C., et al.: Experimental brain ischemia: Protection from irreversible damage with a rapid acting barbiturate (methohexital). Stroke, 4:726–732, 1972.

436. Zervas, N. T., Cosman, E. R., and Cosman, B. J.: A pressure balanced radio-telemetry system for the measurement of intracranial pressure. J. Neurosurg., 47:899–911, 1977.

437. Zwetnow, N. N.: Effects of increased cerebrospinal fluid pressure on the blood flow and on energy metabolism of the brain. Acta Physiol. Scand., suppl. 339:1–31, 1970.

25

NEUROENDOCRINOLOGY

THE PITUITARY GLAND

The pituitary gland, also called the pituitary, the hypophysis, or the hypophysis cerebri, is a complex endocrine gland. It lies in the sella turcica ("Turk's saddle," or fossa hypophysis), a bony depression in the sphenoid bone of the skull. The sella turcica is covered by the diaphragm (diaphragma sellae), a fold of dura mater that is the outermost of the three meninges covering the brain. The dura mater also lines the sella, thus enveloping the pituitary gland. The diaphragm has a foramen through which the pituitary stalk, consisting of neural tissue and blood vessels, runs from the hypothalmus at the base of the brain to that portion of the pituitary gland within the sella. If the foramen of the diaphragm is larger than the pituitary stalk, the arachnoid mater, the middle of the three meninges, may extend downward through the foramen. This arachnoid pouch, filled with cerebrospinal fluid, may become big enough to fill a large portion of the sella and compress the pituitary gland, usually against the inferior posterior portion of the sella, a condition known as "the empty sella syndrome" (see Chapter 100).

The pituitary in the adult male weighs 430 to 625 mg. It is approximately 20 per cent larger in adult females, owing to the larger pars distalis in the female, and increases another 12 per cent during pregnancy. The increase in size associated with pregnancy is probably due to an increase in the size and number of cells producing prolactin. The adult pituitary measures about 10 to 15 mm in transverse diameter, 10 mm in anteroposterior diameter, and 5 to 6 mm in superoinferior diameter.[68]

Embryology and Nomenclature

In vertebrates, the pituitary gland is the result of the union of two endocrine structures derived from separate ectodermal sources (Fig. 25–1). Embryologically, a dorsal hollow evagination (Rathke's pouch) of oral epithelium extends upward and separates from the mother layer to form the adenohypophysis, which joins with a similar hollow process (saccus infundibuli) extending downward but remaining connected to the floor of the diencephalon of the brain, to become the neural lobe, or neurohypophysis. Thus the neurohypophysis retains neural connections with the brain, which are essential to the endocrine function and control of the neurohypophysis. The adenohypophysis, while it joins with and partially envelops the neurohypophysis, has no demonstrable neural connections with the brain but is closely affiliated with the hypothalamus of the brain by the portal blood vessels, down which flows blood from the hypothalamus along the pituitary stalk to the adenohypophysis. The portal blood system, which transports regulatory hormones from the hypothalamus to the adenohypophysis, is as essential to the endocrine functions of the adenohypophysis as the neural connections with the brain are to the endocrine functions of the neurohypophysis.

During embryological development, as Rathke's pouch migrates upward, clusters of cells may separate from the pouch and remain along the migratory tract to be surrounded by sphenoid bone or mucosa and ultimately develop into a small pharyngeal pituitary. There is doubt whether a pharyngeal pituitary has clinically significant endo-

R. V. RANDALL

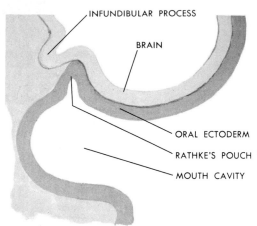

1. BEGINNING FORMATION OF RATHKE'S POUCH
AND INFUNDIBULAR PROCESS

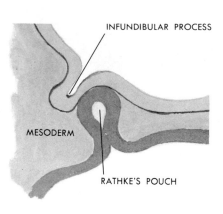

2. NECK OF RATHKE'S POUCH CONSTRICTED
BY GROWTH OF MESODERM

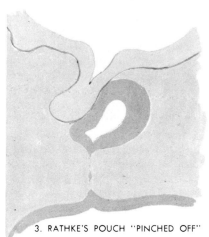

3. RATHKE'S POUCH "PINCHED OFF"

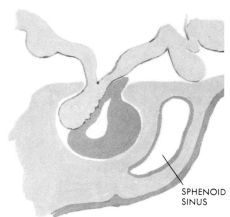

4. "PINCHED OFF" SEGMENT CONFORMS TO
NEURAL PROCESS, FORMING PARS DISTALIS,
PARS INTERMEDIA AND PARS TUBERALIS

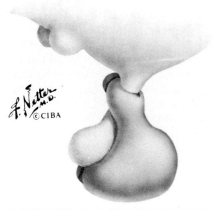

5. PARS TUBERALIS ENCIRCLES INFUNDIBULAR
STALK (LATERAL SURFACE VIEW)

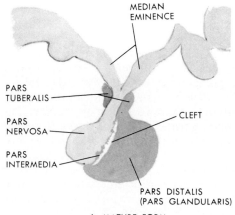

6. MATURE FORM

Figure 25–1   Embryological development of the human pituitary gland. (Copyright 1965 CIBA Pharmaceutical, Division of CIBA-Geigy Corporation. Reprinted by permission from The CIBA Collection of Medical Illustrations by Frank H. Netter, M.D. All rights reserved.)

crine function, although in rare instances ectopic pituitary tissue has been suspected of causing acromegaly.[65]

As Rathke's pouch develops, the anterior portion enlarges to form the pars distalis, the major portion of the anterior lobe of the pituitary (see Fig. 25–1). From the superolateral aspect of Rathke's pouch, two buds of tissue arise and fuse in the midline. As Rathke's pouch meets the neurohypophysis these buds grow upward along and laterally around the superior portion of the neurohypophysis and the pituitary stalk to form the pars tuberalis of the pituitary.

The posterior portion of Rathke's pouch adjacent to the neurohypophysis develops more than the anterior portion and becomes known as the pars intermedia, or intermediate lobe. In man the pars intermedia is present during fetal life and secretes hormones, but after birth it atrophies and becomes a rudimentary, nonsecretory structure, as shown in Figure 25–1, except during pregnancy.[101] The lumen of Rathke's pouch may disappear completely so that the pars distalis and the rudimentary pars intermedia adjoin. Frequently, however, the lumen may persist as a cleft or a series of colloid-filled vesicles or cysts, the function of which is not known. Squamous cell rests are found in about 25 per cent of anterior pituitary glands, primarily in the pars tuberalis.[69] It has been postulated that these cells are the origin of craniopharyngiomas.[55]

As noted earlier, the neurohypophysis depends upon its neural connections with the hypothalamus for its endocrine functions and control. These connections are with two sets of paired nuclei in the hypothalamus, the supraoptic and paraventricular nuclei. The neurohypophysis and its hypothalamic nuclei, the supraoptic and paraventricular nuclei, are regarded as a functioning unit, and the term ''hypothalamico-neurohypophyseal system'' is applied to this unit. There is no analogous term to describe the relationship of the anterior lobe of the pituitary to the hypothalamus by means of the portal blood system.

Blood Supply of the Pituitary Gland

Familiarity with the blood supply of the pituitary gland is essential to understanding the endocrine relationship between the hypothalamus and the anterior lobe of the pituitary. The gland receives its arterial blood supply from two paired arteries, the right and left superior hypophyseal arteries and the right and left inferior hypophyseal arteries, both pairs of which are derived from the internal carotid arteries (Fig. 25–2). The venous drainage of the pituitary is by small efferent veins, which drain into dural sinuses in the dura mater that surrounds the pituitary in the sella turcica. The dural sinuses ultimately drain into the internal jugular veins. On occasion the dural sinuses may be large enough to prohibit operative entry into the sella by the transsphenoidal route.

Each superior hypophyseal artery arises from the internal carotid artery immediately distal to the origin of the thalamic artery and divides into the anterior superior hypophyseal artery and the posterior superior hypophyseal artery. These arteries send branches to the optic nerves, chiasm, and tracts, but the bulk of the arterial blood is directed to the hypothalamus, the median eminence, the upper portion of the pituitary stalk (infundibulum), and the pars tuberalis, with the exception of the flow carried by the trabecular, or loral, artery (artery of trabecula in Figure 25–2), which plunges downward into the anterior lobe of the pituitary.

Capillaries from branches of the paired hypophyseal arteries in the median eminence, upper pituitary stalk, and pars tuberalis drain into a plexus of veins known as the primary plexus of the hypophyseal portal system. The latter, in turn, coalesces into a number of veins known as the long hypophyseal portal veins, which course downward along the anterior portion of the pituitary stalk to the anterior lobe of the pituitary. Upon reaching the anterior lobe, the long portal vessels branch out to form another plexus known as the secondary plexus of the hypophyseal portal system, which supplies blood primarily to the anterior and lateral portions of the anterior lobe. The blood leaves the pituitary by way of the aforementioned efferent veins, draining into the dural sinuses.

The bilateral trabecular, or loral, arteries do not give off branches as they pass through the anterior lobe until they reach the region where the posterior portion of the anterior lobe adjoins the inferior portion of the pituitary stalk. Here they drain into a plexus of veins that coalesce into a series of vessels running downward and known as

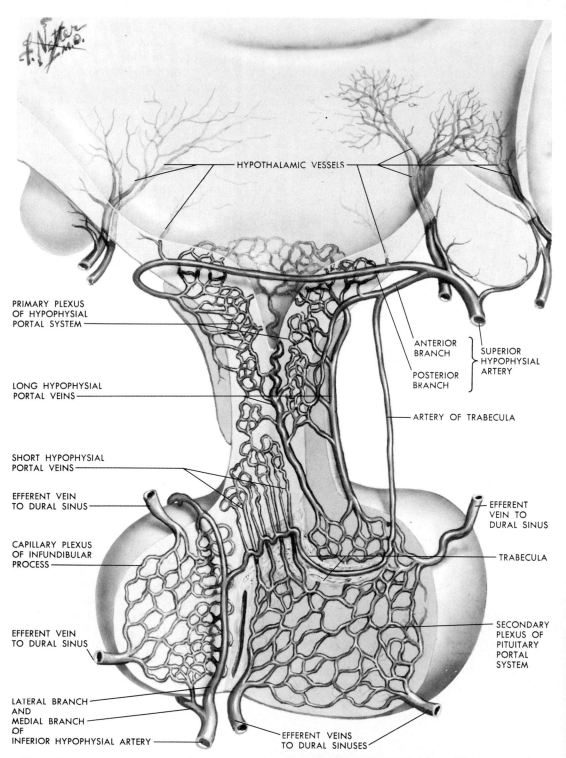

Figure 25-2 Blood supply of the human hypothalamus and pituitary gland. (Copyright 1965 CIBA Pharmaceutical, Division of CIBA-Geigy Corporation. Reprinted by permission from The CIBA Collection of Medical Illustrations by Frank H. Netter, M.D. All rights reserved.)

the short hypophyseal portal veins. Branches from the inferior hypophyseal arteries also contribute to the blood supply entering the short hypophyseal portal veins. These short portal veins empty into that part of the secondary plexus of the pituitary portal system that supplies blood to the posterior portion of the anterior lobe.

The long portal veins and the short portal veins, especially the former, thus supply the blood perfusing the anterior lobe. Little, if any, of the blood supply of the anterior lobe is derived directly from arteries, in contrast to that of the posterior lobe, which is supplied directly by the inferior hypophyseal arteries.

If the pituitary stalk, along with the trabecular arteries, is cut as in an operative stalk section, there will be ischemic necrosis of the anterior lobe. As previously noted, however, the inferior hypophyseal arteries contribute to the blood supply of the short hypophyseal portal veins, and hence, in some instances, when the pituitary stalk and trabecular arteries have been cut, viable tissue may remain in the posterior portion of the anterior lobe.

Recent animal studies, not yet confirmed in man, have shown capillaries running along the posterior aspect of the pituitary stalk, connecting the capillary plexus of the posterior pituitary with that of the median eminence.[91,92] It has been suggested that blood may flow in either direction through these capillaries. It has also been suggested that the short portal vessels do not carry arterial blood anteriorly to the capillary plexus of the anterior lobe, but rather that the capillary plexus of the anterior lobe drains posteriorly through the short vessels into the capillary plexus of the posterior pituitary. These findings postulate a continuous vascular circuit through which blood can flow from the capillary plexus of the median eminence down the long portal vessels to the capillary plexus of the anterior lobe, posteriorly through the short portal vessels into the capillary plexus of the posterior lobe, and up capillaries along the posterior pituitary stalk, back into the capillary plexus of the median eminence. This vascular circuit would be one explanation for the high concentrations of antidiuretic hormone and neurophysin found in the blood of the long portal vessels. It has long been known that antidiuretic hormone can evoke release of adrenocorticotropin (ACTH) by

the anterior lobe, and this circular vascular pathway is a possible route by which antidiuretic hormone could enter into the control of secretion of ACTH.

Structures Adjacent to the Pituitary Gland

The pituitary gland and sella turcica are surrounded by many structures, as shown in Figure 25–3. Tumors of the pituitary gland can grow downward into the sphenoid sinus; upward to press upon the optic chiasm or tracts or nerves, or to impinge upon the hypothalamus or third ventricle; or laterally to invade the cavernous sinus, evoking extraocular motor weakness or paralysis by compromising the third, fourth, or sixth cranial nerve, or pain by impinging upon the ophthalmic or maxillary branches of the fifth nerve. Likewise, tumors or aneurysms arising adjacent to the sella can compromise the function of the pituitary by impinging directly upon the pituitary gland or its blood supply, or by damaging the pituitary stalk, hypothalamus, or long portal vessels that transport regulatory hormones from the hypothalamus to the anterior pituitary. These various mechanical effects of expanding the pituitary tumors are listed in Table 25–1.

THE ADENOHYPOPHYSIS

Cells and Hormones of the Anterior Pituitary

The pars distalis, as demonstrated by staining techniques used in light microscopy, contains three main populations of cells: acidophils or eosinophils, which contain red- or pink-staining granules; basophils, which contain blue- or purple-staining granules; and chromophobes, which are essentially devoid of stainable granules by light microscopy. Granules can be seen by electron microscopy in most of the chromophobe cells. Nevertheless, even with electron microscopy, there remain two types of agranular cells known as follicular cells and stellate cells.[61] The function of these cells is not known. With different staining techniques, however, the pituitary cells can be divided into a number of subgroups, depending upon the type of stain used. This,

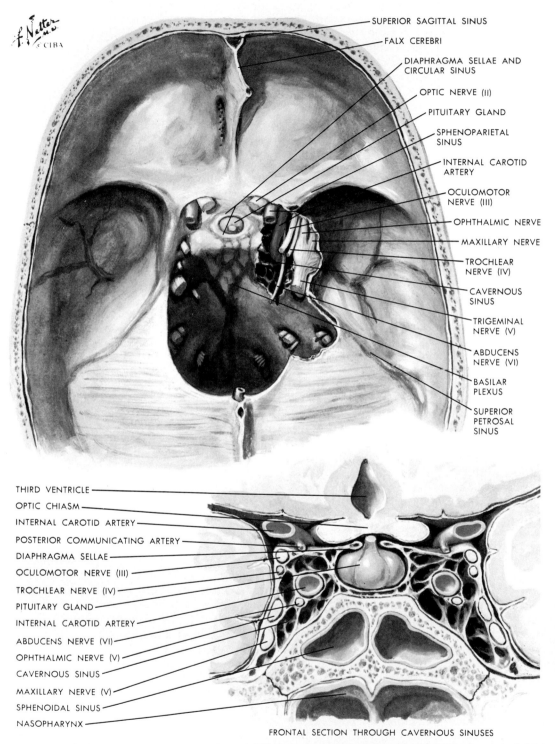

SUPERIOR SAGITTAL SINUS

FALX CEREBRI

DIAPHRAGMA SELLAE AND CIRCULAR SINUS

OPTIC NERVE (II)

PITUITARY GLAND

SPHENOPARIETAL SINUS

INTERNAL CAROTID ARTERY

OCULOMOTOR NERVE (III)

OPHTHALMIC NERVE

MAXILLARY NERVE

TROCHLEAR NERVE (IV)

CAVERNOUS SINUS

TRIGEMINAL NERVE (V)

ABDUCENS NERVE (VI)

BASILAR PLEXUS

SUPERIOR PETROSAL SINUS

THIRD VENTRICLE

OPTIC CHIASM

INTERNAL CAROTID ARTERY

POSTERIOR COMMUNICATING ARTERY

DIAPHRAGMA SELLAE

OCULOMOTOR NERVE (III)

TROCHLEAR NERVE (IV)

PITUITARY GLAND

INTERNAL CAROTID ARTERY

ABDUCENS NERVE (VI)

OPHTHALMIC NERVE (V)

CAVERNOUS SINUS

MAXILLARY NERVE (V)

SPHENOIDAL SINUS

NASOPHARYNX

FRONTAL SECTION THROUGH CAVERNOUS SINUSES

Figure 25–3 Structures adjacent to the human pituitary gland. (Copyright 1965 CIBA Pharmaceutical, Division of CIBA-Geigy Corporation. Reprinted by permission from The CIBA Collection of Medical Illustrations by Frank H. Netter, M.D. All rights reserved.)

TABLE 25–1 MECHANICAL EFFECTS OF PITUITARY TUMORS

Enlargement and erosion of the sella turcica
Cerebrospinal rhinorrhea
Headache
Anterior pituitary failure
Diabetes insipidus
Chiasmal, optic tract, and optic nerve defects
Third, fourth, and sixth cranial nerve palsies
Fifth cranial nerve involvement (pain)
Galactorrhea
Hypothalamic disorders
   Sleep
   Appetite
   Temperature
   Emotions
Increased intracranial pressure
Seizure disorders
Changes in intellect and personality
Brain stem pressure
Obstruction of cavernous sinus
Occlusion of internal carotid artery

©Mayo 1979

The several hormones secreted by the human pars distalis are thought to be produced, stored, and released by cells that are, by the old classification, either acidophilic (A) or basophilic (B) cells, as shown in Table 25–2.

It was formerly believed that in man, beta-melanocyte-stimulating hormone (β_h-MSH, known as melanophore-stimulating hormone, melanotropin, chromatophorotropin, and intermedin) was made and secreted by basophilic pituitary cells. Current thought is that human beta-melanocyte-stimulating hormone is a degradation product of gamma-lipotropin (γ_h-LPH), and that gamma-lipotropin is, in turn, a degradation product of beta-lipotropin. Human beta-lipotropin contains 91 amino acids, and gamma-lipotropin is its 1-58 amino acid sequence. Human beta-melanotropin, which contains 22 amino acids, is the 37-58 amino acid sequence of both beta- and gamma-lipotropin. Beta-lipotropin is also thought to be the precursor of the morphinomimetic peptides, endorphins and enkephalins. Much of the information about the interrelationship among these compounds has been derived from the study of bovine beta-lipotropin, which contains several subunits as follows:

plus the use of a variety of terms to label similar cells, has led to a confusing array of classifications. Fortunately, these classifications have largely been abandoned, and current practice is to name pituitary cells according to the hormones that they produce and secrete, which is determined by immunohistological and electron microscopic techniques.

TABLE 25–2 HORMONE-PRODUCING CELLS OF ANTERIOR PITUITARY

CELL	HORMONE	ABBREVIATION*
GH-producing cell, somatotroph (A)†	Growth hormone, also called somatotropic hormone or somatotropin	GH (also STH)
PRL-producing cell, lactotroph, mammotroph (A)	Prolactin, formerly called luteotropic hormone or luteotropin. Other terms, no longer in vogue, are lactogenic hormone and mammotropin	PRL (formerly LTH)
ACTH-producing cell adrenocorticotroph, corticotroph (B)	Adrenocorticotropic hormone or adrenocorticotropin. Sometimes called adrenocortical-stimulating hormone	ACTH
TSH-producing cell thyrotroph (B)	Thyroid-stimulating hormone or thyrotropin	TSH
FSH-producing cell§ (B)	Follicle-stimulating hormone	FSH
LH-producing cell§ (B)	Luteinizing hormone. In males, sometimes called interstitial cell–stimulating hormone (ICSH)	LH

* Species designation is by lower case letter preceding the abbreviation, e.g., human growth hormone, hGH; bovine thyroid-stimulating hormone, bTSH; ovine prolactin, oPRL.

† By old classifications, hormone-producing cells were acidophilic (A) or basophilic (B).

§ Some workers believe that FSH and LH are produced by the same cell, called a gonadotroph, rather than by separate cells.[93]

© Mayo 1980

The same cell in the anterior pituitary, the lipotroph, is thought to make and release both beta-lipotropin and adrenocorticotropin, which in turn are thought to be derived from a prohormone, "big ACTH."

Scott and Lowry state that alpha- and beta-melanotropins and the corticotropin-like intermediate lobe peptide (CLIP), known also as ACTH (18–39) peptide, have been identified only in animals with a distinct pars intermedia. They believe that the rudimentary nature of the pars intermedia in man accounts for the failure to isolate these compounds from human pituitaries. They further believe that human beta-melanocyte-stimulating hormone is an extraction artifact and that this explains why it has no known physiological function in man.[113] Rees, in a review of the relationship among adrenocorticotropin, lipotropin, and melanotropin, mentions that α-MSH and CLIP are found in the human pituitary during fetal life and during pregnancy when a distinct pars intermedia is present.[101]

The finding that human adrenocorticotropin and beta-lipotropin are secreted on a 1:1 molar basis by normal persons as well as by most patients with pituitary or adrenocortical disease is proving to be of clinical importance. Since human beta-lipotropin is more stable than human corticotropin, and hence easier to assay, the assay for it should become more readily available than has the assay for hACTH. In a further extension of these findings, Jeffcoate and co-workers have found that patients with the ectopic ACTH Cushing's syndrome secrete relatively less gamma-than beta-lipotropin, whereas patients with pituitary ACTH–dependent Cushing's disease secrete relatively more gamma-lipotropin.[51]

Nature and Function of the Hormones of the Anterior Pituitary

Growth hormone, prolactin (PRL) and adrenocorticotropin (ACTH) are polypeptide hormones. Thyroid-stimulating hormone (TSH), follicle-stimulating hormone (FSH), and luteinizing hormone (LH) are glycoproteins, a characteristic shared by chorionic gonadotropin (CG) of placental origin. Each of these glycoproteins, including chorionic gonadotropin, consists of two subunits known as the alpha subunit and the beta subunit. Although the exact structures of the alpha and beta subunits are not completely known, the alpha subunit is thought to have a structure that is identical or similar in all glycoprotein hormones in all species so far studied, while the beta subunits have a different and unique structure in each hormone and in each species. The beta subunit confers upon the hormone immunospecificity and probably specificity for its receptor site. The individual, isolated beta subunit does not possess biological activity, however, but becomes biologically active only when coupled with the nonspecific alpha subunit.

This chapter discusses the clinically relevant activities of the various hormones of the anterior pituitary. Those interested in the research aspects or less clinically relevant details should consult more comprehensive reviews or texts.[6,58,71,128] As an example of such detail, prolactin, which has known effects either directly or indirectly on the breast and gonads, has been shown experimentally to have effects also on fluid and electrolyte metabolism, calcium metabolism, the cardiovascular system, and probably the immune system. It has been shown to increase prostaglandin synthesis and membrane sodium-potassium adenosine triphosphatase activity. Similarly it is known that in addition to stimulating linear growth, growth hormone has many effects on carbohydrate, protein, fat, and electrolyte metabolism. Once a human has attained full stature, however, lack of growth hormone alone does not lead to any clinical syndromes that are recognized at this time. The clinical significance of these various observations is not known.

Growth Hormone

Human growth hormone (hGH) is a single-chain polypeptide of 191 amino acids with two disulfide bridges and a molecular weight of about 21,500 daltons. It is highly species specific, and except for simian growth hormone, no other is effective in man. Unlike some of the other hormones of the anterior pituitary, human growth hormone has no specific target organ but has an effect of virtually every tissue in the body. It is the major hormone that influences linear growth, along with thyroid hormone, insulin, and the sex steroids. Growth is not a direct effect of growth hormone but rather is mediated by substances known as somatomedins. This term is applied to an unknown number of growth hormone–dependent polypeptides that, when activated by growth hormone, directly stimulate growth in responsive tissues. So far, five somatomedins—somatomedin A, somatomedin C, insulin-like growth factor 1, insulin-like growth factor 2, and multiplication-stimulating activity—have been isolated from human plasma. Their molecular weights range between 6000 and 11,000 daltons, and they are thought to be produced in the liver.[20]

Prolactin

Human prolactin (hPRL) is a polypeptide whose amino acid sequence was recently discovered.[115] It consists of 198 amino acid residues with three disulfide bridges, and has a molecular weight of approximately 23,000 daltons. Contrary to expectations, the amino acid sequence differs considerably from those of human growth hormone and human placental lactogen. Human prolactin has only 32 residues (16 per cent) in sequence positions identical with those of human growth hormone and only 26 (13 per cent) in positions identical with those of human placental lactogen.

Prolactin stimulates growth of breast tissues and induces production and secretion of milk. Growth hormone, estrogen, progesterone, and insulin are also known to be necessary for breast development and lactation. During pregnancy, chorionic somatotropin (placental lactogen) contributes to breast enlargement and lactation. In humans, small amounts of prolactin seem to be essential for progesterone production by human granulosa cells, but higher concentrations inhibit progesterone production.[78] Its function in the human male is unknown, but prolactin seems to be essential to normal production of sperm. On the other hand, it has been shown that greater than normal concentrations of prolactin will inhibit 5 alpha-reductase and, hence, the conversion of inactive testosterone to biologically active dihydrotestosterone, which must be present in high concentrations in the testicular tubules for normal spermatogenesis to take place.[70]

Adrenocorticotropic Hormone

Human adrenocorticotropic hormone (hACTH) is a single-chain polypeptide made up of 39 amino acid residues with a molecular weight of 4,567 daltons. ACTH from the various mammalian species studied contains 39 amino acids, with the first 24 and the last 6 being identical in all species, while the differences are in amino acids 25 through 32. The first 20 amino acids are required for full biological activity; the function of the remaining amino acids is not known. Adrenocorticotropin maintains adrenal size and stimulates the adrenal cortex to produce and secrete cortisol and other adrenal steroids, but is not the main regulatory substance for aldosterone, which is primarily under the control of the renin-angiotensin system.

Thyroid-Stimulating Hormone

Human thyroid-stimulating hormone (hTSH) is a glycoprotein with a molecular weight of approximately 28,000 daltons. It stimulates growth of the thyroid gland and stimulates it to produce and secrete thyroid hormone.

The structures of the several human glycoprotein hormones are known. For example, the alpha subunit of human thyroid-stimulating hormone contains 90 amino acid residues with carbohydrate moieties at positions 40 and 75, while the beta subunit contains 112 amino acid residues with a carbohydrate moiety at position 23.

Follicle-Stimulating Hormone

Human follicle-stimulating hormone (hFSH) is a glycoprotein with a molecular weight of about 35,000 daltons and an unknown amino acid content. In females it stimulates the maturation of the ovarian follicle and secretion of estrogens by the follicle. In males it stimulates development of testicular tubules and spermatogenesis.

Luteinizing Hormone

Human luteinizing hormone (hLH) is a glycoprotein with a molecular weight of around 28,000 daltons and 204 amino acid residues. In the female, it induces ovulation in the mature follicle and causes luteinization of the ovarian follicle and the production and secretion of progesterone. In the male, it stimulates the development of the Leydig cells (interstitial cells) of the testes and their production and secretion of testosterone.

Hypothalamic-Pituitary Relationship

In the past, it was thought that the anterior pituitary gland was an autonomously functioning structure secreting thyroid-stimulating hormone (TSH), adrenocorticotropic hormone (ACTH), and the gonadotropic hormones, follicle-stimulating hormone (FSH) and luteinizing hormone (LH), to stimulate the target endocrine glands, namely the thyroid, adrenal cortices, and gonads. The hormonal secretions of these end-organs were thought to exert a negative feedback on the anterior pituitary, thus regulating its secretion of thyrotropin, corticotropin, and follicle-stimulating and luteinizing hormones.

As a result of the pioneering work of Schally and Guillemin and their co-workers, there has evolved the current concept that the anterior pituitary is controlled by releasing and inhibiting substances made in the hypothalamus and secreted into the capillary system in the hypothalamus, whence they are carried by the long portal veins to the anterior pituitary, where they have their effects upon its secretory cells.* There seems to be good evidence for the existence of both a releasing (or stimulating) substance and an inhibiting substance for growth hormone and for prolactin and a releasing substance for thyrotropin, corticotropin, and follicle-stimulating and luteinizing hormones. The last two may well share the same releasing substance, referred to as gonadotropin-releasing hormone (GnRH). Some of these hypothalamic substances have been isolated, characterized, and synthesized. Current convention suggests that the terms "releasing hormone" and "inhibiting hormone" be used to designate substances that have been isolated, characterized, and synthesized, while the terms "releasing factor" and "inhibiting factor" be used to describe substances that have been isolated and shown to be biologically active but whose precise structures are not yet known. All the releasing and inhibiting hormones characterized so far have been simple peptides, or oligopeptides, consisting of three or more amino acids.

The neuronal cells that make the releasing hormones and factors and inhibiting hormones and factors are known as neurosecretory or neuroendocrine cells and lie in the median basal portion of the hypothalamus, which is called the hypophysiotropic area. Once synthesized, these materials migrate down the axons of the neurosecretory cells to their termination in the median eminence of the hypothalamus. Here the

---

* For which they were awarded the Nobel Prize in 1977.

neurosecretory substances are released into the hypothalamic capillary system, which runs into the long portal system down to the anterior pituitary. The hypothalamus is not the only site where these hormones are found. For example, thyrotropin-releasing hormone (TRH) has been isolated from other areas of the brain and spinal cord, and from the placenta.[114] Somatostatin (growth hormone–inhibiting hormone, GHIH) is found in high concentrations in the stomach wall and in the islets of the pancreas as well as in the spinal cord and parts of the brain other than the hypothalamus. The significance of these observations is not understood, but thyrotropin-releasing hormone may be a stimulatory substance with multiple sites of action, and somatostatin, a generalized inhibitory substance.

The secretory control of the hypophysiotropic neuroendocrine cells is influenced by stimuli from virtually all portions of the body including the higher neuropathways, pituitary hormones, and target endocrine gland hormones, as well as metabolic fuels. The final common pathway by which all these stimuli influence the neurosecretory cells of the hypophysiotrophic area is through monoaminergic cells. A number of neurotransmitters in the brain have been identified including dopamine (DA), norepinephrine (NE), serotonin (5-HT), epinephrine, melatonin, acetylcholine (ACh), histamine, and gamma-aminobutyric acid (GABA). Norepinephrine, dopamine, and serotonin are found in greater concentrations in the hypothalamus than in other parts of the brain, and are thought to constitute the final neurotransmitter pathway between the nonneurosecretory neuron cells and the neurosecretory or neuroendocrine cells of the hypothalamus. There is increasing evidence that prostaglandins as well as endorphins and enkephalins also play a mediator role in the secretion of the hypothalamic regulatory hormones. Cyclic AMP has been implicated as a mediator of the actions of the thyrotropin-releasing and gonadotropin-releasing hormones and somatostatin in the anterior pituitary gland.

The following paragraphs represent only a brief outline of the hypothalamic-pituitary relationships in regard to the various pituitary hormones, and the reader is referred to more comprehensive reviews for further information.*

Growth Hormone

Hypothalamic control of growth hormone seems to be mediated through a releasing substance, growth hormone-releasing factor (GHRF) and an inhibiting hormone, which has been variously named growth hormone–inhibiting hormone (GHIH, GIH), somatotropin release–inhibiting hormone (SRIH), somatostatin, and growth hormone release–inhibiting hormone (GHRIH), with "somatostatin" being the preferred term. Growth hormone–releasing activity has been demonstrated in hypothalamic extracts, and the substance has been isolated but not characterized.[100] Somatostatin on the other hand has been characterized and synthesized, and is a tetradecapeptide: H-Ala-Gly-Cys-Lys-Asn-Phe-Phe-Trp-Lys-Thr-Phe-Thr-Ser-Cys-OH. Like some of the other hypothalamic hormones, somatostatin alters the release of hormones other than growth hormone. It inhibits the release of thyrotropin induced by thyrotropin-releasing hormone. It also inhibits release of insulin and glucagon by the islet cells of the pancreas, and has been shown to be effective in the control of labile diabetes. The presence of somatostatin in high concentration in pancreatic islets suggests that it plays a role in the physiological control of the pancreatic secretion of insulin and glucagon. The fact that somatostatin is also found in many areas of the brain other than the hypothalamus—in the spinal cord, and in areas of the gastrointestinal tract other than the pancreatic islets—means there is much to be learned about the functions of this ubiquitous hormone.

The feedback control of growth hormone, although not well understood, is thought to take place at the hypothalamic level and is dependent upon its level in plasma as well as upon metabolic fuels such as glucose and fatty acids, upon steroids such as estrogen, and upon sleep. The level of circulating growth hormone seems to supply a negative feedback to the hypothalamus; that is, when present in excess, it

---

* See references 37–39, 71–75, 90, 102.

suppresses secretion of additional growth hormone.

The monoaminergic control of growth hormone is complex, and there is experimental evidence to suggest that norepinephrine, dopamine, and serotonin all can stimulate growth hormone release. Further, both alpha- and beta-adrenergic receptors play a role in the release of growth hormone. Interestingly, paradoxical effects are seen in acromegaly in that L-dopa, a precursor of dopamine, depresses the elevated levels of growth hormone, whereas it elevates growth hormone levels in the normal person. Apomorphine, a centrally active dopaminergic agent, and bromocriptine, a dopaminergic receptor–stimulating agent, also suppress elevated growth hormone levels in acromegaly. The latter has been used successfully in the treatment of hormonally active acromegaly over a number of months, as has metergoline, an antiserotonin agent.[21,122]

Prolactin

Hypothalamic control of prolactin, unlike that of other anterior pituitary hormones, seems to consist primarily of inhibition. For example, it has long been recognized that pituitary stalk section in the human will result in decreased function of the anterior pituitary and, in some instances, the appearance of galactorrhea secondary to excessive production of prolactin by viable pituitary cells no longer under inhibiting control of the hypothalamus. Experimental transplant of the pituitary to the renal capsule will also result in hypersecretion of prolactin but decreased secretion of the other hormones.

Although prolactin-inhibiting factor (PIF) has been demonstrated in hypothalamic extracts, the substance has not been purified and characterized. On the other hand, it is interesting that the first releasing hormone to be synthesized, the tripeptide thyrotropin-releasing hormone (TRH), is a potent stimulator of prolactin release which, indeed, its administration evokes before thyrotropin is released. A prolactin-releasing factor (PRF) other than thyrotropin-releasing hormone is present in hypothalamic extracts, however, although it has not been characterized, and thyrotropin-releasing hormone is thought not to be the normally occurring prolactin-releasing factor.

The release of prolactin-inhibiting factor is mediated by the hypothalamic catecholamines, dopamine and norepinephrine, and this effect is blocked by dopaminergic blocking agents such as reserpine, methyldopa, phenothiazines (particularly chlorpromazine), pimozide, and the tricyclic antidepressants. Serotonin is also felt to be involved in the control of prolactin secretion, probably by regulating release of prolactin-releasing factor. The administration of 5-hydroxytryptophan, the biological precursor of serotonin, increases serum prolactin levels, and this effect is blocked by the antiserotonin agents, metergoline, methysergide, and cyproheptadine. The secretion of growth hormone is also stimulated by 5-hydroxytryptophan and blocked by the aforementioned antiserotonin agents. There is evidence that dopamine itself, by reaching the anterior pituitary via the portal blood system, can exert direct inhibition on the release of prolactin, and it has been suggested that dopamine and prolactin-inhibiting factor are the same substance. It is not clear at this point exactly what feedback mechanisms control the normal secretion of prolactin.

The ergot alkaloids, especially bromocriptine (2-Br-α-ergocriptine), through their dopaminergic action and also by acting directly on the pituitary, inhibit secretion of prolactin.

Estrogens increase prolactin secretion by the pituitary, while oophorectomy decreases prolactin production, an effect that is reversed by the administration of estrogens. Hypothyroid patients are more responsive to the prolactin-releasing activity of thyrotropin-releasing hormone than are normal persons, while hyperthyroid patients fail to respond to it. Thyrotropin-releasing hormone is thought to act directly on the pituitary gland, and not through the hypothalamus, to evoke release of prolactin.

Thyroid-Stimulating Hormone

Thyrotropin-releasing hormone (TRH) was the first hypothalamic hormone to be characterized and it has a structure consisting of three amino acids: pyro-Glu-His-Pro-NH_2. At this point there is no good evidence that a thyrotropin-inhibiting hormone exists, although as mentioned earlier, somatostatin does inhibit TRH-induced release of thyrotropin. The thyroid hormones themselves, thyroxine and triiodothyronine, play a major role in the controlling the secretion of thyrotropin by a negative feedback mechanism directly at the level of the pituitary, rather than the hypothalamus, by suppressing TRH-mediated release of thyrotropin by the pituitary. There is some suggestion that thyroxine exerts a positive feedback on the hypothalamus and increases the secretion of thyrotropin-releasing hormone.

The role of the neurotransmitters in the secretion of thyrotropin-releasing hormone is not clear, although dopamine and norepinephrine seem to stimulate it, while serotonin inhibits it.

Follicle-Stimulating Hormone and Luteinizing Hormone

Since the secretion of the follicle-stimulating and luteinizing hormones (FSH and LH) occur independently rather than in parallel fashion, it has long been thought that there must be a separate releasing hormone for each of them. A luteinizing hormone-releasing hormone (LHRH) has been characterized and is a decapeptide with the structure: pyro-Glu-His-Trp-Ser-Tyr-Gly-Leu-Arg-Pro-Gly-NH$_2$. This compound has been found to be an excellent releaser of follicle-stimulating hormone as well, although not as effective as in releasing luteinizing hormone, and consequently it is also called gonadotropin-releasing hormone (GnRH). The difference in release of follicle-stimulating and luteinizing hormones by the pituitary in response to gonadotropin-releasing hormone is thought to be related to the positive and negative feedback of the gonadal steroids, particularly estrogens, on the pituitary.

Little is known about the effect of the hypothalamic neurotransmitters on human gonadotropin secretion. It is of interest that the pineal gland secretes melatonin, which has gonadotropin-inhibiting activity in experimental animals. Recently ovine, bovine, and porcine pineal glands have been found to contain gonadotropin-releasing activities that react specifically with the radioimmunoassay for GnRH. Likewise, thyrotropin-releasing hormone has been demonstrated in these same pineal glands. These findings, while startling, are not totally implausible, since somatostatin and thyrotropin-releasing hormone are found in many areas other than the hypothalamus.

Schally and co-workers have synthesized analogues of gonadotropin-releasing hormone that have many times the activity of the normally occurring decapeptide in the release of gonadotropins. They also have synthesized analogues that are inhibitory, probably blocking the pituitary receptor sites for normally occurring gonadotropin-releasing hormone, and that show promise as a nonsteroidal method of contraception.[112]

Adrenocorticotropic Hormone

Although it is known that a great many factors including stress, anesthesia, and hypoglycemia increase adrenocorticotropin (ACTH) production and release, the hypothalamic and neurotransmitter control of corticotropin is less well understood than that of the other pituitary hormones. Corticotropin-releasing factor (CRF) has been repeatedly demonstrated in hypothalamic extracts, and recently has been isolated and partially characterized.[112a] It is well known that antidiuretic hormone (ADH) will evoke a release of corticotropin by the pituitary, but there is good evidence that antidiuretic hormone and corticotropin-releasing factor are distinctly different compounds. For example, in rats serotonin will release corticotropin-releasing factor but has no effect on the neurohypophyseal hormones, vasopressin and oxytocin. On the other hand, dopamine will release some hypothalamic hormones, but not corticotropin-releasing factor. Acetylcholine and serotonin stimulate the release of corticotropin-releasing factor and are perhaps involved in the circadian rhythm of corticotropin, and the antiserotonin agent cyproheptadine has been used in the treatment of Cushing's disease.[57] The data concerning the effect of norepinephrine are confusing, but it appears that norepinephrine and dopamine inhibit secretion of corticotropin-releasing factor. Release of the factor is inhibited by adrenal corticosteroid feedback (long loop) and ACTH feedback (short loop).

Anterior Pituitary Failure

Anterior pituitary failure, also known as hypopituitarism, anterior pituitary insufficiency, Simmonds' disease, Sheehan's syndrome, and hypophyseal cachexia, is characterized by a deficiency of one or more of the hormones secreted by the anterior pituitary gland. The term "unitropic failure" is used when there is a deficiency of a single tropic hormone. Panhypopituitarism, while it actually denotes failure of both the anterior and posterior lobes of the pituitary, by common usage is used interchangeably with the various terms designating anterior pituitary failure. "Simmonds' disease" is synonymous with anterior pituitary failure from any cause, while "Sheehan's syndrome" means anterior pituitary failure secondary to pituitary necrosis developing from shock, hemorrhage, or sepsis associated with childbirth. In rare instances pituitary insufficiency following childbirth may occur even though there is no valid history to suggest that shock, hemorrhage, or sepsis was present at the time.

As noted in the accompanying classification, the causes of anterior pituitary insufficiency fall into two main groups: primary, or idiopathic, failure and secondary failure (Table 25–3).

The signs, symptoms, physical findings, and laboratory findings encountered in anterior pituitary failure are the result of decrease in or lack of production and secretion of growth hormone (GH), pituitary gonadotropins (follicle-stimulating hormone [FSH] and luteinizing hormone [LH]), thryoid-stimulating hormone (TSH), and adrenocorticotropic hormone (ACTH). Currently, it is not clear what role, if any, lack of prolactin (PRL) plays, in pituitary insufficiency. The exact signs, symptoms and laboratory findings present in an adult with pituitary failure will depend upon the severity and duration of the condition and the extent to which the gonads, thyroid, and adrenal cortices (target endocrine glands) have failed.

The syndrome of anterior pituitary failure can be best understood by reviewing the contributions made to this syndrome by the deficiency of growth hormone and the hormones secreted by the target endocrine glands.

Growth Hormone Insufficiency

Although many physiological functions are known to be associated with growth hormone, impaired linear growth (dwarfism) is the one significant finding noted with decreased production of growth hormone in

humans who have not yet reached adult stature. Once a person has completed full linear growth, failure to elaborate growth hormone seems to have no significant clinical implications.

Gonadal Insufficiency

In children, the lack of the gonadotropins, follicle-stimulating hormone (FSH) and luteinizing hormone (LH), leads to the failure of the gonads to develop normally and secrete their hormones. The somatic and sexual changes of puberty do not take place, and secondary sexual characteristics such as growth of sexual hair, growth of genitalia, and maturation of the voice fail

TABLE 25–3 CLASSIFICATION OF CAUSES OF ANTERIOR PITUITARY FAILURE

IDIOPATHIC CAUSES
SECONDARY CAUSES
Trauma
  Accident
  Operation
Therapeutic ablation
  Operation
  Irradiation
Neoplasm
  Primary tumor
    Pituitary adenoma
    Craniopharyngioma
    Meningioma
    Epidermoid
    Ectopic pinealoma
    Glioma
    Chordoma
    Oncocytoma
    Hamartoma
    Myoblastoma*
    Sphenoid sinus tumor
    Miscellaneous
  Metastasis
Vascular disease
  Postpartum necrosis (Sheehan's syndrome)
  Hemorrhage
  Thrombosis
  Aneurysm
  Vasculitis
Infectious disease
  Abscess
  Granulomatous disease
  Meningitis
  Aqueductal stenosis
Systemic disease
  Sarcoidosis
  Histiocytosis X
  Hemochromatosis
  Lymphoma, leukemia, and related diseases
  Autoimmune endocrine failure
Developmental anomaly
  Aqueductal stenosis
  Arachnoid cyst
  Basal encephalocele

© Mayo 1979

* Granular cell tumor of the neurohypophysis.

to appear. Enlargement of the breasts and menarche do not take place in girls, and there is a failure of spermatogenesis in boys. If growth hormone and the other tropic hormones of the pituitary (thyrotropin and adrenocorticotropin) are elaborated normally in the absence of gonadotropins, linear growth will continue beyond the usual time of epiphyseal closure, and a eunuchoid body habitus results.

In adults who develop gonadal insufficiency, there is a partial reversal or regression of the changes that took place during sexual maturation. In men, the earliest evidence of gonadotropic failure is loss of libido and potentia. Concurrently there are prostatic atrophy (a sensitive index of testicular failure) and failure of spermatogenesis, and later, a decrease in the rate of growth of the beard. In women, there are loss of libido and cessation of menses. Atrophy of the breasts is not common, although the nipples may lose their pigmentation. Galactorrhea may occur in either sex if the pituitary failure is the result of a prolactin-producing pituitary adenoma or a suprasellar lesion that impinges upon the hypothalamus or the portal blood system flowing from the hypothalamus to the anterior pituitary. In both sexes, failure of the gonads is accompanied by thinning or loss of axillary and pubic hair as well as loss of hair from the trunk and extremities, but not the scalp. The skin becomes pale and atrophic, and the complexion may acquire a yellowish tinge frequently with fine freckles, particularly over the face. Transient hot flushes may occur in either sex as the gonads fail.

Thyroid Insufficiency

Some patients with anterior pituitary failure that includes thyrotropin deficiency and secondary hypothyroidism will have the typical appearance and other characteristics of primary myxedema such as myxedematous skin, myoedema, slowed tendon reflexes, and hypercholesterolemia. The majority of patients with secondary thyroid failure do not present these manifestations, however, despite the failure being severe and of long duration. In either instance, as the thyroid fails, the patient experiences intolerance to cold, a decrease in perspiration, and dryness of the skin.

Patients who have unitropic thyrotropin failure have the usual physical signs associated with primary myxedema.

Adrenal Cortical Insufficiency

Failure of the adrenal cortices leads to weakness, poor resistance to infection, and inability to cope with stress in a normal fashion. Lack of adrenal cortical hormones also contributes to the loss of sexual hair.

Hypoglycemia may be found in patients with severe pituitary failure, and although several hormonal factors play a role in this hypoglycemia, it is primarily the result of lack of adrenal cortical hormones and is readily corrected by the administration of physiological doses of adrenal corticosteroids such as cortisone.

Generalized symptoms such as apathy, fatigue, and lack of strength are nonspecific findings that cannot be ascribed to the failure of any specific target gland and are probably the result of the comprehensive debility associated with advanced pituitary insufficiency. On the other hand it is amazing how rapidly these symptoms, along with the nonspecific generalized muscular and joint aching, which is occasionally seen with advanced pituitary insufficiency, will improve within 24 to 36 hours after starting physiological replacement doses of adrenal corticosteroids.

Unitropic (Monohormonal) Hypopituitarism

Unitropic failure may be idiopathic or familial. In either instance it often is not clear whether the defect lies in the pituitary or in the hypothalamus, but such distinctions undoubtedly will become clearer in the future as the releasing hormones that are available at present (TRH and GnRH) are more widely used and as releasing hormones for other pituitary hormones become available.

The various syndromes of unitropic failure of growth hormone, thyrotropin, adrenocorticotropin, and follicle-stimulating and luteinizing hormones are not reviewed here in detail. They are of practical interest to the neurosurgeon only in that seemingly unitropic failure in an adult, who otherwise appears normal, may merely be the first manifestation of what will ultimately become complete failure of the anterior pituitary as the secretions of its other hormones fails with progression of some underlying lesion. This is particulary true in young women who have never undergone menarche or who have had a menarche and have subsequently become amenorrheic.

Laboratory Studies in Anterior Pituitary Failure

In pituitary failure the lack of secretion of tropic hormones (TSH, ACTH, FSH, and LH) by the anterior pituitary results in a decrease in the function of the target endocrine glands, namely the thyroid, the adrenal cortices, and the gonads, and inability of the anterior pituitary to increase its production of tropic hormones when challenged—that is, lack of pituitary reserve. Currently it is possible to measure both the tropic hormones and the hormones produced by the target endocrine glands. Likewise, it is possible to measure the "nontropic" hormones of the pituitary, namely growth hormone and prolactin.

When failure of one or more of the target endocrine glands is demonstrated, the physician must decide whether the cause is failure of the target gland or glands (primary failure) or failure due to anterior pituitary insufficiency (secondary failure). If there is primary failure of a target gland, the production of the appropriate tropic hormone should be increased by the anterior pituitary and the target gland should not respond to the exogenous administration of that hormone. On the other hand, if secondary failure of a target gland is present, production of the tropic hormone should be decreased or absent and the target gland should respond to its administration. In actual practice it is only in the exceptional case that one needs to administer the appropriate tropic hormone to differentiate between primary and secondary failure of a target gland. In primary failure, measurement of the tropic hormone is useful because there is usually a clear-cut separation between the normal range and the higher values found with failure of the target gland. For example, an elevation of the thyrotropin level is one of the most sensitive indicators of early primary thyroidal failure. On the other hand, the distinction between low-normal and abnormally low values for tropic hormones is not at all clear-cut, and there is a large overlap between their levels in normal persons and in patients with anterior pituitary failure. This is quite analogous to the uptake of radioio-

TABLE 25–4   ANTERIOR PITUITARY FAILURE PITUITARY AND TARGET HORMONES

HORMONES		STIMULATION TESTS		
Pituitary	Serum (Plasma) Value	Drug	Normal Response	Response in Pituitary Tumor*
Growth-hormone (GH)	Normal–borderline low	Insulin	↑	0 ± ↑
		Arginine	↑	0 ± ↑
		Propranolol-Glucagon	↑	0 ± ↑
		L-dopa	↑	0 ± ↑
Prolactin (PRL)	Normal–borderline low	Thyrotropin-releasing hormone (TRH)	↑	0 ± ↑
		Chlorpromazine	↑	0 ± ↑
Thyroid-stimulating hormone (TSH)	Normal–borderline low	TRH	↑	0 ± ↑
Adrenocorticotropin (ACTH)	Normal–borderline low	Insulin	↑	0 ±
Follicle-stimulating hormone (FSH) and luteinizing hormone (LH)	Normal–borderline low	Gonadotropin-releasing hormone (GnRH)	↑	0 ± ↑
		Clomiphene	↑	0 ± ↑
TARGET				
Thyroxine	Borderline low ↓	Thyrotropin-releasing hormone (TRH)	↑	0 ± ↑
Corticosteroids	Borderline low ↓	Insulin	↑	0 ±
Testosterone	Borderline low ↓	GnRH	↑	0 ± ↑
Estrogens	Borderline low ↓	Clomiphene	↑	0 ±

* When pituitary tumor does not make hormone being tested.
Key: ↑ increased, ↓ decreased, ± equivocal, 0 no response.

© Mayo 1979

dine by the thyroid, which is not helpful in differentiating normal thyroid function from hypothyroidism because there is too much overlap between these two states.

When anterior pituitary failure is moderately severe or in the advanced state, the physical findings plus measurement of the hormones produced by the target glands will usually confirm the diagnosis. When there is doubt, as in early pituitary failure, the stimulation tests that challenge pituitary reserve may be helpful. Table 25–4 is a guide to these tests. Because of limitations of space, details concerning the performance of these tests and the nuances of interpretation are left to standard textbooks of endocrinology such as those by Williams, and by Labhart, and the text on endocrine laboratory tests by Alsever and Gotlin.[1,58,128] The texts by Martin and co-workers and by Martin and Besser are especially outstanding in this regard.[71,72]

As noted in Table 25–4, administration of a releasing hormone, in some instances, may evoke a normal release of the tropic hormone by the pituitary even though there may be some deficiency of the circulating target hormone stimulated by this tropic hormone. The precise mechanism is not understood, but it may be that the pituitary cells that make the tropic hormone are not being maximally stimulated or that the pituitary tumor may be impairing the passage of the endogenous releasing hormone along the portal veins from the hypothalamus to the anterior pituitary.

Electrolytes

Since patients with pituitary failure have essentially normal aldosterone production, they usually do not have hyponatremia, hypochloremia, or hyperkalemia as can patients with primary adrenal failure. Patients with severe pituitary failure, however, readily develop hyponatremia and hypochloremia with illnesses that are manifested by vomiting and diarrhea. Also, patients with severe anterior pituitary failure are unable to excrete a water load normally, and thus are subject to water intoxication, which is readily reversed by the administration of adrenal corticosteroids.

Plasma Glucose

Typically the plasma or blood glucose of patients with untreated pituitary insuffi-

ciency is normal, although often in the lower portion of the normal range. Patients with severe, untreated anterior pituitary failure, however, may have hypoglycemia, which at times is symptomatic and can be fatal, and which is readily corrected or prevented by the administration of adrenal corticosteroids. When hypoglycemia is present in a patient with a pituitary tumor, the clinician should always be alert to the possibility that the patient may have multiple endocrine adenomatosis (MEA-I syndrome) with one or more insulin-producing pancreatic islet cell tumors.[5,59]

Peripheral Blood Counts

Hemoglobin and the erythrocyte count are usually normal in patients with mild pituitary insufficiency. Prolonged severe pituitary insufficiency may, however, result in a moderate to severe normochromic, normocytic anemia, particularly in males. Moderate elevation of the sedimentation rate (30 to 50 mm per hour) may also be present. These abnormalities are readily reversed by giving the patient hormonal replacement therapy. A mild eosinophilia of more than 5 per cent may also be present, but disappears when the patient is given adrenal corticosteroids.

Other Features of Anterior Pituitary Failure

When pituitary failure results from a tumor in or around the sella turcica, the usual symptoms and findings listed in Table 25–2 may develop. Encroachment upon the hypothalamico-neurohypophyseal system may result in diabetes insipidus. As anterior pituitary failure progresses, however, there will be an amelioration of the polyuria and polydipsia, although the inability to concentrate urine will remain (Fig. 25–4). The clinician may be misled into believing that the subsidence of the polyuria and polydipsia is an indication that the patient is improving, while in fact the situation is deteriorating because of the development of progressive anterior pituitary failure.

With progressive anterior pituitary failure, as seen with an enlarging tumor, there is usually first a loss of production of pituitary gonadotropins (FSH and LH), then of thyrotropin, and finally of adrenocorticotropin. This sequence is not inviolable; the adrenal cortices may fail before the thyroid,

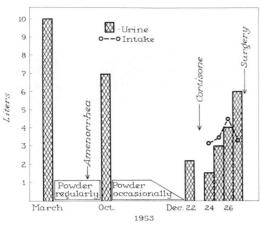

Figure 25–4 Decrease in polyuria of diabetes insipidus with the development of anterior pituitary failure. Large doses of cortisone prior to operation evoked a significant polyuria. Powder, posterior pituitary powder. (From Clark, E. C., Dodge, H. W., Jr., and Randall, R. V.: Therapeutic problems in diabetes insipidus. J.A.M.A., *163*:341–344, 1957. Copyright 1957, American Medical Association. Reprinted by permission.)

and either may fail before the gonads, although it is unusual for them to do so. It is not clear where growth hormone and prolactin fit in this scheme of events. If, however, the lesion is one that results in increased elaboration of prolactin, the secretion of this hormone will increase as the other pituitary hormones fail.

Whenever pituitary failure is caused by a nonfunctioning pituitary adenoma, a growth hormone–producing pituitary adenoma, or a prolactin-producing pituitary adenoma, the presence of multiple endocrine adenomatosis (MEA-I syndrome), especially that involving the parathyroid glands and insulin-producing islet cells of the pancreas, must be considered in addition to the pituitary.[5,59]

When pituitary insufficiency is secondary to a systemic disease such as sarcoidosis, histiocytosis X, metastatic tumor, or the like, one should expect to find the signs, symptoms, and physical findings typically associated with the primary disease.

One of the major pitfalls in dealing with a patient with anterior pituitary failure is to establish that diagnosis and then, on failing to find an etiological factor, to assume that it is primary (idiopathic) in origin. Pituitary insufficiency that occurs in adults is almost invariably secondary in origin rather than idiopathic. It should be recognized that in anterior pituitary failure, evidences of pituitary dysfunction may, by months or years, precede other manifestations of a tumor in or around the sella or of some systemic disease. The author has followed patients for as long as 8 to 10 years before the underlying cause became evident, although this is less likely to occur nowadays with better ways of looking for tumors, such as polycyclic tomography of the sella, bilateral carotid angiography, and computed tomography of the head.

In general, pituitary insufficiency is slowly progressive and may be compatible with life for many years. Such patients, however, are sensitive to stress, and relatively mild febrile illnesses or operative procedures may precipitate a pituitary crisis manifested by rapidly progressive weakness, fever, hypotension, collapse, and death if untreated.

Pituitary apoplexy (abrupt anterior pituitary failure) may be precipitated by a hemorrhage into the normal pituitary gland (most commonly seen in patients with diabetes mellitus), by hemorrhage into a pituitary tumor, or by pituitary necrosis secondary to postpartum shock (Sheehan's syndrome), any one of which may result in sudden death if not recognized and promptly treated.[108]

Replacement Therapy for Anterior Pituitary Failure

Growth Hormone Replacement

Although growth hormone has many known physiological effects, its administration is not essential to the optimal treatment of adult patients with anterior pituitary failure. This is fortunate, because only human growth hormone and simian growth hormone are effective in humans, and the supply of the human hormone for treating dwarfed, growth hormone–deficient, growth hormone–responsive persons is available in only limited quantities.

A number of treatment schedules with growth hormones have been proposed for children dwarfed from lack of it, and although the optimal dose has not been clearly defined, the usual treatment consists of two units of hormone given subcutaneously three times a week. Many patients receiving growth hormone develop antibodies to the material, but this rarely results in failure to respond to the treatment. Interestingly enough, some patients receiving growth hormone develop hypothyroidism, for unknown reasons, which disappears when administration of the hormone is discontinued.

When growth hormone is unavailable, anabolic steroids, which are weak androgens, may be helpful. The author has usually used oxandrolone (Anavar, Searle) 0.1 to 0.15 mg per kilogram per 24 hours divided into two or three oral doses. This must be monitored carefully to avoid excessive progression of skeletal age and premature closure of the epiphyses. The physician should be aware also of the possible undesirable androgenic effects in females and the possible changes in liver function that may occur.

Thyroid Replacement

Effective thyroid replacement is attained by giving 0.15 mg of levothyroxine sodium in a single dose each day. An occasional patient will require 0.2 or even 0.3 mg a day, or a smaller dose of 0.1 mg per day. The two guides to the appropriate dose are the response of the patient and the level of serum thyroxine. It must be kept in mind that the administration of estrogenic materials increases thyroxine-binding globulin, while androgens reduce it. Interestingly enough, children usually require and tolerate essentially the same dose as adults.

Adrenal Corticosteroid Replacement

Since the adrenal cortices in the normal adult make 20 to 30 mg of hydrocortisone per day, replacement consists of giving this substance orally in two or three divided doses or an equivalent amount of a related compound such as cortisone or prednisone. Since hydrocortisone is the compound normally made by the human adrenal cortices, the author has used this compound in recent years rather than prednisone as formerly when there was a greater price differential between the two. The usual plan is to have the patient take 15 to 20 mg of hydrocortisone each morning and 10 mg in the late afternoon or early evening, or else 10 mg three times a day: morning, around noontime, and late afternoon or early evening. Some patients who take the last dose late in the evening just before retiring may complain of difficulty in sleeping.

Some authors advocate the use of as much as 37.5 or 50 mg of hydrocortisone or cortisone a day, but the author believes this is excessive, and some patients given these doses develop undesirable side effects such as mild hypercortisonism or personality changes. One must also wonder whether such doses may not accelerate the normal skeletal demineralization that occurs as people grow older.

Growing children are acutely sensitive to excessive amounts of adrenal corticosteroids and respond with a slowing or cessation of linear growth. As a consequence, the author gives preadult patients a total of only 7.5 to 10 mg of hydrocortisone a day in two or three divided doses and carefully monitors their growth as well as the adequacy of the daily dose.

All patients taking adrenal corticosteroids are advised, in the event of a minor febrile illness, to double their intake of steroids and notify their physician at once. Patients are asked to keep on hand a supply of parenteral steroid that can be given in the event of a sudden, stressful illness until they can obtain medical help. A convenient form is a packet consisting of a disposable needle and a syringe containing a 1-ml solution of 4 mg of dexamethasone sodium phosphate (Decadron phosphate, Merck Sharp & Dohme). Patients are also asked to tell physicians caring for them that in the event of an operation, severe illness, or other undue physical stress they should be given large doses of parenteral adrenocortical steroids. It is also advisable for such patients to wear a bracelet or necklace inscribed with the facts that they have pituitary insufficiency, are taking replacement therapy, and need to be given parenteral steroids. The Medic Alert necklace or bracelet is most satisfactory.*

Gonadal Replacement

For males, androgens can be given intramuscularly, orally, or buccally. The intramuscular preparations are more effective and less expensive for equivalent androgenic effects than the oral or buccal preparations. The author prefers to use testosterone enanthate in sesame oil (Delatestryl, Squibb) or testosterone cypionate in cot-

---

* Medic Alert Foundation, P. O. Box 1009, Turlock, California 95380.

tonseed oil (Depo-Testosterone, Upjohn) in doses of 200 mg intramuscularly every three weeks. The former has the advantage of being available prepackaged, 200 mg in a disposable syringe with a needle. An occasional patient may need an injection every two weeks, while some patients may go as long as four weeks or a month between injections. A member of the family is usually instructed in the intramuscular administration of this material in the buttocks, but some patients prefer to give the material themselves into the large anterior thigh muscles.

The intramuscular preparations do not seem to carry the risk of cholestatic jaundice that the oral and buccal preparations do, although such occurrence with the latter is infrequent and reversible once the material has been stopped.

Androgens preferably are not started in the hypogonadal adolescent male as long as the epiphyses of the long bones are open and the patient has not reached an acceptable height. The epiphyses will close at an older age than normally, but if there is also a deficiency of growth hormone, the rate of growth will be less than average. As a consequence, there may be an emotional conflict between his desire for more height and his desire for sexual maturation. If one is obligated to start treatment with testosterone under such circumstances, 75 to 100 mg of testosterone enanthate or cypionate is given intramuscularly once a month until the epiphyses have closed, at which time the dose is increased to 200 mg every three weeks. Growth is monitored every six months by measuring height and roentgenograms of the epiphyses of the wrist for skeletal maturation.

For females, adequate replacement therapy can be given orally, and it is not necessary to use intramuscular estrogens. The estrogenic materials are given cyclically to induce withdrawal bleeding should there be enough build-up of the endometrial mucosa, and to relieve breast fullness and tenderness if such take place. In adults, conjugated estrogens (such as Premarin, Ayerst), 0.625 or 1.25 mg per day are given for the first 21 days of each month or for three of every four weeks; diethylstilbestrol, 0.1 mg daily is given on the same schedule; or ethinyl estradiol (Estinyl, Schering; Lynoral, Organon) 0.01 or 0.2 mg daily on the same

schedule. If irregular uterine bleeding occurs, then 5 to 10 mg of a progesterone preparation such as medroxyprogesterone acetate (Provera, Upjohn) may be given orally at the rate of 10 mg every day during the third week of estrogen therapy. A convenient form of giving combined estrogen and progesterone therapy is to use one of the birth control pills containing both substances.

Precautions similar to those described for using sex steroid therapy in the adolescent male must be observed in the adolescent female. Once the epiphyses are closed it may be helpful to give two or three times the usual maintenance dose of estrogenic materials for up to one year and add progesterone in an attempt to obtain optimal development of the breasts and external genitalia. If there is poor development of sexual hair, a cautious trial of small doses of androgens (2 mg of fluoxymesterone [Halotestin, Upjohn] orally every one or two days) for a period of six to nine months can be used. This must, however, be monitored carefully to prevent excessive androgenism.

While the patient is taking estrogens, she should be on the lookout for thrombophlebitis, the development of hypertension, and other side effects ascribed to estrogens in birth control pills. Although the author does not have statistical data, it is his impression that women with anterior pituitary failure who receive estrogens are less likely to develop these side effects than are normal women who are given estrogens.

Mineralocorticoids

Since the production of aldosterone by the adrenal cortex is primarily under the control of the renin-angiotensin system rather than adrenocorticotropin, the administration of a mineralocorticoid is usually not necessary in the treatment of patients with secondary adrenal failure as it is in patients with primary adrenal failure (Addison's disease). Nonetheless, an occasional patient with anterior pituitary failure (usually secondary to a tumor in the suprasellar region), despite adequate treatment with thyroid, adrenal cortical, and gonadal replacement therapy, may exhibit mineralocorticoid deficiency mainfested by decreased values for serum sodium and chlorides, increased value for serum potassium, and hypotension. This deficiency is readily corrected by the oral administration of 0.1 mg of fludrocortisone acetate (Florinef Acetate, Squibb) each day.

Schedule for Studying Patients to Detect Anterior Pituitary Failure

DAY ONE

Routine studies. Hematological studies; blood chemistry determinations; sedimentation rate, x-rays of chest; electrocardiogram, and urinalysis (overnight "concentrated" specimen to exclude nonpolyuric diabetes insipidus, as described under Other Features of Anterior Pituitary Failure).

Special studies. X-rays of skull and polycyclic tomograms of sella with posteroanterior and lateral views with cuts every 2 to 3 mm; ophthalmoscopy and perimetric examination of the visual fields; blood analyses for corticosteroids (8:00 A.M. and 4:00 P.M.), PRL, GH, ACTH, TSH, LH, FSH, testosterone or estrogens, and total thyroxine.*

Start 24-hour urine collection at 7:00 or 8:00 A.M. for evaluation of 17-ketosteroids and 17-hydroxycorticosteroids (or 17-ketogenic steroids), and pituitary gonadotropins (requires 48-hour urine specimen).

DAY TWO

A.M.: Insulin hypoglycemia test (after completion of 24-hour urine collection for adrenal steroids).† Patient is given crystalline zinc insulin intravenously, 0.05 unit per kilogram of body weight, *after* determination that the baseline value for plasma glucose is not in the hypoglycemic range. Blood for glucose, GH, corticosteroids, and ACTH measurement is obtained at 30, 60, 90, and 120 minutes after insulin is given. *The patient must be watched closely for possible hypoglycemia.*

Note: Some clinicians prefer to avoid possible severe hypoglycemia from insulin and use a propranolol-glucagon provocative test to study GH

and ACTH responsiveness. Blood for determination of GH, ACTH, and corticosteroid levels is obtained at 7:00 A.M. and the patient is given orally 40 mg of propranolol hydrochloride (Inderal, Ayerst). At 9:00 A.M. the patient is given 1.0 mg of glucagon intramuscularly (Glucagon for Injection, Lilly). Blood is obtained at 11:00 A.M. and again at 12:00 noon for GH, ACTH, and corticosteroid evaluations.

P.M. Computed tomographic scans of head, with contrast medium, with particular attention to suprasellar-hypothalamic region, if x-rays of head and polycyclic tomograms of sella are normal.

DAY THREE

A.M. LHRH (GnRH) test (after completion of 48-hour urine collection for measurement of pituitary gonadotropins).† Patient is given 100 μg LHRH intravenously. Blood for FSH and LH tests is obtained at 0, 30, and 60 minutes.

P.M. TRH test.† Patient is given 400 μg TRH intravenously. Blood for TSH and PRL determinations is obtained at 0, 30, and 60 minutes.

Note: Some clinicians give an intravenous mixture containing insulin, TRH, and LHRH in the foregoing doses and measure glucose, GH, corticosteroids, ACTH, TSH, PRL, FSH, and LH at 0, 15, 30, 60, 90, and 120 minutes.

DAY FOUR

Bilateral carotid angiography with magnification and subtraction views or pneumoencephalography, or both, if preceding studies have not revealed the cause of the anterior pituitary failure. If, after these studies, the cause of the anterior pituitary failure is not evident, then periodic reevaluation of the patient is indicated, in addition to treatment of pituitary insufficiency.

Hyperfunction of the Anterior Pituitary

In the normal human, the anterior pituitary secretes growth hormone (GH), prolactin (PRL), adrenocorticotropic hormone (ACTH), thyroid-stimulating hormone (TSH), follicle-stimulating hormone (FSH), and luteinizing hormone (LH). Pituitary tumors secreting each of these hormones have been described. There are also so-called "nonfunctioning" chromophobe adenomas of the pituitary, which manifest themselves by signs and symptoms related to the fact that they are space-occupying lesions (see Table 25–1). The term "nonfunctioning" may be a misnomer because studies by electron microscopy suggest that the

---

* Separation between values for PRL, GH, ACTH, TSH, LH, and FSH that are in lower portion of normal range and values present in pituitary failure is poor but helpful in diagnosing overproduction of one or more of these hormones by a pituitary tumor.

† If desired. The author, in the interest of economy, usually does not do releasing hormone studies or provocative studies with insulin or propranolol and glucagon in the routine evaluation of patients with anterior pituitary failure. Decisions about hormonal replacement therapy are based on clinical findings and laboratory tests of thyroid, gonadal, and adrenal function, i.e., values for serum thyroxine and testosterone or estrogens, blood corticosteroids, and urinary 17-ketosteroids and 17-ketogenic steroids.

cells of such tumors usually contain secretory elements, and it is entirely possible that some of these tumors may be secreting substances that are unknown at this time.

Pituitary tumors that secrete thyroid-stimulating hormone or gonadotropin are relatively rare, while those that secrete growth hormone, adrenocorticotropin, or prolactin are relatively common. It was previously thought that the growth hormone–secreting tumors were the most common, causing either acromegaly or, in the preadult, gigantism, while those secreting adrenocorticotropin and causing Cushing's disease were less common, and those secreting prolactin the least common. As methods for assaying prolactin are being used more widely, however, it is evident that prolactin-secreting pituitary tumors are the most common of all. The frequency of these various neoplasms will not be known until a large number of them have been studied both before and after removal, by measuring blood values for the various pituitary hormones, and by immunohistological studies of the removed tissues or other techniques to determine exactly what hormones their cells are producing. For example, it is entirely possible that a pituitary tumor could be producing prolactin, yet studies before operation would reveal normal values in the blood and normal dynamics for the hormone, since some prolactin-producing tumors may respond normally when stimulation or suppression tests are done. The true secretory nature of the tumor would not be revealed until immunohistological studies were done on the tumor's cells after its removal. This would be somewhat analogous to a thyroxine-producing adenoma of the thyroid that produces enough thyroxine to suppress partially or completely the normal thyroid gland, but not enough to elevate the circulating thyroxine levels in the blood above the normal range.

Growth Hormone–Secreting Pituitary Tumors

These tumors cause acromegaly in adults or, in preadults, gigantism followed by acromegalic changes if the tumor continues to secrete excessive amounts of growth hormone after the epiphyses of the long bones have closed. With rare exceptions, the author believes that all patients with excessive production of growth hormone have GH-secreting pituitary tumors. In recent years there has been little evidence to suggest that eosinophilic hyperplasia of the pituitary exists, although this used to be a popular diagnosis years ago. Nonetheless, the theory of eosinophilic hyperplasia must remain open, because until recently the majority of patients with acromegaly or gigantism were not operated upon, but either they were given radiation therapy or no treatment was directed at the pituitary, and autopsy studies in large series of acromegalic patients are nonexistent. There have been several reports of patients with acromegaly associated with an extrapituitary tumor (pulmonary carcinoid) that was thought to be producing growth hormone and in whom the acromegalic syndrome regressed after the tumor had been removed.[19,119] The author has seen an acromegalic woman in whom the acromegaly regressed after the removal of an islet cell tumor of the pancreas.[11] The tumor was thought but not proved to be secreting a growth hormone–releasing substance. Subsequently, Leveston and co-workers showed that a growth hormone–releasing substance was secreted by a metastatic carcinoid tumor in an 18-year-old man with gigantism, and Frohman and co-workers demonstrated a similar substance in a bronchial carcinoid tumor removed from a patient with acromegaly.[36,63,131] Frohman and co-workers have since isolated and partially characterized a peptide with growth hormone–releasing activity from the tumors of these three patients.[35]

The basic defect giving rise to the growth hormone–producing pituitary tumor in acromegaly and gigantism is not known. Current thoughts are that the tumor either arises de novo or results from a hypothalamic disorder giving rise to an excessive production of growth hormone–releasing factor by the hypothalamus, a decreased production of growth hormone–inhibiting hormone (somatostatin) by the hypothalamus, or an imbalance between these two hypothalamic regulatory substances.

The signs and symptoms of acromegaly

are discussed in Chapter 98 and in standard texts.[58,96,128] The following discussion of this syndrome may apply to gigantism as well.

At times the physician may be faced with one of two problems when dealing with patients having or suspected of having acromegaly. The first is to establish a diagnosis when early mild acromegaly is suspected but the classic signs and symptoms are not present. The second is one in which the patient has the obvious signs and symptoms of acromegaly, but it is not evident whether the disease is hormonally active. One should assume that a patient with acromegaly who has not previously received treatment for the condition has hormonally active acromegaly. It was once thought that "burned-out acromegaly," that is, acromegaly that spontaneously has become hormonally inactive, was common. Now that it is possible to measure serum growth hormone, it has become evident that burned-out acromegaly is uncommon, and that it is possible for a patient to have hormonally active acromegaly even though there is coexisting anterior pituitary failure secondary to the expanding growth hormone–producing pituitary tumor.[94] Even when dealing with a patient with acromegaly who has previously received treatment directed to the pituitary, one must determine whether the treatment has been effective or the process continues to be hormonally active.

Laboratory Examination

In addition to the usual studies such as roentgenograms of the skull, polycyclic tomograms of the sella, examination of the visual fields, and measurement of pituitary and end-organ hormones, usually done in patients having or suspected of having pituitary tumors, the following procedures are helpful in assessing the acromegalic patient.

SERUM GROWTH HORMONE. The single most useful laboratory procedure in the diagnosis of hormonally active acromegaly is measurement of serum growth hormone. With rare exceptions to be mentioned later, patients with active acromegaly have increased values for serum growth hormone. In the author's institution the normal basal range is, for females, 10 ng per milliliter or less, and for males 5 ng per milliliter or less. The normal range may vary in different laboratories, and as is true of all laboratory tests, the physician must be familiar with the normal range in the laboratory he uses. Some normal females and patients of either sex who are taking estrogens or L-dopa, are not under basal conditions, or have hypoglycemia at the time the blood samples are obtained may have elevated values for growth hormone. Severe food deprivation, notably anorexia nervosa, will elevate the values. In these instances and in the normal person with values in the basal range, the growth hormone decreases to zero or less than 1 ng per milliliter with hyperglycemia. Hence, the standard test is to do a three- or five-hour glucose tolerance test measuring both glucose and growth hormone values immediately before and at one-hourly intervals following the administration of glucose. In the normal person, the values for growth hormone fall to zero or less than 1 ng per milliliter in 30 to 60 minutes. In some normal patients, toward the end of a glucose tolerance test, particularly one continued for five hours, the value for glucose may fall below 50 to 55 mg per 100 ml and there may be a reciprocal rise in growth hormone to 15 to 20 ng or so. This is a normal response to the relative hypoglycemia. In hormonally active acromegaly, the response of growth hormone during the glucose tolerance test varies; the values may (1) fall toward but not to normal, (2) remain unchanged, (3) vary in a random fashion, or (4) rise.

In patients who have been successfully treated for acromegaly and whose values for growth hormone have returned to normal, the value frequently will not be depressed normally in response to hyperglycemia during a glucose tolerance test. This suggests that while the hypersecretion of growth hormone has been successfully treated, an underlying hypothalamic defect or imbalance is still operative, or there may still be a functioning remnant of the tumor.

The level of serum growth hormone is not a good index to the rate of progression of the syndrome as judged by changes in soft tissues and abnormalities in other laboratory tests. It should also be recognized that, on the basis of other criteria, hormonally active acromegaly may be present even though basal values for growth hormone are normal. The values, however, will not be depressed normally during a glucose tolerance test. This suggests that either the hormone is utilized or degraded at a greater than normal rate or the pituitary tumor is secreting either a biologically active hormone that differs structurally from normal growth hormone (against which the assay is devised) or biologically active fragments of hormone that are not fully detected by the hGH immunoassay. Arnaud and associates have demonstrated an analogous situation in patients with parathormone-producing tumors.[3] Thus, the physician must use other criteria, which are discussed in the following paragraphs, when values for growth hormone do not confirm the clinical impression or hormonally active acromegaly, and must not allow the normal hormone levels to deter him from prescribing appropriate treatment of the acromegaly when other findings indicate that the disease process is hormonally active.

PROLACTIN. It has been recognized for many years that some patients, both female and male, with acromegaly also have galactorrhea. Ezrin, Kovacs and associates, using immunohistological and electron microscopic techniques, have shown that some growth hormone–producing pituitary tumors associated with acromegaly also contain tumor cells that are distinct from the growth hormone–producing cells and that produce prolactin.[16,117] The possibility that the some tumor cells lines may produce and secrete both growth hormone and prolactin has not, however, been ruled out. Not unexpectedly, one patient with acromegaly and galactorrhea-amenorrhea was found to have two pituitary adenomas, one secreting growth hormone and the other, prolactin.[124]

Whenever galactorrhea is present in a patient with acromegaly, the value for serum prolactin is usually but not always increased. Patients may, however, have acromegaly and elevated prolactin values and not have galactorrhea. The frequency of hyperprolactinemia in acromegaly differs in various reports, but has been observed to be as great as 40 per cent.[32,33]

INORGANIC PHOSPHATE. Before the immunoassay for growth hormone became available, the serum inorganic phosphate level was used as a guide to activity, being elevated in many patients with hormonally active acromegaly. It is now known that many patients with active acromegaly have normal serum inorganic phosphate values. Patients with coexisting acromegaly and primary hyperparathyroidism (multiple endocrine adenomatosis) usually have serum inorganic phosphate values within the normal range or, rarely, below the normal range, unless renal failure is present.

CALCIUM. Hormonally active acromegaly can increase the serum calcium 0.5 to 1.0 mg per 100 ml above the normal range, but with higher values the presence of coexisting primary hyperparathyroidism (multiple endocrine adenomatosis) must be suspected and ruled out.[5,59] Serum parathormone is normal in those patients who have elevation of the serum calcium content from active acromegaly. Measurement of serum parathormone in patients with acromegaly and hypercalcemia is useful in distinguishing between those who have acromegaly alone and those who have acromegaly and primary hyperparathyroidism.[97]

Hypercalciuria of 450 to 700 mg per 24 hours is not unusual in active acromegaly. These values are greater than expected in primary hyperparathyroidism alone. When the urinary calcium is over 900 to 1000 mg per 24 hours, one should strongly suspect the presence of primary hyperparathyroidism in addition to active acromegaly.

ALKALINE PHOSPHATASE. Some patients with active acromegaly have an elevated serum alkaline phosphatase level that returns to normal when the acromegaly is rendered inactive. When this abnormality is found, one must always rule out the additional possibility of coexisting primary hyperparathyroidism with bony involvement.

GLUCOSE. The frequency of hyperglycemia and diabetes mellitus in active acromegaly varies according to different reports. In recent years, as patients with active acromegaly have been studied more carefully, particularly with glucose tolerance tests, it has become evident that the frequency of diabetes mellitus is lower than previously suspected, and the author's current estimate is that a positive glucose tolerance test occurs in about 20 to 25 per cent of patients with active acromegaly.

If hypoglycemia is found, the presence of

a coexisting insulin-producing islet cell adenoma or adenomas of the pancreas should be ruled out.[5,59]

BASAL METABOLIC RATE. The basal metabolic rate may be elevated by more than 50 to 70 per cent by active acromegaly. The reason for this is not known, but the rate returns to normal after successful treatment of the acromegaly. It is interesting that patients with severe anorexia nervosa may have growth hormone values greater than 100 ng per milliliter, yet they often will have basal metabolic rates as low as 45 to 50 per cent below normal.

URINARY ADRENAL STEROIDS. Urinary 17-ketosteroids and 17-hydroxycorticosteroids (or 17-ketogenic steroids) are usually normal in active acromegaly, although the levels may be elevated, particularly those of the urinary 17-ketosteroids. In the latter instances, the plasma corticosteroids are normal, and the adrenals respond normally to testing with metyrapone or dexamethasone.

SOMATOMEDIN. Clemmons and co-workers have shown that the level of somatomedin C in the blood is increased in hormonally active acromegaly, returns to normal when the acromegaly is in remission, and is a better guide to the hormonal activity than is the level of growth hormone.[15]

CREATININE CLEARANCE. The renal creatinine clearance may be increased in active acromegaly, probably because of increased renal size. This test is no longer commonly used as an index of hormonal activity in acromegaly.

COSTOCHONDRAL EPIPHYSES. Normally, the epiphyses of the ribs in humans close in the third decade of life.[52] In patients with active acromegaly, however, the costochondral junction remains open and continues to show active endochondral bone formation beyond the third decade, and in younger acromegalic patients endochondral formation will be greater than that in normal persons of the same age. The costochondral junction closes when active acromegaly is rendered inactive.[53] This test was occasionally used as an autobioassay of growth hormone activity before the advent of the radioimmunoassay.

URINARY HYDROXYPROLINE. The urinary excretion of hydroxyproline is increased in hormonally active acromegaly and returns to normal when the acromegalic process is rendered quiescent. This test is rarely used now that it is possible to measure serum or plasma growth hormone.

CARPAL TUNNEL SYNDROME. One study suggests that approximately one third of patients with active acromegaly have a carpal tunnel syndrome in one or both hands along with the typical findings on electromyography.[89] Patients with active acromegaly and carpal tunnel syndrome frequently state that the symptoms of this syndrome, like the hyperhidrosis so commonly present in active acromegaly, disappear within several days after successful removal of the pituitary tumor, and this may be the first clue to a decrease in the level of growth hormone after operation.

SPINAL FLUID EXAMINATION. The value for cerebrospinal fluid human growth hormone will be well above 1 ng per milliliter when there is suprasellar extension of a hormonally active pituitary tumor associated with acromegaly.[46,66] Computed tomography is, in the author's experience, a more helpful test because it will reveal not only suprasellar extension of such a tumor but also the magnitude of the extension

Potential Pitfalls in Active Acromegaly

There are several potential pitfalls in dealing with patients who have or are suspected of having active acromegaly.

FAILURE TO IDENTIFY THE PITUITARY TUMOR. A normal appearing sella on standard roentgenographic views of the skull (anteroposterior, posteroanterior, and stereoscopic lateral views) does not rule out the presence of a pituitary tumor. In the acromegalic patient, the increased amount of bone in the calvarium and the enlarged mastoid and paranasal sinuses often make it difficult to identify the bony limits of the sella. Spiral or polycyclic tomographic posteroanterior and lateral views of the sella with serial cuts every 2 to 3 mm will frequently demonstrate a small pituitary tumor that is not appreciated on the standard views. If these studies are not diagnostic, bilateral carotid angiography with magnification and subtraction views should be done. With this procedure tumors as small as 3 or 4 mm in diameter may be identified.[95] Keeping in mind the rare occurrence of ectopic production of growth hormone or growth hormone–releasing substance by a tumor outside the pituitary, the physician should assume that all patients with acromegaly have a pituitary tumor.[19,119] If the acromegaly is active, no effort should be spared to demonstrate the tumor, because it is desirable, except in unusual circumstances, to treat the tumor in an attempt to make the acromegaly hormonally inactive.

FAILURE TO APPRECIATE HORMONAL ACTIVITY OF ACROMEGALY. As mentioned earlier, hormonally active acromegaly is usually associated with elevated values for serum or plasma growth hormone that are not suppressed with hyperglycemia. It is possible, however, to have hormonally active acromegaly in the presence of normal values for growth hormone. In such instances, the hormone values do not undergo normal suppression with hyperglycemia, as described in the preceding section on laboratory diagnosis. The physician should use the other criteria just discussed when the values for growth hormone do not confirm the clinical impression of active acromegaly.

FAILURE TO RECOGNIZE EARLY ACROMEGALY. This is a difficult problem for which there is no satisfactory solution. As in other diseases, there is a spectrum of acromegaly from frank, classic acromegaly to subclinical acromegaly wherein growth hormone values are elevated but there has not been time for the usual physical stigmata to develop. It is, therefore, appropriate to use growth hormone studies to screen all patients with newly diagnosed pituitary tumors and patients suspected of having acromegaly. A single elevated value, especially in females, is not sufficient evidence that active acromegaly is present, but is an indication for further investigation with a three- or five-hour glucose tolerance test.

Differential Diagnosis of Acromegaly and Gigantism

Fortunately, there are few conditions that can be confused with excessive production of growth hormone. In children, cerebral gigantism may be mistaken for gigantism from excessive growth hormone. Patients with cerebral gigantism, however, have normal sellas and, more importantly, normal values for serum growth hormone.

In adults, the only situation that is usually mistaken for acromegaly is the rare condition of pachydermoperiostosis, a form of inherited hypertrophic osteoarthropathy.[104] Patients with pachydermoperiostosis have thick skin with marked wrinkling of the forehead, enlarged hands and wrists and feet and ankles, marked generalized hyperhidrosis, and may have clubbing of fingers and toes. Pachydermoperiostosis is usually mistaken for acromegaly unless the physician is familiar with the former syndrome. Patients with pachydermoperiostosis have normal sellas, and the few the author has studied have had normal growth hormone values. Roentgenograms of the hands and wrists show the typical changes of hypertrophic osteoarthropathy and should lead to the correct diagnosis.

Normal persons with large bones and prominent frontal sinuses (acromegaloid appearance) may be difficult to differentiate from persons with mild early acromegaly. The former, of course, should have normal values for growth hormone and normal growth hormone dynamics. It should be emphasized again, however, that the finding of a normal appearing sella turcica on routine roentgenographic views of the skull is not sufficient evidence to exclude a microadenoma of the pituitary. Polycyclic tomographic posteroanterior and lateral views of the sella must be done.

While Paget's disease is often included in the differential diagnosis of acromegaly, confusion between the two conditions is rare and readily settled by skeletal roentgenograms.

Treatment of Acromegaly

The various methods of treatment listed in Table 25–5 are applicable to acromegaly.

Currently in this country, treatment of acromegaly usually consists of operation or radiation therapy, or a combination of the two. In the author's experience, the transsphenoidal approach has proved superior to the transfrontal approach in dealing with patients with acromegaly, and in his institution, the transfrontal approach is used only when there is lateral extension or a large suprasellar extension of the tumor. Some patients with such extension are treated with a combination transfrontal and transsphenoidal operation.

Radiation therapy is available in the form of conventional high-voltage x-ray therapy, linear accelerator, ^{60}cobalt, and cyclotron

TABLE 25–5 OPTIONS OF MANAGEMENT OF PITUITARY TUMORS

Observation
Operation
  Transfrontal approach
  Transsphenoidal approach
    Conventional microsurgery
    Cryosurgery
    Radiofrequency surgery (thermocoagulation)
    Direct ultrasonic irradiation
  Combination of transfrontal and transsphenoidal approaches
Radiation
  Conventional radiation
    Orthovoltage (high-voltage) x-rays
    ^{60}Cobalt
    Linear accelerator
  Intrasellar implantation of radioactive isotopes
    ^{90}Yttrium
    ^{198}Gold
    Other isotopes
  Heavy-particle radiation (cyclotron)
    Alpha particles
    Protons
    Other particles
Chemotherapy
  Varies with type of pituitary tumor (see text)
Combinations of operation, radiation, and chemotherapy

© Mayo 1979

radiation; and implantation of radioactive isotopes, usually radioactive yttrium or gold. In selected cases to be treated by radiation therapy alone, the most effective of these forms is cyclotron radiation, which is available at the Massachusetts General Hospital in Boston and the Lawrence Radiation Laboratory at the Donner Laboratories of the University of California in Berkeley.[56,62]

Various forms of chemotherapy have been employed in the past such as large doses of estrogenic substances in the form of diethylstilbestrol, 5 to 25 mg orally a day; androgens such as testosterone enanthate or cypionate, 200 mg intramuscularly two or three times a week; medroxyprogesterone, 10 to 20 mg orally every six hours; and chlorpromazine, 25 mg orally three times a day; but none of these has proved very effective. Somatostatin will lower growth hormone levels in acromegalic patients, but has not been approved for use in this country and is not practical for long-term treatment because it is given intravenously or by a protamine-zinc preparation that has a duration of action of five to six hours.[7,130]

Currently, the most promising chemotherapeutic agents seem to be bromocriptine (2-Br-α-ergocriptine, Parlodel, Sandoz), which is thought to depress growth hormone secretion in acromegalic patients by stimulating dopaminergic neurons, and metergoline, which is an antiserotonin agent.[21,122] At this point, it is not clear what effect these compounds have on tumor growth. These materials are not available in the United States for clinical use in the treatment of acromegaly.

Currently, the author's approach to patients with active acromegaly is to remove the tumor transsphenoidally and follow this with 4500 to 5000 rads radiation therapy with a linear accelerator if the tumor is found to be invading the sellar floor, a cavernous sinus, or the diaphragm; if the tumor is larger than a microadenoma (more than 10 mm in diameter); or if the levels of serum growth hormone do not return to normal following the transsphenoidal operation. Some, but not all, patients will respond to conventional radiation therapy alone, but unfortunately, it is not possible at this time to separate, in advance, those who will respond from those who will not. If radiation therapy alone is to be used, the author prefers cyclotron radiation.

If a patient with active acromegaly has coexisting primary hyperparathyroidism and the serum calcium is above 11.0 mg per 100 ml (in the author's institution the normal range is 8.9 to 10.1 mg per 100 ml), parathyroid operation to correct the hyperparathyroidism should be undertaken before operating upon the pituitary tumor. Likewise, any coexisting pheochromocytomas should be removed before pituitary operation.

Schedule for Studying Patients
With Acromegaly or Gigantism
Secondary to GH-Producing
Pituitary Tumor

DAY ONE

Routine studies. Hematological studies; blood chemistry, including calcium, inorganic phosphate, alkaline phosphatase, glucose, creatinine or urea, sodium, and potassium; x-rays of the chest; urinalysis; and electrocardiogram.

Special studies. X-rays of the skull and polycyclic tomograms of the sella with posteroanterior and lateral views with cuts every 2 to 3 mm; ophthalmoscopy and perimetric examination of the visual fields; blood tests for corticosteroids (8 A.M. and 4 P.M.), GH, PRL, ACTH, TSH, FSH, LH, testosterone or estrogens, total thyroxine, and somatomedin; and x-rays of the hand, particularly useful in patients with gigantism to determine the status of the epiphyses, and of the feet to measure the thickness of the fatty heel pad (if desired).

Start 24-hour urine collection for evaluation of 17-ketosteroids and 17-hydroxycorticosteroids (or 17-ketogenic steroids); calcium; pituitary gonadotropins (requires 48-hour collection); and, if patient is hypertensive, metanephrines and aldosterone (pheochromocytoma and aldosteronoma have been reported to occur in acromegalic patients).

Day Two

A.M. If initial serum calcium level is elevated, repeat calcium, phosphorus and alkaline phosphatase tests and obtain blood for parathormone determination. A three- or five-hour glucose tolerance test with GH determinations.
P.M. CT scan of head with contrast medium.

Day Three

Blood tests for calcium and phosphorus if initial calcium level elevated. Excretory urogram (intravenous pyelogram) if patient is hypertensive. Special studies desired by physician.

Day Three or Day Four

If CT scan of head fails to reveal the tumor, bilateral carotid angiography with magnification and subtraction views, pneumoencephalography, or both may be needed.

Cushing's Disease

The term "Cushing's syndrome" is used here to designate the typical disease complex described originally by Cushing. There are several different causes of Cushing's syndrome. The term "Cushing's disease" designates only a specific form of Cushing's syndrome, namely that disease caused by pituitary ACTH–dependent hyperplasia of the adrenal cortices.

Current thought is that Cushing's disease is probably a hypothalamic disorder. Whether this results from an excess of corticotropin-releasing factor (CRF), a deficiency of corticotropin-inhibiting factor (CIF), if such exists, or an imbalance of these two factors is not known. It is well known that higher areas of the central nervous system may alter the function of the pituitary-adrenocortical axis, because it is not unusual to find that patients under severe physical or emotional stress have increased levels of plasma corticosteroids and urinary corticosteroids.

At present, it is not known whether all patients with Cushing's disease have pituitary adenomas producing excess adreno-corticotropin or whether some may have hyperplasia of the corticotropin-producing basophilic cells of the pituitary.

Space does not permit a review of the typical signs, symptoms, and laboratory findings in Cushing's syndrome. These are readily available in standard texts.[58,128]

Laboratory Diagnosis of Cushing's Syndrome and of Cushing's Disease

The diagnosis of Cushing's syndrome is established by documenting an increased secretion of adrenal corticosteroids that is not normally suppressible by methods such as the following:

The standard screening test for differentiating normal persons from those with Cushing's syndrome is the overnight dexamethasone suppression test. Blood for baseline plasma corticosteroid determination is obtained at 8:00 A.M. on the first day. At 11:00 P.M. that evening the patient is given 1 mg of dexamethasone orally. The next morning a second blood sample is taken at 8:00 A.M. for measurement of plasma corticosteroids. In the normal person, the value for plasma corticosteroids on the second day should be less than 50 per cent of the first day's value. Persons who are suspected of having Cushing's syndrome should be investigated further, however, even though their response to the overnight dexamethasone test is normal. Likewise, an abnormal response, while usually indicative of Cushing's syndrome, is not necessarily diagnostic, and further studies are indicated before the diagnosis can be made with certainty (Table 25–6).

Once a diagnosis of Cushing's syndrome has been made, the next step is to determine which type of Cushing's syndrome the patient has, and to do so one must differentiate between: (1) pituitary ACTH–dependent hyperplasia of the adrenal cortices (Cushing's disease), (2) benign adrenal cortical adenoma, (3) adrenal cortical carcinoma, (4) Non-ACTH-dependent adenomatous hyperplasia of both adrenal cortices, and (5) ectopic ACTH secretion by a nonpituitary neoplasm, the most common being carcinoma of the lungs. Other tumors are carcinomas of the thymus and pancreas, bronchial carcinoids, and pheochromocytoma. Tumors from almost every other organ system have, however, been reported to secrete ectopic ACTH, including

TABLE 25–6 DIFFERENTIATION OF CUSHING'S SYNDROME

TYPE OF CUSHING'S SYNDROME	DEXAMETHASONE SUPPRESSION*		METYRAPONE TEST*	ACTH (PLASMA)	IODOCHOLESTEROL SCANNING	
	2 MG	8 MG			Bilateral Visualization	Unilateral Visualization
Pituitary-ACTH dependent hyperlasia of the adrenal cortices (Cushing's disease)	0	+	+	+	+	
Benign adrenal cortical adenoma	0	0	0	0		+
Adrenal cortical carcinoma	0	0	0	0		±
Non-ACTH-dependent adenomatous hyperplasia of the adrenal cortices	0	0	0	0	+	
Ectopic ACTH secretion by non-pituitary neoplasm	0	0	0,+	+++	+	

* See text for interpretation of tests.

© Mayo 1979

the thyroid, gonads, prostate, kidney, and gastrointestinal tract. Hence an extensive investigation may be necessary to locate the tumor. Whole body CT scans with contrast medium of the chest, abdomen, and pelvis have been most helpful in locating small tumors. At times, however, the tumor may be too small to be detected initially, and subsequent investigations may be necessary to locate the responsible neoplasm.

Differentiation of Cushing's disease from other types of Cushing's syndrome is accomplished by dexamethasone tests, the metyrapone test, and measurement of adrenocorticotropin as shown in Table 25–6. Scans of the adrenal areas using [131]I-19-iodocholesterol or NP-59 are helpful in determining which gland is involved when a benign adrenal cortical adenoma is present, but not as helpful in differentiating among the other types of Cushing's syndrome.[64,111]

Treatment of Cushing's Disease

Only the treatment of Cushing's disease (pituitary ACTH–dependent hyperplasia of the adrenal cortices) is considered here, since the other forms of Cushing's syndrome fall outside the realm of neurosurgery and do not respond to operative procedures on the pituitary. Hence, it is essential that the diagnosis of Cushing's disease be firmly established, and that other forms of Cushing's syndrome be excluded before the patient is committed to any form of treatment (see Table 25–6).

Currently, there are several ways of treating Cushing's disease: (1) operation for removal of the corticotropin-producing pituitary adenoma, usually by the transsphenoidal route; (2) radiation therapy to the pituitary area by one of the methods listed in Table 25–5 for the treatment of pituitary tumors; (3) chemotherapy; (4) various combinations of operation for removal of a pituitary tumor, radiation therapy directed to the pituitary, and chemotherapy; and (5) bilateral total adrenalectomy. Radiation therapy by conventional high-voltage x-ray, linear accelerator, or [60]cobalt is often effective in controlling Cushing's disease. The author has used radiation therapy alone in patients in whom the disease was mild but not in those in whom it was severe. Subsidence of the disease following successful irradiation takes at least several months, and the patient with advanced Cushing's disease may have severe or fatal complications of the disease before responding to radiation. Cyclotron therapy has been used with good success by both the Boston group and the group in Berkeley, California.[56,62] Implantation of radioactive yttrium or gold is not being used as widely as in the past.

Of the various chemotherapeutic agents used to treat Cushing's disease, the most successful one available in the United States seems to be cyproheptadine (Periactin, Merck Sharp & Dohme).[57] This is used in doses of 4 to 8 mg every six hours and seems to be effective in about 50 per cent of patients. Cyproheptadine has not been in use long enough to show whether permanent reversal of the Cushing's disease will take place after long-term treatment with this drug, as may happen, for example, when some patients with Graves' disease are treated with antithyroid drugs. Also, the effects of cyproheptadine on the growth of ACTH-producing pituitary tumors is not known.

Transsphenoidal operation is the treatment of choice for Cushing's disease and hence is advised for all patients with this disorder, with certain exceptions to be mentioned later, when a tumor can be demonstrated by polycyclic tomography of the sella and carotid angiography with magnification and subtraction techniques. Standard roentgenographic views (anteroposterior, posteroanterior, and lateral) alone are not adequate to diagnose or exclude the presence of a small pituitary adenoma.

Salassa and colleagues, at the author's institution, recently reported that a clinical remission occurred in 16 of 18 patients with Cushing's disease who underwent transsphenoidal operation.[110] In the future, the author may well suggest a transsphenoidal procedure to look for a pituitary tumor in those patients who have Cushing's disease even though a tumor cannot be demonstrated preoperatively, if his experience and that elsewhere suggests that most patients with Cushing's disease do indeed have pituitary tumors. With the angiographic techniques used at his institution, tumors as small as 3 to 4 mm in diameter can be identified, but it is uncertain whether these techniques can reveal smaller tumors.

Postoperative Assessment

It is helpful to assess adrenal function during the postoperative period in all patients who have had transsphenoidal removal of a pituitary tumor as the initial treatment for Cushing's disease. In order to do this the patient should be given a short-acting adrenal corticosteroid such as prednisolone phosphate (Hydeltrasol, Merck Sharp & Dohme) intramuscularly, 40 mg before operation and 20 to 40 mg every six to eight hours for the first few days after operation until he can be given an oral adrenal corticosteroid. One week or so after operation the evening dose of adrenal corticosteroid is omitted, and blood is drawn the next morning for measurement of plasma corticosteroids and adrenocorticotropin. The oral adrenal corticosteroid can then be restarted. If the plasma corticosteroid value is below normal or zero, this suggests that the ACTH-producing pituitary tumor has been successfully removed. Thereafter, to prevent adrenal insufficiency, the patient should be given continuous replacement treatment. Four to six months later, when the pituitary gland has begun to recover from suppression by the excessive preoperative endogenous adrenal corticosteroids, an attempt can be made to reduce gradually and stop exogenous replacement therapy. This must be done cautiously because the pituitary-adrenal axis may remain suppressed for up to two years.[110]

If the value for plasma corticosteroid in the immediate postoperative period is still at or near the preoperative levels, then further testing should be done to determine whether part of the pituitary tumor is still present and active (dexamethasone suppression tests are described in the schedule for investigation of the disease). In those patients with continued severe Cushing's disease, bilateral total adrenalectomy can be performed a week or so later. Those patients with mild or moderate Cushing's disease can be given cyproheptadine, 4 to 8 mg orally every six hours, and radiation therapy to the region of the pituitary. Bilateral total adrenalectomy can be performed at a later date if the disease is not satisfactorily controlled by radiation therapy or if it progresses to a severe degree before enough time has elapsed (four to six months) to allow radiation therapy to control it. Reoperation on the pituitary tumor can also be considered.

Special Considerations in the Treatment of Cushing's Disease

OBVIOUS PITUITARY TUMOR. Even though an obvious pituitary tumor is detected early in the work-up of a patient with Cushing's syndrome, one should still do the necessary testing to establish the diagnosis of Cushing's disease (pituitary ACTH–dependent hyperplasia of the adrenal cortices) on the off chance that the patient might have Cushing's syndrome from some other reason plus an incidental pituitary tumor that plays no role in the Cushing's syndrome.

BILATERAL TOTAL ADRENALECTOMY AS TREATMENT OF CHOICE. There are situations in which bilateral total adrenalectomy should be considered in the treatment of Cushing's disease.

The patient with severe Cushing's disease is placed at considerable risk, including that of death, if transsphenoidal operation on the pituitary tumor is not successful in reducing the output of adrenocorticotropin by the tumor and, hence, reversing the hyperactivity of the adrenal glands. There is a good chance of this happening in the patient who has a large pituitary tumor (more than 25 mm in diameter) or a moderate-sized one (11 to 25 mm), but it is less likely to happen in patients who have microadenomas (less than 10 mm in diameter), in whom the chances for complete removal of the adenoma are greater.

When there is a good possibility that the size of the pituitary tumor makes complete removal by the transsphenoidal or transfrontal route unlikely, it is preferable to do a bilateral total adrenalectomy initially, which will immediately reverse the Cushing's disease, and then a few weeks later to proceed with removal of the pituitary tumor. Operation upon the pituitary tumor is then followed by radiation therapy when appropriate, that is, when the surgeon thinks he may not have removed the entire tumor or the plasma ACTH values remain elevated following operation.

Schedule for Investigating Patients With Cushing's Syndrome

DAY ONE

Routine studies. Hematological studies; blood chemistry, including sodium, potassium, glucose, creatinine or urea evaluations; x-rays of the chest; x-rays of the thoracic and lumbar spine to detect osteoporosis; urinalysis; and electrocardiogram.

Special studies. X-rays of the skull and posteroanterior and lateral polycyclic tomograms of the sella; blood tests for corticosteroids or cortisol, 11-deoxycortisol, ACTH and beta-lipotropin at 8 A.M. and 4 P.M.; start 24-hour urine collection for determination of 17-ketosteroids, free cortisol, and 17-ketogenic steroids or 17-hydroxycorticosteroids at 7 or 8 A.M.

DAY TWO

Obtain blood for measurement of corticosteroids or cortisol, 11-deoxycortisol, ACTH, and beta-lipotropin at 8 A.M. and 4 P.M. Start another 24-hour urine collection for determination of 17-ketosteroids, free cortisol, and 17-ketogenic steroids or 17-hydroxycorticosteroids at 7 or 8 A.M.

If x-rays of skull and polycyclic tomograms of sella suggest the presence of a pituitary tumor, obtain perimetric examination of visual fields and blood tests for GH, PRL, TSH, FSH, LH, testosterone or estrogens, and total thyroxine.

DAY THREE

Complete 24-hour urine collection at 7 A.M. or 8 A.M. CT scan of head with and without contrast medium if pituitary tumor is suspected.

Start three-day 2-mg dexamethasone test, giving 0.5 mg dexamethasone orally at 2 A.M., 8 A.M., 2 P.M., and 8 P.M.

DAY FOUR

Continue dexamethasone, 0.5 mg orally at 2 A.M., 8 A.M., 2 P.M., and 8 P.M.

DAY FIVE

Continue dexamethasone, 0.5 mg orally at 2 A.M., 8 A.M., 2 P.M., and 8 P.M.

Blood tests for corticosteroids or cortisol, 11-deoxycortisol, ACTH, and beta-lipotropin at 8 A.M. and 4 P.M.

Start 24-hour urine collection for measurement of 17-ketosteroids, free cortisol, and 17-ketogenic steroids or 17-hydroxycorticosteroids at 7 or 8 A.M.

DAY SIX

Give 0.5 mg dexamethasone at 2 A.M.

Complete 24-hour urine collection at 7 or 8 A.M.

Start three-day 8-mg dexamethasone test, giving 2 mg dexamethasone orally at 8 A.M., 2 P.M., and 8 P.M.

DAY SEVEN

Continue dexamethasone, 2 mg orally at 2 A.M., 8 A.M., 2 P.M. and 8 P.M.

DAY EIGHT

Continue dexamethasone, 2 mg orally at 2 A.M., 8 A.M., 2 P.M., and 8 P.M.

Blood tests for corticosteroids or cortisol, 11-deoxycortisol, ACTH, and beta-lipotropin at 8 A.M. and 4 P.M.

Start 24-hour urine collection for measurement of 17-ketosteroids, free cortisol, and 17-ketogenic steroids or 17-hydroxycorticosteroids at 7 or 8 A.M.

DAY NINE

Give 2 mg dexamethasone orally at 2 A.M.

Complete 24-hour urine collection at 7 or 8 A.M.

No further adrenal testing on this day.

DAY TEN

Start metyrapone, 500 or 750 mg orally every four hours at midnight, 4 A.M., 8 A.M., noon, 4 P.M., and 8 P.M. Blood pressure and pulse are to be measured and the patient's responses checked each time metyrapone is given or if the patient should develop weakness, fever, nausea, or vomiting.

If it is planned to do an adrenal scan, NP-59 (6β-^{131}I-iodomethylnorcholesterol), or ^{131}I-19-iodocholesterol can be given after blocking the patient's thyroid (to protect against ^{131}iodine uptake) by giving 10 drops of Lugol's solution the day before and again the morning of the scan. NP-59 is the preferred scanning agent because a reliable scan can be obtained one or two days after it is given as opposed to a lapse of five to seven days or longer for ^{131}I-iodocholesterol. Continue Lugol's solution, 10 drops a day for two or three more days.

DAY ELEVEN

Continue metyrapone, 500 or 750 mg orally at midnight, 4 A.M., 8 A.M., noon, 4 P.M., and 8 P.M.

Obtain blood for measurement of corticosteroids or cortisol, 11-deoxycortisol, ACTH, and beta-lipotropin at 8 A.M. and 4 P.M.

Start 24-hour urine collection for determination of 17-ketosteroids, cortisol, and 17-ketogenic steroids or 17-hydroxycorticosteroids at 7 or 8 A.M.

DAY TWELVE

Give metyrapone, 500 or 750 mg orally at midnight and 4 A.M.

Complete 24-hour urine collection at 7 or 8 A.M.

If testing shows that patient does not have Cushing's disease (pituitary ACTH–dependent hyperplasia of the adrenal cortices), a bolus nephrotomogram is done in an attempt to demonstrate an adrenal tumor. Adrenal scanning, as mentioned for day ten, may settle the question without the need for a bolus nephrotomogram. A CT whole body scan with and without contrast medium can be helpful in differentiating bilateral adrenal hyperplasia from an adrenal cortical tumor. If Cushing's syndrome secondary to ectopic ACTH secretion by a nonpituitary neoplasm is suspected on clinical grounds or on results of testing as outlined in Table 25–6, then a search for a neoplasm should be undertaken. A whole body CT scan with contrast medium of the chest, abdomen, and pelvis may be most helpful in locating such a tumor.

Special Considerations and Interpretation of Results

The metyrapone test should be done under close observation in the hospital because, if the patient has a benign adrenal cortical adenoma, adrenal cortical carcinoma, or non-ACTH-dependent adenomatous hyperplasia of adrenal cortices, the enzymatic block of 11-beta hydroxylation imposed by the metyrapone may stop production of cortisol by the tumor or adenomatous hyperplasia. Consequently, the patient may slip into adrenal collapse because the normal adrenal cortical tissues are atrophic from prolonged suppression by excessive corticosteroids made by the adrenal cortical tumor or adenomatous hyperplasia. The patient's blood pressure, pulse, and temperature should be monitored carefully, and if he develops nausea, vomiting, weakness, fever, or other difficulty, the test should be terminated by drawing blood for corticosteroid or cortisol and 11-deoxycortisol determinations, and immediately thereafter giving large doses of adrenal corticosteroids such as 40 mg of prednisolone phosphate (Hydeltrasol, Merck Sharp & Dohme) intravenously and 20 mg intramuscularly at the same time. The patient will need careful observation for a minimum of 24 hours because the enzymatic block may persist that length of time or longer after the metyrapone has been discontinued.

There are a number of ways of doing the metyrapone test. The author prefers to give 500 mg of metyrapone orally every 4 hours for 48 hours.* In Cushing's disease, there will be a two- to fivefold increase in the urinary 17-hydroxycorticosteroids (or 17-ketogenic steroids). The plasma corticosteroids and cortisol will show little or no increase or even a decrease, while there will be a five- to tenfold increase or more in 11-deoxycortisol. Patients with benign adrenal cortical adenoma, adrenal cortical carcinoma or non-ACTH-dependent adenomatous hyperplasia of the adrenal cortices do not respond to metyrapone and there will be a decrease in the plasma corticosteroids and cortisol and the urinary 17-ketosteroids and 17-hydroxycorticosteroids (or 17-ketogenic steroids), but a rise in 11-

---

* More recently (1979–1980) the author has been using a short metyrapone test. Blood for 11-deoxycortisol determination is drawn at 8 A.M. That evening at 11 P.M. the patient is given 3.0 gm of metyrapone orally. At 8 A.M. the next morning, blood is again drawn for measurement of 11-deoxycortisol. Normal persons and patients with pituitary ACTH–dependent adrenal hyperplasia (Cushing's disease) will have a fivefold or greater increase in 11-deoxycortisol. Patients with benign cortical adenoma, adrenal cortical carcinoma, or non-ACTH-dependent adenomatous hyperplasia of the adrenal cortices will have no or, at most, up to a twofold increase in 11-deoxycortisol.

deoxycortisol. Patients with ectopic secretion of adrenocorticotropin by a nonpituitary neoplasm usually do not respond to metyrapone, although some do.

When doing the dexamethasone test, some physicians prefer to give dexamethasone for two days, while others prefer to give it for three days at each of the two dose levels. When the normal person is given 0.5 mg of dexamethasone every six hours ("2-mg test") for three days, the urinary 17-hydroxycorticosteroids (or 17-ketogenic steroids) will decrease to less than 4 mg per 24 hours, or less than half the baseline value. The plasma corticosteroids will also decrease to less than 50 per cent of the baseline values and often to or near zero. There is, however, no danger of the patient's going into adrenal collapse, because he is receiving dexamethasone, a potent adrenal corticosteroid. Patients with all types of Cushing's syndrome, including Cushing's disease, fail to show normal suppression with this dose of dexamethasone. With 2 mg of dexamethasone every six hours ("8-mg test") for three days, patients with Cushing's disease will have a more than 50 per cent reduction in the values of plasma corticosteroids and urinary 17-hydroxycorticosteroids (or 17-ketogenic steroids. There is, however, an occasional patient with Cushing's disease in whom suppression will not occur with the 8-mg dexamethasone test, and the metyrapone test is useful in separating such patients with Cushing's disease from those with other forms of Cushing's syndrome. There has been a rare patient with Cushing's disease who has not responded in the expected fashion to metyrapone, but the author has not seen anyone with Cushing's disease who failed to respond to both the metyrapone test and the 8-mg dexamethasone test.

Nelson's Syndrome (Nelson-Salassa Syndrome)

This syndrome as originally defined consisted of pituitary tumors secreting large amounts of adrenocorticotropin (ACTH) and beta-melanocyte-stimulating hormone (beta-MSH) that were thought to occur following bilateral total or subtotal adrenalectomy for Cushing's disease.[87,109] The secretion of adrenocorticotropin was not suppressed by the usual dexamethasone suppression tests, and because of the large amount of beta-melanotropin and adrenocorticotropin secreted, the patients became highly pigmented. The pituitary tumors, while slow-growing and relatively innocuous in many patients, were aggressive, highly invasive of adjacent structures, and sometimes malignant with metastases in other patients. Now that the high frequency of pituitary tumors in patients with Cushing's disease has become evident, it seems likely that the tumors of the Nelson-Salassa syndrome are merely a continuum of the pituitary tumors present prior to adrenalectomy, which become recognized later only after further growth in the months or years following the operation.

Treatment

In patients with the Nelson-Salassa syndrome (the term being used in its original context to describe a pituitary tumor presenting following adrenalectomy) the tumor should be removed transsphenoidally, since it is not possible to distinguish tumors that will have a relatively uneventful course from those that will become highly aggressive. If the tumor has already spread laterally or superiorly so that it is not resectable transsphenoidally, a transfrontal approach is used, and this may be combined with a secondary transsphenoidal procedure as well. If the tumor is more than a microadenoma in size (10 mm) or if the levels of adrenocorticotropin in the blood do not fall to normal, the operation is followed by radiation therapy.

If the patient continues to secrete excessive corticotropin following operation and radiation therapy, a trial of cyproheptadine (Periactin, Merck Sharp & Dohme) in doses of 8 mg every six hours is warranted. If there is a good reduction in the level of ACTH, then an attempt can be made to treat the patient with a smaller dose of cyproheptadine. As mentioned earlier, experience is too limited to know how effective this treatment will be in permanent control of such tumors.

Thyrotropin-Secreting Pituitary Tumors

Currently, 10 patients with thyroid-stimulating hormone (TSH)–producing tumors and hyperthyroidism have been reported.*

---

* See references 27, 28, 44, 45, 50, 60, 67, 81, 88.

One of the patients initially reported by Faglia and associates has been restudied by Reschini and co-workers.[28,103] The usual findings have been those typical of a pituitary tumor, such as an enlarged or eroded sella and visual field defects. The patients have had evidences of hyperthyroidism with increased metabolic rate, elevated serum thyroxine level, or abnormal values on other tests for circulating thyroid hormone such as protein bound iodine or butanol extractable iodine, and an increased uptake of [131]iodine by the thyroid. In addition, these patients have had an inappropriately elevated level of thyrotropin in the serum. (Characteristically, the serum level is decreased in other forms of hyperthyroidism, such as Grave's disease, toxic nodular goiter [Plummer's disease], increased circulating thyroxine associated with thyroiditis, or excessive intake of exogenous thyroid.)

Dynamic studies in patients with thyrotropin-producing pituitary tumors have been few, but of five tested with thyrotropin-releasing hormone (TRH), three failed to respond with an increase in serum thyrotropin, while two did respond. In seven patients undergoing a T3 suppression test, thyroid-stimulating hormone showed no decrease in two, partial decrease in three, and good suppression in two. The heterogeneity of these responses is not understood. One patient was given somatostatin, which resulted in a decrease in serum thyrotropin, a finding that is seen in both normal individuals and those with primary hypothyroidism.

Pituitary tumors have also been found in patients with long-standing hypothyroidism and are thought to result from loss of negative feedback from the thyroid, like those that occur in experimental animals following long-term administration of antithyroid drugs.[61,79] Some of these patients have had galactorrhea and have been responsive to the administration of thyroid. The relationship between such patients and those with the overlapping syndrome of galactorrhea, precocious menstruation, and enlarged sella in hypothyroid children is not clear.[125]

Gonadotropin-Secreting Pituitary Tumors

Nine gonadotropin-secreting pituitary tumors have been reported.* Most of the patients had had long-standing hypogonadism and pituitary tumors that secreted follicle-stimulating hormone (FSH). It is possible that such tumors could readily go undetected because of the dearth of clinical symptoms associated with increased gonadotropin levels in the presence of gonadal failure.

The production of only luteinizing hormone (LH) by a pituitary tumor has not been reported. Snyder and Sterling, however, reported a 51-year-old man with an enlarged sella, chiasmal defect, elevated serum follicle-stimulating and luteinizing hormone level, and increased serum testosterone. The serum follicle-stimulating and luteinzing hormones increased following the administration of gonadotropin-releasing hormone (GnRH). Interestingly, the patient also had increased serum prolactin.

Treatment of Thyrotropin- and Gonadotropin-Secreting Pituitary Tumors

Pituitary tumors that secrete follicle-stimulating or luteinizing hormones or thyrotropin should be handled by the same methods used in treating tumors that secrete growth hormone, adrenocorticotropin, or prolactin (see Table 25–5). The one notable exception would be a patient with a thyrotropin-secreting pituitary tumor in whom operation, radiation, or a combination of the two failed to eradicate the tumor and the excessive production of hormone continued to cause thyrotoxicosis. Under such circumstances, the hyperthyroidism should be readily controlled by the administration of a therapeutic dose of [131]iodine.

Polysecretory Pituitary Adenomas

The presence, occasionally, of galactorrhea in a patient with acromegaly has been recognized for decades, but it was not known whether the pituitary tumor in such patients was secreting prolactin in addition to growth hormone. This has been shown to be the case in some tumors, now that it is possible to measure prolactin. Recently, Corenblum and co-workers have shown by electron microscopy and immunostains that such tumors are composed of two cell lines, one secreting growth hormone and the other, prolactin.[16]

More recently, Horn and co-workers reported a 22-year-old woman with a pituitary

---

* See references 2, 10, 18, 34, 41, 54, 77, 118, 129.

tumor who had hyperthyroidism, galactorrhea, and amenorrhea. Appropriate histological study of the tumor showed two cell lines—one producing thyrotropin and the other, prolactin.[49]

As mentioned earlier, a pituitary adenoma secreting both follicle-stimulating hormone and luteinizing hormone has been described by Snyder and Sterling. Interestingly, the serum prolactin was also increased. It was not clear to the authors whether the excess prolactin was being secreted by the tumor cells or by prolactin-secreting cells in normal pituitary tissue that were no longer under the influence of prolactin-inhibiting factor because of interference by the tumor with its flow through the portal blood system from the hypothalamus to the anterior pituitary.

In view of these reports, it seems advisable to measure serum prolactin and follicle-stimulating and luteinizing hormones in all patients with a pituitary tumor, since the hypersecretion of such hormones may not be readily evident on clinical grounds. The hypersecretion of growth hormone, adrenocorticotropin, or thyrotropin should cause characteristic clinical manifestations. However, the presence of a pituitary tumor secreting thyrotropin could easily be overlooked, should the clinician mistakenly think that the hyperthyroidism was caused by a primary thyroidal dysfunction such as Grave's disease or toxic nodular goiter (Plummer's disease).

Hyperprolactinemia

The most common type of pituitary tumors are those that secrete prolactin (PRL), hyperprolactinemia being reported in 70 per cent in one series of patients with pituitary tumors.[2] It has been estimated that only about 30 per cent of patients with such tumors have galactorrhea, which incidentally, occurs in males as well as in females. It is not known why some patients with hyperprolactinemia become galactorrheic while others do not. The occurrence of galactorrhea does not seem to be related to the level of serum prolactin.

The physician should be aware that the finding of hyperprolactinemia in a patient with a pituitary tumor does not necessarily mean that the tumor is secreting prolactin, although this is usually the case. A non-prolactin-secreting pituitary tumor or tumors arising in other structures may impinge upon that part of the hypothalamus that makes and releases prolactin-inhibiting factor, or on the portal blood system carrying the inhibiting factor from the hypothalamus to the anterior pituitary, thereby releasing the normal prolactin-secreting cells of the pituitary from its restraining influence and resulting in hyperprolactinemia.

Besides prolactin-secreting pituitary tumors, there are many other causes of galactorrhea, as shown in Table 25–7. Hyperprolactinemia has also been described in patients who had hyperplasia of the prolactin-producing cells of the anterior pituitary gland.[77]

In the past, the eponyms "Del Castillo," "Chiari-Frommel," and "Forbes-Albright" have been applied to syndromes in the following context. The Del Castillo syndrome refers to amenorrhea and galactorrhea in a nulliparous woman without evidence of a pituitary tumor. The Chiari-Frommel syndrome is amenorrhea and galactorrhea occurring postpartum in a woman without evidence of a pituitary tumor. The Forbes-Albright syndrome is the occurrence of amenorrhea and galactorrhea in a woman with a pituitary or suprasellar tumor. The term "Forbes-Albright syndrome" is not applied to those patients with acromegaly and amenorrhea and galactorrhea because, for many decades before Forbes and co-workers wrote their description of what is now known as the Forbes-Albright syndrome, it had been recognized that patients with acromegaly might have amenorrhea and galactorrhea. As the present-day techniques for identifying microadenomas of the pituitary have evolved, it has become evident that most patients with the Del Castillo and Chiari-Frommel syndromes actually have small prolactin-secreting pituitary tumors, and the syndromes, as originally described, may not exist. Certainly, all patients with the so-called Del Castillo or Chiari-Frommel syndromes in whom initial investigation fails to reveal a pituitary tumor should be followed carefully and reinvestigated periodically for the possible presence of a pituitary tumor. Gould and co-workers state that in 24 female patients with galactorrhea associated with a tumor in or near the sella, the interval between the onset of galactorrhea and discovery of the tumor ranged up to 18 years. Eight of these patients had an initial history compatible with the Del Castillo syndrome, and eight others had one compatible with the Chiari-Frommel syndrome.[42]

While many patients with hyperprolactinemia have no symptoms related to the excessive secretion of prolactin, some are symptomatic. In addition to galactorrhea, there may be gonadal dysfunction in either sex. Women may have irregular menses and anovulation or amenorrhea, while men may have decreased potency and libido and oligospermia or azoospermia.

Females

The spectrum of findings related to hyperprolactinemia in women seems to range from no effects through galactorrhea with no changes in menses or fertility, anovulatory regular menses with or without ga-

---

TABLE 25-7 CONDITIONS ASSOCIATED WITH HYPERPROLACTINEMIA*

CENTRAL NERVOUS SYSTEM DISORDERS AND DISTURBANCES
Tumor
  Pituitary tumor
    Chromophobe adenoma
    Eosinophil (acidophil) adenoma
    Basophil adenoma
  Craniopharyngioma
  Pinealoma
  Astrocytoma
  Meningioma
  Other primary tumors
  Hemangioma
  Metastasis to hypothalamus
Hyperplasia of prolactin-producing pituitary cells
Operative procedures
  Stalk section
  Resection of intrasellar or suprasellar tumor
Sheehan's syndrome
Empty sella syndrome
Pseudotumor cerebri
Arachnoiditis and encephalitis
Tabes dorsalis
Syringomyelia
Pneumoencephalography
Psychiatric illness
Pseudocyesis
Sarcoidosis
Histiocytosis X

OTHER ENDOCRINE RELATIONSHIPS
Primary hypothyroidism
  Without sellar enlargement
  With sellar enlargement
Hyperthyroidism
Adrenal carcinoma
Adrenal cortical hyperplasia
Polycystic ovaries
Chorionepithelioma of testis
Multiple endocrine adenomatosis (neoplasias)
Ovarian resection
Hysterectomy
Dilatation and curettage
Ectopic tumor production of prolactin
  Hypernephroma
  Bronchogenic carcinoma

DISTURBANCES OF THORACIC WALL
Stimulation of nonpuerperal female or male breasts
Unilateral mastectomy

Mammoplasty
Thoracic operations
Trauma
Atopic dermatitis
Herpes zoster

HEPATIC CIRRHOSIS

RENAL FAILURE

DRUG RELATED
Hormones
  Estrogen-progesterone combination
    During administration
    After withdrawal
  Progesterone
  Androgen
Psychotropic drugs
  Phenothiazines
    Chlorpromazine (Thorazine, Largactil)
    Thioridazine (Mellaril)
    Methotrimeprazine (Levoprone)
    Trimeprazine (Temaril)
    Piperazine nucleus
      Prochlorperazine (Compazine)
      Thiopropazate (Dartal)
      Fluphenazine (Prolixin, Sevinol)
      Perphenazine (Trilafon)
      Thioproperazine (Mayeptil)
      Trifluoperazine (Stelazine)
  Tricyclic antidepressants
    Imipramine (Tofranil)
    Amitriptyline (Elavil, Tryptizol)
  Butyrophenones
    Haloperidol (Haldol, Aloperidine)
    Droperidol (Innovar)
  Chlorprothixene (Taractan, Truxal)
  Antianxiety drugs
    Meprobamate (Equanil, Miltown)
    Chlordiazepoxide (Librium)
  Antihypertensive drugs
    Methyldopa (Aldomet)
    Reserpine (Serpasil)
  Histamine H2 receptor antagonists
    Cimetidine (Tagamet)
  Opiates
    Morphine
    Methadone
    Enkephalins
    Endorphins

---

* Adapted from Table 2–II *in* Gould, B. K., Randall, R. V., Kempers, R. D., and Ryan, R. J.: Galactorrhea. Springfield, Ill., Charles C Thomas, 1974.

lactorrhea, and ovulatory or anovulatory irregular menses with or without galactorrhea to amenorrhea (primary or secondary) with or without galactorrhea.

The mechanisms whereby hyperprolactinemia causes disturbances in menses and ovulation have not been fully elucidated. In general, such patients have low-normal levels of serum follicle-stimulating hormone, low-normal or low levels of luteinizing hormone, and low-normal or low estrogen values, but have a normal or exaggerated response to the administration of gonadotropin-releasing hormone (GnRH, HRH).[14,82] It is known that prolactin suppresses the normal pulsatile secretion of luteinizing hormone by the pituitary.[9] In vitro studies by McNatty and co-workers have shown that although physiological amounts of prolactin are essential for the secretion of progesterone by the granulosa cells of the human graafian follicle, increased concentration of prolactin suppresses secretion of progesterone, which can lead to amenorrhea.[78] Also, Glass and associates found that when patients with hyperprolactinemia were given estrogens, they failed to respond normally with a release of luteinizing hormone, which is essential for ovulation.[40] Thus, excessive prolactin in humans seems to have a suppressive effect on the hypothalamus as well as an ovarian steroidogenesis.

Males

In men, the spectrum of findings ranges from no effects through galactorrhea with no change in libido or potentia, gynecomastia (occasionally), and decreased libido and potentia with or without galactorrhea to oligospermia or azoospermia, with or without galactorrhea.

Magrini and co-workers have found that prolactin inhibits the enzyme 5-alpha reductase that converts hormonally inert testosterone to hormonally active dihydrotestosterone.[70] Through this mechanism, prolactin could produce not only hypoandrogenism but also oligospermia and azoospermia, since a high concentration of dihydrotestosterone in the tubules is essential for spermatogenesis.

The foregoing findings, noted in conjunction with hyperprolactinemia in both females and males, make it prudent to measure the amount of circulating prolactin in the blood of seemingly normal women with unexplained infertility, irregular menses, or amenorrhea; and in all men with unexplained decrease in libido and potentia or oligospermia or azoospermia or any combination of these. The finding and successful removal of a prolactin-producing tumor makes it likely that fertility will be restored in either sex if the tumor has not permanently disrupted pituitary function. It will be interesting to learn, as more data become available, what percentage of patients with hyperprolactinemia have gonadal dysfunction. In retrospect, certainly, many patients with pituitary tumors whose gonadal dysfunction was thought to be due simply to impaired secretion of gonadotropins undoubtedly had hyperprolactinemia that was not appreciated at the time because they did not have galactorrhea.

Diagnosis

The diagnosis of a prolactin-producing pituitary tumor is made either by finding hyperprolactinemia during the investigation of a patient with a pituitary tumor, or by finding hyperprolactinemia in a patient who is investigated because of galactorrhea or infertility or both, irregular menses or amenorrhea in a woman, or galactorrhea and decreased libido and potentia or oligospermia or azoospermia in a man. Not unlike the experience with acromegalic patients, symptoms attributable to hyperprolactinemia in a few of the author's patients who had normal prolactin values prior to operation were reversed by removal of a pituitary adenoma. At this point, the author is not certain whether the finding of normal prolactin values in such patients is an artificial situation because, in his institution the current ranges for prolactin are up to 23 ng per milliliter in normal females and up to 20 ng per milliliter in males. The upper limits, while defined by the usual statistical methods, may need revision as data on normal persons increase. The other possibilities are that the rate at which prolactin disappears from the blood may be greater than normal in these patients, or more likely, their tumors may be producing an analogue or fragments of prolactin that are biologically active but not as efficiently measured by the prolactin assay as is normal prolactin.

Treatment

The usual modalities of treatment listed in Table 25–5 have been used in the treatment of patients with pituitary tumors and hyperprolactinemia. The author's experience with conventional high-voltage radiation therapy, [60]cobalt, and linear accelerator has been similar to that in patients with acromegaly—not completely satisfactory.

Some patients with amenorrhea, galactorrhea, and infertility have had cessation of galactorrhea, return of menses, and one or more pregnancies following radiation therapy. The interval between radiation therapy and return of menses and fertility was two to three years in some patients, while in others it was a matter of only four to six months. The majority of patients, however, have not had the desired results —cessation of galactorrhea and return of menses and fertility—and furthermore it is not possible to predict which patient will respond satisfactorily to radiation and which will not.

Prolactin-producing pituitary tumors should be removed transsphenoidally when feasible, or by the transfrontal or the combined transsphenoidal and transfrontal approach if there is lateral extension or extensive suprasellar extension. Radiation therapy with linear accelerator is given those patients in whom the tumor has invaded the floor of the sella, a cavernous sinus, or the diaphragm of the sella, or in whom the serum prolactin does not return to normal in the postoperative period. Patients who have had a satisfactory operative result have had a return of menses as rapidly as a few days after operation, but in most instances not until after several weeks to several months. Menses have returned in some cases even though the levels for serum prolactin have not returned to normal, but these patients have not been followed long enough to know whether fertility has been restored.

CHEMOTHERAPY. Many types of hormonal treatment have been used in patients with amenorrhea and galactorrhea, and the one attribute common to all these forms of treatment has been failure in most instances to alter the syndrome.[42] More recently L-dopa and some of the ergot alkaloids have been tried. The most noteworthy results have been achieved with bromocriptine (2-Br-α-ergocriptine, Parlodel, Sandoz). In most patients it will effectively decrease serum prolactin, bringing about cessation of galactorrhea and a return of menses and fertility.[123] Del Pozo of Switzerland stated that he knows of 1276 pregnancies occurring after bromocriptine was given to previously infertile women.[22] This effective form of treatment is clinically available in the United States only on a limited basis and not for treating infertility.

The studies of Delitala and associates in Italy showed that metergoline, a specific antiserotonin agent that suppresses the release of prolactin, may be of therapeutic use in conditions associated with hyperprolactinemia accompanied by amenorrhea and galactorrhea.[21] The effect of bromocriptine and metergoline on the growth of prolactin-producing pituitary tumors is not, however, entirely known. McGregor and co-workers have reported that a patient had regression of the extrasellar extension of a locally invasive prolactin-secreting tumor and a decrease in serum prolactin while being treated with bromocriptine.[76] Subsequently, Wass and co-workers reported a reduction in tumor size in five patients treated with bromocriptine alone. Three patients had prolactin-producing pituitary tumors, and two patients had acromegaly and hyperprolactinemia.[126] Also, little is known about the rate of growth of these tumors when untreated. They must grow at different rates in different patients, because some patients present with amenorrhea or galactorrhea or a combination of the two and have large pituitary tumors extending beyond the confines of the sella, while others who have had similar symptoms for a similar length of time have tumors as small as 3 or 4 mm in diameter. The author is following eight patients who, on the basis of the presence of amenorrhea and galactorrhea, hyperprolactinemia, an abnormal sella consistent with a pituitary microadenoma, and in two instances, a tumor that has been demonstrated by carotid angiography, are presumed to have such tumors. These patients have not wished to have transsphenoidal operations. They have been followed for two to three years, during which there has been no change in the abnormal findings noted on posteroanterior and lateral polycyclic tomographic views of the sella and their visual fields have remained normal. These patients have been advised not to use birth control pills for contraception, because while it is known that estrogenic materials will increase the secretion of prolactin by the normal pituitary, the effect of estrogenic substances (contained in the combination birth control pills) on prolactin-producing pituitary tumors, if any, is not known. Current plans are to attempt to remove these tumors as soon as feasible and at a time while they are still small, the risk of postoperative pituitary failure is minimal, and the chance of reducing the hyperprolactinemia is good.

COMBINED ABLATIVE THERAPY AND CHEMOTHERAPY. It is clear that bromocriptine is frequently successful in reducing circulating prolactin and restoring menses and fertility in women with prolactin-producing pituitary tumors. Because pregnancy is known to increase the size of the normal pituitary and is thought to increase the size of pituitary tumors, operation or some other form of ablative therapy is indicated in patients whose infertility is caused by a prolactin-producing pituitary tumor. If this fails to reduce abnormal prolactin levels and restore fertility, then treatment with a prolactin-suppressing chemotherapeutic agent such as bromocriptine seems warranted. At the time of this writing, the second step is not possible in the United States because bromocriptine and other effective prolactin-suppressing agents are not approved for clinical use to restore fertility.

Early Diagnosis and Treatment of Pituitary Tumors

The author's current efforts in dealing with patients suspected of having functioning pituitary tumors are directed toward the earliest possible detection of these tumors so they can be removed transsphenoidally. The objectives are threefold: reversal of the endocrine abnormalities caused by the tumor, preservation or restoration of normal pituitary function, and prevention of the mechanical effects of a growing space-occupying tumor (see Table 25–1).

Realization of these objectives requires familiarity with the early signs, symptoms, and laboratory and roentgenographic abnormalities caused by these tumors. Investigation of patients suspected of having acromegaly or gigantism, or Cushing's disease, and patients suspected of having hyperprolactinemia must be thorough. This means serum prolactin studies must be performed in women with infertility, irregular menses, amenorrhea or galactorrhea (or both), and in men with decreased libido and potentia, hypoandrogenism, and oligospermia or azoospermia with or without galactorrhea. Polycyclic tomographic posteroanterior and lateral roentgenographic studies of the sella and bilateral carotid angiography with magnification and subtraction techniques are necessary, and in appropriate instances when a pituitary tumor is strongly suspected, should be followed by a transsphenoidal exploration of the pituitary despite negative roentgenographic studies.

Present laboratory, roentgenographic, and operative techniques allow one to undertake such an aggressive approach with a high degree of success.

Incidental Microadenomas of the Pituitary

Small pituitary tumors ranging in diameter from less than 1 mm to 8 to 10 mm are not an uncommon finding at postmortem examination of patients who had no recognizable endocrine abnormality. The finding of incidental adenomas is not unique to the pituitary. They are also found in the thyroid and adrenal cortex as well as in other endocrine glands. Costello, working with Kernohan, made serial sections of pituitaries removed at postmortem examination from a thousand patients without evidence of endocrine disease. Of these 1000 pituitary glands, 22.4 per cent contained a microadenoma. A few of them contained two or even three microadenomas.[17] A microscopic section of one of these pituitaries harboring an adenoma, made available by Kernohan, is showed in Figure 25–5.

The significance of these small pituitary tumors is still unclear. It is not known whether for one reason or another they become active, begin to grow and secrete hormones, and become what we clinically recognize as pituitary tumors. As yet immunohistological and electron microscopic studies have not been done on such tumors to show whether they are producing hormones in amounts too small to manifest themselves either clinically or by elevation of the circulating levels of those hormones.

These small, incidental pituitary tumors are of more than theoretical interest. It is conceivable that the neurosurgeon, upon

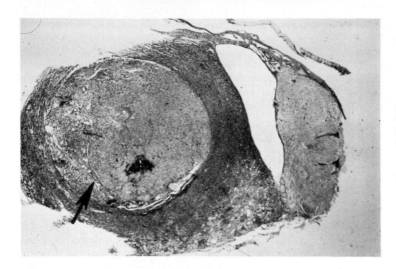

Figure 25–5   Incidental chromophobe adenoma of a human pituitary. Arrow points to the adenoma in the anterior lobe. Posterior lobe lies in right-hand side of photomicrograph. 7 ×. (Courtesy of James W. Kernohan, M.D., Mayo Clinic.)

entering the pituitary in an attempt to remove a functioning pituitary microadenoma, might encounter one of these incidental adenomas that was totally unrelated to the syndrome under treatment and remove it, thinking that he was removing the hyperfunctioning tumor responsible for the syndrome. Interestingly, McKeel and Jacobs reported a patient with hyperprolactinemia, amenorrhea, and galactorrhea who had a pituitary adenoma large enough to cause chiasmal compression. Immunostains failed to disclose prolactin, growth hormone, or thyrotropin in the tumor cells, but the surrounding pituitary tissue contained large clusters of hyperplastic cells that, by immunostain, were shown to be prolactin-producing cells.[77] It is not clear from this brief report whether the tumor might have interfered with the long portal blood system and prevented prolactin-inhibiting factor from reaching the anterior pituitary, thus allowing the prolactin-secreting cells to secrete unchecked, or whether the adenoma may have been secreting a prolactin-releasing substance.

HYPOTHALAMICO-NEUROHYPOPHYSEAL SYSTEM

The neurohypophysis, which consists of the infundibular process (known also as the posterior lobe, neural lobe, and pars nervosa) and the infundibulum (that part of the pituitary or neural stalk extending from the floor of the diencephalon, through the diaphragma sellae, to the neural lobe) along with the paired supraoptic nuclei and paraventricular nuclei in the hypothalamus, constitutes the hypothalamico-neurohypophyseal system. The supraoptic nuclei and paraventricular nuclei are made up of neurosecretory cells whose axons run parallel to one another and pass via the infundibulum to the posterior lobe, where they terminate in contact with capillaries in that structure. Some axons from the supraoptic nuclei terminate in the median eminence and in the stalk, and it is thought that these axons can store and release antidiuretic hormone in the absence of the neural lobe (Fig. 25–6). In the human, the hypothalamico-neurohypophyseal system produces two hormones: antidiuretic hormone (also known as ADH or vasopressin) and oxytocin. These hormones are nonapeptides that were both isolated and synthesized by du Vigneaud and associates. Their structure is given in Figure 25–7.* The human and most other mammals make arginine vasopressin, while the pig and closely related mammals make lysine vasopressin. The biological activity of these compounds depends upon integrity of the disulfide bonds between the two cysteine components in positions 1 and 6.

Antidiuretic hormone (ADH) is made pri-

---

* Originally these compounds were designated "octapeptides," the two cysteine ("hemicystine") amino acid residues being considered to be a single amino acid, cystine. Each of these "octapeptides" contains nine amino acid residues when the two cysteines are counted individually as shown in Figure 25–7. Hence, the term "nonapeptide" is now generally used to describe antidiuretic hormone and oxytocin, and is in keeping with the current terminology of polypeptides.

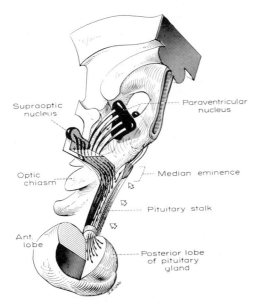

Figure 25–6 Schematic drawing of the human hypothalamico-neurohypophyseal system. Antidiuretic hormone (vasopressin) is made primarily in the supraoptic nuclei and migrates down axons from the nuclei to the posterior pituitary. As indicated by the arrows, some of the axons are thought to terminate in the median eminence and pituitary stalk, and to store and release antidiuretic hormone in the absence of the posterior lobe. (From Randall, R. V.: Diabetes insipidus. In Davis' Encyclopedia of Medicine, Surgery, Specialties. Vol 4. Philadelphia, F. A. Davis Company, 1963, pp. 501–504. Reprinted by permission.)

marily in the supraoptic nuclei, and oxytocin in the paraventricular nuclei. As each of these compounds is formed, it is made in combination with a polypeptide with a molecular weight of approximately 10,000 daltons, known as a neurophysin. Currently there is no unanimity concerning the nomenclature and number of neurophysins

produced in different mammals, including man, but it would appear that in man the neurophysin coupled with oxytocin and the neurophysin coupled with antidiuretic hormone differ in structure. The exact role of neurophysins is not known, but they probably facilitate transport of the relatively small and soluble nonapeptides from the hypothalamic nuclei down the axons of the cells until they are freed from the neurophysins as both are released into the bloodstream. Some ectopic tumors that produce antidiuretic hormone also produce neurophysin.[43]

The secretion of neurophysins by the neurohypophysis is stimulated by nicotine and by estrogen. The neurophysin secreted following the administration of nicotine is called nicotine-stimulated neurophysin (NSN); that secreted following the administration of estrogenic substances is called estrogen-stimulated neurophysin (ESN). The two compounds are similar, but not identical, polypeptides. In man, NSN has been shown to be associated with vasopressin, and ESN is presumed to be associated with oxytocin. The actions of the neurophysins, if any, once they have been separated from vasopressin and oxytocin as they are secreted into the bloodstream, are not known. Likewise, the physiological significance of the effect of estrogenic substances on the neurohypophysis is not known.[106,107]

Recent studies in animals have shown that there are axons running from the supraoptic and paraventricular nuclei to the floor of the third ventricle and to the median eminence, in addition to the long-recognized pathways between these nuclei and the neurohypophysis.[132] Presumably vaso-

$$S\text{———————}S$$
$$|\qquad\qquad\qquad\qquad\qquad|$$
Cys-Tyr-Phe-Glu(NH$_2$)-Asp(NH$_2$)-Cys-Pro-Arg*-Gly(NH$_2$)

1 2 3 4 5 6 7 8 9

ANTIDIURETIC HORMONE (VASOPRESSIN)

* Lysine substituted for arginine in porcine family

$$S\text{———————}S$$
$$|\qquad\qquad\qquad\qquad\qquad|$$
Cys-Tyr-Ileu-Glu(NH$_2$)-Asp(NH$_2$)-Cys-Pro-Leu-Gly(NH$_2$)

1 2 3 4 5 6 7 8 9

OXYTOCIN

Figure 25–7 Amino acid sequence of the hormones of the human hypothalamico-neurohypophyseal system: antidiuretic hormone (vasopressin) and oxytocin.

pressin, oxytocin, and the neurophysins can be secreted into the cerebrospinal fluid in the ventricular system and into the long portal blood vessels in the median eminence as well as into the blood at the level of the neurohypophysis. Vasopressin in high concentrations has been demonstrated in the portal blood draining into the anterior pituitary. The significance of all these findings is not known, but the discovery of large amounts of vasopressin in the portal system reawakens interest in two areas. First, the supraoptic–median eminence pathway may be the route by which vasopressin is redirected when the neurohypophysis is damaged or destroyed. Second, vasopressin may play a role in the regulation of secretion of adrenocorticotropin. It has long been known that the administration of vasopressin will evoke the secretion of ACTH by the anterior pituitary.[106] At the moment, however, it seems unlikely that vasopressin is the long-recognized but as yet uncharacterized corticotropin-releasing factor (CRF).[112]

Oxytocin affects primarily the smooth muscle of the uterus and the mammary glands and, in the latter organs, forces milk from the alveolar channels (milk ejection). It also has some antidiuretic activity. Because oxytocin and its effects lie outside the domain of neurosurgery, this hormone is not considered further, the remainder of this portion of the text being devoted to antidiuretic hormone.

Antidiuretic hormone plays a major role in the regulation of the metabolism of water by the body.[26,99] Normally, each day, the human kidneys form about 180 liters of glomerular filtrate. Less than 1 per cent of this, or approximately 1500 ml, is excreted as urine. Approximately 85 per cent of the water in the glomerular filtrate is resorbed in the proximal tubules and loops of Henle, and approximately 14 per cent is resorbed by the distal tubules and collecting ducts under the influence of antidiuretic hormone. With partial or complete absence of the hormone, large amounts of glomerular filtrate that normally would be resorbed in the distal tubules and collecting ducts are execreted as dilute urine.

Current thoughts on the action of antidiuretic hormone are that the molecule does not enter into the target cells, the renal tubular cells, but interacts with a specific receptor site on their peritubular surface membrane. This in turn activates adenylate cyclase, which catalyzes the formation of cyclic AMP (adenosine 3′,5′-cyclic monophosphate) from adenosine triphosphate (ATP). Cyclic AMP activates protein kinase, which phosphorylates specific membrane proteins controlling the porosity (permeability) of the luminal plasma membrane, thereby increasing the porosity of the membrane and the rate at which water flows from the tubular lumen across the cell membrane into the cells of the tubular wall. The action is opposed by prostaglandins E_1 and E_2, probably by decreasing the concentration of cyclic AMP in the cell.[24,25,134]

The release of antidiuretic hormone by the hypothalamico-neurohypophyseal system is primarily under the control of plasma osmoreceptors that are thought to be located in or near the supraoptic nuclei. When plasma osmolality increases, the osmoreceptors signal the hypothalamico-neurohypophyseal system to release antidiuretic hormone, thereby enhancing renal tubular reabsorption of water, which reduces plasma osmolality. A decrease in plasma osmolality reduces or stops release of the hormone, thereby promoting renal excretion of water, which increases plasma osmolality. In normal persons a reduction in plasma osmolality to a mean of 281.7 mOsm per liter results in maximal diuresis, whereas a rise to a mean of 287.3 mOsm per liter initiates a release of antidiuretic hormone. Hence, the difference between values for plasma osmolality that result in diuresis or antidiuresis is only 5.6 mOsm.[84]

Changes in plasma volume and blood pressure also alter the release of antidiuretic hormone. A decrease in plasma volume is detected by the stretch receptors in the left atrial wall. This, in turn, reduces tonic inhibitory impulses from the atrium along the vagus nerve, which results in the release of the hormone by the hypothalamico-neurohypophyseal system. An increase in plasma volume, by increasing the atrial inhibitory impulses, leads to diuresis by inhibiting the hormone's release. Baroreceptors in the carotid arteries and aorta respond to a reduction in blood pressure by evoking release of antidiuretic hormone.

Many other factors have an effect on the release of vasopressin.[85] Pain, emotional stress, and vomiting stimulate it, as do cholinergic and beta-adrenergic stimulation, whereas alpha-adrenergic stimulation inhibits it. Many pharmacological agents, among them nicotine, morphine, barbiturates, chlorpropamide, clofibrate, carbamazepine, vincristine, cyclophosphamide, and some tricyclic antidepressants stimulate release of antidiuretic hormone; diphenylhydantoin, ethanol, chlorpromazine, reserpine, and two narcotic antagonists, oxilorphan and butorphanol, inhibit it. Some of these pharmacological agents are used in the treatment of diabetes insipidus and the syndrome of inappropriate secretion of antidiuretic hormone.

Neurohypophyseal Diabetes Insipidus

Neurohypophyseal diabetes insipidus is caused by a deficiency of antidiuretic hormone secondary to impairment of the hypothalamico-neurohypophyseal system and is characterized by excessive thirst (polydipsia) and excretion of large amounts of dilute urine (polyuria). The administration of antidiuretic hormone (ADH) will temporarily relieve the polydipsia and polyuria. Other medications, as discussed under treatment, will alleviate these symptoms when they are relatively mild.

Differential Diagnosis of Neurohypophyseal Diabetes Insipidus

When searching for the cause of a patient's polyuria, one must consider a number of other entities in addition to neurohypophyseal diabetes insipidus. The more common ones are given in Table 25–8.

Of all the causes listed, only neurohypophyseal diabetes insipidus and psychogenic polydipsia are relieved by the administration of antidiuretic hormone (ADH).

TABLE 25–8 CAUSES OF POLYURIA

Neurohypophyseal diabetes insipidus
Psychogenic polydipsia
Diabetes mellitus
Familial nephrogenic diabetes insipidus
Hypercalcemia
Hypokalemia
Chronic renal disease
Methoxyflurane (Penthrane, Abbott) anesthesia
Lithium carbonate
Demeclocycline (Declomycin, Lederle)
Obstructive uropathy
Multiple myeloma
Sickle cell anemia
Amyloidosis

© Mayo 1979

The other conditions fail to respond because the renal tubules and collecting ducts are unresponsive to the hormone. Along with a reduction in polyuria, the patient with neurohypophyseal diabetes insipidus who is given antidiuretic hormone will also have a concurrent reduction in thirst. The patient with psychogenic polydipsia who is so treated may or may not have a concurrent reduction in thirst. Hence, patients with psychogenic polydipsia who are given long-acting antidiuretic hormone in the form of pitressin tannate in oil or DDAVP may develop water intoxication if their excessive thirst continues concurrently with an ADH-induced reduction in urinary volume.

Establishing the Diagnosis of Diabetes Insipidus

The various causes of polyuria and polydipsia, are usually readily differentiated by a detailed history including inquiry into family history and exposure to medications and anesthesia; a complete physical examination; and routine studies including x-rays of the chest and head, CT scan with contrast medium of the suprasellar-hypothalamic area, hematological studies, blood chemistry screening, and urinalysis.

When the initial work-up suggests that the patient has neurohypophyseal diabetes insipidus, the diagnosis is then established by demonstrating that he is unable to concentrate urine normally or defend the serum or plasma osmolality during water deprivation, and that the polyuria and polydipsia respond to the administration of antidiuretic hormone.

When dealing with an outpatient who seems to have mild neurohypophyseal diabetes insipidus, the author has the patient refrain from drinking water or eating from supper to 7 or 8 A.M. the next morning. The patient is instructed to empty the bladder upon going to bed and at 7 or 8 A.M. the next morning. The latter voiding is saved, and its osmolality is measured (other voidings between supper and 7 or 8 A.M. are discarded). The patient is also instructed not to eat or drink fluids during this period but, if thirsty, to rinse out the mouth and discard the water. He is also told that, should he develop excessive thirst or become weak, he may drink water and record the time and amount. Immediately following the 7 or 8

A.M. voiding, blood is drawn, and the serum osmolality is measured. In patients with neurohypophyseal diabetes insipidus, urine osmolality is usually less than 300 mOsm per liter (specific gravity less than 1.010) and serum osmolality greater than 300. The next step is to demonstrate that the patient's polyuria and polydipsia will respond to the administration of antidiuretic hormone. This can be done by instructing the patient in the use of lysine-8-vasopressin nasal spray (Diapid, Sandoz) or, as the author usually does, by administering 0.5 to 1.0 ml pitressin tannate in oil (if it seems likely that the patient does not have psychogenic polydipsia). With these two steps the author has had little occasion to use the test described by Hickey and Hare or any of the many modifications thereof, such as that by Carter and Robbins, wherein the hypothalamico-neurohypophyseal system is challenged to release antidiuretic hormone by increasing the osmolality of the blood with intravenously administered hypertonic saline.[12,48]

It should be realized that diabetes insipidus is usually not an "all-or-none" phenomenon. Patients are often seen when there is partial impairment of the hypothalamico-neurohypophyseal release of antidiuretic hormone, with the result that they have mild polyuria and polydipsia but still retain some ability to concentrate urine when deprived of water. While patients with psychogenic polydipsia should theoretically respond to water deprivation the way normal persons do, in actual practice many such patients do not. The presumed reason for this is that prolonged, excessive intake of water and polyuria result in a "washout" of the normal renal medullary hypertonicity. As renal medullary hypertonicity decreases, the ability to concentrate urine decreases. Hence, a simple overnight water-fast may not result in normal urinary concentration, although the patient is usually able to defend the serum osmolality successfully enough so that the value on the morning following the water-fast usually does not exceed 300. If the fluid intake of such patients is restricted to normal amounts for five to seven days, renal medullary hypertonicity is restored and, along with this, the ability to concentrate urine normally during water deprivation.

There are two points that help in differentiating neurohypophyseal diabetes insipidus from psychogenic polydipsia. Measurement of random or morning urinary and serum osmolalities is useful because in the patient with diabetes insipidus urine osmolality usually is less than 300 and serum osmolality greater than 300, while in the patient with psychogenic polydipsia urine osmolality usually is less than 300, (a random specimen) or greater than 300 (an overnight water-fast specimen), and serum osmolality is 285 or less. Also, the patient with neurohypophyseal diabetes insipidus gives a history of excessive intake of fluids and excessive urination, both of which vary little in volume day after day except during the onset of the syndrome when there may be a progressive increase in these volumes until a plateau is reached. On the other hand, the volumes of fluid ingested and excreted by the patient with psychogenic polydipsia characteristically show marked variations from day to day and week to week, and may be normal for weeks or months.

If a patient has severe polyuria (in excess of 4 to 5 liters of urine a day) and polydipsia, water deprivation should be done only under close observation in the hospital and beginning about 7 or 8 A.M. rather than overnight so the patient can be closely watched. Patients who have severe neurohypophyseal diabetes insipidus, when denied water, can rapidly become dehydrated and hypovolemic. In such patients a water-fast of five hours will usually suffice to establish the diagnosis. During this time all urine passed is measured, the patient is weighed hourly, and the fast is terminated (after obtaining appropriate blood and urine samples) if the patient has difficulty before five hours.

Once the diagnosis of neurohypophyseal diabetes insipidus has been established, the physician must then look for the cause of the syndrome (Table 25–9).

The causes of neurohypophyseal diabetes insipidus can be divided into two major categories: primary, involving pathological changes that are poorly understood; and secondary, resulting from damage to the hypothalamico-neurohypophyseal system by trauma, tumor, or other insult. In two large series of cases, 59 of 124 (48 per cent) and 32 of 100 (32 per cent) of cases of diabetes insipidus were primary.[8,99] It is important to realize that an initial diagnosis of primary diabetes insipidus can be made with

TABLE 25-9 CLASSIFICATION OF CAUSES OF NEUROHYPOPHYSEAL DIABETES INSIPIDUS

PRIMARY CAUSES
  Familial
  Idiopathic
SECONDARY CAUSES
  Trauma
    Accidental
    Operative
  Neoplasm
    Primary
      Pituitary adenoma
      Craniopharyngioma
      Meningioma
      Epidermoid
      Ectopic pinealoma
      Chordoma
      Glioma
      Oncocytoma
      Hamartoma
      Myoblastoma
      Miscellaneous
    Metastatic
  Vascular diseases
    Postpartum necrosis (Sheehan's syndrome)
    Hemorrhage
    Aneurysm
    Hemangioma
  Infectious disease
    Abscess
    Granulomatous disease
    Meningitis
    Encephalitis
  Systemic disease
    Sarcoidosis
    Histiocytosis X
    Lymphoma, leukemia, and related diseases
    Wegener's granulomatosis
  Hypoxemic encephalopathy

© Mayo 1979

confidence only if the condition has been present for a number of years or if other members of the family are involved, because polyuria and polydipsia may precede other evidences of underlying disease by months or even by many years. The author has seen patients in whom the cause of the diabetes insipidus did not become evident until 8 to 12 years after the onset of polyuria and polydipsia. With present diagnostic techniques, including computed tomography of the head with contrast medium, lesions such as hypothalamic tumors are less likely to go undetected for long periods.

Treatment of Neurohypophyseal Diabetes Insipidus

Antidiuretic Hormone

Since neurohypophyseal diabetes insipidus is the result of a deficiency of antidiuretic hormone, administration of the hormone is the logical but not the only treatment. Several forms of the drug are available for clinical use.

POSTERIOR PITUITARY POWDER, USP. Posterior pituitary powder is available in capsules containing ⅔ grain of powder. The powder is applied to the nasal mucosa through which its active principle, antidiuretic hormone, is absorbed. The powder is applied by blowing it onto the nasal mucosa by means of a plastic insufflator, available from the pharmacist. If the patient inhales vigorously while insufflating the powder, it may go beyond the nose into the upper respiratory tract, causing sneezing, coughing, and occasionally wheezing. An alternate method of applying the powder, which usually avoids these undesirable effects, is to place the powder from the capsule on the tip of the little finger and apply it directly to the nasal mucosa by gently dabbing the mucosa with the finger. The patient must be cautioned against rubbing the powder vigorously against the nasal mucosa because this will lead to trauma, bleeding, and decreased absorption of the hormone.

The antidiuretic effect of the powder lasts only two to eight hours, depending upon the severity of the diabetes insipidus. Each patient must find out for himself the amount of powder needed and how frequently it must be used to obtain satisfactory relief from symptoms. When the patient first begins to use the posterior pituitary powder, he is instructed to insufflate it into both nostrils in the morning upon arising, at midmorning, noontime, midafternoon, late afternoon, early evening, bedtime, and each time he arises during the night to void. The amount of powder and the frequency of application can be increased or decreased according to the severity of the symptoms. The polyuria and polydipsia themselves do not pose a hazard to the patient's health as long as he has access to water. The symptoms are, however, an inconvenience and, of course, will interrupt the patient's sleep. Because the cost of pituitary powder has risen steeply in the past several years, the patient is advised to use the smallest amount of powder necessary to control the symptoms satisfactorily. As a general rule, most patients find that if the 24-hour urinary volume, while the diabetes insipidus is untreated, is greater than 4 to 5 liters, posterior pituitary powder usually does not provide adequate symptomatic relief, and the long-acting, intramuscular vasopressin tannate in oil or DDAVP is necessary.

Unfortunately, antidiuretic hormone is inactivated if the material is swallowed. The powder may be compressed into buccal tablets, which are inserted in the cheek between the teeth and the buccal mucosa, where they slowly disintegrate, the active principle being absorbed through the buccal mucosa. Buccal tablets are not available commercially but can be made up by a pharmacist into compressed tablets containing 100 mg of powder each. In the author's experience, patients usually do not like this form of administration because the tablets take 20 to 60 minutes to disintegrate and have an objectionable taste. Also, three or more tablets may be needed during each 24-hour period, and this method of treatment is less economical than the application of powder to the nasal mucosa.

SYNTHETIC LYSINE-8-VASOPRESSIN. Synthetic antidiuretic hormone (Diapid, Sandoz) is available for clinical use as an aqueous solution in plastic squeeze bottles that are used to insufflate a fine spray of the medication onto the nasal mucosa. Each squeeze bottle contains 8.0 ml of an aqueous solution of lysine-8-vasopressin, 50 IU per milliliter. This solution is used in the same fashion as posterior pituitary powder, and the duration of effect is similar. Most patients find that the contents of a plastic squeeze bottle will last anywhere from several days to a week or longer, depending upon the severity of the diabetes insipidus. Lysine-8-vasopressin is not available in aqueous form for parenteral use, nor is the synthetic compound available in a long-acting form.

AQUEOUS VASOPRESSIN. Aqueous vasopressin (Aqueous Pitressin, Parke, Davis) is available as a solution containing 20 pressor units per milliliter and comes in ampules of 0.5 and 1.0 ml. When given subcutaneously or intramuscularly in doses of 5 to 10 pressor units, this material has an antidiuretic effect lasting two to eight hours. When given parenterally in these doses, aqueous vasopressin may cause angina pectoris in patients with coronary disease, and frequently causes abdominal cramps, because it is a smooth muscle stimulant. It can also be administered as a spray onto the nasal mucosa or by placing the solution on a pledget of cotton that is inserted into the nose or vagina. When given by any of these routes, aqueous vasopressin, like the posterior pituitary powder and lysine-8-vasopressin, has a duration of action of two to eight hours. Consequently, the use of parenteral solutions of aqueous vasopressin is not convenient for long-term treatment, and the author uses it primarily to treat patients during the acute onset of diabetes insipidus following operative procedures in or around the pituitary and hypothalamus.

VASOPRESSIN TANNATE IN OIL. Vasopressin tannate in oil (Pitressin Tannate in Oil, Parke, Davis) comes in ampules containing 5 pressor units in 1.0 ml of peanut oil. The active material is suspended in the oil, and it is essential that the contents of the ampule be mixed thoroughly before being withdrawn into the needle and syringe. The preparation is given intramuscularly, and an injection of 0.5 to 1.0 ml will have an antidiuretic effect lasting approximately one to four days. For the majority of patients, 1.0 ml will produce an antidiuretic effect for approximately 48 hours. Since the use of this form of antidiuretic hormone requires repeated injections, the patient is instructed in the technique necessary to administer the material at home with disposable syringes and needles. It is imperative that the material be injected intramuscularly and not subcutaneously because, when given subcutaneously, it is poorly absorbed and results in tender nodules that may persist for an indefinite period. The patient is advised to wait until the polyuria and polydipsia just return before taking the next dose. This will prevent an excessive antidiuretic effect with its inherent danger of water intoxication. After the patient has used the material for a few weeks, he can pretty well predict when the antidiuretic effect of the previous injection will wear off. Rather than administer the material at an inconvenient time or place, patients usually carry posterior pituitary powder or synthetic lysine-8-vasopressin to use after the effect of an injection has worn off and until they can reach home to take the next one. Patients frequently mention that different batches of vasopressin tannate in oil vary slightly in duration of effect.

DDAVP. Analogues of antidiuretic hormone may have greater or lesser antidiuretic and vasopressor activities than the hormone has.[105] Deamination of the first amino acid residue (cysteine) of vasopressin increases its antidiuretic effect, while the introduction of the D form of the amino acid in position 8 (lysine or arginine) reduces its pressor effects. Using this information, chemists have synthesized DDAVP (1-deamino-8-d-arginine-vaso-pressin), which has an antidiuretic effect lasting approximately 8 to 20 hours and minimal pressor effects.*

DDAVP comes in a plastic squeeze bottle containing 2.5 ml of an aqueous solution of 0.1 mg per milliliter. It is administered by placing one end of a small flexible plastic tube (supplied with bottle) over the nipple of the bottle and squeezing the nipple until the solution has reached the desired dosage mark. The end of the tube containing the solution is placed into a nostril, the other end is placed in the mouth, and the solution is then blown onto the nasal mucosa. DDAVP has an effect lasting 8 to 20 hours or longer, depending upon the severity of the diabetes insipidus. The usual dosage is 0.05 to 0.2 ml, one to three times a day. When a single dose is used, it is given in the evening to give maximal effect during the sleeping hours. In more severe diabetes insipidus, an additional dose will be required in the morning, and sometimes a third dose at noon or in the early afternoon. As with posterior pituitary powder and lysine-8-vasopressin, the patient must adjust the amount and frequency of applications to suit his needs.

Other Forms of Treatment

BENZOTHIAZIDE COMPOUNDS. Other compounds have been found to have a beneficial effect upon neurohypophyseal diabetes insipidus. Chlorothiazide, which is known to be beneficial in the treatment of nephrogenic diabetes insipidus, has been found to have a similar effect in neurohypophyseal diabetes insipidus. Subsequently other benzothiazide compounds and other potent diuretics such as ethacrynic acid and triamterene have been found to have a similar effect. The mechanism by which these agents control diabetes insipidus is not completely understood, but their natriuretic action is believed to play an important role. When given to non-edematous subjects, these compounds cause a sustained,

moderate depletion of sodium, chloride, and water. This is thought to result in a more complete reabsorption of glomerular filtrate in the proximal tubule, while the diuretic concurrently decreases the resorption of sodium in the distal tubule. Thus a smaller volume of fluid with a higher solute concentration is eventually excreted.

These diuretic agents are of use only in treating patients with relatively mild diabetes insipidus. When chlorothiazide (Diuril, Merck Sharpe & Dohme) is given in doses of 500 mg approximately every 12 hours to a patient with a 24-hour urinary volume of approximately 3500 to 4000 ml in the untreated state, the urinary volume will be reduced by approximately one third. Because chlorothiazide and related thiazide compounds may lead to potassium depletion, the author prefers to use a combination of diuretics such as one consisting of hydrochlorothiazide and triamterene (Dyazide, Smith Kline & French, each capsule containing 25 mg of hydrochlorothiazide and 50 mg of triamterene) at a dosage of one capsule approximately every 12 hours.

CHLORPROPAMIDE. Chlorpropamide (Diabinese, Pfizer) will reduce the urinary volume in patients with diabetes insipidus. It is not entirely clear whether it acts solely by augmenting the renal effect of the antidiuretic hormone which is released by the hypothalamico-neurohypophyseal system in small but inadequate amounts in patients with partial neurohypophyseal diabetes insipidus, or whether it also has a central effect leading to release of small amounts of the hormone by the hypothalamico-neurohypophyseal system. The magnitude of its effect is similar to that of the diuretic agents in that it is useful only in patients with mild neurohypophyseal diabetes insipidus. The author does not use chlorpropamide in treating patients with diabetes insipidus because it can lead to serious hypoglycemia, and thus poses a hazard that does not exist with the diuretics.

CLOFIBRATE. Clofibrate (Atromid-S, Ayerst) will ameliorate mild neurohypophyseal diabetes insipidus to about the same extent as the diuretics and chlorpropamide. It has a number of side effects. The usual dose for treating diabetes insipidus is 500 mg approximately every 12 hours.

CARBAMAZEPINE. Carbamazepine (Tegretol, Geigy), which is used as an anticonvulsant and for the treatment of trigeminal

---

* DDAVP (Desmopressin Acetate, Ferring Pharmaceuticals, Inc., Malmo, Sweden) is available from Centerchem Products, Inc., 475 Park Avenue South, New York, N.Y., 10016.

neuralgia and glossopharyngeal neuralgia, will also ameliorate mild neurohypophyseal diabetes insipidus. It has a number of side effects.

Management of Patients With Chronic Neurohypophyseal Diabetes Insipidus

In treating a patient with chronic neurohypophyseal diabetes insipidus, it is preferable to start by using posterior pituitary powder or lysine-8-vasopressin nasal spray. Since the urinary volume is to some extent determined by the solute load handled by the kidneys, limiting the intake of sodium chloride is helpful. If these measures do not control the diabetes insipidus adequately, Dyazide, one capsule approximately every 12 hours, is given in addition to the posterior pituitary powder or lysine-8-vasopressin nasal spray. If symptomatic relief is still not obtained, it will be necessary to use intramuscular pitressin tannate in oil or DDAVP according to the directions given earlier. Fortunately, neurohypophyseal diabetes insipidus is usually mild enough in most patients so that it can be controlled satisfactorily without recourse to vasopressin tannate in oil, which is a relatively inconvenient method of treating a patient over a period of years, or DDAVP.

Neurohypophyseal Diabetes Insipidus in the Neurosurgical Patient

The neurosurgeon may be called upon to deal with neurohypophyseal diabetes insipidus in two situations. The first is when a patient with pre-existing diabetes insipidus is undergoing a neurosurgical procedure, and the second is when acute diabetes insipidus occurs in the patient who had undergone a procedure in or around the pituitary and hypothalamus. These situations, while somewhat analogous, pose essentially different problems and are discussed separately.

Pre-Existing Diabetes Insipidus

When a patient with pre-existing diabetes insipidus is to undergo an operative procedure, the neurosurgeon should know what form of treatment has been used. If the patient has been using one of the diuretics, potassium depletion must be ruled out or, if present, must be corrected before the operation. If chlorpropamide has been used, this should be discontinued several days before the procedure because of the potential, relatively long hypoglycemic effect associated with this drug. If vasopressin tannate in oil has been used, the patient will know how long each injection lasts, and this information will be a useful guide to the postoperative treatment.

The administration of large doses of adrenal glucocorticoids may increase the severity of the polyuria until the dosage is reduced to a maintenance level or the medication is discontinued in the postoperative period. Of particular interest in this regard is the patient who initially develops diabetes insipidus, which is then followed by the onset of pituitary insufficiency, which in turn may reduce the urinary volume of the diabetes insipidus to a normal amount. The administration of adrenal glucocorticoids prior to an operation will cause a sudden return of the polyuria and polydipsia (see Fig. 25–4).

Regardless of the type of treatment the patient has been using to control the disorder, the best way to handle diabetes insipidus during a neurosurgical procedure is to administer vasopressin tannate in oil the day before the operation and in the postoperative period until the patient's condition has become stabilized and he can return to the form of treatment used before the operation, assuming it was another method than vasopressin tannate in oil. The patient is given 1.0 ml of vasopressin tannate in oil intramuscularly the afternoon or evening before the operative procedure, and again each time the antidiuretic effect of the preceding injection has begun to wear off. The vasopressin tannate in oil is not administered on a predetermined schedule, but rather one waits for the effect to begin to wear off before giving the next dose, thereby avoiding the possible hazards of water retention and water intoxication, especially when the patient is being given intravenous fluids.

Acute Postoperative Neurohypophyseal Diabetes Insipidus

Classic studies on experimental animals have demonstrated three patterns of diabetes insipidus after damage to the hypothalamico-neurohypophyseal system.[30] Three patterns of postoperative neurohypophyseal diabetes insipidus, similar to those

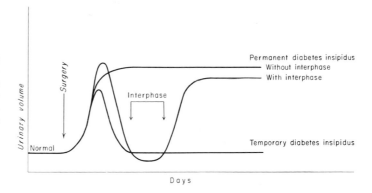

Figure 25–8 Schematic curves showing patterns of onset of postoperative diabetes insipidus in man. (From Randall, R. V.: Medical problems associated with pituitary operations. Med. Clin. N. Amer., *46*:1037–1043, 1962. Reprinted by permission.)

seen in experimental animals, have been observed in man following procedures on or near the pituitary or hypothalamus: (1) transient diabetes insipidus, (2) triphasic diabetes insipidus, and (3) permanent diabetes insipidus without an interphase (Fig. 25–8).[98]

Transient diabetes insipidus begins anywhere up to four days after operation and may last as long as five or six days. During this time the kidney is unable to concentrate urine. Following the transient polyuria the urinary volume returns permanently to normal or nearly normal amounts and there is a return of normal or nearly normal ability to concentrate urine.

Triphasic diabetes insipidus is characterized by transient polyuria and polyuria followed by a return of urinary volume to normal or less than normal, which in turn is followed by permanent polyuria. The initial polyuria and polydipsia may start any time up to several days after operation, and during this phase the kidneys are unable to form concentrated urine. The urinary volume then returns to normal or subnormal, and the urine is highly concentrated. This period of normal or subnormal urinary volume is known as the interphase and lasts from part of a day to up to 8 to 10 days. This is then followed by permanent polyuria and polydipsia. The patient is vulnerable to water intoxication during the interphase, and intravenous fluids must be given with caution.

Permanent diabetes insipidus begins anywhere up to six days after operation and continues indefinitely without an interphase.

Animal studies have shown that transient diabetes insipidus is due to minimal injury to the hypothalamico-neurohypophyseal system, such as a small cut in the stalk, from which a rapid and complete, or nearly complete, recovery is made.[30] For reasons that are not clear there is temporary failure of the hypothalamico-neurohypophyseal system to release antidiuretic hormone, thus resulting in the transient polyuria. In all three patterns of diabetes insipidus, the intake of fluids roughly parallels the urinary excretion, and the urinary concentration is inversely proportional to the urinary volume. A similar mechanism is postulated for the transient phase of the triphasic pattern. The interphase is thought to be due to uncontrolled release of stored antidiuretic hormone in the neurohypophysis.[86] Once this is exhausted, permanent diabetes insipidus ensues. In the experimental animal, the triphasic pattern is created by placing in the median eminence a lesion that severs all the fibers carrying vasopressin to the lower portion of the median eminence, pituitary stalk, and posterior pituitary. After the transient phase, during which the hormone is not released, there is then thought to be uncontrolled release of the stored substance in the areas distal to the lesion. Once this is used up, permanent diabetes insipidus ensues. If a lesion is placed distal to the median eminence in the pituitary stalk, there will be transient diabetes insipidus followed by a return of the urinary volume to or nearly to normal. The return of normal or nearly normal urinary volume is thought to coincide with resumption of function by the remaining intact ADH-releasing axons running from the supraoptic nuclei to above the site of the lesion. If, in the experimental animal, a lesion is placed through the median eminence and all the distal neurohypophyseal tissue is removed, immediate and permanent diabetes insipidus results because the separated portion of the hypothalamico-neurohypophyseal portion is no longer present to release the stored hormone and cause an interphase. Limited pathological studies in man suggest that analogous lesions are responsible for the three patterns in man.[4]

Because the body is unable to excrete large amounts of urine during the interphase, and because it is impossible during the first few days following the onset of postoperative diabetes insipidus to predict whether the condition will be transient or permanent, or whether an interphase will intervene in the case of permanent diabetes insipidus, it is not desirable to give large amounts of long-acting vasopressin. Hence, to prevent a patient who is developing an interphase from entering this phase with excessive amounts of both exogenous and endogenous antidiuretic hormone, the author treats all patients during the initial onset of diabetes insipidus with aqueous vasopressin or no more than 0.5 ml of vasopressin tannate in oil, which generally has an effect lasting 24 hours or less. He does not give the next dose of vasopressin, be it aqueous or in oil, until the polyuria has briefly returned. By this method it is possible to tell within a few days whether the patient has transient or permanent diabetes insipidus (with or without an interphase) and avoid water intoxication. Treatment of permanent diabetes insipidus is started when the polyuria and polydipsia return after an interphase or when it becomes evident that there is to be no interphase. Permanent diabetes insipidus emerging from either pattern is treated as outlined earlier.

To facilitate fluid replacement and early recognition of the onset of postoperative diabetes insipidus, patients who undergo operation in or near the pituitary or hypothalamus have an indwelling urinary catheter in place for the first few days following operation, and the urinary volume and specific gravity or osmolality of the urine are determined every hour. During this time the patient is usually in a neurosurgical intensive care unit for careful observation and for the almost constant nursing care that is required. Once the patient leaves the intensive care unit, the urinary catheter is removed, and the intake and output of fluids and the urinary specific gravity or osmolality continue to be monitored on a 12- or 24-hour basis.

One will occasionally see a patient who has postoperative diabetes insipidus but lacks a thirst drive. This situation is characterized by the excretion of essentially normal volumes of urine, but of low specific gravity or osmolality, and an intake of normal amounts of fluid even though the patient has free access to fluids. If uncorrected this will result in hyperosmolality of the serum with the sodium concentration rising to 180 mEq per liter or more, and the patient may become somnolent or comatose. Treatment consists of administering fluids and antidiuretic hormone, being careful to avoid overtreatment and resultant water intoxication.

Inappropriate Secretion of Antidiuretic Hormone

The secretion of antidiuretic hormone (ADH) is "appropriate" when it responds normally to the usual controlling mechanisms, namely serum osmolality and blood volume. Secretion that occurs independently of these controlling mechanisms is called "inappropriate" and may lead to

TABLE 25–10 CONDITIONS ASSOCIATED WITH SYNDROME OF INAPPROPRIATE SECRETION OF ANTIDIURETIC HORMONE

IDIOPATHIC CAUSES	CENTRAL NERVOUS SYSTEM DISEASE
MALIGNANT TUMORS (ECTOPIC ADH)	Acute polyneuropathy
Lung	Brain abscess
Thymus	Brain trauma
Pancreas	Brain tumor
Duodenum	Primary and metastic
Ureter	Delirium tremens
Prostate	Encephalitis
Lymphoma	Guillain-Barré syndrome
Others	Meningitis
DRUGS	Peripheral neuropathy
Antidiuretic hormone	Psychosis
Carbamazepine	Subarachnoid hemorrhage
Chlorpropamide	Tuberculosis
Clofibrate	**MISCELLANEOUS CAUSES**
Cyclophosphamide	Intrathoracic tumors
Diuretics	Lung abscess
Narcotics	Lymphoma
Nicotine	Pneumonia
Oxytocin	Porphyria
Phenothiazides	Positive-pressure breathing
Vincristine	Pulmonary tuberculosis
	Trauma
	Status asthmaticus

© Mayo 1979

signs and symptoms that are known as the syndrome of inappropriate antidiuretic hormone secretion (SIADH).

The syndrome is characterized by (1) decreased serum sodium and osmolality, but increased total body water, extracellular fluid volume, and plasma volume (edema does not occur, and a sodium load is promptly excreted despite the increased serum sodium, and consequently, the administration of hypertonic saline alone is not appropriate treatment); (2) urinary osmolality greater than serum osmolality (the urine is less than maximally dilute, and its osmolality is inappropriately high for the serum osmolality); (3) increased glomerular filtration rate and normal or decreased blood urea nitrogen and urea; and (4) absence of renal, cardiac, hepatic, or adrenal disease. The condition may be masked if the intake of water is minimal. Likewise, renal sodium wasting may not occur if the intake of sodium is restricted.

Etiology

Inappropriate secretion of antidiuretic hormone may be idiopathic or associated with a number of seemingly unrelated non-neoplastic and neoplastic conditions shown in Table 25–10.

Differential Diagnosis

The syndrome of inappropriate secretion of antidiuretic hormone must be differentiated from a number of other conditions. The administration of mannitol can result in hyponatremia, hypovolemia, and hypo-osmolality. Similar findings may occur in patients whose intake of sodium is deficient and out of proportion to the intake of water or loss of sodium, but this combination is most frequently seen postoperatively in the patient whose intake is primarily by the intravenous route or who has vomiting, nasogastric suction, or diarrhea. Such patients have dehydration and azotemia, neither of which is seen in inappropriate secretion of antidiuretic hormone. Excessive salt wasting and depletion due to renal tubular disease or Addison's disease may lead to a similar picture.

The hyponatremia found in some patients with anterior pituitary failure, although not fully understood, seems to be unrelated to excessive secretion of vasopressin and clears rapidly with the administration of hydrocortisone or one of the related compounds. In patients with myxedema, serum osmolality may be low and urinary osmolality increased. Although this has been thought to be secondary to inappropriate secretion of antidiuretic hormone, the relationship has not been firmly established. Some think the phenomenon to be due to a decrease in volume of glomerular filtrate and solute delivered to the distal renal tubules.

Treatment of Inappropriate Secretion of Antidiuretic Hormone

The treatment of the syndrome is determined by the severity of the symptoms and by the underlying cause. If the patient has asymptomatic hyponatremia, restriction of fluid intake will suffice to keep the hyponatremia from worsening and becoming symptomatic. On the other hand, if the patient has hyponatremia severe enough (usually below 115 mEq of sodium per liter) to result in somnolence, loss of consciousness, or convulsions, then rapid corrective measures must be taken. If the syndrome results from a self-limited condition such as a lung abscess or pneumonia, or one correctible by withdrawal of a causative medication (see Table 25–10), then treatment is merely a matter of tiding the patient over until the situation has been corrected. If inappropriate secretion of antidiuretic hormone is the result of secreting malignant tumor, removal of the tumor will correct the situation. If, however, the tumor cannot be removed or there are metastases remaining after the primary tumor has been removed, then the syndrome will continue unabated.

In addition to restricting the intake of water to 500 to 800 ml per 24 hours and attempting to correct the underlying cause, the following methods of treatment have been used.

Hypertonic Saline

The administration of hypertonic saline, usually as a 3 per cent solution, has been advocated in the past but is now usually used only when other measures have failed. Since the patient already has increased total body water and extracellular fluid volume, although without edema, the administration of hypertonic saline expands the extracellular fluid volume and can result in the rapid onset of pulmonary edema. Also, since sodium loads are rapidly excreted in the urine, the administration of sodium by either the intravenous or oral route fails to increase the total body sodium permanently.

Diphenylhydantoin

The administration of 500 mg of diphenylhydantoin sodium (Dilantin sodium, Parke, Davis) intravenously at a rate no faster than 50 mg per minute will increase the free water clearance by the kidneys for a period of several hours. Fichman and Bethune found that diphenylhydantoin evoked an improvement in water handling in patients who had the syndrome from causes other than a hormone-secreting malignant tumor but did not work in a patient with a bronchogenic carcinoma that produced antidiuretic hormone. Diphenylhydantoin when given orally was not effective in any of their patients.[29] On the other hand, Tanay and co-workers reported that 100 mg of diphenylhydantoin orally three times a day successfully controlled the syndrome in a patient with basilar skull fracture.[121]

Demeclocycline

Demeclocycline (Declomycin [HC1] and Declomycin [base], Lederle) can cause nephrogenic diabetes insipidus and for this reason has been used in the treatment of the syndrome of inappropriate antidiuretic hormone secretion.[13,23] Singer and Rotenberg found that 1200 mg of demeclocycline daily in four oral doses of 300 mg each severely impaired renal concentrating ability in each of five patients within three weeks' time.[116] This form of treatment is obviously applicable to subacute and chronic disorders rather than acute ones. Treatment with demeclocycline has the advantage of not requiring restriction of the intake of fluids. Since its effect on the renal tubules is reversible, it would seem to be the current treatment of choice for long-term treatment, although of course, long-term treatment with any antibiotic carries the risk of superimposed infections.

Lithium Carbonate

Lithium carbonate, like demeclocycline, can evoke nephrogenic diabetes insipidus by making the renal tubules resistant to endogenous antidiuretic hormone. White and Fetner found that 300 mg of lithium carbonate orally every eight hours caused a decrease in urinary excretion of sodium and an increase in the plasma osmolality within nine days and, like demeclocycline, obviated the need for restriction of fluid intake.[127] Since lithium carbonate has a number of toxic effects that are related to its blood level, the patient must be carefully monitored. Forrest and co-workers reported that only 12 per cent of patients treated with lithium carbonate developed nephrogenic diabetes insipidus, and hence, its application to the treatment of inappropriate antidiuretic hormone secretion would seem to be limited.[31]

Diuretic Plus Electrolyte Replacement

Currently the most effective way of treating the acute symptoms of inappropriate secretion of antidiuretic hormone is the method advocated by Hantman and associates.[47] They used furosemide (Lasix, Hoechst) to induce diuresis and replaced the urinary losses of sodium and potassium, which were measured hourly, with an infusion of 3 per cent hypertonic sodium chloride to which appropriate amounts of potassium chloride were added. A single dose of furosemide of 1 mg per kilogram of body weight was administered intravenously, and subsequent doses of furosemide were administered as necessary to obtain the desired negative fluid balance. With this treatment they were successful in raising the serum sodium level within several hours. Their paper should be reviewed in detail before such treatment is attempted.

Narcotic Antagonists

Two morphine antagonists, oxilorphan and butorphanol, when injected into rats cause an increase in urinary volume and a decrease in urinary osmolality. They seem to inhibit the release of antidiuretic hormone by the hypothalamico-neurohypophyseal system by interfering with the osmotic feedback that regulates it, but they do not interfere with its renal tubular action. Each has been used successfully in treating a patient with a central (neurohypophyseal) syndrome of inappropriate secretion of vasopressin, but ineffectively in a patient in whom the disorder was caused by an oat-cell carcinoma of the lung.[80,83]

Analogues of Antidiuretic Hormone

Since analogues of antidiuretic hormone have been made that are more effective than the natural hormone (as described earlier in the section on DDAVP), it would seem likely that analogues that have minimal or no antidiuretic activity could be synthesized and used to block the renal binding sites for the hormone, thus negating its effect. Unfortunately, the syndrome occurs so infrequently that nobody, apparently, has been motivated to synthesize analogues of this type for clinical use.

USE OF ADRENAL CORTICOSTEROIDS IN THE NEUROSURGICAL PATIENT

The use of adrenal corticosteroids in special situations (pseudotumor cerebri, cerebral edema, and the like) is covered in the sections of this text dealing with these subjects. Administration of adrenal corticosteroids is essential to those patients who are taking or who have recently been taking cortisone or one of the related steroids in doses that may suppress the pituitary-adrenal axis and who are undergoing neurosurgical procedures. They also are essential for patients who have adrenocortical insufficiency from Addison's disease, bilateral total adrenalectomy for Cushing's disease, or pituitary failure, and for those who are undergoing procedures, such as resection of a pituitary tumor, hypophysectomy, or section of the pituitary stalk, that may lead to pituitary insufficiency.

Adrenal Cortical Suppression From Exogenous Adrenal Corticosteroids or Corticotropin

Adrenal corticosteroids should be given to patients who have received cortisone or one of the related compounds daily in physiological or larger quantities by intramuscular injections or divided oral doses for a week or more within the preceding three months. "Physiological quantities" are considered to be 25 mg of cortisone acetate per 24 hours, or the equivalent dose of one of the related compounds such as 20 mg of hydrocortisone, 5 mg of prednisone or prednisolone, 4 mg of triamcinolone, 0.75 mg of dexamethasone or the like, or ACTH (when given daily for treatment rather than testing of adrenal function). When the patient has received suppressive doses of adrenal corticosteroids for a number of months, one should anticipate that adrenal suppression may persist for as long as 6 to 12 months after the corticosteroids have been stopped. All such patients should be protected against possible postoperative adrenal insufficiency by the administration of cortisone or one of the related steroids. Any one of the following plans of treatment will provide adequate protection.

1. Cortisone acetate (not *hydro*cortisone acetate), 200 mg intramuscularly approximately 48 hours before operation, the same dose approximately 24 hours before operation, and again on the morning of operation.

2. Cortisone acetate, 200 mg intramuscularly the day before operation, again on the morning of operation, and in addition, 40 mg of prednisolone sodium phosphate (Hydeltrasol, Merck Sharp & Dohme) intramuscularly one hour before operation.

3. Cortisone acetate, 200 mg intramuscularly to act as a long-acting depot plus 40 mg of prednisolone sodium phosphate intramuscularly one hour before operation. Prednisolone sodium phosphate is given in the same dose intramuscularly six to eight hours later. An intravenous infusion containing 40 mg of prednisolone sodium phosphate or 100 mg of sodium hydrocortisone hemisuccinate can be used if the intravenous route is preferred. The initial intravenous adrenal corticosteroids are given over a period of three to four hours and followed by a similar continuous intravenous dose every 8 to 12 hours until the stress of the procedure has passed.

Oral adrenal corticosteroids are not used initially because of their relatively short duration of action, the chance that they may be lost by vomiting, and the frequent inability of the patient to take oral medications in the immediate postoperative period. Barring complications, the administration of adrenal corticosteroids can be discontinued within one or two days after operation unless the patient has had long-term adrenal corticosteroid therapy prior to operation or has pre-existing pituitary or adrenal insufficiency, operatively induced pituitary insufficiency, or a chronic condition such as active rheumatoid arthritis, asthma, or certain hematological disorders in which abrupt cessation of adrenal corticosteroids might result in exacerbation of the disease. Because large doses of adrenal corticosteroids such as cortisone and hydrocortisone have a sodium-retaining effect, intravenous saline must be used cautiously while the patient is receiving large amounts of these substances (more than 75 mg per day). In the case of the patient with Addison's disease or the one whose adrenal glands have been removed for Cushing's disease, daily intramuscular doses of cortisone of 75 mg or more will provide adequate electrolyte retention. Once the daily dose has been reduced below 75 mg, an electrolyte-retaining hormone such as 0.1 mg fludrocortisone acetate (Florinef Acetate, Squibb) should be given orally each day in addition to the daily dose of cortisone.

Should circulatory collapse occur during the operation or in the immediate postoperative period, the patient is given an intravenous infusion of 40 mg of prednisolone sodium phosphate or 100 mg of sodium hydrocortisone hemisuccinate over a period of 15 to 20 minutes in addition to the usual treatment for shock.

Special Considerations

For patients who are undergoing a transsphenoidal procedure for a microadenoma of the pituitary, the method of preparation with adrenal corticosteroids may be altered for two reasons. The first reason is that patients who have microadenomas of the pituitary, except those with Cushing's disease, are likely to have normal pituitary function (insofar as the pituitary-adrenal axis is concerned) following the operation. To determine whether the patient has good adrenal function after the operation all adrenal corticosteroids are stopped and the serum corticosteroids, or urinary (17-ketogenic steroids) or 17-hydroxycorticosteroids (or both) are measured before the

patient is dismissed from the hospital. The second reason concerns patients with Cushing's disease in whom an attempt is being made to control the disease by removing the corticotropin-producing pituitary tumor. If one can be assured that the tumor has been completely removed and the excessive production of corticotropin has ceased, the patient is sent home, and maintenance doses of adrenal corticosteroids are continued until they can eventually be reduced and stopped. On the other hand, if one has not been successful in stopping the overproduction of ACTH, the Cushing's disease will continue unabated, and additional treatment to control it must be undertaken, as described in the section on postoperative assessment in Cushing's disease.

If valid evaluations are to be made in the immediate postoperative period, long-acting intramuscular adrenal corticosteroids cannot be used in the preoperative preparation of the patient. Instead, the patient is given 40 mg of prednisolone sodium phosphate intramuscularly one hour prior to the procedure. An intramuscular dose of 20 to 40 mg is repeated every six to eight hours for the first two or three postoperative days until the patient can be given an oral adrenal corticosteroid preparation. When the stress of the procedure has regressed, the afternoon dose is omitted, and blood is obtained at 8 A.M. and 4 P.M. the next day for determination of plasma corticosteroids and, in addition, in the patient with Cushing's disease, for determination of corticotropin and beta-lipoprotein. In the case of the patient who has been operated upon for a non-adrenocorticotropin-producing pituitary tumor, finding plasma corticosteroids to be within the normal range is indicative of essentially normal adrenal function. If the values are in the borderline range or low, then the patient is given maintenance oral adrenal corticosteroids until evaluation of adrenal function at a later date. In the patient with Cushing's disease, a low level or absence of plasma corticosteroids would be presumptive evidence that the patient is in remission and could then be given replacement adrenal corticosteroids until suitable testing at a later date. Should the plasma corticosteroid value be normal or elevated, however, the overnight suppression test described earlier should be done to see whether the disease is still active. Confirmatory evidence would be detectable adrenocorticotropin and beta-lipoprotein in the blood, and further therapy should then be undertaken.

REFERENCES

1. Alsever, R. N., and Gotlin, R. W.: Handbook of Endocrine Tests in Adults and Children. Chicago, Year Book Medical Publishers, Inc., 1975.
2. Antunes, J. L., Housepian, E. M., Frantz, A. G., et al.: Prolactin-secreting pituitary tumors. Ann. Neurol., 2:148–153, 1977.
3. Arnaud, C. D., Goldsmith, R. S., Bordier, P. J., et al.: Influence of immunoheterogeneity of circulating parathyroid hormone on results of radioimmunoassays of serum in man. Amer. J. Med., 56:785–793, 1974.
4. Bahn, R. C., and Randall, R. V.: Unpublished data.
5. Ballard, H. S., Frame, B., and Hartsock, R. J.: Familial multiple endocrine adenoma–peptic ulcer complex. Medicine (Balt.), 43:481–516, 1964.
6. Besser, G. M., ed.: The Hypothalamus and Pituitary. Clinics Endocr. Metab., 6:1–281, 1977.
7. Besser, G. M., Mortimer, C. H., McNeilly, A. S., et al.: Long-term infusion of growth hormone release inhibiting hormone in acromegaly: Effects on pituitary and pancreatic hormone. Brit. Med. J., 4:622–627, 1974.
8. Blotner, H.: Primary or idiopathic diabetes insipidus: A systemic disease. Metabolism, 7:191–200, 1958.
9. Bohnet, H. G., Dahlen, H. G., Wuttke, W., et al.: Hyperprolactinemic anovulatory syndrome. J. Clin. Endocr., 42:132–143, 1976.
10. Bower, B. F.: Pituitary enlargement secondary to untreated primary hypogonadism. An. Intern. Med., 69:107–109, 1968.
11. Caplan, R. H., Koob, L., Abellera, R. M., et al.: Cure of acromegaly by operative removal of an islet cell tumor of the pancreas. Amer. J. Med., 64:874–882, 1978.
12. Carter, A. C., and Robbins, J.: The use of hypertonic saline in the differential diagnosis of diabetes insipidus and psychogenic polydipsia. J. Clin. Endocr., 7:753–766, 1947.
13. Cherrill, D. A., Stote, R. M., Birge, J. R., et al.: Demeclocycline treatment in the syndrome of inappropriate antidiuretic hormone secretion. Ann. Intern. Med., 83:654–656, 1975.
14. Child, D. F., Nader, S., Mashiter, K., et al.: Prolactin studies in "functionless" pituitary tumours. Brit. Med. J., 1:604–606, 1975.
15. Clemmons, D. R., Van Wyk, J. J., Ridgway, E. C., et al.: Evaluation of acromegaly by radioimmunoassay of somatomedin-C. New Eng. J. Med., 301:1138–1142, 1979.
16. Corenblum, B., Sirek, A. M. T., Horvath, E., et al.: Human mixed somatotrophic and lactotrophic pituitary adenomas. J. Clin. Endocr. 42:857–863, 1976.
17. Costello, R. T.: Subclinical adenoma of the pituitary gland. Amer. J. Path., 12:205–215, 1936.
18. Cunningham, G. R., and Huckins, C.: An FSH and prolactin-secreting pituitary tumor: Pituitary dynamics and testicular histology. J. Clin. Endocr., 44:248–253, 1977.
19. Dabek, J. T.: Bronchial carcinoid tumor with acromegaly in two patients. J. Clin. Endocr., 38:329–333, 1974.
20. Daughaday, W. H.: Hormonal regulation of growth by somatomedin and other tissue growth factors. Clinics Endocr. Metab., 6:117–135, 1977.
21. Delitala, G., Masala, A., Alagna, S., et al.: Growth hormone and prolactin release in acromegalic patients following metergoline administration. J. Clin. Endocr., 43:1382–1386, 1976.
22. del Pozo, E.: Personal communications, 1980.
23. De Troyer, A., and Demanet, J.-C.: Correction of antidiuresis by demeclocycline. New Eng. J. Med., 293:915–918, 1975.
24. Dousa, T. P.: Cellular action of antidiuretic hormone in nephrogenic diabetes insipidus. Mayo Clin. Proc., 49:188–199, 1974.
25. Dousa, T. P.: Drugs and other agents affecting the renal adenylate cyclase system. *In* Martinez-Maldonado, M., ed.: Methods in Pharmacology. Vol. 4A. New York, Plenum Publishing Corp., 1976, pp. 293–331.
25a. du Vigneaud, V.: Hormones of the posterior pituitary gland: Oxytocin and vasopressin. *In* The Harvey Lectures 1954–1955. New York, Academic Press Inc., 1956.
26. Edwards, C. R. W.: Vasopressin and oxytocin in health and disease. Clinics Endocr. Metab., 6:223–259, 1977.
27. Emerson, C. H., and Utiger, R. D.: Hyperthyroidism and excessive thyrotropin secretion. New Eng. J. Med., 287:328–333, 1972.
27a. Ezrin, C., Kovacs, K., and Horvath, E.: Pituitary tumors causing prolactin hypersecretion and other adenomas. Med. Clin. N. Amer., 62:393–408, 1978.
28. Faglia, G., Ferrari, C., Neri, V., et al.: High plasma thyrotropin levels in two patients with pituitary tumour. Acta Endocr., 69:649–658, 1972.
29. Fichman, M. P., and Bethune, J. E.: The role of adrenocorticoids in the inappropriate antidiuretic hormone syndrome. Ann. Intern. Med., 68:806–820, 1968.
30. Fischer, C., Ingram, W. R., and Ranson, S. W.: Diabetes insipidus and the neurohormonal control of water balance: A contribution to the structure and function of the hypothalamico-hypophyseal system. Ann Arbor, Edwards Brothers, Inc. 1938.
31. Forrest, J. N., Jr., Cohen, A. D., Torretti, J., et al.: On the mechanism of lithium-induced diabetes insipidus in man and the rat. J. Clin. Invest., 53:1115–1123, 1974.
32. Franks, S., Jacobs, H. S., and Nabarro, J. D. N.: Prolactin concentrations in patients with acromegaly: Clinical significance and response to surgery. Clin. Endocr. (Tokyo), 5:63–69, 1976.
33. Frantz, A. G., Kleinberg, D. L., and Noel, G. L.: Studies on prolactin in man. Recent Prog Hormone Res., 28:527–573, 1972.
34. Friend, J. N., Judge, D. M., Sherman, B. M., et al.: FSH-secreting pituitary adenomas: Stimulation and suppression studies in two patients. J. Clin. Endocr., 43:650–657, 1976.

35. Frohman, L. A., Szabo, M., Berelowitz, M., et al.: Partial purification and characterization of a peptide with growth hormone-releasing activity from extrapituitary tumors in patients with acromegaly. J. Clin. Invest., 65:43–54, 1980.

36. Frohman, L. A., Szabo, M., Stachura, M. E., et al.: Growth hormone-releasing activity in an extract of a bronchial carcinoid tumor associated with acromegaly. Clin. Res., 26:702A, 1978.

37. Ganong, W. F., and Martini, L., eds.: Frontiers in Neuroendocrinology, 1969. New York, Oxford University Press, 1969.

38. Ganong, W. F., and Martini, L., eds.: Frontiers in Neuroendocrinology, 1973. New York, Oxford University Press, 1973.

39. Ganong, W. F., and Martini, L., eds.: Frontiers in Neuroendocrinology. Vol 5. New York, Raven Press, 1978.

40. Glass, M. R., Shaw, R. W., Butt, W. R., et al.: An abnormality of oestrogen feedback in amenorrhea-galactorrhea. Brit. Med. J., 3:274–275, 1975.

41. Gordon, S. J., and Moses, A. M.: Multiple endocrine organ refractoriness to trophic hormone stimulation. A patient with an enlarged sella turcica and increased FSH secretion. Ann. Intern. Med., 63:313–316, 1965.

42. Gould, B. K., Randall, R. V., Kempers, R. D., et al.: Galactorrhea. Springfield, Ill., Charles C Thomas, 1974.

43. Hamilton, B. P. M., Upton, G. V., and Amatruda, T. T., Jr.: Evidence for the presence of neurophysin in tumors producing the syndrome of inappropriate antidiuresis. J. Clin. Endocr., 35:764–767, 1972.

44. Hamilton, C. R., Jr., and Maloof, F.: Acromegaly and toxic goiter. Cure of the hyperthyroidism and acromegaly by proton-beam partial hypophysectomy. J. Clin. Endocr., 35:659–664, 1972.

45. Hamilton, C. R., Jr., Adams, L. C., and Maloof, F.: Hyperthyroidism due to thyrotropin-producing pituitary chromophobe adenoma. New Eng. J. Med., 283:1077–1079, 1970.

46. Hanson, E. J., Jr., Miller, R. H., and Randall, R. V.: Suprasellar extension of tumor associated with increased cerebrospinal fluid activity of growth hormone. Mayo Clin. Proc., 51:412–416, 1976.

47. Hantman, D., Rossier, B., Zohlman, R., et al.: Rapid correction of hyponatremia in the syndrome of inappropriate secretion of antidiuretic hormone. Ann. Intern. Med., 78:870–875, 1973.

48. Hickey, R. C., and Hare, K.: The renal excretion of chloride and water in diabetes insipidus. J. Clin. Invest., 23:768–775, 1944.

49. Horn, K., Erdhart, F., Fahlbusch, R., et al.: Recurrent goiter, hyperthyroidism, galactorrhea and amenorrhea due to a thyrotropin and prolactin-producing pituitary tumor. J. Clin. Endocr., 43:137–143, 1976.

50. Jailer, J. W., and Holub, D. A.: Remission of Graves' disease following radiotherapy of a pituitary neoplasm. Amer. J. Med., 28:497–500, 1960.

51. Jeffcoate, W. J., Gilkes, J. J. H., Rees, L. H., et al.: The use of radioimmunoassays for human β-lipotropin. Endocrinology, 100:suppl.:215, 1977.

52. Jones, D. R., Bahn, R. C., Randall, R. V., et al.: The human costochondral junction. I. Patients without primary growth disturbance. Mayo Clin. Proc., 44:324–329, 1969.

53. Jones, D. R., Bahn, R. C., Randall, R. V., et al.: The human costochondral junction. II. Patients with acromegaly. Mayo Clin. Proc., 44:330–334, 1969.

54. Kelly, L. W.: Ovarian dwarfism with pituitary tumor. J. Clin. Endocr., 23:50–53, 1963.

55. Kernohan, J. W., and Sayre, G. P.: Tumors of the pituitary gland and infundibulum. In Atlas of Tumor Pathology, Section X, Fascicle 36. Armed Forces Institute of Pathology, 1956, pp. 60–76.

56. Kjellberg, R. N., and Kliman, B.: A system for therapy of pituitary tumors. In Kohler, P. O., and Ross, G. T., eds.: Diagnosis and Treatment of Pituitary Tumors. New York, American Elsevier Publishing Co, Inc, 1973, pp. 234–252.

57. Krieger, D. T., Amorosa, L., and Linick, F.: Cyproheptadine-induced remission of Cushing's disease. New Eng. J. Med., 293:893–896, 1975.

58. Labhart, A., ed.: Clinical Endocrinology. New York, Springer-Verlag, 1974.

59. Labhart, A.: The pluriglandular syndromes. In Labhart, A., ed.. Clinical Endocrinology. New York, Springer-Verlag, 1974, pp. 1007–1008.

60. Lamberg, B.-A., Ripatti, J., Gordin, A., et al.: Chromophobe pituitary adenoma with acromegaly and TSH-induced hyperthyroidism associated with parathyroid adenoma: Acromegaly and parathyroid adenoma. Acta Endocr. (Kobenhaon), 60:157–172, 1969.

61. Landolt, A. M.: Ultrastructure of human sella tumors: Correlations of clinical findings and morphology. Acta Neurochir. (Wien), suppl. 22, 1975.

62. Lawrence, J. H., Tobias, C. A., Linfoot, J. A., et al.: Heavy-particle therapy in acromegaly and Cushing disease. J.A.M.A. 235:2307–2310, 1976.

63. Leveston, S. A., Lee, Y.-C., Jaffe, B. M., et al.: Massive GH and ACTH hypersecretion associated with a metastatic carcinoid tumor. Endocrinology 102:suppl.:371, 1978.

64. Liberman, L. M., Beierwaltes, W. H., Conn, J. W., et al.: Diagnosis of adrenal disease by visualization of human adrenal glands with ^{131}I-19-iodocholesterol. New Eng. J. Med., 285:1387–1393, 1971.

65. Lindholm, J., Korsgaard, O., and Rasmussen, P.: Ectopic pituitary function. Acta Med. Scand., 198:299–302, 1975.

66. Linfoot, J. A., Garcia, J. F., Wei, W., et al.: Human growth hormone levels in cerebrospinal fluid. J. Clin. Endocr., 31:230–232, 1970.

67. Linquette, U., Herlant, U., Fossati, P., et al.: Adénome hypophysaire a cellules thyrotropes avec hyperthyroïdie. Ann. Endocr. (Paris), 30:731–740, 1969.

68. Locke, W., and Schally, A. V.: The Hypothalamus and Pituitary in Health and Disease.

Springfield, Ill., Charles C Thomas, 1972, pp. 11–12.

69. Luse, S. A., and Kernohan, J. W.: Squamous cell nests of pituitary gland. Cancer, *8*:623–628, 1955.

70. Magrini, G., Ebiner, J. R., Burchardt, P., and Felber, J. P.: Study on the relationship between plasma prolactin levels and androgen metabolism in man. J. Clin. Endocr., *43*:944–947, 1976.

71. Martin, J. B., Reichlin, S., and Brown, G. M.: Clinical Neuroendocrinology. Philadelphia, F. A. Davis, 1977.

72. Martini, L., and Besser, G. M., eds.: Clinical Neuroendocrinology. New York, Academic Press, 1978.

73. Martini, L., and Ganong, W. F., eds.: Neuroendocrinology. Vols. I and II. New York, Academic Press, 1966.

74. Martini, L., and Ganong, W. F., eds.: Frontiers in Neuroendocrinology, 1971. New York, Oxford University Press, 1971.

75. Martini, L., and Ganong, W. F., eds.: Frontiers in Neuroendocrinology. Vol. 4. New York, Raven Press, 1976.

76. McGregor, A. M., Scanton, M. F., Hall, K., et al.: Reduction in size of a pituitary tumor by bromocriptine therapy. New Eng. J. Med., *300*:291–293, 1979.

77. McKeel, D. W., Jr., and Jacobs, L. S.: Non-adenomatous pituitary mammotroph hyperplasia in patients with pathologic hyperprolactinemia. Endocrinology, *100*:suppl.:124, 1977.

78. McNatty, K. P., Sawyers, R. S., and McNeilly, A. S.: A possible role for prolactin in control of steroid secretion by the human Graafian follicle. Nature, *250*:653–654, 1974.

79. Melnyk, C. S., and Greer, M. A.: Functional pituitary tumor in an adult possibly secondary to long-standing myxedema. J. Clin. Endocr., *25*:761–766, 1965.

80. Miller, M., and Moses, A. M.: Drug-induced states of impaired water excretion. Kidney Int., *10*:96–103, 1976.

81. Mornex, R., Tommasi, M., Cure, M., et al.: Hyperthyroïdie associée à un hypopituitarisme au cours de l'évolution d'une tumeur hypophysaire sécrétant TSH. Ann. Endocr. (Paris), *33*:390–396, 1972.

82. Mortimer, C. H., Besser, G. M., McNeilly, A. S., et al.: Interaction between secretion of gonadotropins, prolactin, growth hormone, thyrotrophin and corticosteroids in man: the effects of LH/FSH-RH, TRH and hypoglycaemia alone and in combination. Clin. Endocr., *2*:317–326, 1973.

83. Moses, A. M.: Diabetes insipidus and ADH regulation. Hosp. Pract., *12*:37–44, 1977.

84. Moses, A. M., and Miller, M.: Osmotic influences on the release of vasopressin. *In* Greep, R. O., Astwood, E. B., Knobil, E., and Sawyer, W. H., eds.: Handbook of Physiology. Sec. 7, Vol. 4, The Pituitary Gland and Its Neuroendocrine Control, Part 1. Washington. American Physiological Society, 1974, pp. 225–242.

85. Moses, A. M., Miller, M., and Streeten, D. H. P.: Pathophysiologica and pharmaco-

logic alterations in the release and action of ADH. Metabolism, *25*:697–721, 1976.

86. Mudd, R. H., Dodge, H. W., Jr., Clark, E. C., et al.: Experimental diabetes insipidus: A study of the normal interphase. Mayo Clin. Proc., *32*:99–108, 1957.

87. Nelson, D. H., Meakin, J. W., Dealy, J. B., Jr., et al.: ACTH-producing tumor of the pituitary gland. New Eng. J. Med., *259*:161–164, 1958.

88. O'Donnel, J., Hadden, D. R., Weaver, J. A., et al.: Thyrotoxicosis recurring after surgical removal of a thyrotropin-secreting pituitary tumor. Proc. Roy. Soc. Med., *66*:441–442, 1973.

89. O'Duffy, J. D., Randall, R. V., and MacCarty, C. S.: Neuropathy (carpal-tunnel syndrome) in acromegaly: A sign of endocrine overactivity. Ann. Intern. Med., *78*:379–383, 1973.

90. Okerlund, M. D., and Greenspan, F. S.: Clinical studies of thyrotropin and thyrotropin-releasing-hormone. Pharmacol. Ther. B, *2*:79–94, 1977.

91. Page, R. B., and Bergland, R. M.: The neurohypophyseal capillary bed: 1. Anatomy and arterial supply. Amer. J. Anat., *148*:345–357, 1977.

92. Page, R. B., and Munger, B. L., and Bergland, R. M.: Scanning microscopy of pituitary vascular casts. Amer. J. Anat., *146*:273–301, 1976.

93. Phifer, R. F., Midgley, A. R., and Spicer, S. S.: Immunohistologic and histologic evidence that follicle-stimulating hormone and luteinizing hormone are present in the same cell type in the human pars distalis. J. Clin. Endocr., *36*:125–141, 1973.

94. Plummer, A. L., Randall, R. V., and Riggs, B. L.: Active acromegaly with anterior pituitary failure. Metabolism, *18*:469–475, 1969.

95. Powell, D. F., Baker, H. L., Jr., and Laws, E. R., Jr.: The primary angiographic findings in pituitary adenomas. Radiology, *110*:589–595, 1974.

96. Randall, R. V.: Acromegaly. *In* Conn, H. F., and Conn, R. B., eds.: Current Diagnosis 5. Philadelphia, W. B. Saunders Co., 1977, pp. 757–763.

97. Randall, R. V., Arnaud, C. D., Scholz, D. A., et al.: Hypercalcemia and acromegaly: Differential diagnosis using parathyroid hormone radioimmunoassay. Ric. Sci., *2*:suppl. 1:Abst. 92, 1975.

98. Randall, R. V., Clark, E. C., Dodge, H. W., Jr., et al.: Polyuria after operation for tumors in the region of the hypophysis and hypothalamus. J. Clin. Endocr. *20*:1614–1621, 1960.

99. Randall, R. V., Clark, E. C., Dodge, H. W., Jr., et al.: Diabetes insipidus: Current concepts in the production of antidiuretic hormone: Clinical and experimental observations (Exhibit). Postgrad. Med., *29*:97–107, 1961.

100. Redding, T. W., and Schally, A. V.: The purification of a growth hormone-releasing factor from porcine hypothalamic tissue. Endocrinology (suppl.), *100*:231, 1977.

101. Rees, L. H.: ACTH, lipotropin and MSH in health and disease. Clinics Endocr. Metab., *6*:137–153, 1977.

102. Reichlin, S., Baldessarini, R. J., and Martin, J.

B., eds.: The Hypothalamus. New York, Raven Press, 1978.

103. Reschini, E., Giustina, G., Cantalamessa, L., et al.: Hyperthyroidism with elevated plasma TSH levels and pituitary tumor: Study with somatostatin. J. Clin. Endocr., 43:924–927, 1976.

104. Rimoin, D. L.: Pachydermoperiostosis (idiopathic clubbing and periostosis): Genetic and physiologic considerations. New Eng. J. Med., 272:923–931, 1965.

105. Robinson, A. G.: DDAVP in the treatment of central diabetes insipidus. New Eng. J. Med., 294:507–511, 1976.

106. Robinson, A. G.: Neurophysins and their physiologic significance. Hosp. Pract., 12:57–63, 1977.

107. Robinson, A. G.: The neurophysins in health and disease. Clinics Endocr. Metab., 6:261–275, 1977.

108. Rovit, R. L., and Fein, J. M.: Pituitary apoplexy: A review and reappraisal. J. Neurosurg., 37:280–288, 1972.

109. Salassa, R. M., Kearns, T. P., Kernohan, J. W., et al.: Pituitary tumors in patients with Cushing's syndrome. J. Clin. Endocr. 19:1523–1539, 1959.

110. Salassa, R. M., Laws, E. R., Carpenter, P. C., et al.: Transsphenoidal removal of pituitary microadenoma in Cushing's disease. Mayo Clin. Proc., 53:24–28, 1977.

111. Sarkar, S. D., Beierwaltes, W. H., Ice, R. D., et al.: A new and superior adrenal scanning agent, NP-59. J. Nucl. Med., 16:1038–1042, 1975.

112. Schally, A. V., and Arimura, A.: Physiology and nature of hypothalamic regulatory hormones. In Martini, L., and Besser, G. M., eds.: Clinical Neuroendocrinology. New York, Academic Press, 1977, pp. 1–42.

112a. Schally, A. V., Arimura, A., Redding, T. W., et al.: Purification of corticotropin releasing factor from porcine hypothalamic. Endocrinology (suppl.), 100:95, 1977.

113. Scott, A. P., and Lowry, P. J.: Adrenocorticotropic and melanocyte-stimulating peptides in the human pituitary. Biochem. J., 139:593–602, 1974.

114. Shambaugh, G. E., III, Kubek, M., and Wilber, J. F.: Placenta: A newly identified source of thyrotropin-releasing hormone (TRH). Endocrinology, 100:suppl.:Abst T–24, 1977.

115. Shome, B., and Parlow, A. F.: Human pituitary prolactin (hPRL): The entire linear amino acid sequence. J. Clin. Endocr. Metab. 45:1112–1115, 1977.

116. Singer, I., and Rotenberg, D.: Demeclocycline-induced nephrogenic diabetes insipidus. Ann. Intern. Med., 79:679–683, 1973.

117. Sirek, A. M. T., Corenblum, B., Horvath, E., et al.: A new look at pituitary adenomas: Structure elucidating function. Can. Med. Asso. J., 114:225–229, 1976.

118. Snyder, P. J., and Sterling, F. H.: Hypersecretion of LH and FSH by a pituitary adenoma. J. Clin. Endocr., 43:544–550, 1976.

119. Sönksen, P. H., Ayres, A. B., Braimbridge, M., et al.: Acromegaly caused by pulmonary carcinoid tumors. Clin. Endocr. (Oxford), 5:503–513, 1976.

120. Symon, L., Ganz, J. C., and Burston, J.: Granular cell myoblastoma of the neurohypophysis. Report of two cases. J. Neurosurg., 35:82–89, 1971.

121. Tanay, A., Yust, I., Peresecenchi, G., et al.: Long-term treatment of the syndrome of inappropriate antidiuretic hormone secretion with phenytoin. Ann. Intern. Med., 90:50–52, 1979.

122. Thorner, M. O., Chait, A., Aitken, M., et al.: Bromocriptine treatment of acromegaly. Brit. Med. J., 1:299–303, 1975.

123. Thorner, M. O., McNeilly, A. S., Hagan, C., et al.: Long-term treatment of galactorrhea and hypogonadism with bromocriptine. Brit. Med. J., 2:419–422, 1974.

124. Tolis,-G., Bertrand, G., Carpenter, S., et al.: Acromegaly and galactorrhea-amenorrhea with two pituitary adenomas secreting growth hormone or prolactin. Ann. Intern. Med., 89:345–348, 1978.

125. Van Wyk, J. J., and Grumbach, M.: Syndrome of precocious menstruation and galactorrhea in juvenile hypothyroidism: An example of hormonal overlap in pituitary feedback. J. Pediat., 57:416–435, 1960.

126. Wass, J. A. H., Thorner, M. O., Charlesworth, M., et al.: Reduction of pituitary tumor size in patients with prolactinomas and acromegaly treated with bromocriptine with or without radiotherapy. Lancet, 2:66–69, 1979.

127. White, M. G., and Fetner, C. D.: Treatment of the syndrome of inappropriate secretion of antidiuretic hormone with lithium carbonate. New Eng. J. Med., 292:390–392, 1975.

128. Williams, R. H., ed.: Textbook of Endocrinology. 5th Ed. Philadelphia, W. B. Saunders, Co., 1974.

129. Woolf, P. D., and Schenk, E. A.: An FSH-producing pituitary tumor in a patient with hypogonadism. J. Clin. Endocr., 38:561–568, 1974.

130. Yen, S. S. C., Siler, T. M., and DeVane, G. W.: Effect of somatostatin in patients with acromegaly. New Eng. J. Med., 290:935–938, 1974.

131. Zafar, M. S., Mellinger, R. C., Fine, G., et al.: Acromegaly associated with a bronchial carcinoid tumor: Evidence for ectopic production of growth hormone-releasing activity. J. Clin. Endocr., 48:66–71, 1979.

132. Zimmerman, E. A., and Robinson, A. G.: Hypothalamic neurons secreting vasopressin and neurophysin. Kidney Int., 10:12–24, 1976.

133. Zusman, R. M., Keiser, H. R., and Handler, J. S.: A hypothesis for the molecular mechanism of action of chlorpropamide in the treatment of diabetes mellitus and diabetes insipidus. Fed. Proc., 36:2728–2729, 1977.

134. Zusman, R. M., Keiser, H. R., and Handler, J. S.: Vasopressin-stimulated prostaglandin E biosynthesis in the toad bladder. J. Clin. Invest., 60:1339–1347, 1977.

26

NUTRITION AND PARENTERAL THERAPY

The importance of maintaining body fluid homeostasis following trauma or operation has been emphasized for more than four decades. Kerpel-Fronius, in 1935, distinguished between the two "pure" types of dehydration, the first being due to water depletion alone, and the second resulting from the depletion of electrolytes.[22] Nadal, Pedersen, and Maddock and Marriott aided in the clinical differentiation of these two types of dehydration by defining the characteristic symptoms and physical findings of each.[26,32] The work of Moore and Ball in 1952 further elucidated the metabolic reactions occurring in response to trauma.[31] Even though physicians are now increasingly aware of the occurrence of metabolic, fluid, and electrolyte disturbances in the post-traumatic or postoperative period, occasions still arise when the clinical patterns or laboratory findings prove to be confusing, and this often results in failure to give the patient proper replacement therapy.

During the past 40 years a large body of evidence has been reported that indicates the metabolic response to head injury, cerebral disease, or cerebral operation is similar to that occurring after general body trauma, usually differing only in the degree of response. It has been established without question that cerebral areas are involved in body fluid and metabolic homeostasis.[55]

HISTORICAL BACKGROUND

Lewy and Gassman were among the earliest investigators to establish a relationship between central nervous system lesions and electrolyte and metabolic regulation.[24]

They found that unilateral stimulation and subsequent destruction of the paroptic ganglion of cats was followed by an increase of blood chlorides with a decrease in urinary chloride. There was no effect upon the blood sugar. They also noted that unilateral stimulation and subsequent destruction of the periventricular nucleus was associated with an increase of the blood sugar with no effect upon the blood chloride. Since that time numerous reports have been made noting the association of electrolyte and metabolic abnormalities occurring in patients with cerebral lesions.

Allott was the first to associate cerebral lesions with hypernatremia and hyperchloremia in the absence of renal disease.[1] He reported five cases in which hypernatremia, hyperchloremia, and azotemia occurred with decreased urinary excretion of sodium and chloride. Three of his patients had ruptured aneurysms of the anterior cerebral artery, one a recent cerebral infarct, and the other a tumor of the choroid plexus.

Sweet and his colleagues found gastrointestinal hemorrhages, hyperglycemia, azotemia, hyperchloremia, and hypernatremia following lesions of the frontal lobe in humans.[48] They presented data on four patients and suggested that these changes occurred with lesions confined to the anterior portion of the frontal lobes. Wolfman and Schoch reported the case of a patient with closed head trauma and midbrain injury who developed hypernatremia, hyperchloremia, azotemia, and hypochloruria.[53] They felt this most likely resulted from water depletion in a comatose patient. MacCarty and Cooper also found hypernatremia, hyperchloremia, hypochloruria, ure-

E. F. WOLFMAN, JR., AND R. E. HODGES

mia, and moderate hypopotassemia in a patient in whom both anterior cerebral arteries were ligated proximal to the site of the anterior communicating artery during the removal of a pituitary adenoma.[25] These authors reported upon two additional cases that same year and suggested that cerebral dysfunction concerned with the control of water balance might be responsible for their findings.[7]

Cooper and Crevier, in 1952, reviewed 14 cases of marked hypernatremia or hyperchloremia or both associated with cerebral lesions and added four additional cases.[6] Although they did not elucidate upon the mechanisms involved, they suggested they were neurogenic in origin and perhaps caused by damage to cerebral osmoreceptor mechanisms. They further noted that the cerebral lesions associated with these disturbances usually involved the frontal lobes or hypothalamus.

Simultaneous with the aforementioned documentation of hypertonicity of the extracellular fluid, other reports of "cerebral salt-wasting" were being presented. Peters and associates, in 1950, described three cases of excessive sodium excretion in the presence of hyponatremia.[37] The cerebral lesions associated with these disturbances were encephalitis, stroke, and bulbar poliomyelitis. Cort, in 1954, described similar findings in a patient with a glioma of the thalamus.[9]

In addition to the marked derangement of the extracellular electrolytes that occurred in association with cerebral lesions, like disturbances were found in protein and carbohydrate metabolism. The work of Lewy and Gassman established experimentally a relationship between the brain and glucose metabolism.[24] Sweet and his associates found a severe hyperglycemia without acetonuria occurring in a patient 15 days following bilateral frontal lobotomy.[48] Wolfman and Schoch further noted urinary nitrogen excretions ranging between 27 and 34 gm per 24 hours in their patient with a midbrain injury.[53]

These basic reports served to call attention to a relationship between the central nervous system and body fluid, electrolyte, and metabolic homeostasis and to alert the clinician to severe derangements that may occur in association with operation, trauma, or disease of the brain.

METABOLIC RESPONSE TO CRANIOCEREBRAL TRAUMA

McLaurin and co-workers and Wise, as well as others, have well documented the metabolic changes occurring in patients with craniocerebral injury and have found that in general these changes are similar to those occurring in patients responding to general body trauma or operation.[28,29,52] The metabolic response to trauma or operation includes the following:

1. Increased body protein losses and urine nitrogen excretion.
2. Increased urinary excretion of potassium.
3. Increase in blood sugar.
4. Decreased urinary excretion and decreased serum concentration of sodium and chloride.
5. Decreased body weight.
6. Decreased renal excretion of water.

It has long been assumed that the increased output of adrenal steroids (17-hydroxycorticosteroids and aldosterone) occurring in response to the stress of operation or trauma is responsible for these electrolyte, carbohydrate, and protein metabolic changes. Antidiuresis has been attributed to pain, emotion, and anesthesia producing central stimulation leading to an increased output of antidiuretic hormone.

Sodium

Sodium retention usually begins on the day of operation or injury and lasts between two and four days. The degree of sodium retention may range from minimal to maximal and is related to a number of factors: the status of the functional or circulating extracellular fluid volume before injury or operation, increased output of adrenal cortical steroid hormones, and the area of the brain injured.

Although decreased renal excretion of sodium is a well-known feature of the postoperative and post-traumatic state, the mechanisms responsible for this retention have not yet been clearly defined. There is evidence that the changes in sodium excretion observed under these circumstances can occur *independently* of variation in the supply of adrenal cortical hormones. In normal individuals the renal excretion of sodium is directly related to the functional or circulating extracellular fluid volume.[44,46] Sodium retention that occurs postoperatively also relates directly to a diminution of the effective extracellular fluid volume.[43] Randall and Papper have offered further evidence that the postoperative and post-traumatic retention of sodium is due to a contraction of the circulating extracellular fluid volume, rather than to an augmented output of adrenal cortical steroids.[38] These workers, studying healthy young males before and after major orthopedic procedures, found that the usual postoperative sodium and chloride retention could be prevented if extracellular fluid losses were restored.

There is now experimental evidence that sodium retention can be due to a cerebral lesion per se. Because of the earlier findings of hypernatremia occurring in patients with lesions of the frontal lobes or hypothalamus, Wolfman and co-workers have studied the correlation of retention of sodium and chloride, edema of the contralateral leg, and a negative nitrogen balance with a destructive lesion in the precommissural septum.[55] When the precommissural septum was spared, no metabolic derangements were detected.

On the basis of balance studies of humans and experimental animals subjected to craniocerebral injury or operation, the following conclusions may be reached:

1. Sodium retention does occur in most patients for two to three days, is followed by diuresis and then equilibrium.

2. During this phase of sodium retention the serum sodium tends, paradoxically, to decrease, probably owing to water retention.

3. The magnitude of retention is related to both the degree of trauma and the area of the brain injured, i.e., the precommissural septum or its connections.[27,55]

Potassium

Immediately following cerebral operations or trauma, negative potassium balances are common for one or two days, but seldom of enough magnitude to assume clinical significance. It is, therefore, seldom necessary to administer potassium under these circumstances unless extrarenal losses, i.e., diarrhea or vomiting, are occurring. A serum potassium level of less than 3.5 mEq. per liter indicates an extracellular potassium deficit. It should be remembered that serum potassium levels can be misleading and a deficit of total body potassium can be present despite normal serum concentrations of this ion. This can occur when acidosis is present and a shift of potassium occurs from the cells into the circulating extracellular fluid. Under these circumstances the serum potassium concentration may be found to be normal or high, associated with decreased total body potassium. Alkalosis, on the other hand, is associated with a movement of potassium from the extracellular compartment into the cells, resulting in a hypokalemia without loss of potassium from the body. The electrocardiogram is more accurate in detecting serum potassium abnormalities than are serum levels. Low flat T waves, prolonged Q-T intervals, and a depressed RS-T segment are characteristic of hypokalemia. In contrast, hyperkalemia is indicated by tall peaked T waves, absence of P waves, aberrant QRS complexes, and an idioventricular rhythm. Potassium intoxication is most often seen with the cerebral salt-losing syndrome, diabetic coma, or acute renal insufficiency.

Nitrogen

Nitrogen losses are a common accompaniment of craniocerebral trauma, operation, or disease and have been considered to result from a response to stress. Recently, James and co-workers have questioned whether protein catabolism is the process that changes primarily in stress, and suggested that a fall in protein synthesis may be more important.[21] O'Keefe and associates investigated this thesis by infusing ^{14}C-leucine to measure the synthesis and breakdown roles of body protein before and after abdominal operations in four patients.[34] They found that the postoperative loss of nitrogen was associated with a consistent decrease in protein synthesis. Their results suggest that the previously described catabolic response to operation and trauma may be due to a decrease in protein synthesis rather than to an acute increase in body protein breakdown. The usual losses in the neurosurgical patient are similar to those following other major general operative procedures, approximately 10 gm per day, and this catabolic condition lasts from 7 to 10 days. Patients, after cerebral injury or cerebral operations, however, are apt to excrete massive amounts of urinary nitrogen in a manner closely paralleling that of burn patients. The excretion of up to 34 gm of nitrogen per day has been reported and this amounts to an endogenous body protein breakdown or failure of synthesis of over 200 gm per day.[53] The situations under which this degree of negative nitrogen balance occurs do not relate directly to the degree of trauma sustained, but are related more to the specific areas of the brain involved. This is confirmed by experiments of Wolfman and associates in which monkeys were subjected first to unilateral and then bilateral destruction of the precommissural septum without hemispherectomy.[56] Sodium and chloride retention and negative nitrogen balances again occurred even though this operation was traumatically a much less extensive operation than hemispherectomy.

Although there is no evidence that the usual period and degree of negative nitrogen balance jeopardizes the patient's postoperative convalescence, it would seem wise to attempt to minimize the effects of massive body protein loss, i.e., in excess of 100 gm of body protein per day. The catabolism of large quantities of body protein delivers to the kidneys excessive amounts of urea for excretion. The resultant osmotic diuresis, forced diuresis caused by the osmotic attraction for water of the large quantities of urea being excreted, may produce marked losses of body water. Administration of a high protein diet (1.5 to 2.0 gm protein per kilogram body weight per day) combined with enough calories to meet metabolic demands (2000 to 2500 calories per day) will reduce the negativity of the nitrogen balance sustained and may even produce a positive nitrogen balance.[40]

In summary, negative nitrogen balance is seldom prolonged or excessive, and usually no attempts are necessary to minimize or reverse these losses in the usual neurosurgical patient. One must always be alert for massive losses or situations characterized by chronic negative nitrogen balance (paraplegia). In these latter instances a high protein, high caloric diet, and anabolic steroids may be required to avoid complications.

Water

The response of the neurosurgical patient subjected to craniotomy or craniocerebral trauma is not unlike that of other surgical patients in regard to postoperative water retention. The usual response is that of retaining water for 12 to 36 hours following craniotomy and perhaps somewhat longer following cranial trauma.[27,58] The response in each instance is presumably caused by the release of antidiuretic hormone from the posterior lobe of the pituitary gland after activation of the supraopticohypophyseal tract. McLaurin found that water retention does occur and that it closely coincides with the period of sodium retention, but different mechanisms are responsible for each.[27] He noted a lack of dependency of water retention on salt metabolism because water balance statistically correlated with sodium balance only on the third postoperative day. Oliguria does not occur if diabetes insipidus is produced by a lesion of the pituitary, the infundibulum, or the supraoptic nucleus of the hypothalamus.

Hormones

The hormonal response of patients to brain injury or operation is also similar to that in other surgical patients. Following injury or operation, the pituitary secretes increased amounts of adrenocorticotropic hormone, which acts upon the adrenal glands to increase their output of the adrenal steroid hormones. Of these, the 11-oxy-17-hydroxycorticosterone known also as cortisol, compound F, or hydrocortisone, is produced in greatest amounts. This hormone is largely responsible for the increased nitrogen excretion, decreased glucose tolerance, and alteration in the formed elements of the blood (decreased lymphocytes, decreased eosinophiles) and involution of lymphoid tissue. It has only a moderate effect on the postoperative retention of sodium and excretion of potassium. Aldosterone, the most potent of the adrenal mineral corticoids, is produced in smaller quantities and is probably primarily responsible for the postoperative electrolyte changes previously mentioned. There is some evidence to suggest that aldosterone cannot account for *all* these changes. For example, postoperative sodium retention has been reported in patients with Addison's disease who have undergone subsequent operations while receiving constant dosages of steroids.[38] There is little question that aldosterone is intimately involved in the regulation of the extracellular fluid volume. Barrter has demonstrated that aldosterone secretion decreased if the extracellular fluid volume was increased, regardless of the associated intracellular volume changes, and increased with a contraction of the extracellular fluid volume.[2] Some evidence exists that suggests aldosterone secretion is under the control of volume receptors in the afferent renal arterioles, which respond to changes in the renal arterial pressure and blood flow.[11] A decreased renal arterial blood pressure or flow has been found to increase the release of renin from the juxtaglomerular cells, causing the formation of angiotensin II, and this substance stimulates the secretion of aldosterone by the adrenal glands. Similarly, an increase in pressure results in a decreased secretion of aldosterone. Probably none of the metabolic responses to operation are regulated entirely by hormones, but rather these substances serve as catalysts to the metabolic and other phenomena occurring.

FLUID AND ELECTROLYTE DERANGEMENTS IN THE NEUROSURGICAL PATIENT

The metabolic responses to cerebral injury and operation are usually unnoticed and most often are of little clinical significance. There are, however, instances in which marked derangements occur and must be recognized and treated if severe sequelae are to be avoided. Often these metabolic abnormalities are of a temporary nature, and if fluid and electrolyte homeostasis can be maintained during the acute phase, the patient will subsequently recover. The electrolyte aberrations encountered can be classified simply as hypertonicity or hypotonicity of the extracellular fluid (Table 26–1).

Hypertonicity of the Extracellular Fluid

Severe hypertonicity of the extracellular fluid has often been observed in patients with cerebral lesions.* Although the etiological mechanisms are largely unknown, enough information is available to permit treatment of these patients in a rational manner. The degree of hypertonicity of the extracellular fluid reported in patients with cerebral lesions has seldom been noted in those without cerebral disease. Most of the reported cases of hypernatremia and hyperchloremia, with or without azotemia, hyperglycemia, and hypokalemia, have had lesions either in the frontal lobes or in the hypothalamus or both.[1,6,7,19,25,35,48,53,57] There are no available data to indicate the frequency of hypertonicity occurring in as-

* See references 1, 5–7, 13, 17, 19, 25, 33, 35, 48, 49, 53, 54, 57.

TABLE 26–1 DIFFERENTIAL DIAGNOSIS OF HYPERTONIC EXTRACELLULAR FLUID

	COMA PER SE		DIABETES INSIPIDUS WITH THIRST LOSS OR COMA		"OSMOREGULATORY" DEFECT	
	Early	Late	Early	Late	Early	Late
24-hour urine volume	Oliguric	Increased	Increased	Increased	Normal	Oliguric to increased
Urine specific gravity	Increased	Increased	Decreased	Decreased	Decreased to normal	May be increased
Urine osmolality	Increased	Increased	Decreased	Decreased	Decreased to normal	May be increased
Urinary NaCl	Normal to increased	Decreased to absent	Normal	Normal	Decreased to normal	Normal to increased
Dry mouth and membranes	Present	Severe	Present	Severe	Absent	Minimal
Blood pressure	Normal	Hypotension	Normal to mild hyper-tension	Shock	Normal	Normal
Proper treatment	Water	Water	Water and Pitressin	Water and Pitressin	Water	Water

sociation with cerebral disease, but it has most usually been encountered under the following circumstances: (1) after closed head injury with midbrain involvement; (2) after removal of a craniopharyngioma or a chromophobic adenoma of the pituitary gland; and (3) after rupture of an aneurysm of the anterior cerebral artery.[54]

Since awareness of the potential for this complication to develop is essential to early diagnosis in all the foregoing clinical situations, serum electrolytes should be determined routinely after trauma or an operation. Measurement of the 24-hour fluid intake and urine output is also mandatory. In this manner the onset of the metabolic abnormality can be detected and corrective measures instituted early. The hyperosmolal or hypertonic condition has been observed most often in the following three groups of patients: the comatose patient per se; the patient with diabetes insipidus and coma or the patient with diabetes insipidus and the concomitant loss of the sensation of thirst; and the patient with "osmoregulatory" defects.

The Comatose Patient Per Se

Coma may result from trauma or operation. It is usually necessary to maintain these patients on parenteral fluids for prolonged periods, and many clinicians prefer to limit the quantity of fluids administered to minimize the possibility of producing cerebral edema. In normal subjects, complete fluid restriction does not result in hypertonicity of the extracellular fluid. Nadal and co-workers withheld all fluids from a normal subject for four days without producing significant extracellular fluid hypertonicity.[32] Thirst, however, became marked, and this necessitated the administration of oral fluids.

There are several reasons why the comatose patient is more likely to develop a hyperosmolal extracellular fluid than normal persons. First, since he is unable to express the thirst of which he would complain if conscious, water deficits can progress to more advanced stages without recognition than in patients with an intact thirst mechanism. The thirst mechanism is presumably actuated by losses of intracellular and extracellular fluid and not by the degree of hypertonicity of the extracellular fluid itself.[47]

The regulation of the tonicity of the extracellular fluid, in the early stages of water depletion, is dependent upon two physiological processes: renal excretion of sodium and chloride ions equivalent to the deficit of body water, and maximal water reabsorption. As water deprivation continues, the kidneys, presumably under the influence of antidiuretic hormone, continue to reabsorb water. In addition, sodium and chloride ions are reabsorbed, and the urine is concentrated maximally in a compensatory attempt to prevent further depletion of the volume of extracellular fluid. Since obligatory water losses continue in the absence of an adequate intake of water, and since reabsorption of sodium and chloride ions is maximal under these circumstances, the extracellular fluid becomes hypertonic. The comatose patient, unable to express thirst, may progress to the late stages of dehydration before the disproportion between fluid intake and output is recognized. Second, patients with cerebral damage may excrete massive amounts of urinary nitrogen. Such quantities of urinary nitrogen, excreted largely as urea, produce an osmolal diuresis, increasing obligatory urinary water losses. Third, some patients, i.e., those with midbrain damage, lose control of the mechanisms regulating body temperature. Consequently, marked elevations in body temperature result in large losses of body water. Finally, with midbrain damage, hyperpnea, with or without polypnea, is commonly seen and serves to greatly increase the quantity of water vaporized from the lungs. Therefore, since water requirements may be increased in comatose patients, dehydration and associated hyperosmolality of the extracellular fluid may develop rapidly if adequate quantities of water are not given.

Many comatose patients excrete large urinary volumes, frequently as high as 3000 ml daily.[53] Regardless of the volume of urine excreted, however, if the extracellular fluid is hypertonic, the urine specific gravity or osmolality will be high unless diabetes insipidus or chronic renal disease is present. Excretion of a large volume of highly concentrated urine does not indicate adequate body hydration, but merely represents the least urinary volume in which the contained solute load can be excreted—obligatory losses.

Since the hypernatremia occurring under

these circumstances is due to a primary water depletion, the early physical examination of the patient reveals little in the way of positive findings. The greatest absolute water losses are sustained from the intracellular compartment (70 per cent) and only about 7 per cent of the total losses are derived from the plasma volume. Consequently, the physical findings are minimal early and the diagnosis is best confirmed by detecting serum hypertonicity and the high urinary specific gravity or osmolality. As the body water deficit increases, dryness of the mouth, tongue, and mucous membranes will be present. In more advanced stages, hypotension may result from the reduction in total circulatory blood volume (Table 26-1).

Proper therapy will correct the dehydration, and the quantities of fluid necessary to achieve this are determined by correlating the urinary specific gravity or osmolal concentration with the amount of fluid administered. When water balance is re-established, concentrations of the serum electrolytes will decrease and the urine will become more dilute. Patients who are extremely dehydrated, with associated hyperpyrexia or large obligatory urinary losses, frequently require 4000 to 6000 ml of water daily. Water may be administered intravenously as 5 per cent dextrose in water, but cerebral edema is less likely to occur if it is given slowly into the gastrointestinal tract via a small caliber nasogastric tube.

The ideal fluid for replacement not only supplies adequate quantities of water but also contains enough calories to minimize endogenous protein catabolism, thus reducing the associated osmolal diuresis. For this reason, intravenous solutions of 10 per cent glucose given slowly serve well. If replacement therapy is to be given by way of the intestinal tract, many commercial formulas are available. Many of the commercial formulas cause diarrhea; Youmans has suggested one that seldom does.[59] It is a blended mixture of the regular hospital diet of the day. The low incidence of diarrhea and other complications probably is due to the fact that the gastrointestinal tract is accustomed to this diet. In preparing the blended diet, only the bones and decorations are removed. The remainder is pulverized in a blender. Enough water is added to increase breakfast to 400 ml, lunch to

1000 ml, and dinner to 1000 ml. The tube feeding is begun in small amounts, 10 to 30 ml each two hours as the intravenous fluids are decreased. Ten milliliters of water is injected in one quick bolus after each feeding. This method is used to clear the feeding tube. Gradually the feeding is increased until 200 ml is given each two hours throughout the day and night. It is important to give the feeding in 200 ml boluses rather than larger doses that may distend the stomach and increase the probability of regurgitation and aspiration of the gastric contents. Experience has shown that if the patient develops diarrhea on this diet, one of the more likely causes is an unauthorized change in the diet by the personnel in the kitchen. In order to decrease the work of blending the diet, such items as milk, raw eggs, or emulsified fat have been substituted for the regular hospital diet. A check with the kitchen personnel can identify and remedy the problem.

A patient receiving nasogastric tube feeding requires the addition of sodium chloride in the same amount as a normal patient. The diet kitchen personnel must be kept informed of this need. Periodic checks of the serum electrolytes are necessary to insure that adequate sodium and potassium are included in the diet. Additional discussion of nasogastric and gastrotomy feedings is given in Chapter 77.

As the accumulated water deficit is being corrected, replacement of electrolytes may also be required since, in the early stages of water depletion, electrolytes have been excreted by the kidneys in a compensatory attempt to maintain isotonicity of the extracellular fluid.[36] Later, even though the extracellular fluid is hypertonic, the total body quantities of sodium and chloride are reduced. The quantity of electrolytes that must be replaced can be estimated by determining the serum electrolyte concentrations and correlating these values with the urinary excretion of the same ions; a persistently positive sodium or chloride balance occurring while the serum levels of these electrolytes are decreasing indicates the need for larger quantities to be administered.

Interestingly, the clinical condition of patients who have been presumed to have hopeless cerebral damage frequently improves with correction of the dehydration and return of the concentrations of the extracellular electrolytes to normal.

Diabetes Insipidus Associated with Loss of Thirst Sensation or Coma

Patients with diabetes insipidus excrete large urinary volumes of low specific gravity or osmolality. These individuals usually do not become dehydrated because the thirst mechanism, actuated by intracellular and extracellular fluid losses, serves as a compensatory device.[47] If, however, because of cerebral injury, the sensation of thirst is not present or the patient is comatose and unable to express thirst, dehydration may occur within 24 to 48 hours unless an adequate amount of exogenous water is supplied. If the necessary supplies of water are lacking, the extracellular fluid becomes concentrated; severe hypertonicity develops more rapidly in this type of patient than in the comatose patient per se who is still able to concentrate urine.

In patients with diabetes insipidus, the osmolality of the urine is usually less than that of the serum. Examination of the mouth shows dryness of the mucous membranes. If the patient is conscious, dysphagia may be present. A 2- to 5-pound loss of body weight may occur in a 24-hour period of time. Occasionally, increasing lethargy or coma in a previously conscious patient results from hypertonicity of the extracellular fluid. Later, sudden circulatory collapse and profound shock may follow a gradual but marked decrease in the total circulating blood volume. Unless appropriate therapeutic measures are immediately undertaken, most of these patients die in ''irreversible shock.''

Appropriate management of these cases is contingent upon early recognition of this abnormality and correction of the fluid deficits. Since there is insufficient antidiuretic hormonal activity, administration of vasopressin (Pitressin) will prevent the large losses of body fluid that might otherwise occur. Vasopressin may be given either intramuscularly or intravenously. The most commonly used preparation is Pitressin tannate in oil, which is administered intramuscularly. The amount of this drug required and the frequency with which it is administered varies with each patient. It must be given cautiously, and the patient's response carefully evaluated. The average duration of action of Pitressin tannate in oil is 48 hours. If the patient is highly sensitive to Pitressin, or if it is given too frequently or in excessive amounts, water intoxication may occur. Fluids must be given cautiously after Pitressin therapy has been instituted, and the specific gravity, or osmolality, and volume of the urine should be determined daily. If the urinary specific gravity rises and then returns to low levels, more Pitressin must be given. Contrariwise, if oliguria occurs, fluid administration should be limited so that excessive retention of fluid and subsequent water intoxication do not occur.

In the later stages of dehydration, if shock occurs, fluids must be given rapidly to restore the circulating blood volume. If the administered fluids are to be retained, then Pitressin must also be given. Under these circumstances intravenous aqueous Pitressin is preferred, since its action is immediate and of short duration, and cumulation of the drug will not occur. If Pitressin tannate in oil is administered to a hypotensive patient, absorption occurs slowly and usually only after large quantities of fluid have been given. Consequently, significant water retention may occur 24 to 48 hours later and cause water intoxication. Once hypotension has been corrected and the extracellular fluid volume restored, periodic intramuscular Pitressin tannate in oil serves well for maintenance.

The type and quantity of solutions to be replaced are similar to those recommended for the comatose patient per se. If the patient is conscious, oral administration is preferred. If the patient is comatose, replacement may be given enterally via a nasogastric tube of small caliber. If more than 4000 or 5000 ml of fluid must be administered daily, the intravenous route should also be used to prevent troublesome diarrhea. By titrating the dosage of Pitressin with the volume of fluid given, it is possible to correct the deficits of body fluid. With proper titration of Pitressin and intravenous and oral fluid, the patient should excrete a 24-hour urinary volume of 1000 to 1500 ml; this urine should have a specific gravity of approximately 1.010 to 1.015.

Patients with "Osmoregulatory" Defects

Although there is no conclusive evidence to indicate the presence of osmoreceptors in the human diencephalon, Verney has presented indirect evidence that favors the presence of osmoreceptors in that portion of the dog brain supplied by the internal carotid arteries.[50] If osmoreceptors do exist in human beings, they should respond to small deviations in the concentration of the extracellular electrolytes. Presumably, increases in the tonicity of the extracellular fluid may normally be prevented by an osmoregulatory response to small increases in the concentration of the extracellular electrolytes. This response may be manifested by either an increased renal excretion of sodium and chloride ions or an inhibition of urine flow or both. If a defect in osmoregulatory function exists, then relatively small deficits of body water could cause hypertonicity of the extracellular fluid, since compensatory urinary losses of sodium and chloride would not occur or because antidiuresis does not result. It is possible, then, that the severe hypertonicity of the extracellular fluid that is observed in certain patients with cerebral damage is related to a disturbance of some osmoregulatory system that is operative in individuals without cerebral disorders. Such a thesis would explain those cases of extreme extracellular fluid hypertonicity occurring in the absence of clinical signs of dehydration.[6]

The development of hyperosmolality of the extracellular fluid in association with an inadequate supply of water may occur even more rapidly in individuals with postulated osmoregulatory defects than in persons in the other two groups. Since minor deficits of water remain uncompensated, hypernatremia or hyperchloremia or both may develop within 48 hours after injury or operation.

Osmoregulatory defects should be suspected in patients who fail to regain consciousness after head injury or cerebral operation, even though other more common causes exist. The diagnosis can be made by determining the serum electrolyte values and correlating them with urinary concentration. A low urinary osmolality or specific gravity associated with hypertonicity of the extracellular fluid is highly suggestive. For reasons yet unexplained, hyperchloremia usually precedes the hypernatremia. In the early stages of development of this pattern, urinary volumes appear adequate, usually ranging from 1000 to 5000 ml daily; urinary specific gravity is low. Later, after the serum becomes more hypertonic, the urine becomes more concentrated; it is not uncommon to find the specific gravity to be 1.020 to 1.035 or the osmolality to exceed 1200 mOsm per liter. In some instances it appears that osmoregulatory response to *moderate changes* in serum osmolality is impaired; when osmolal changes in the serum become great enough, some compensatory response occurs.

Treatment is aimed at correcting the fluid deficits and establishing a positive water balance. The amount of fluid required varies, but approximately 3000 ml daily is sufficient if adequate calories are given to lessen endogenous catabolism of nitrogen and subsequent osmolar diuresis. The fluids may be given either orally as a liquid formula or intravenously in the form of 10 per cent glucose or invert sugar. Again, serum electrolyte levels and urinary concentration serve as a guide to the quantity of fluid required. Once water balance has been established, a progressive fall in the serum electrolyte and urinary concentrations will be noted. To avoid cerebral edema one should attempt to lower the serum electrolyte concentrations gradually over an interval of several days rather than attempting to correct the entire water deficit in a 24-hour period. Concomitant with a return of the serum electrolytes to normal values, improvement in the patient's clinical condition usually occurs.

Hypotonicity of the Extracellular Fluid

Hyponatremia, hypochloremia, hyperchloruria, and hypernatruria may also be seen in association with cerebral disease, injury, or operation, but less commonly than the hypertonic state. Hyponatremia may result from excessive loss of sodium from the body, an excessive or abnormal retention of body water, the overadministration of electrolyte-free solutions, and any combination of these factors.

Excessive Loss of Body Sodium

Any patient who has been on prolonged diuretic therapy or sodium restriction may have serious depletion of the total body sodium and would be especially susceptible to postoperative hypotonicity of the extracellular fluid. Patients with liver disease or adrenal insufficiency may likewise become hypotonic.

Excessive Retention of Body Water

Peters and co-workers observed a number of patients with cerebral hyponatremia.[37] They identified this entity as cerebral salt-wasting and postulated that the brain lesion decreased the renal tubular reabsorption of sodium either indirectly by depressing adrenocortical function or directly by way of the renal nerves. Welt and associates, in 1952, reported two additional cases and, since these patients excreted large amounts of potassium when given desoxycorticosterone acetate, concluded the salt wastage was due to the impaired proximal renal tubular reabsorption of sodium.[51] In 1954 Cort described a patient with a glioma of the thalamus with hyponatremia.[9] In 1957, Schwartz's group found hyponatremia in two patients with carcinoma of the bronchus that was unlike that due to sodium depletion, since large volumes of intravenous hypertonic saline produced only transient elevations of the plasma protein.[42] Furthermore, in both cases the urine remained persistently hypertonic to the plasma, suggesting an excessive secretion of antidiuretic hormone. Since there was no evidence of adrenal or renal disease, it was assumed that the hyponatremia resulted from an excessive retention of water induced by the hypersecretion of antidiuretic hormone. The term "inappropriate secretion" was used to indicate that the hormone was secreted despite hyponatremia and the lack of any known stimulus to the neurohypophysis. Carter and co-workers performed balance studies on two patients with cerebral hyponatremia.[4] One of these had a metastatic brain carcinoma and the other a basilar skull fracture. They found that in each instance the hyponatremia resulted from water retention rather than from significant salt wastage. Their studies suggested that the water retention resulted from a persistently high secretion of antidiuretic hormone, but the manner in which the cerebral injury produced this result was not determined. Initially in both patients the secretion of antidiuretic hormone appeared to be autonomous of both osmotic and volume control. In one of their patients the secretion of antidiuretic hormone in the later stages appeared to be under the control of extracellular volume, but remained independent of plasma osmolality. It has been postulated also that the expanded extracellular fluid volume causes increased sodium excretion by inhibiting aldosterone secretion and increasing the glomerular filtration rate. Today the syndrome of inappropriate secretion of antidiuretic hormone is a well-documented sequela of head injury.[10]

Overadministration of Electrolyte-Free Solutions

Probably the most common cause of hyponatremia in the neurosurgical patient is the injudicious administration of glucose solutions in the immediate postoperative or post-traumatic period. Water intoxication results when the hyponatremia is marked enough to produce clinical symptoms. Postoperative hyponatremia is a well-known sequela following other major surgical procedures. It is particularly important to recognize hyponatremia in neurosurgical patients because the signs and symptoms closely mimic those of postoperative intracranial hemorrhage or other complications. Furthermore, hyponatremia postoperatively produces cerebral edema and increased intracranial pressure. Since water diffuses freely across the capillary and cell membranes, most of any excess water administered becomes intracellular and, consequently, water intoxication is due to intracellular water rather than to any measurable changes in extracellular electrolytes.

The signs and symptoms of hypotonicity of the extracellular fluid vary, depending upon its cause, the rate with which it develops, and whether or not there is associated intracerebral disease or injury. If total body sodium depletion is contributory to the hyponatremia, there will be a more marked associated decrease in the circulating blood volume. Under these circumstances symptoms of hypovolemia such as tachycardia, weakness, decreased peripheral venous filling, peripheral vasoconstriction, oliguria, and hypotension will be present. The severity of the symptoms relates directly to the extent of the hypovolemia produced by the salt deficit. The most common type of hyponatremia occurring in the neurosurgical patient is dilutional with only minor electrolyte deficits and, depending upon its severity, produces the symptom complex referred to as water intoxication. The more rapidly the serum electrolyte concentration is lowered, the more severe the symptoms. The brain is most sensitive to osmolal changes while the blood-brain barrier is slowly permeable to sodium. Consequently, with rapid decreases in the extracellular fluid tonicity due to overhydration, the brain imbibes water because it contains a relative excess of sodium, and this produces cerebral swelling. The cerebral swelling is responsible for the neurological symptoms produced. These vary from subtle manifestations of apprehension, restlessness, depression, and irritability to confusion, disorientation, delirium, seizures, lethargy, coma, and death. Objective findings include serum hypotonicity, elevated cerebrospinal fluid pressure, and decreased voltage and frequency of electroencephalographic activity. Symptoms seldom appear until the serum sodium concentration is less than 128 to 130 mEq per liter. Since the symptoms produced by hyponatremia are not distinguishable from those due to intracranial hematoma, serum sodium concentration and serum osmolality should be determined before re-exploration of suspected postoperative intracranial hemorrhage.

Treatment of hypotonicity depends upon its cause. Since the surgeon may confuse the symptoms with postoperative or post-traumatic complications, all measures should be employed to prevent the development of hypotonicity. This may be done in most circumstances by the intravenous administration of only sufficient 5 per cent glucose, after injury or operation, to provide for an adequate urinary volume. In general, 1500 ml of 5 per cent glucose will suffice to cover insensible losses and water of vaporization and to provide enough urine to clear metabolic wastes from the body. The urine specific gravity should be monitored simultaneously and, in a glucose-free, protein-free, 24-hour urine sample, should be kept in the 1.015 to 1.020 range. If water intoxication does occur, one can raise the tonicity of the extracellular fluid by either the addition of electrolytes or the restriction and removal of water. Not all hyponatremic states require aggressive treatment, and the use of hypertonic salt solutions should be reserved for those situations in which central nervous system signs are present. A patient in whom a hyponatremia is found by examination of the serum sodium should be treated by water restriction and isotonic electrolyte administration if electrolyte replacement is important (i.e., if total body sodium is reduced).

When central nervous system signs are present, immediate treatment with hypertonic salt solutions is indicated. The type of solution employed depends upon the acid-base balance of the patient. Disturbances in acid-base balance are best diagnosed by determining both the serum bicarbonate level and the serum pH. If neither acidosis nor alkalosis is present, therapy can be initiated by the intravenous administration of 500 ml of a solution containing 250 ml of ⅓ molar sodium lactate and 250 ml of 3 per cent sodium chloride. If acidosis is present, 500 ml of ⅓ molar sodium lactate should be given. Conversely, if the patient is alkalotic, then 500 ml of 3 per cent sodium chloride is administered. Infusion time should be one and one half hours. Hypertonic solutions are effective because they remove water from the cells, thus reducing intracellular edema as well as expanding the extracellular fluid volume. Certain precautions should be observed during their administration. A central hyperpyrexia may result from the too rapid withdrawal of fluid from the brain. Therefore, the body temperature should be monitored and, if it exceeds 102° to 103° F, administration should be slowed or discontinued. In elderly patients or those with borderline cardiac status, monitoring of the central venous pressure is advisable so as not to expand the extracellular fluid volume too rapidly.

PARENTERAL NUTRITION

Some patients may be unable to ingest an oral diet in the post-traumatic or postoperative period, and parenteral therapy must be employed. During this interval the metabolic derangements previously mentioned may occur, and careful attention must be given to the metabolic state of the patient. Simple screening techniques such as recording the 24-hour fluid intake and urinary output, and determination of the urine specific gravity and body weight provide helpful guides to clinical management. Ideally, biochemical evaluation of the serum and urine should be obtained preoperatively or in the immediate post-traumatic period and be repeated periodically until the well-being of the patient is evident.

The aim of parenteral therapy is to maintain metabolic homeostasis and to correct any deviations that may occur. In the past it has been impossible to maintain adequate body nutrition by the parenteral route alone over long periods. In recent years, however, much progress has been made in this field until at the present time numerous reports have indicated that appropriate parenteral fluid therapy can achieve and maintain metabolic homeostasis even for a prolonged time.[3,12,20,23]

Total Parenteral Nutrition

Patients who have an obvious contraindication to enteral feeding, e.g., bowel fistula, peritonitis, intra-abdominal abscess, or the like, should be considered for total parenteral nutrition (TPN). Indeed, many who are able to tolerate only small amounts of food by mouth or by gavage feedings may benefit from parenteral feeding.

Whether enteral or parenteral feedings are to be given, it is helpful to estimate a reasonable target level of nutrients based upon the patient's normal weight for his or her height. Such information can be obtained from a standard height-weight table such as the Metropolitan Life Insurance Company's tables or the Home Economics Report.[18] A simpler method for approximating a patient's weight is to allow 105 pounds for the first 5 feet of height and an additional 5 pounds for each additional inch of height. Thus, the weight of a patient 5'10" tall would be estimated at 105 pounds + 50 pounds = 155 pounds. Body weight should be converted to kilograms (lb/2.2); in this case 70 kg. A reasonable target level for energy is 35 kcal per kilogram of body weight, or 2450 kcal for this hypothetical patient. The recommended protein allowance is 0.8 gm per kilogram, or 56 gm.[39] Many surgeons prefer to give more generous amounts of protein, such as 1.0 or 1.5 gm per kilogram. The excess does no harm in the absence of azotemia, in which it may create an undesirable osmotic load to be excreted by the kidneys.

Problems associated with total parenteral nutrition are attributable largely to neglect of a few simple but important principles. These include:

1. Make changes slowly in the amount of fluid, energy sources, or amount of protein given daily. If only a few hundred kilocalories daily has been given as isotonic dextrose, *don't* attempt to increase to the full target level of nutrients at one time. It is preferable to start with a fourth of the target amount and increase stepwise at one to three day intervals until the desired level is reached.

2. Monitor the patient's vital and metabolic signs closely. Daily measurements of the body weight, fluid intake, urine output, fecal or fistula drainage, nasogastric suction, and vital signs are essential. Urine should be collected fractionally four times daily and tested for the presence of glucose and acetone. Serum electrolyte, glucose, and urea levels should be measured daily for the first three to six days, then twice weekly thereafter. Other biochemical measurements including total serum protein, albumin, calcium, phosphorus, bilirubin, creatinine, uric acid, and four enzymes should be performed twice weekly for the first week or two, then once each week. Hematological studies including hemoglobin determination, erythrocyte count, hematocrit, white blood cell count, and differential count are done twice weekly for the first two weeks, then once a week thereafter. Prothrombin time and activated partial thromboplastin time should be measured every week. If the patient is anemic, measurements of serum levels of iron, folic acid, and vitamin B-12 are obtained and repeated when necessary.

3. The greatest hazard of total parenteral nutrition therapy is sepsis, and consequently, staff members caring for these patients must maintain a constant vigil to prevent contamination of the feeding unit, which consists of the bottle of solution, tubing, filter, and intravenous catheter. Each phase of patient care, from catheter insertion to changing of bottles, tubing, and dressings, must follow a scrupulous routine. The unit should not be invaded for any reason, including administration of medications, drawing of blood, or measurement of venous pressure.

Methods and Precautions

The hypertonic solution of dextrose, amino acids, vitamins, and minerals is too irritating to infuse into a peripheral vein where the flow of blood is relatively sluggish. For this reason a central venous catheter is required to introduce the hypertonic solution into a larger caliber vein where the flow of blood is abundant. The favored infusion site is the subclavian vein on either side. Percutaneous puncture is performed by placing the patient in a Trendelenburg position with a folded or rolled sheet between the scapulae allowing the shoulders to fall backward. The skin surrounding the proposed puncture site is prepared by shaving, defatting with acetone, and scrubbing with an iodine preparation such as Betadine for five minutes. The area is then isolated with sterile drapes; the operator wears a surgical mask and sterile gloves. The patient is instructed in the Valsalva maneuver and is advised to keep his head turned away from the operator and his ipsilateral arm at his side. After local anesthesia with procaine has been administered, the operator places his index finger in the suprasternal notch and, with a 14-gauge needle on a syringe, punctures the skin just below the midpoint of the clavicle. The needle, directed at the finger in the suprasternal notch, is kept parallel with the inferior surface of the clavicle. The bevel of the needle is directed toward the heart. When the needle is near the subclavian vein the patient is asked to perform a Valsalva maneuver while the needle is advanced into the distended vein. Once venous blood is aspirated, the syringe is elevated toward the head to position the tip of the needle close to the heart. The catheter is then inserted and threaded into the superior vena cava. The catheter is advanced to the needle hub and both catheter and needle are withdrawn until the needle comes out of the skin. At this point the tip of the catheter lies approximately 1 to 2 cm above the right auricle. A needle guard is placed over the needle to prevent damage to the catheter, which is then sutured to the skin. An isotonic solution of saline or glucose is infused through the catheter as soon as it is inserted. An x-ray must be taken to locate the position of the catheter (which is x-ray opaque) *before* the hypertonic nutrient solution is infused. The catheter site is then cleaned again with Betadine, and Betadine ointment is placed on the skin about the catheter entry site. A square of sterile gauze is applied, and the surrounding skin is sprayed with tincture of benzoin. An elastic dressing (Elastoplast) is placed over the gauze, and the edges are taped securely.

This dressing permits the evaporation of perspiration, thus avoiding maceration of the skin.[16] In infants and small children, the jugular vein is often used. The proximal end of the catheter is tunneled subcutaneously to the occipital region to permit attachment of the infusion tubing and sterile dressings.

Once the position of the catheter has been verified and the hypertonic infusion begun, a routine of preventive care is undertaken. The team consisting of a physician, nurse, and pharmacist evaluates the patient for evidence of fluid overload or osmotic diuresis, metabolic imbalance (especially hyper- or hypoglycemia, hypophosphatemia, or electrolyte imbalance), and infection. If fever occurs, efforts must be made to identify the cause. At the same time, the bottle of infusion fluid, the connecting tubing, and the filter are replaced, and cultures are made from the fluid and filter. If fever persists beyond 24 hours and cannot be otherwise explained, the catheter should be removed and material from the tip cultured for bacteria and fungi. If blood and catheter tip cultures are positive for the same organism, the infection is deemed "catheter-related." If, on the other hand, the catheter is sterile, but cultures from blood and an abscess or sinus grew out the same organism, the infection was not related to the catheter. Often in a patient with septicemia, the blood cultures, the infection source, *and* the catheter will grow the same organism. This represents secondary seeding of the catheter. Nonetheless, an infected catheter must be removed and another catheter placed in the opposite side. Copeland and associates found that patients with neoplastic disease had a catheter contamination rate of only 7.5 per cent despite their high rate of sepsis and impaired resistance to infection.[8] These workers attributed this low rate of infection, even in high-risk patients, to the meticulous care provided by a team of experts. The catheter site dressings were changed under sterile conditions three times weekly, and great care was taken to avoid any source of contamination of the total parenteral nutrition unit (bottle, tubing, filter, and catheter).

Results of Therapy

Following the pioneering work of Dudrick, total parenteral nutrition has been increasingly utilized for the management of critically ill patients.[12] The overall results have been good, and most patients gain weight, achieve positive nitrogen balance, and begin to restore depleted levels of hemoglobin, albumin, and other plasma proteins. Although wound healing has been improved in experimental animals, this has been more difficult to evaluate in human patients.[45]

Most reported patients receiving total parenteral nutritional therapy have had disease or injury of the digestive tract, but there are reports of those with head injuries who have benefited from this type of management.[30] The ultimate choice of whether to feed an unconscious patient parenterally or by gavage should be an individual one.

Parenteral feeding represents a significant advance in patient care, but it is far from perfect. In addition to mechanical hazards and the risk of infection, there is the potential for producing metabolic derangements and deficiencies of essential nutrients. Essential fatty acid deficiency can be avoided by giving infusions of fat emulsion.[14] Deficiencies of trace minerals also occur and are more difficult to avoid because, at present, there is no commercial preparation containing these elements that is approved for parenteral use.[15] Finally, there is evidence that available vitamin preparations are less than ideal in terms of nutrient balance.[41] These and other factors suggest that most neurosurgical patients should be fed enterally by nasogastric gavage or by gastrostomy if possible. Parenteral feeding should be reserved for those in whom enteral feeding is inadequate or impractical and should be used only to maintain the nutritional and metabolic balance of the patient until oral feedings can be resumed.

REFERENCES

1. Allott, E. N.: Sodium and chloride retention without renal disease. Lancet, *1*:1035–1037, 1939.
2. Barrter, F. C.: The role of aldosterone in normal homeostasis and in certain disease states. Metabolism, *5*:369–383, 1956.
3. Beal, J. M., Payne, M. A., Gilder, H., Johnson, G., Jr., and Carver, W. L.: Experience with administration of an intravenous fat emulsion to surgical patients. Metabolism, *6*:673–681, 1957.
4. Carter, N. W., Rector, F. C., Jr., and Seldin, D. W.: Hyponatremia in cerebral disease resulting from the inappropriate secretion of antidiuretic hormone. New Eng. J. Med., *264*:67–72, 1961.
5. Cooper, I. S.: Disorders of electrolyte and water metabolism following brain surgery. J. Neurosurg., *10*:389–396, 1953.
6. Cooper, I. S., and Crevier, P. H.: Neurogenic hypernatremia and hyperchloremia. J. Clin. Endocr., *12*:821–830, 1952.
7. Cooper, I. S., and MacCarty, C. S.: Unusual electrolyte abnormalities associated with cerebral lesions. Proc. Mayo Clin., *26*:354–358, 1951.
8. Copeland, E. M., MacFadyen, B. V., Jr., and Dudrick, S. J.: Prevention of microbial catheter contamination in patients receiving parenteral hyperalimentation. Southern Med. J., *67*:303, 1974.
9. Cort, J. H.: Cerebral salt wasting. Lancet, *1*:752–754, 1954.
10. Davis, B. P., and Matukas, V. J.: Inappropriate secretion of antidiuretic hormone after cerebral injury. J. Oral Surg., *34*:609–615, 1976.
11. Davis, J. O.: Aldosterone and angiotensin. Interrelationships in normal and diseased states. J.A.M.A., *188*:1062–1068, 1964.
12. Dudrick, S. J., Wilmore, D. W., Vars, H. M., and Rhoads, J. E.: Can intravenous feeding as the sole means of nutrition support growth in the child and restore weight loss in an adult? Ann. Surg., *169*:974–984, 1969.
13. Engstrom, W. W., and Liebman, A.: Chronic hyperosmolarity of the body fluids with a cerebral lesion causing diabetes insipidus and anterior pituitary insufficiency. Amer. J. Med., *15*:180–186, 1953.
14. Fleming, C. R., Hodges, R. E., and Hurley, L. S.: A prospective study of serum copper and zinc levels in patients receiving total parenteral nutrition. Amer. J. Clin. Nutr., *29*:70, 1976.
15. Fleming, C. R., Smith, L. M., and Hodges, R. E.: Essential fatty acid deficiency in adults receiving total parenteral nutrition. Amer. J. Clin. Nutr., *29*:976, 1976.
16. Goldmann, D. A., Maki, D. G., Rhame, F. S., Kaiser, A. B., Tenney, J. H., and Bennett, J. Y.: Guidelines for infection control in intravenous therapy. Ann. Intern. Med., *79*:848, 1973.
17. Gordon, G. L., and Goldner, F.: Hypernatremia, azotemia and acidosis after cerebral injury. Amer. J. Med., *23*:543–553, 1957.
18. Hathaway and Foard, 1960. Heights and Weights of Adults in the United States, Home Economics Research Report No. 10, ARS, USDA. *Quoted in* American College of Surgeons (Ballinger, W. F., Collins, J. A., Drucker, W. R., Dudrick, S. J., and Zeppa, R., eds.): Manual of Surgical Nutrition. Philadelphia, W. B. Saunders Co., 1975, p. 228.
19. Higgins, G., Lewin, W., O'Brien, J. R. P., and Taylor, W. H.: Metabolic disorders in head injury. Hyperchloremia and hypochloremia. Lancet, *1*:1295–1300, 1951.
20. Holden, W. D., Krieger, H., Levey, S., Abbott, W. E.: The effect of nutrition on nitrogen metabolism in the surgical patient. Ann. Surg., *146*:563–579, 1957.
21. James, W. P. T., Millward, D. J., and Garlick,

P. J.: Insulin and Glucon to reduce catabolic response to burns. Lancet, *1*:1078, 1971.

22. Kerpel-Fronius, E. Ö.: Über die Beziehungen Zwischen Salz- und Wasserhaushalt bei experimentellen Wasserverlusten. Z. Kinderheilk., *57*:489–504, 1935.

23. Larsen, V., and Brockner, J.: The effect of pre- and postoperative parenteral nutrition on the nitrogen balance following major surgery. Acta Chir. Scand., Suppl., *357*:247–251, 1966.

24. Lewy, F. H., and Gassman, F. K.: Experiments on the hypothalamic nuclei in the regulation of chloride and sugar metabolism. Amer. J. Physiol., *112*:504–510, 1935.

25. MacCarty, C. S., and Cooper, I. S.: Neurologic and metabolic effects of bilateral ligation of the anterior cerebral arteries in man. Proc. Mayo Clin., *26*:185–190, 1951.

26. Marriott, H. L.: Water and Salt Depletion. Springfield, Ill., Charles C Thomas, 1950.

27. McLaurin, R. L.: *In* Covencss, W. E., and Walker, A. E., eds.: Head Injury. Conference Proceedings. Philadelphia, J. B. Lippincott Co., 1966, Chapter 11.

28. McLaurin, R. L., King, L., Elam, E. B., and Budde, R. B.: Metabolic response to craniocerebral trauma. Surg. Gynec. Obstet., *110*: 282–288, 1960.

29. McLaurin, R. L., King, L., Tutor, F. T., and Knowles, H., Jr.: Metabolic response to intracranial surgery. Surg. Forum, *10*:770–773, 1960.

30. McNamara, J. J., Molot, M. D., Wissman, D., Collins, C., and Stremple, J. F.: Intravenous hyperalimentation. An important adjunct in the treatment of combat casualties. Amer. J. Surg., *122*:70, 1971.

31. Moore, F. D., and Ball, M. R.: The Metabolic Response to Surgery. Springfield, Ill., Charles C Thomas, 1952.

32. Nadal, J. W., Pedersen, S., and Maddock, W. G.: Comparison between dehydration from salt loss and from water deprivation. J. Clin. Invest., *20*:691–703, 1941.

33. Natelson, S., and Alexander, M. O.: Marked hypernatremia and hyperchloremia with damage to the central nervous system. A.M.A. Arch. Int. Med., *96*:172–175, 1955.

34. O'Keefe, S. J. D., Sender, P. M., and James, W. P. T.: "Catabolic" loss of body nitrogen in response to surgery. Lancet, *2*:1035–1038, 1974.

35. Peters, J. P.: The role of sodium in the production of edema. New Eng. J. Med., *239*:353–362, 1948.

36. Peters, J. P.: Water balance in health and disease. *In* Duncan, G. C.: Diseases of Metabolism. 2nd Ed. Philadelphia, W. B. Saunders Co., 1947, pp. 271–346.

37. Peters, J. P., Welt, L. G., Sims, E. A. H., Orloff, J., and Needham, J. A.: Salt-wasting syndrome associated with cerebral disease. Trans. Ass. Amer. Physicians, *63*:57–64, 1950.

38. Randall, R. E., and Papper. S.: Mechanism of postoperative limitation in sodium excretion: The role of extracellular fluid volume and of adrenal cortical activity. J. Clin. Invest., *37*:1628–1641, 1958.

39. Recommended Dietary Allowances, 8th Ed. Washington, D.C., Committee on Dietary Allowances, Food and Nutrition Board, National Research Council, National Academy of Sciences, 1974.

40. Rhoads, J. E.: Protein nutrition in surgical patients. Fed. Proc., *11*:659–665, 1952.

41. Ryan, J. H., Jr.: *In* Fischer, J. E., ed.: Complications of Parenteral Nutrition. Total Parenteral Nutrition. Boston, Little, Brown & Co., 1976, pp. 94–95.

42. Schwartz, W. B., Bennett, W., Curelop, S., and Bartler, F. C.: A syndrome of renal sodium loss and hyponatremia probably resulting from inappropriate secretion of antidiuretic hormone. Amer. J. Med., *23*:529–542, 1957.

43. Shires, T., Williams, J., and Brown, F.: Acute changes in extracellular fluid associated with major surgical procedures. Ann. Surg., *154*: 803–810, 1961.

44. Smith, H. W.: Salt and water volume receptors. Amer. J. Med., *23*:623–652, 1957.

45. Steiger, E., Allen, T. R., Daly, J. M., Vars, H. M., and Dudrick, S. J.: Beneficial effects of immediate post operative total parenteral nutrition. Surg. Forum, *22*:89, 1971.

46. Strauss, M. B.: Body Water in Man: The Acquisition and Maintenance of the Body Fluids. Boston, Little, Brown & Co., 1957.

47. Strauss, M. B.: Body Water in Man. Boston, Little, Brown & Co., 1957, pp. 29–49.

48. Sweet, W. H., Cotzias, G. C., Seed, V., and Yakovlev, P. I.: Gastrointestinal hemorrhages, hyperglycemia, azotemia, hyperchloremia, and hypernatremia following lesions of the frontal lobe in man. (1947). Ass. Res. Nerve. Dis. Proc., *27*:795–831, 1948.

49. Ulmann, T. D.: Hyperosmolarity of the extracellular fluid in encephalitis. Amer. J. Med., *15*: 885–890, 1953.

50. Verney, E. B.: Croonian Lecture: Antidiuretic hormone and factors which determine its release. Proc. Roy. Soc. London, s.B. *135*:25–105, 1947.

51. Welt, L. G., Seldin, D. W., Nelson, W. P., German, W. J., and Peters, J. P.: Role of the central nervous system in metabolism of electrolytes and water. Arch. Int. Med., *90*:355–378, 1952.

52. Wise, B. L.: Fluids and Electrolytes in Neurological Surgery. Springfield, Ill., Charles C Thomas, 1965.

53. Wolfman, E. F., Jr., and Schoch, H. K.: Water depletion in the comatose patient. Univ. Mich. Med. Bull., *17*:73–82, 1951.

54. Wolfman, E. F., Jr., Coon, W. W., and Kahn, E. A.: The recognition and management of severe hypertonicity of the extracellular fluid associated with cerebral lesions. Surgery, *47*:410–416, 1960.

55. Wolfman, E. F., Jr., Coon, W. W., and Schwartz, S.: Sodium retention following experimental lesions of the precommissural septum in the monkey. J. Surg. Res., *6*:2–18, 1966.

56. Wolfman, E. F., Jr., Coon, W. W., and Sloan, C.: Unpublished data.

57. Wolfman, E. F., Jr., Coon, W. W., Reifel, E., Iob, V., and McMath, M.: Severe hypertonicity of the extracellular fluid associated with cerebral lesions. Surgery, *47*:929–939, 1960.

58. Wynn, V., and Rob, C. G.: Water intoxication: Differential diagnosis of the hypotonic syndromes. Lancet, *1*:587–594, 1954.

59. Youmans, J. R.: Personal communication.

27

PULMONARY CARE
AND COMPLICATIONS

Acute respiratory failure is a common complication of serious illness, trauma, and operation. The problem is of particular importance in neurosurgical patients because of the frequency with which consciousness is impaired and the sensitivity of the central nervous system to hypoxia, hypercarbia, hypocarbia, acidosis, and alkalosis. Since blood gas determinations became clinically available, and owing to the impetus of the military medical experience in Viet Nam, a wealth of clinical and laboratory investigation has gone far toward defining the syndrome and the causes of acute respiratory failure.*

Acute respiratory failure is a condition in which gas exchange is impaired at the alveolar level, usually in a patient with previously healthy lungs. It is associated with a large number of clinical conditions and hence has been described under a large number of synonyms (congestive atelectasis, fat embolism, oxygen intoxication, post-traumatic pulmonary insufficiency, pump lung, respirator lung, shock lung, white lung, and many others). Because the diverse events of fat embolism, head injury, pulmonary embolism, and airway obstruction are different, not all would agree to lumping these processes under one name.[44,60]

Chronic obstructive respiratory disease, cardiac failure, and lung infection are excluded by definition, although if pre-existing, they may precipitate and complicate acute respiratory failure.

The relationship of central nervous system disease and cardiopulmonary complications has a long and interesting history, for which the reader is referred to the comprehensive review of Rossi and Graf.[61] A serious problem in interpretation has been the separation of acute pulmonary edema from the syndrome of acute respiratory failure. A variety of experimental manipulations of the central nervous system have produced acute pulmonary edema, and yet it rarely follows central nervous system disease clinically. Conversely, despite much laboratory and clinical investigation, it is not clear that acute respiratory failure following central nervous system disease differs in any material way from that associated with other trauma or disease. The authors use the term "acute respiratory failure" as a general description, not as the name of a specific syndrome, and recognize different etiologies.

Neurosurgical patients may suffer from (1) generalized hypoventilation due to central nervous system depression or disease, (2) direct chest and lung injury, (3) obstruction of either proximal or distal airways, (4) interstitial pulmonary edema, (5) failure of lung circulation, (6) disproportion or inhomogeneity of ventilation and perfusion, or a combination of these problems. This chapter examines the pulmonary anatomy and physiology necessary to an understanding of lung function, the pathophysiology of acute respiratory failure, its etiology and clinical course as encountered in neurological surgery, useful diagnostic procedures, suggestions for therapy (plus a representative case in which the reader may do the necessary analysis), and the complications resulting from the condition.

From the hundreds of articles that are available, references have been chosen that

---

* See references 11, 23, 37, 40, 43, 52, 54, 66, 67.

C. E. BRACKETT AND R. C. BONE

will provide more detailed, authoritative, and recent material. The pulmonary complications of trauma (including chest injury, airway management, and pulmonary embolism) are discussed in Chapter 77.

NORMAL RESPIRATION

The function of the lung is to add oxygen to the venous blood and remove carbon dioxide from it. The heart and circulation transport the oxygen to the peripheral organs and remove carbon dioxide from them. The lungs also have important filtering and metabolic functions. In order to identify and treat abnormal changes in the lung, it is necessary to understand the pertinent anatomy and physiology. Weibel discusses the morphology in detail, and Comroe and associates, Nunn, and Peters similarly discuss the physiology of the lung.[19,46,47,68] A concise and complete review of the essentials of respiratory physiology is presented by West.[69]

Anatomy
Thorax

The thoracic skeleton consists of the sternum anteriorly, the vertebrae posteriorly, and the ribs. The thorax is shaped like a cone and on inspiration moves in an axis that increases its anterior, posterior, and transverse diameters. The muscles of respiration include the diaphragm and the intercostal and accessory muscles of respiration. The diaphragm is the principal muscle of inspiration. Each hemidiaphragm is innervated by the ipsilateral phrenic nerve, which has its origins from the ventral horn cells at spinal levels C3 to C5. The intercostal muscles are innervated by their corresponding intercostal nerves. Thus an injury to the spinal cord below C5 will paralyze intercostal muscles but will leave the diaphragm intact. If the diaphragm is paralyzed, it moves paradoxically (passively) with respiration.

Lung

The right lung has three lobes (upper, middle, lower). The left lung has two lobes (upper and lower). The right lung has 10 and the left lung 8 bronchopulmonary segments. Knowledge of the distribution of the segmental bronchi and the bronchopulmonary segments is important in describing the location of pulmonary lesions accurately and is thus important in radiological interpretation and in bronchoscopy. The two main bronchi arise at the tracheal bifurcation. The right main bronchus is shorter than the left and deviates less from the vertical axis of the trachea. Because of the position of the right bronchus, aspirated material and intratracheal tubes are more likely to lodge in the right than in the left lung. The bronchi divide through 16 subdivisions into lobar and segmental bronchi and terminal bronchioles. These make up the conducting airways and have no gas exchange function. The mouth, pharynx, and conductory airways constitute the anatomical dead space (V_{DAN}), which equals 150 cc.

The respiratory zone of the lung is composed of respiratory bronchioles and alveoli, is of short length (5 mm), and makes up nearly all of the 2500-cc lung volume.

Mucus secreted by goblet cells in the airways is constantly moved upward by the cilia. Damage to this important elevator mechanism leads to failure to clear secretions, bacteria, and foreign bodies, and promotes atelectasis.

The 300,000,000 alveoli are lined by type I pneumocytes without organelles and type II pneumocytes that secrete organelles into the alveolus to form surfactant, a lipoprotein. The alveolus is inherently unstable, tending to collapse because of the surface tension of its moist surface. This tendency is opposed by surfactant. Damage to surfactant or its producing pneumocytes leads to alveolar collapse.[8]

The septum of the alveolus contains capillaries and an interstitial space continuous with the interstitial space of the airway and blood vessels. The capillary is closely applied to the alveolar surface so that the gas diffusion distance is short.[26] The interstitial space provides lymphatic drainage for the lung. Distention of the interstitial space with water makes the lung stiff, less compliant, and difficult to ventilate; it ordinarily does not interfere with gas diffusion until late in the process of swelling.

Vascular Supply

The lungs have a double arterial supply. The bronchial arteries carry blood to the supporting tissues of the lung, particularly the bronchi, and are not concerned with gas exchange. The right and left pulmonary arteries are concerned with gas exchange and carry deoxygenated blood from the right ventricle as far as the respiratory bronchioles. The pulmonary capillaries drain into the pulmonary venules, which form the pulmonary veins, to empty into the left atrium. The pulmonary arteries and veins constitute a thin-walled, low-pressure system without precapillary sphincters. The pulmonary veins in man are thin-walled but may have constrictive properties. They are poorly responsive to nerve stimulation. It is suggested that these features make the circulation of the blood very gravity-dependent; this has important clinical implications.

Innervation

Changes in resistance to air flow occur mainly in the large and medium-sized bronchi, whose diameter is controlled by the smooth muscle in the wall. The smooth muscle is constricted by the vagus, acetylcholine, and histamine, and dilated by sympathetic stimulation and drugs such as epinephrine. The bronchial musculature is also reflexly controlled by receptors in the trachea and large bronchi, so with aspiration, bronchospasm may be an important part of acute respiratory distress.

The vessels of the lung are innervated by the vagus nerve and the second to fifth sympathetic ganglia; thus they have both adrenergic and cholinergic innervation. The degree to which pulmonary vessels are responsive to stimulation in man as opposed to experimental animals is controversial at present. This makes extrapolation of animal work (particularly in dogs) to the human hazardous. The vessels are responsive to oxygen tension, so that low oxygen tension causes vasoconstriction and shunting of blood from nonventilated areas, while high oxygen tensions cause dilation and may lead to excess of perfusion over ventilation and thus venous admixture. The vessels are also responsive to circulating catecholamines and locally produced histamine, prostaglandins, and other humoral substances.

Physiology

The symbols used in respiratory physiology and their definitions are given in Table 27–1. Table 27–2 contains the necessary calculations for clinical application of cardiopulmonary physiology in caring for the critically ill patient.

Mechanics of Breathing

During normal inspiration (tidal volume, V_T = 7 cc per kilogram or about 500 cc) the diaphragm (C3–C5) moves downward, and the intercostals (T1–T12) move the chest wall up and forward. The lateral dimension of the chest expands passively. During hyperinflation ($V_T > 7$ cc per kilogram) these movements are increased and accessory muscles (scalene and sternocleidomastoid) are brought into play. With spinal cord paralysis at C5, the resultant diaphragmatic tidal volume will be reduced to 150 to 300 cc. With an anatomical dead space of 150 cc, little alveolar ventilation will take place.

Expiration is normally passive, but during hyperventilation, e.g., in head injury and decerebration, may become active. This may be detected by noting active abdominal muscle contraction during expiration. The unwanted result is a decreased functional residual capacity (FRC, the volume of gas remaining after normal expiration).

During normal ventilation, chest expansion produces a negative pleural pressure, causing expansion of the lung, but during artificial ventilation, air enters the lung under pressure positive to the atmosphere, influenced by the elastic properties of the chest wall and lung. Owing to pressure differentials and multiple bronchial branching, air flow is both laminar and turbulent to the respiratory zone, where pressure changes are so slight that gas exchanges by diffusion. The major resistance to air flow occurs in the proximal airways, especially the medium-sized bronchi. Distribution of inspired gas varies because of differences in the shape and elasticity of the thorax, so the bottom of the lung is better ventilated than the top. The terminal airways close at low lung volumes. This tendency to closure is increased by tracheal irritation, anoxia, histamine, and cholinergic drugs. In acute respiratory failure, the closing volume (the volume at which these airways close) is markedly increased; that is, the terminal airways close while the lung is still inflated above residual volume. This closure has important therapeutic implications. The lung is very distensible, and the compliance (volume change per unit of pressure change) is approximately 200 cc per centimeter of water. Static compliance (compliance of lung parenchyma) is decreased by

TABLE 27-1 SYMBOLS USED IN CARDIOPULMONARY PHYSIOLOGY

SYMBOL*	DEFINITION	EXAMPLES
Primary Symbols		
V	Gas volume	V_A = volume of alveolar gas
$\dot{V}$	Gas volume per unit time	V_T = tidal volume
P	Gas pressure	$\dot{V}$ = minute volume
$\bar{P}$	Mean gas pressure	$\dot{V}_{O_2}$ = oxygen consumption per minute
F	Fractional concentration in dry gas phase	$P_{A_{O_2}}$ = alveolar oxygen pressure
(f)	Respiratory frequency (breaths per unit time)	$\bar{P}_{c_{O_2}}$ = mean capillary oxygen pressure
D	Diffusing capacity	$F_{I_{O_2}}$ = fractional concentration of oxygen in inspired gas
R	Respiratory exchange ratio	D_{O_2} = diffusing capacity for oxygen (milliliters of oxygen per millimeter of mercury per minute)
Q	Volume of blood	$R = \dot{V}_{CO_2}/\dot{V}_{O_2}$
$\dot{Q}$	Volume flow of blood per unit time	Q_C = volume of blood in pulmonary capillaries
C	Concentration of gas in blood phase	$\dot{Q}_C$ = blood flow through pulmonary capillaries per minute
S	Per cent saturation of hemoglobin oxygen or carbon dioxide	$C_{a_{O_2}}$ = milliliters of oxygen per milliliter of arterial blood
		$S_{V_{\bar{v}}}$ = saturation of hemoglobin with oxygen in mixed venous blood
Subscripts		
I	Inspired gas	$F_{I_{CO_2}}$ = fractional concentration of carbon dioxide in inspired gas
E	Expired gas	V_E = volume of expired gas
A	Alveolar gas	$\dot{V}_A$ = alveolar ventilation per minute
T	Tidal gas	V_T = tidal volume
D	Dead space gas	V_D = volume of dead space gas
B	Barometric	P_B = barometric pressure
a	Arterial blood	$P_{a_{CO_2}}$ = partial pressure of carbon dioxide in arterial blood
v	Venous blood	$P_{V_{O_2}}$ = partial pressure of oxygen in mixed venous blood
c	Capillary blood	$P_{c_{CO}}$ = partial pressure of carbon monoxide in pulmonary capillary blood

* - Dash above any symbol indicates a mean value.
 · Dot above any symbol indicates a time derivative.

TABLE 27–2   FORMULAS FOR CLINICAL APPLICATION OF CARDIOPULMONARY PHYSIOLOGY

Alveolar air equation

$$PA_{O_2} = FI_{O_2} (PB - 47) - \frac{Pa_{CO_2}}{R}$$

On 100 per cent oxygen
$$PA_{O_2} = (PB - PH_2O) FI_{O_2} - Pa_{CO_2}$$
Alveolar-arterial gradient ($\Delta A - a$)
$$\Delta A - a = PA_{O_2} - Pa_{O_2}$$
Arterial/alveolar ratio (a/A)

$$a/A = \frac{Pa_{O_2}}{PA_{O_2}}$$

Arterial oxygen content (Ca_{O_2})
$$Ca_{O_2} - .003\ Pa_{O_2} + 1.39\ (Hb)(Sa_{O_2})$$
Mixed venous oxygen content ($C\bar{v}_{O_2}$)
$$C\bar{v}_{O_2} = .003\ P\bar{v}_{O_2} + 1.39\ (Hb)(S\bar{v}_{O_2})$$
Coefficient of oxygen delivery (COD)

$$COD = \frac{Ca_{O_2}}{Ca_{O_2} - C\bar{v}_{O_2}}$$

Shunt ($\dot{Q}s/\dot{Q}T$)
If Pa_{O_2} is over 150 mm of mercury, the hemoglobin is fully saturated; use equation 1.
Equation 1

$$\frac{\dot{Q}s}{\dot{Q}T} = \frac{(.003)(PA_{O_2} - Pa_{O_2})}{C(a - \bar{v})_{O_2} + (.003)(PA_{O_2} - Pa_{O_2})}$$

If the Pa_{O_2} is less than 150 mm of mercury, the hemoglobin is not fully saturated and equation 2 must be used.
Equation 2

$$\frac{\dot{Q}s}{\dot{Q}T} = \frac{(.003)(PA_{O_2} - Pa_{O_2}) + (Hb)(1.39)(DSa_{O_2})^*}{(.003)(PA_{O_2} - Pa_{O_2}) + Hb\ (1.39)(DSa_{O_2}) + (Ca_{O_2} - C\bar{v}_{O_2})} \times 100$$

*DSa_{O_2} = Desaturation of arterial blood (1-saturation)

The ratio of physiological dead space to tidal volume is a measure of wasted ventilation.

$$\frac{VD}{VT} = \frac{Pa_{CO_2} - P\bar{E}_{CO_2}}{Pa_{CO_2}}$$

edema, vascular distention, fibrosis, and other factors that increase the stiffness of the lung tissue, and by reduced elasticity of the chest wall. Resistance to air flow is increased by obstruction of the airways by, e.g., secretions, airway collapse, or spasm, which results in decreased dynamic compliance.

Ventilation

When a normal breath is taken (tidal volume, V_T = 500 cc), anatomical dead space (V_{DAN}) occupies 150 cc, leaving 350 cc for distribution to the alveoli (alveolar volume, V_A). At 15 breaths per minute, a minute volume (V_M) of 7500 cc delivers 2250 cc to dead space and 5250 cc to the alveoli (V_A). Doubling the rate (30 breaths per minute) at the same tidal volume will deliver 4500 cc to dead space and 10,500 cc to the alveoli, while doubling tidal volume (V_T = 1000) at a rate of 15 breaths per minute will deliver 2250 cc to dead space and 12,750 cc to alveolar ventilation. The disadvantage of tachypneic, low-tidal-volume hyperventilation and the advantage of slow, large-tidal-volume ventilation in increasing alveolar ventilation can be seen.

The volume of gas in the lung after normal expiration is the functional residual capacity (FRC). In acute respiratory failure this is reduced by atelectasis, airway closure, hemorrhage, edema, and forced expiration.

It is important to realize that although the anatomical dead space is small (150 cc), the physiological dead space may be very large (up to 2500 cc) owing to ventilated areas of the lung that have no effective blood supply, e.g., in pulmonary embolism.

Oxygen and carbon dioxide flow from and to the alveolus and the capillary by diffusion, carbon dioxide about 20 times as fast as oxygen. Under normal conditions, mixed venous blood (Pv_{O_2} = 40) is reoxygenated to Pa_{O_2} of 100 mm of mercury in a fraction of its course along the pulmonary capillary. This means that the diffusion reserve of the lung is large and is rarely a problem in acute respiratory failure. The problem is, of course, even less for carbon dioxide.

Perfusion

The pulmonary vasculature is a low-pressure circuit of thin-walled vessels in which the capillaries are so richly applied to the alveolar wall that blood flows almost in a sheet.[28] The total volume of the pulmonary capillaries is only about 70 to 100 cc. The vascular pressures are (in millimeters of mercury): right atrium 5/3, pulmonary artery 25/8, pulmonary veins 8/4, and left atrium 5. The thin-walled vessels increase in diameter as the lung expands, but may decrease if the alveolar pressure rises with artificial ventilation, e.g., posititive end-expiratory pressure. This is particularly true of the alveolar capillaries, arterioles, and veins. The resistance of the pulmonary circuit is very slight. Increasing pulmonary artery pressure will open previously closed capillaries, and previously open capillaries will be distended. Because of these characteristics, blood flow in the lung is very gravity-dependent; i.e., is greater in basal regions when the person is upright, in posterior regions when he is supine, and in the dependent lung when he lies on his side.

The effect of pulmonary vessel innervation is weak. Pulmonary arterioles sensitively constrict at alveolar oxygen tensions below 70, however, thus shunting blood from hypoxemic areas of the lung. Conversely, hyperoxygenated areas of the lung are associated with vascular distention.

Ventilation-to-Perfusion Relationships

For optimum gas exchange, there must be an appropriate relation of ventilation to perfusion ($\dot{V}/\dot{Q}$) of the alveolus (Fig. 27–1). If ventilation fails, oxygen is not added to or carbon dioxide abstracted from the mixed venous blood, and hence Pa_{O_2} falls and Pa_{CO_2} rises. If the circulation fails, the alveolus has a relatively high Po_2 (no oxygen being abstracted) and a zero CO_2; it is a dead space unit (no gas exchange). These alveoli that receive no circulation make up

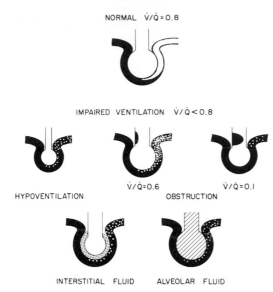

NORMAL $\dot{V}/\dot{Q} = 0.8$

IMPAIRED VENTILATION $\dot{V}/\dot{Q} < 0.8$

HYPOVENTILATION

$\dot{V}/\dot{Q} = 0.6$ $\dot{V}/\dot{Q} = 0.1$

OBSTRUCTION

INTERSTITIAL FLUID   ALVEOLAR FLUID

Figure 27–1 Ventilation-perfusion relationships. Normally mixed venous blood ($P\bar{v}_{O_2} = 40$ mm of mercury, *shown in black*) is ventilated to Pa_{O_2} of 80 mm of mercury (*white*). The effect of alveolar hypoventilation, secretions, interstitial pulmonary edema, and alveolar high-protein edema is incomplete oxygenation of venous blood. Interstitial edema decreases alveolar ventilation; it does not interfere with diffusion except terminally.

the physiological dead space, which may become very large in disease and may add greatly to the work of breathing. They do not, however, lower the oxygen tension.

West has shown that normally, because of the shape and action of the thorax and lung, ventilation increases from the top to the bottom of the lung.[69] Owing to gravity, however, the perfusion increases even more rapidly from top to bottom. In addition, the alveolar pressure exceeds pulmonary artery pressure at the top of the lung, cutting off blood flow and producing useless alveolar dead space. In mid zone, pulmonary artery pressure exceeds alveolar pressure, which in turn is greater than venous pressure; hence, flow depends on pulmonary artery–alveolar pressure differences. At the bottom of the lung, both pulmonary artery and venous pressures exceed alveolar pressure, and flow is determined by ordinary arterial-venous pressure differences. Thus, at the top of the lung, ventilation exceeds perfusion ($\dot{V}/\dot{Q} > 1$), and the area tends to be a ventilatory dead space. At the bottom of the lung, perfusion exceeds ventilation, and the lung resembles a shunt lung ($\dot{V}/\dot{Q} < 1$). When ventilation is

less than perfusion, the venous blood is not fully oxygenated, and admixture of this unoxygenated blood with normally oxygenated blood is called venous admixture or right-to-left shunt. (The word "shunt" is used for convenience.) Similar considerations apply to the supine patient, in whom the large dependent posterior lung surface tends to have low ventilation-to-perfusion ratios. When the patient is on his side, the top lung tends to be a dead space lung and the dependent lung a shunt lung. This is the reason for turning patients frequently. In acute respiratory failure, depending on its cause, the lung contains scattered areas of dead space lung and shunt lung. Thus, in pulmonary embolism, the affected area of the lung may be dead space lung, while with secretions or edema, ventilation is impaired and shunting results. The shunt areas contribute most to hypoxemia, however, since they are the areas that are hyperperfused, while the dead space areas are hypoperfused. Thus, the shunt areas contribute most blood to the circulation, and this blood is nonventilated mixed venous blood of low Po_2.

Normally, only a small amount of nonventilated blood is anatomically shunted, (bronchial arteries, thesbian veins). If ventilation is impaired (by secretions, airway collapse, edema) mixed venous blood is not fully oxygenated and, mixing with normally oxygenated blood, lowers Pa_{O_2} (see Fig. 27–1). This is the commonest mechanism of hypoxemia in acute respiratory failure and cannot be corrected by giving 100 per cent oxygen, since the oxygen cannot reach the nonventilated blood. Pa_{CO_2} is not elevated because when the carbon dioxide level starts to rise, medullary chemoreceptors increase the rate of ventilation and carbon dioxide is eliminated through nonshunt areas of the lung. Typically, in acute respiratory failure, Pa_{O_2} is low because of shunting and Pa_{CO_2} is also low owing to hyperventilation.

Impairment of ventilation that causes shunting is due to secretions, airway collapse, or alveolar septal edema from fluid overload or capillary damage with loss of fluid to the interstitial space.

In generalized hypoventilation, as opposed to shunting, Pa_{O_2} is low and Pa_{CO_2} is elevated because carbon dioxide elimination is reduced.

The important clinical implication of the foregoing is that in acute respiratory failure, therapy must be directed toward improving ventilation of the lung, not toward raising inspired oxygen tensions.

Gas Transport

The atmosphere is made up of nitrogen, oxygen, water vapor, carbon dioxide, rare gases, and pollutants. Atmospheric carbon dioxide, rare gases, and pollutants may be ignored in gas calculations. The atmosphere is approximately 20 per cent oxygen and 80 per cent nitrogen. At sea level barometric pressure of 760 mm of mercury, the partial pressure of oxygen is thus 20 per cent of $760 - 47$ (water vapor pressure) or 142 mm of mercury. In the alveolus and blood, the partial pressure of carbon dioxide is 45 and Pa_{O_2} is approximately 100 mm of mercury. If one breathes 100 per cent oxygen, nitrogen is washed out, and the alveolar and arterial partial pressure of oxygen is 668 mm of mercury ($760 - 47$ [water vapor] $- 45$ [CO_2]). This theoretical figure is not reached in the normal lung because of anatomical shunt and ventilation-perfusion inhomogeneities, so a figure of 550 to 600 mm of mercury is more common.

Blood carries 0.3 cc of oxygen per 100 cc physically dissolved in the plasma and 20.8 cc of oxygen per 100 cc combined with hemoglobin, which normally is 98 per cent saturated. The shape of the oxygen dissociation curve insures continuing high saturation despite falls in partial pressure of oxygen.[68] In conditions of acidosis (increased tissue metabolism, fall in pH, rises in Pco_2 and temperature) the curve is shifted to the right and oxygen unloading at the periphery is enhanced. Alkalosis shifts the curve to the left with increased retention of oxygen by the red cell.

Volume transport of oxygen and carbon dioxide is clearly dependent on blood flow and red cell mass. Oxygen availability is expressed as cardiac output times oxygen content. In addition, adequate tissue blood flow is essential for adequate delivery of oxygen to and removal of carbon dioxide from the tissues. Furthermore, if blood flow is deficient, products of metabolism and tissue damage (lactic acid, potassium ion, enzymes) are not removed and acidosis results. Thus, ischemic anoxia is more damaging than hypoxemic anoxia. Knowledge of cardiac output and pulmonary and peripheral tissue blood flow are important in evaluating tissue oxygenation.

At the tissue, oxygen diffuses from the capillaries through the tissue according to the solubility and diffusion pressure characteristics. If the intracellular pressure of oxygen falls below 3 mm of mercury because of increased metabolic activity or increased diffusion distance secondary to edema, tissue hypoxia ensues, aerobic metabolism ceases, and anaerobic metabolism commences with the production of lactic acid, tissue acidosis, increased capillary permeability, and other destructive effects. Oxygen supply to the tissue may be inadequate because of pulmonary disease (low Pa_{O_2}), anemia (low oxygen content), or low blood flow secondary to low cardiac output or peripheral vascular obstruction.

Since all oxygen is not abstracted from the blood, the oxygen in mixed venous blood presented to the lungs normally has a pressure of 45 mm of mercury. This assay provides a useful index of tissue oxygenation.

Carbon dioxide, 20 times as soluble as oxygen, is carried to the lung in dissolved form as bicarbonate and combined with hemoglobin and other proteins.

Regulation of Ventilation

The body has peripheral and central chemoreceptors sensitive to low Po_2, low pH, or elevated Pco_2. The peripheral receptors are located in the carotid and aortic bodies and respond rapidly to changes in arterial blood by increasing the rate and depth of ventilation via impulses over the glossopharyngeal and vagus nerves to the medullary respiratory center. The peripheral receptors are most important in responses to hypoxemia, while the central receptors located in the ventral surface of the medulla predominate in the ventilatory response to carbon dioxide. They respond to changes in pH of the surrounding cerebrospinal fluid brought about by changes in the carbon dioxide level. They do not respond to hypoxemia.

The airways contain a number of mechanical and chemical receptors that may cause sneezing, coughing, changes in respiratory rate and volume, and bronchoconstriction. The lung also contains stretch receptors in the airway smooth muscle; when these are stretched by large tidal volumes, respiration slows. Type J receptors are thought to lie in the capillary and to respond to increase in fluid pressure.

Voluntary respiration is governed by the cerebral cortex within limits, while automatic respiration is governed by the three brain stem respiratory centers: the pneumotaxic center in the rostral pons, the apneustic center in the pontine reticular formation, and the dorsal and ventral components of the medullary center, the dorsal being of predominant importance. The dorsal medullary center has primary connections with the ninth and tenth cranial nerves, and probably serves as the primary center for respiratory rhythmicity.

Specific types of breathing abnormality have been reported in animal and some human studies with lesions in these nuclei.[20,49,50] Cheyne-Stokes respiration has been associated with lesions at the level of the basal ganglia; forced hyperventilation with midbrain or collicular level lesions, often in association with decerebration; apneustic breathing with pontine lesions; ataxic or grossly irregular breathing with medullary lesions; and apnea with low medullary, high cervical lesions. Others have not found reliable correlation of lesion site and respiratory abnormality in patients.[45] One problem in the human is the lack of knowledge of the precise neurological lesion in most cases, whether anatomical or biochemical.

Descending voluntary respiratory neurons course with the corticospinal paths, while fibers carrying impulses for automatic control lie medial to the ventral spinothalamic pathways. Bilateral cervical cordotomy may thus interrupt automatic respiration, so that the patient can breathe while awake but is apneic when asleep (Ondine's curse).[31,32] The reviews of Berger and co-workers and others should be consulted for further details of regulation of respiration.[5-7,38,55]

ACUTE RESPIRATORY FAILURE

Pathophysiology

Pathological changes in patients with acute respiratory failure are varied. Clearly the pathology of pulmonary contusion, gastric aspiration, sepsis, severe shock, throm-

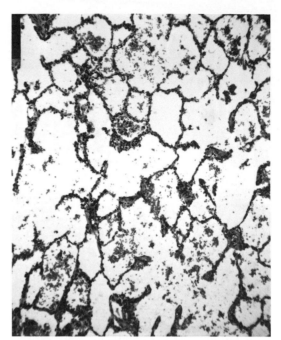

Figure 27–2 Early changes in acute respiratory failure. There are focal thickening of the alveolar septa by edema, and mononuclear cells and leukocytes in the capillaries; red cells are present in the alveoli. Hematoxylin and eosin, 100 ×. (Courtesy of Dr. Richard Sabonya, M.D., Department of Pathology and Oncology, University of Kansas Medical Center.)

boembolism, and fat embolism will vary in specific ways. There are, however, a series of changes that are seen in most forms of acute respiratory failure and that are common in neurosurgical patients, after both trauma and operation.*

In the early stages the lungs appear normal, but microscopic examination shows early interstitial edema and platelet, leukocyte, and fibrin thrombi. Within 6 to 18 hours, the lung appears congested with scattered petechial hemorrhages, and microscopically there are increased interstitial edema, periarteriolar hemorrhages, and vascular congestion (Fig. 27–2). This is soon followed at 18 to 48 hours by increased interstitial and alveolar edema, microatelectasis, transudation of red cells and confluent hemorrhage, and hyperplasia of granular pneumocytes (Fig. 27–3). The lung is heavy and hemorrhagic. At 48 to 72 hours, severe atelectasis, widespread hemorrhage, and hyaline membrane formation

---

* See references 10, 21, 27, 35, 43, 56, 66.

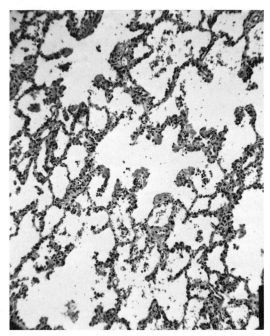

Figure 27–3 Moderate changes at 18 to 48 hours show continuing edema, alveolar hemorrhage with macrophages, hypertrophy of pneumocytes, and early hyaline membranes. Hematoxylin and eosin, 100 ×. (Courtesy of Dr. Richard Sabonya, M.D., Department of Pathology and Oncology, University of Kansas Medical Center.)

duction in ventilation and will be reflected by an increase in airway resistance.

If the capillary is damaged by hypoxia or products of tissue injury, there is separation of the endothelial cells and loss first of fluid and then of protein to the interstitial space. The problem is made worse by the administration of the large volumes of crystaloid needed for blood volume restitution in shock. If colloid (plasma) is used at a stage when protein is being lost, the problem will only be worsened, since water will follow the plasma into the alveolar septum. Because the capillary is closely applied to the alveolar wall, diffusion will not be impaired, but the turgid thickened septum makes the alveolus difficult to ventilate and leads to alveolar and terminal airway collapse.[26] There is thus a tendency toward progressive microatelectasis and progressive failure of ventilation. Progressively higher pressures are needed to open the alveolus, which then remains open for a shorter portion of each pressure cycle. While the patient breathes room air, inert slowly diffusible nitrogen tends to hold the alveolus open, but if nitrogen is washed out

are seen (Fig. 27–4). Bacterial pneumonia usually supervenes. If the patient survives, diffuse fibrosis may result.

Physiologically, these changes mean that as capillary permeability is altered and fluid and protein escape to the alveolar septum, the lung becomes stiffer, static compliance decreases, there is a tendency to alveolar and terminal airway collapse, the functional residual capacity diminishes, and fewer alveoli are ventilated. Coincident with this there is vascular distention. Since all these events occur more in the dependent portions of the lung, the combination of progressive failure of alveolar ventilation and vascular congestion produces ventilation-perfusion inhomogeneity, or shunting, that is the cause of hypoxemia. Progressively higher pressures are needed to ventilate the lung, and the work of breathing is increased. With local damage, surfactant is lost, further increasing the tendency to alveolar collapse. There is usually an increase in cardiac output and a rise in pulmonary artery pressure and resistance.

The addition of secretions and bronchoconstriction will further contribute to re-

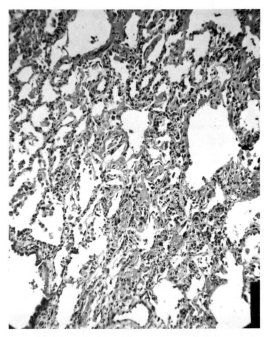

Figure 27–4 Late severe changes with atelectasis, extensive proliferation of granular pneumocytes, hyaline membrane formation, and intra-alveolar fibrin. Hematoxylin and eosin, 100 ×. (Courtesy of Dr. Richard Sabonya, M.D., Department of Pathology and Oncology, University of Kansas Medical Center.)

by breathing 100 per cent oxygen, oxygen is readily absorbed by the blood, partially open alveoli collapse, and shunting occurs. This has been described by Markello and is a very important reason to avoid the use of high oxygen concentrations in acute respiratory failure.[42,51] The production of progressive absorption microatelectasis in the sick lung is the important reason for the toxicity of oxygen in acute respiratory failure. Furthermore, the shunted blood is not exposed to the high concentration of oxygen. The only rise in blood oxygen is through the small increase in dissolved oxygen from the normal alveoli.

The amount of difficulty with oxygenation may be estimated by calculation of the alveolar-arterial gradient and by measurement of the shunt. The measurement of shunt on 100 per cent oxygen is a very sensitive and useful measure, as described in Diagnostic Methods (see Table 27–2 for formulae). Shapiro and Peters and West give more details.[63,69]

The predominant pathophysiological effects of acute respiratory failure are decreasing compliance due to small airway obstruction and collapse, alveolar septal edema, alveolar atelectasis, and shunting of venous blood that produces venous admixture and hypoxemia. Hypoxemia and rising carbon dioxide levels produce tachypnea, resultant hypocarbia, and the common clinical picture of hypoxemia, hypocarbia, and alkalosis.

Etiology

It is emphasized that the term "acute respiratory failure" is used here in a general sense, not to designate any specific etiology or pathological changes. It describes a series of events that commonly follows diverse kinds of influences on and injuries to the lung. It excludes chronic pulmonary and cardiac disease except as they may be pre-existing and complicate the clinical problem.

It is convenient to consider acute respiratory failure as it relates to traumatic and nontraumatic situations, i.e., after head and associated injuries and in the preoperative, operative, and postoperative settings.

Under its various synonyms, the clinical aspects of acute respiratory failure have been the subject of numerous reviews to which the reader is referred for detailed discussion.* Respiratory problems in the patient with multiple injuries and their management are discussed in Chapter 77. The following is a brief summary of some features of their etiology and clinical course, excluding chest injuries from discussion.

As one considers the diverse causes of acute respiratory failure, it is useful to remember that oxygenation can be adversely affected by only four mechanisms: failure of ventilation, failure of circulation, production of lung edema, and failure of respiratory control.

The conditions that set these mechanisms in motion nearly all occur in both the trauma patient and the elective operative patient. Acute respiratory failure is a preventable disease. It is easier to prevent than treat. Prevention depends on very early recognition before the gross changes of acute respiratory failure are present.

Failure of Ventilation

Airway Obstruction

Upper airway obstruction by foreign objects causes severe respiratory stridor or complete obstruction of breathing with rapid hypoxemia, hypercarbia, cyanosis, bradycardia, cardiac failure, and death. Lesser degrees of obstruction are produced by slack tongue and jaw, secretions, overdistention of the cuffs of endotracheal tubes, and angulation of tracheostomy tubes. Endotracheal tubes may enter the right main stem bronchus, with resulting occlusion and collapse of the left lung. On occasion, the tube may ride in and out of the right bronchus with respiration or motion of the neck but may appear to be in a safe position on chest x-ray. This condition can be diagnosed by fiberoptic bronchoscopy. Occlusion of the lower conducting airways usually results from secretions, mucous plugs, and airway or interstitial edema.

The terminal respiratory airways in the dependent portion of the lung have a tendency to close.[1,25] This is reflected in the re-

---

* See references 11, 23, 36, 37, 40, 43, 48, 52–54, 56, 60, 61, 66, 67.

duced functional residual capacity and the tendency toward shunting seen in acute respiratory failure and during anesthesia, immobility, and prolonged monotonous controlled ventilation without sighing. The propensity to terminal airway closure increases with age and with pulmonary congestion, overhydration, and hypocarbia. Thus any patient who is immobile because of central nervous system injury, drugs, or anesthesia, and subject to monotonous ventilation without sighing, may be susceptible to terminal airway closure and reduction in alveolar ventilation and functional residual capacity. Since this occurs in the dependent portion of the lung where perfusion is normally in excess of ventilation and where excess fluid accumulates, shunting results. In the supine patient, the posterior aspect of the lung is involved, while with the patient on the side, the dependent lung tends to be a shunt lung and the superior lung tends to be a dead space lung. This is the important reason for changing position frequently and avoiding monotonous ventilation by introducing large-volume sighs.

Use of a high inspired oxygen concentration ($FI_{O_2} > 50$ per cent) leads to progressive alveolar collapse, particularly in partially closed, hard to ventilate alveoli.[42] In addition, 100 per cent oxygen may be toxic to the cilia and paralyze the mucous elevator mechanism.

Aspiration

Aspiration of saliva and gastric contents occurs in patients who are unconscious from all causes including anesthesia.[16] The incidence rate is high (75 per cent) after trauma. In unconscious or ill patients, immobility, depression of reflexes (particularly from drugs), gastric dilation, and nasogastric or gastrostomy feedings all may be sources of aspiration. The tracheal burn of aspirated gastric juice is short lived and must be diagnosed promptly by fiberoptic bronchoscopy. It should be remembered that fasting patients may have large amounts of gastric juice to aspirate. Aspiration leads to edema, atelectasis, and pneumonia that is often due to gram-negative organisms. Tracheostomy with or without a cuff interferes with normal swallowing and leads to aspiration, while the use of oral endotracheal tubes may be associated with a lower incidence of aspiration.[17]

Decreased Compliance

As the lung becomes stiff, the alveolus is more difficult to ventilate. This means that higher pressures are needed to open the alveolus, which remains open for only a very short time at the peak of the pressure cycle. This leads to a tendency to collapse, especially if oxygen instead of nitrogen-containing air is breathed, as previously described. Aside from chest injuries and pain that restricts ventilation, the commonest cause of ventilatory failure due to decreased compliance is interstitial edema secondary to capillary damage or fluid overload.

Generalized Hypoventilation

Respiratory drive can fail or become ineffective because of injuries to the brain stem, drug overdosage, section of descending respiratory fibers during bilateral high cervical cordotomy, cervical cord injuries, and neuromuscular diseases such as myasthenia gravis.[31,32,50] Generalized decrease in ventilation leads to hypoxemia, hypercarbia, and acidosis in contrast to the usual hypocarbia and alkalosis of acute respiratory failure. The condition can be readily identified by measuring the tidal volume and analyzing the blood gases. Even in cervical cord injury, however, in which diaphragmatic breathing can deliver a tidal volume of only 150 to 300 cc and vital capacity is seriously reduced, the changes of acute respiratory failure usually supersede those of generalized hypoventilation so that shunting becomes a problem and hypoxemic tachypnea may lead to respiratory alkalosis rather than acidosis.

Failure of Circulation

The circulation may fail because of hypovolemia, cardiac failure, or pulmonary macroembolism or microembolism. Studies have shown that shock lung is probably not due to hypoperfusion but to the products of tissue injury that are filtered by the lung.[10,11] Thus, in trauma and during operations, precautions should be taken to filter blood being used for transfusion adequately. The problem of thrombophlebitis and pulmonary embolism is considered in Chapter 77. The maintenance of cardiac output in consonant relationship with volume of ventilation is important. Ordinarily, 5000 cc of air passes through the lung per minute and the cardiac output is 5000 cc; $\dot{V}/\dot{Q} = 1.0$. If ventilation fails and cardiac output increases, then the ratio of gas volume to volume flow of blood ($\dot{V}/\dot{Q}$) is less than 1.0 and conditions favor shunting. If circulation fails, then insufficient blood is delivered to the lung to be oxygenated, a large part of the lung may be dead space (ventilated, not perfused), circulation is inadequate to deliver oxygen to the periphery, and tissue ischemia may result. It is thus important to restore ventilation and perfusion to normal levels as quickly as possible and to avoid accumulation of the by-products of prolonged peripheral tissue ischemia that are so toxic to the lung.

The relation of cerebral injury and increased intracranial pressure to respiratory failure and pulmonary edema is reviewed by Rossi and Graf.[61] The evidence suggests that: (1) Neurosurgical patients share the same pulmonary problems as other patients. (2) Acceleration injury or sudden severe increase in intracranial pressure causes sympathetic discharge and release of catecholamines, which increase cardiac output, produce peripheral vasoconstriction and fluid shift to the pulmonary bed, and cause pulmonary venular constriction, all favoring interstitial pulmonary edema and its consequences.[9,23] These effects, however, are seen experimentally at intracranial pressures not commonly encountered clinically (100 to 200 mm of mercury). The facts are that fulminating pulmonary edema is rare in neurosurgical patients, being usually associated with arteriovenous aneurysm or bleeding in the hypothalamus or roof of the fourth ventricle. (3) The more common findings with moderate increases in intracranial pressure are increase in cardiac output, tachypnea, decrease in functional residual capacity, and hypoxemia due to shunting. In this neurosurgical patients resemble other patients with acute respiratory failure. Despite numerous clinical and laboratory studies, the exact relation between intracranial injury and pressure and pulmonary changes is still not clear in the clinical situation. The complexity of the changes occurring in the human situation makes definitive studies difficult.

Production of Lung Edema

During conditions of immobility, fluid accumulates in the dependent portions of the lung, as described previously, making the lung less compliant and more difficult to ventilate.[26,58,59]

During traumatic or operative shock, a number of substances are released that adversely affect the pulmonary vessels. The release of catecholamines produces pulmonary venular constriction and increased pressure in the capillary. Peripheral vasoconstriction shifts the fluid load from the peripheral circulation to the pulmonary bed, increasing hydrostatic pressure. A number of enzymes (including histamine, bradykinin, and serotonin) released during shock also have deleterious effects on the pulmonary vessels. The products of tissue destruction and ischemia are filtered by the lung and are vasodestructive. Two very important aspects are, first, production of microemboli of platelets, leukocytes, and fibrin from intravascular coagulation associated with shock and, second, the early onset of sepsis with release of endotoxin.[27] Fat emboli are reduced to fatty acids, which destroy the capillary endothelium. A further very important factor is the introduction in transfusions of particulate matter that acts as microemboli.

These factors all tend to damage the capillary endothelium, causing the loss first of water and then of protein to the alveolar septum. In the early phase of only water loss, the septal lymphatics can adequately transport excess septal water. When the process leading to capillary damage continues unrecognized, protein is lost and there is a marked increase in septal edema that swamps the lymphatic mechanism.

A final factor in production of interstitial edema is the introduction of excess crystalloid during operative maintenance or resuscitation from trauma. This fluid accumulates in the dependent lung, with resulting loss of compliance and shunting.

Control of water balance and prevention of interstitial edema are a very important part of the management of acute respiratory failure.

Failure of Respiratory Control

Lesions in the brain stem cause tachypnea, irregular breathing, ataxic breathing, or cessation of respiration. In addition, decerebration is associated with forced expiration, which reduces functional residual capacity.

Damage to automatic respiratory spinal pathways during cordotomy produces sleep apnea. Damage to both voluntary and automatic spinal pathways in cervical cord injury below C4 produces generalized hypoventilation, but the immobility and other factors soon cause the onset of all the features of acute respiratory failure: low ventilation, interstitial edema, shunting, and infection.[4]

In summary, whatever the clinical problem—head injury or elective neurosurgical procedure—there are certain factors that predispose to the development of acute respiratory failure: (1) unconsciousness with immobility and loss of protective reflexes, (2) aspiration, (3) airway obstruction, (4) terminal airway closure, (5) decreased ventilation, (6) decreased functional residual capacity, (7) microembolization of pulmonary vessels, (8) pulmonary venular constriction, (9) interstitial pulmonary edema, (10) decreased compliance, (11) pulmonary shunting (venous admixture), (12) hypoxemia, (13) reflex tachypnea and hyperventilation, (14) hypocarbia, (15) increased physiological dead space, and (16) increase in work of breathing.

The therapeutic requirements are: (1) maintenance of open airways to alveoli; (2) maintenance of adequate alveolar ventilation; (3) maintenance of adequate circulation; (4) prevention of embolization; (5) prevention of pulmonary edema; and (6) prevention of complication, especially infection.

Clinical Course of Acute Respiratory Failure

Since Moore's description of the four stages of the clinical presentation of shock lung, a number of authors have presented modifications.[11,37,43,52-54] Caution should be exercised, since acute respiratory failure secondary to fat embolism may progress differently from that associated with disseminated intravascular coagulation or head injury. Nevertheless, one can make a few generalizations regarding the typical course of acute respiratory failure, recognizing that there will be wide variations depending on the combination of clinicopathological conditions present.

Stage of Injury: 0 to 6 Hours

In the first six hours, the lungs are clear to auscultation and x-ray examination. Head injury may produce respiratory irregularity or tachypnea. Tachycardia, fever, elevated white count, and blood sugar may reflect sympathetic discharge with elevated catecholamine levels. If blood pressure is low owing to other injuries, large volumes of crystalloid, colloid, or blood products may be administered. In the confusion of ambulance pick-up, emergency room care, transfer to a tertiary care emergency room, x-ray, and operation, very large amounts of fluid may be given inadvertently through multiple intravenous channels. Well tolerated in the normal person, these resuscitative fluids may produce severe edema in the lung and brain whose vessels are damaged by injury. Unfiltered transfusions and tissue injuries introduce microemboli of blood elements, fibrin, fat, and collagen into the lung vessels.

Stage of Apparent Stability: 6 to 24 Hours

Tachypnea with low, normal, or high tidal volume is associated with mildly depressed or normal arterial oxygen tension (Pa_{O_2}, 80 to 100 mm of mercury) with the patient receiving an increased concentration of oxygen (FI_{O_2}) by mask. The cardiac output may be high, physical examination may be normal, and x-ray may be normal or show only vascular congestion.

Stage of Respiratory Failure: 24 to 48 Hours

Hyperventilation ensues with increased respiratory work, functional residual capacity decreases, and there is increasing hypoxemia despite increasing inspired oxygen concentration and progressive decrease in arterial carbon dioxide tension due to hyperventilation. Pulmonary shunting is present with increased alveolar-arterial gradient. Pulmonary edema is reflected by decrease in static compliance, and terminal airway closure from edema and secretions is reflected in decreased dynamic compliance. Physical examination shows rales and rhonchi, x-ray shows diffuse fleecy exudate, especially in the dependent lung. Respiratory alkalosis shifts the oxygen dissociation curve to the left as unloading of oxygen is decreased and tissue hypoxia is increased.

Terminal Stage: 48 Hours Onward

There are increasing hypoxia resistant to high inspired oxygen concentrations, progressive consolidation, and inability to ventilate the lung despite high ventilation pressures. Onset of infection, progressive consolidation of the lung apparent on physical and x-ray examination, and tissue hypoxia are evidenced by decreasing level of consciousness, bradycardia and arrhythmia, and renal failure.

Stage of Recovery

If recovery ensues, there may be no changes, or pulmonary fibrosis and limited pulmonary function may follow.[34]

Predisposing Factors

In patients undergoing elective neurosurgical procedures, a number of factors may produce pulmonary complications. Preoperatively a history of heavy smoking, asthma, chronic obstructive pulmonary disease, intercurrent infection, or diseases associated with reduced ventilation (arthritis, Parkinson's disease, pain) will all predispose to postoperative complications. Cardiac failure, a history of myocardial infarction, angina, arrhythmia, or abnormal cardiac or electrocardiographic findings also predispose to complications leading to pulmonary failure.[18] Poor technique during installation of intravenous lines and tracheal tubes paves the way for later infection.

During operation, factors predisposing to postoperative pulmonary complications are: excessive dosage of narcotics, barbiturates, or long-lasting agents that produce prolonged postoperative narcosis; paralysis of sympathetic vascular tone with use of excess fluid volumes to compensate for peripheral vasodilation, which on postoperative recovery of vascular tone produces central fluid overload; use of large amounts of unfiltered blood; monotonous tidal ventilation without sighs that leads to a decrease in functional residual capacity; and use of dry nonhumidified gas that leads to airway drying, ciliary paralysis, infection, and postoperative airway obstruction. The use of high oxygen concentrations to compensate for faulty anesthetic practices or to maintain artificially high Pa_{O_2} leads to closure of dependent alveoli and decrease in functional residual capacity. The practice of flushing the lungs with 100 per cent oxygen at the end of the operation and during transport to the recovery room is also harmful.

In the recovery room, the patient is usually awakened but soon drifts back to a semi-anesthetized state. He is frequently given supplemental oxygen instead of being forced to take deep tidal breaths. He is not turned—in short, all the factors leading to failure of ventilation and hypoxemia due to shunting are present. Continued administration of unrecognized large fluid volumes leads to edema. Sloppy technique of suctioning and pulmonary therapy guarantees later pulmonary sepsis.

The best treatment of acute respiratory failure is prevention. Clinical personnel must be aware of the insidious onset of the syndrome and the difficulty of its treatment once it is fully developed. Avoidance of the aforementioned adverse factors and careful monitoring for *early* signs of pulmonary difficulty will go far to prevent acute respiratory failure.

Diagnostic Studies

In the evaluation of pulmonary competence over time, the methods of physical diagnosis and radiological examination continue to be of prime importance. Because the key to the treatment of acute respiratory failure is prevention, it is essential to obtain warning of impending pulmonary failure before it reaches the stage of irreversible damage. The important changes are mechanical: failure of ventilation, fluid overload, and nonhomogeneous ventilation-perfusion relations. Monitoring procedures should make possible the early recognition of these changes.

There are many tests of pulmonary function that are appropriate to the pulmonary disease laboratory but not suitable to the intensive care unit in which the neurosurgical patient finds himself. Those of importance that are attainable in the clinical setting are: (1) physical examination (including fiberoptic bronchoscopy); (2) radiological examination; and assessment of (3) respiratory rate (RR), (4) tidal volume (VT) and derived minute volume ($\dot{V}$), (5) vital capacity (VC) or forced expiratory volume in one second (FEV_1), (6) physiological dead space (VD) or the ratio of dead space ventilation to total ventilation (VD/VT), (7) static and dynamic compliance, (8) cardiac output ($\dot{Q}$), (9) systemic arterial blood pressure (SABP), (10) pulse rate (PR), (11) pulmonary artery and wedge pressure (PPA and Pw), (12) hemoglobin (Hb), (13) arterial and mixed venous blood gases (Pa_{O_2}, $P\bar{v}_{O_2}$, Pa_{CO_2}, $P\bar{v}_{CO_2}$, and pH), (14) inspired oxygen (FI_{O_2}) and expired carbon dioxide ($F\bar{E}_{CO_2}$), (15) intake and output and daily weight of the patient, and (16) serum and urinary electrolyte levels and osmolalities.

Physical Examination

The presence of rales, rhonchi, and dullness to percussion are late signs of acute respiratory failure. Nevertheless, physical examination is important in detecting chronic pulmonary disease preoperatively and detecting failure of ventilation, airway obstruction, hemopneumothorax, and pleuritic reactions in the trauma patient. Physical examination, in correlation with radiological and physiological studies, is also important in following the course of treatment. An extension of the physical examination is bronchoscopy with the flexible fiberoptic bronchoscope, which permits direct visualization of the airways for gastric burns, secretions, edema, and mucous plugs.

Radiological Examination

The chest x-ray reflects only late changes in acute respiratory failure except for showing pre-existing disease preoperatively and the presence of lung injury in the trauma victim. It is very useful, however, in following the course of treatment, particularly of edema, pneumonia, and airway obstruction.[24]

The film should be examined for position of the artificial airway, it being remembered that the tube may ride in and out of the right main stem bronchus with respiration or movement of the neck. The size of the inflated cuff should be studied to avoid overdistention. Search should be made for mediastinal air to identify tracheal injury during trauma or intubation or later from cuff erosion. Late films should be examined for evidence of tracheal stenosis from prolonged intubation or cuff injury. Search should be made for atelectasis indicating obstruction of large or small airways (Fig. 27–5). Pulmonary contusion may be difficult to differentiate from aspiration or obstruction, since what appears to be contusion may disappear in hours with adequate ventilation (Fig. 27–6). The findings of aspiration are generally more diffuse and reflect the secondary changes in the lung from irritation by gastric contents (Fig. 27–7B). These changes may lead directly into those of bacterial pneumonia if untreated.

The chest film may give evidence of distention of the pulmonary vessels and indirect evidence of pulmonary edema (Fig. 27–8).

An especially important role of chest radiography is to distinguish pneumothorax

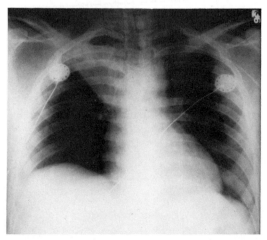

Figure 27–5 Right upper lobe atelectasis secondary to mucous plugging. Fiberoptic bronchoscopy is ideal for diagnosing and treating this problem.

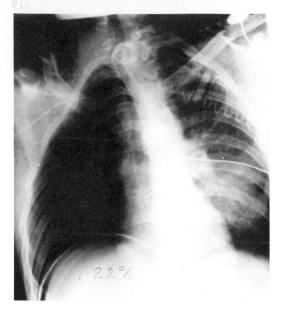

Figure 27–6 Segmental atelectasis, diagnosed as pulmonary contusion and associated with a 22 per cent shunt, cleared within four hours with adequate ventilation.

from trauma—from intubation or subclavian venous catheterization—and from the barotrauma associated with high-pressure machine ventilation (see Fig. 27–7A).

Isotope lung scanning is useful for studying the ventilation-perfusion relationship and confirming the presence of pulmonary emboli.

Since acute respiratory failure is preventable and treatment must center around prevention, the unconscious or traumatized neurosurgical patient must be closely monitored from the time of accident onward. Observations of physiological function give the earliest and most sensitive indications of impending respiratory complications.

Respiratory Rate

The earliest response of peripheral receptors to a fall in Pa_{O_2} or of the medullary receptors to a rise in Pa_{CO_2} is an increase in respiratory rate. The normal range is 10 to 16 breaths per minute, and a rate over 20 per minute should be viewed as indicating potential trouble, particularly if there is a trend upward. Rates over 30 per minute indicate severe respiratory distress and produce severe hypocarbia. The rhythm of respiration may give some clue to the location of the neurological lesion in certain cases: Cheyne-Stokes breathing with lesions at the level of the basal ganglia, hyperventilation with decerebration at collicular levels,

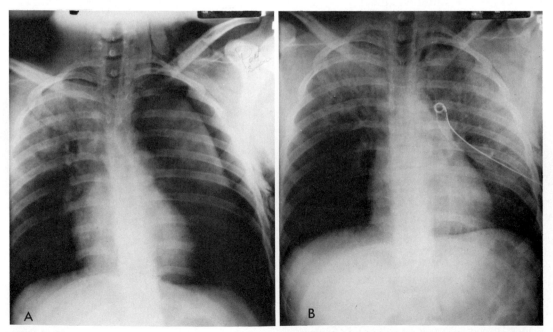

Figure 27–7   *A.* Chest injury with left pneumothorax and evidence of aspiration or contusion on the right. *B.* Following correction of the pneumothorax by chest tube, evidence of severe bilateral aspiration remains. The lungs are cleared with volume and positive end-expiratory pressure ventilation.

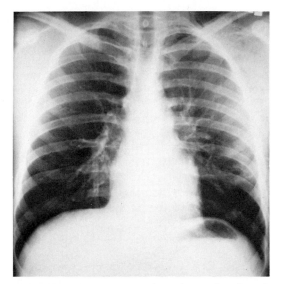

Figure 27–8 Vascular congestion and early pulmonary edema, particularly of the left upper lobe.

and irregular or ataxic ventilation with disorders at medullary levels.[50]

Tidal Volume

As pointed out previously, slow, large-tidal-volume breathing (7 to 15 cc per kilogram) is necessary for adequate alveolar ventilation. Low-tidal-volume, tachypneic ventilation diverts too much volume to dead space ventilation and results in poor diffusion of the alveolar gas. Measurement of tidal volume is necessary for the calculation of dead space. The tidal volume is easily measured with a Wright or similar respirometer (Fig. 27–9).

The product of rate and tidal volume gives the minute volume, a useful measure of total ventilation. Large minute volumes warn of severe hypocarbia and increased respiratory work, which may lead to exhaustion.

Vital Capacity and Forced Expiratory Volume in One Second

The maximum volume that can be exhaled after maximum inspiration is the vital capacity (VC), and the amount exhaled in the first second is the forced expiratory volume in one second (FEV_1); the latter is normally 80 per cent of the former. They are useful measures of the conscious patient's ability to expand the lungs. They are particularly useful pre- and postoperatively, in patients with cervical cord injuries, and during weaning from the ventilator. Of course, they do not measure how long the patient will be able to sustain adequate pulmonary drive. Even if vital capacity is adequate, the patient must be watched for exhaustion.

Physiological Dead Space

This represents wasted ventilation and added respiratory work. It is due to nonperfusion or poor perfusion of alveoli and may be calculated by measurement of tidal volume and arterial and mixed expired carbon

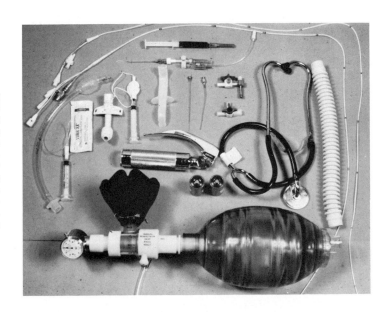

Figure 27–9 Equipment useful in treating acute respiratory failure. At the bottom, a self-inflating bag with a Rudolf valve to vary inspired oxygen concentration (FI_{O_2}) and a Wright respirometer to measure tidal volume. At top center is the arterial catheter with rubber stoppered side arm on the stopcock for taking arterial samples and the Sorenson Intraflow continuous-flush device. At left, plastic tracheal tubes with high-volume, low-pressure cuffs and Swan-Ganz catheters.

dioxide tension. It is usually expressed as the ratio of dead space to total ventilation:

$$\frac{V_D}{V_T} = \frac{Pa_{CO_2} - P\bar{E}_{CO_2}}{Pa_{CO_2}}$$

Static and Dynamic Compliance

Volume change per unit of pressure change is compliance, a useful measure of the elastic properties of a body. The compliance of the normal lung is about 200 cc per centimeter of water. If one follows the pressure dial on a ventilator, he notes a rapid rise of airway pressure to a peak at the end of inspiration and a rapid fall to resting pressure with each tidal volume. This peak pressure is a combination of the elastic properties of the thorax and the flow-restrictive properties of the airway. Since it is a combination of factors, it may be best termed dynamic characteristic rather than dynamic compliance.[12,13] If the outflow of the ventilator is occluded momentarily (by pinching the tubing or dialing in "expiratory retard"), the descending limb of the pressure curve will show a momentary plateau at which no air is flowing. This plateau pressure divided into the tidal volume gives the static compliance, the inverse of the thoracic elastance without air flowing. If one ventilates the lung at various tidal volumes and records the peak and plateau pressure for each volume, he can quickly plot dynamic and static curves, the former a measure of airway resistance and the latter a measure of lung stiffness (Fig. 27–

10).[12,13] Lung compliance alone without the chest wall factor can also be measured by recording esophageal pressures via an esophageal balloon as representative of pleural pressure and the pressure gradient from the airway to the esophagus taken as transpulmonary pressure. This method is more cumbersome than the simple method of using the ventilator described by Bone, which is as follows:

1. Explain the procedure to the patient if he is awake.

2. Insure adequate tracheal tube cuff pressure during the procedure to prevent leaks.

3. Dial in expiratory retard on the ventilator.

4. Select a series of volume settings to be used, such as 7, 10, 13, and 16 cc per kilogram body weight or 300, 500, 700, 900, 1100, 1300 cc.

5. For each volume, record spirometer volume, peak airway pressure, and plateau pressure. When positive end-expiratory pressure (PEEP) is being used, its pressure must be subtracted from peak and plateau pressures before charting. The compliance of the tubing is about 3 cc per centimeter of water. Thus:

$$\text{Static compliance} = \frac{\text{spirometer volume} - \text{tube volume}}{\text{plateau pressure} - \text{PEEP}}$$

6. Repeat this step for each volume setting selected.

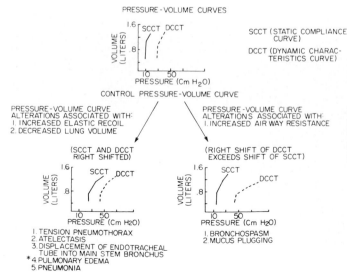

Figure 27–10 Normal and abnormal static and dynamic curves with notation of associated lung changes and clinical conditions associated with each. SCCT, static compliance curve; DCCT, dynamic characteristics curve.

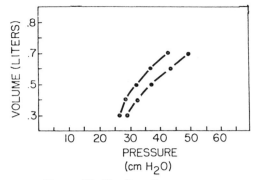

Figure 27–11 Compliance curves.

7. If at any setting, the pressure suddenly increases markedly, do not go to larger volumes, as barotrauma could result.

8. Remove expiratory retard.

9. Readjust cuff pressure.

10. Check ventilator completely.

11. Chart data on graph (Fig. 27–11). (Six such charts can be printed on an 8- by 11-inch sheet.)[12,13]

Inspection of Figure 27–10 indicates that conditions affecting the airway shift the dynamic curve to the right and flatten it (higher pressure per volume increase). Those conditions producing increased lung and thoracic stiffness shift both the static and dynamic curves to the right and flatten both. If the patient is hypoxemic and the compliance curves are normal, then pulmonary embolism should be suspected.

The factors that are important clinically in acute respiratory failure (atelectasis, edema, secretions, bronchospasm) produce mechanical changes in the elasticity of the lung and thorax, which can be measured by doing the foregoing compliance measurements. The great advantage of the method is that it requires no special equipment, takes only a few minutes, and can be done routinely by the respiratory therapist. The serial curves give early warning of decreasing compliance and an indication of whether the disease is in the airways, the lung parenchyma, or the circulation.[13] Further, the point at which the pressure curve breaks to the right indicates the optimum volume for inflation tidal volume; beyond this, inordinate pressure is required.

Cardiac Output

Today, serial cardiac output values are most easily determined by the thermal dilution method. It or the cardiac index gives a useful measure of the adequacy of central and peripheral blood flow. Adequate blood flow is an essential aspect of oxygen delivery, given by the formula:

$$\text{Oxygen delivery} = \text{cardiac output} \times Ca_{O_2}$$

Inadequate flow is associated with tissue hypoxia, anaerobic metabolism, and acidosis, factors that are very destructive to tissue capillaries.

Systemic Arterial Blood Pressure

Arterial blood pressure is an indicator of adequacy of cardiac output, fluid volume, and peripheral vascular tone. When hypotension ensues, the patient must be examined to determine which of the three components has failed. It is important to remember that in cervical cord injury the associated sympathetic paralysis leads to vasodilation with hypotension but normal tissue perfusion.

Pulse Rate

Failure of adequate cardiac filling causes reflex tachycardia, as does increased sympathetic activity with head injury. Bradycardia is an ominous indicator of severe anoxia as well as of severe posterior fossa pressure.

Pulmonary Artery and Pulmonary Wedge Pressure

The central venous pressure is a guide to adequate volume and to cardiac failure. The pulmonary artery pressure is an indicator of pulmonary hypertension with acute respiratory failure or of right ventricular failure. The wedge pressure corresponds to left atrial pressure and may be used to document an element of left atrial hypertension in pulmonary edema. These measurements require the use of a Swan-Ganz catheter, which may also be used for thermal dilution determinations of cardiac output. While these measurements may be available only in well-organized intensive care units, they do add very useful information about the critically ill patient.[30]

Hemoglobin

Serial hemoglobin measurements are needed to provide data about the oxygen content of the blood, since most of the volume of oxygen is carried to the tissues combined with hemoglobin. Depending on dilutional factors, the hemoglobin content also gives a rough estimate of red cell volume.

Arterial and Venous Blood Gases

The development of reliable clinical instrumentation for blood gas analysis has made possible the physiological evaluation of pulmonary complications. While oxygen is carried in bulk combined with hemoglobin, it is delivered to the tissue by its partial pressure in the blood, and this in turn is a reflection of the oxygen available to be delivered from the hemoglobin. Similar considerations apply to carbon dioxide. The ready measurement of gas pressures rapidly and reliably from small volumes of blood makes possible not only diagnosis but continuous assessment of results of treatment. One must be familiar with the errors of sampling, transport, and machine analysis. In particular, it is critical to know the fractional concentration of inspired oxygen ($F_{I_{O_2}}$) with each analysis. A Pa_{O_2} of 80 mm of mercury on room air ($F_{I_{O_2}} = 0.2$) is normal, but on 100 per cent oxygen ($F_{I_{O_2}} = 1.0$) or even 40 per cent oxygen, indicates serious pulmonary difficulty. Without the $F_{I_{O_2}}$ being known, a Pa_{O_2} of 80 mm of mercury indicates an adequate level for tissue oxygenation but tells nothing of the pulmonary situation.

The mixed venous oxygen ($P\bar{v}_{O_2}$) is obtained from a right atrial or pulmonary artery catheter and is an indicator of tissue oxygen utilization and blood flow. It is also needed for calculation of right-to-left shunt.

Inspired Oxygen and Expired Carbon Dioxide Concentrations

The importance of the inspired oxygen concentration ($F_{I_{O_2}}$) has been noted. The expired carbon dioxide concentration ($F\bar{e}_{CO_2}$ or $P\bar{e}_{CO_2}$) is useful as a measure of adequacy of ventilation and is used in the physiological dead space equation.

Not all of the foregoing measurements will be available to the neurosurgeon. Those that are important, however, and that can be done in any intensive care unit prepared to care for the seriously ill patient are: (1) physical examination; (2) radiologic examination; and determination of (3) respiratory rate, (4) tidal volume, (5) vital capacity, (6) static compliance and dynamic characteristics, (7) systemic arterial blood pressure, (8) pulse rate, (9) central venous or right atrial pressure, (10) hemoglobin concentration, (11) arterial blood gas levels, (12) inspired oxygen concentration, and (13) serum and urinary electrolyte concentrations and osmolalities.

Treatment of Acute Respiratory Failure

The previous sections have explored the problems associated with acute respiratory failure and emphasized the many factors that lead to inadequate alveolar ventilation and consequent hypoxemia secondary to right-to-left shunting and gas volume–to–blood volume ($\dot{V}/\dot{Q}$) inhomogeneities in relation to time. A logical treatment plan must be based on physiological principles and must not only consider the provision for adequate levels of peripheral oxygenation but must also insure that the treatment is restoring the lung itself to normal. Maintenance of normal oxygen tension by increasing the inspired oxygen concentration in the face of progressive lung failure is the worst kind of management.

The key to successful treatment of acute respiratory failure is *prevention*. This means that everyone must be aware of which patients are at risk and which conditions predispose to acute respiratory failure, and take measures to prevent its occurrence. It is a tribute to those who have brought about the recognition of this entity that the full-blown irreversible syndrome is rarely seen at present in well-equipped intensive care services.

Prevention

Elective Neurosurgical Procedures

The patient with normal lungs should be told preoperatively what his postoperative situation will be and given instruction and practice in deep breathing and, if necessary, incentive spirometry. He should avoid prolonged immobility preoperatively if possible. If he is a heavy smoker or has chronic lung disease, then several days of non-smoking, bronchodilator and mucolytic medication, chest therapy, drainage, and incentive spirometry deep breathing should precede any anesthesia. A complete evaluation and possible period of treatment by specialists in pulmonary disease may be in order before the operation. Infection if present must be treated appropriately.

During operation, anesthetic levels should be adjusted to be as low as possible at the end of the procedure to avoid postoperative narcosis, monotonous ventilation should be avoided, low concentrations of oxygen should be used to avoid reduction of functional residual capacity, gas should be humidified, and careful intubation and intravenous technique should be insisted upon to avoid later infection. Deep breathing should be instituted as soon as possible upon arrival in the recovery room, the patient should be turned frequently, and the sitting position should at least be alternated with the supine as soon as possible. If necessary, incentive spirometry should be started as soon as the patient can cooperate.

Trauma

A constant danger for the unconscious patient is aspiration. Hence, the unconscious trauma patient should be intubated with a nasal or oral tube of the largest convenient size with an integral low-pressure cuff, and the cuff should be inflated to just audible occlusion. The aim is to keep the cuff pressure below 20 mm of mercury to prevent tracheal erosion. Then if respirations are inadequate (less than 7 cc per kilogram) the patient should be ventilated with a self-inflating bag at about 15 times per minute, using about 50 per cent oxygen if possible. The volume of these bags is about 1000 cc, ideal for the purpose in the adult. The airway should be suctioned if necessary. Bleeding must be stopped and blood pressure restored by fluid administration (see Chapter 77). These measures must be instituted as soon as possible after the accident—preferably at the scene and by well-trained ambulance personnel.

Management of Acute Respiratory Failure

The fundamental rules of treatment are that it be begun as soon as possible, that it be based on physiological principles, and that it be terminated as soon as possible to avoid long-term complications such as in-

fection.[57] What are the indications for treatment?

PHYSICAL EXAMINATION. Tachypnea, dullness to percussion in the dependent lung, noisy breathing, rales, and friction rub are late signs of respiratory embarrassment. In any unconscious patient, the likelihood of impending difficulty should be anticipated.

RADIOLOGICAL EXAMINATION. Increased bronchovascular markings, infiltrates, pleural fluid or air indicate progressive respiratory failure.

RESPIRATORY RATE. Any rate over 20 breaths per minute is abnormal, and over 30 signifies severe problems.

TIDAL VOLUME. A measured volume of less than 7 cc per kilogram is inadequate. With developed acute respiratory failure, a tidal volume of 10 to 15 cc per kilogram may be needed.

VITAL CAPACITY. If the normal vital capacity of 70 cc per kilogram drops to 20 cc per kilogram or less, ventilatory assistance will be needed. Forced expiratory volume (FEV_1), which normally is 80 per cent of the vital capacity may also be used.

COMPLIANCE. Measurements shifted to the right as shown in Figure 27–10 indicate need for fluid restriction, increased ventilation, or airway clearance.

BLOOD PRESSURE. A rising blood pressure is a late sign of acute respiratory failure. A low pressure may indicate cardiac failure, low blood volume, or vasodilation due to cervical cord injury.

BLOOD GASES. A Pa_{O_2} below 70 mm of mercury indicates respiratory difficulty. If the Pa_{CO_2} is above 45 mm of mercury, there is generalized hypoventilation, as from drug overdose or muscle paralysis. If a Pa_{O_2} below 70 is associated with a Pa_{CO_2} below 35 mm of mercury, then the usual problems of acute respiratory failure—atelectasis and edema—are present and treatment is indicated. A volume-regulated ventilator should be used. The Bennett MA-1 has been found reliable and convenient. The usual procedure, subject to modifications in the individual case, is as follows:

1. Intubate the patient as described.
2. Check the position of the tube by auscultation and x-ray.
3. Ventilate by bag, with 50 per cent oxygen if necessary.
4. Check for aspiration—by fiberoptic bronchoscopy if necessary. If it is present,

lavage with saline, aspirate, and take specimens for culture as deeply as possible. Give methylprednisolone, 2 mg per kilogram every six hours for two days, then 2 mg per kilogram per day for two days.

5. Install an arterial catheter, attach a sterile three-way stopcock with a sterile rubber cap on a side arm through which samples may be drawn. To the stopcock attach a Sorenson continuous-flush Intraflow attached to a pressure fluid reservoir. This system is never opened, and its use prevents infection (see Fig. 27–9).

6. Measure the respiratory rate and tidal volume with a respirometer (see Fig. 27–9).

7. If the patient is breathing spontaneously, set the tidal volume at 10 cc per kilogram, or about 800 cc, and the rate guarantee at 10 per minute.

8. Set the inspired oxygen concentration ($F_{I_{O_2}}$) at 50 per cent; be sure the humidifier is functioning well.

9. Install a central venous pressure catheter or a Swan-Ganz pulmonary artery catheter, depending on the severity of the problem.

10. Measure dynamic and static compliance as described.[13]

11. Assess cardiac output if possible.

12. Put $F_{I_{O_2}}$ at 100 per cent for 15 minutes and repeat blood gas determinations. Return $F_{I_{O_2}}$ to 50 per cent. (Even this short exposure to 100 per cent oxygen will produce some atelectasis, so its use should be minimized). Calculate the shunt.

13. If the Pa_{O_2} on 50 per cent oxygen is 150 to 250 mm of mercury, gradually reduce the $F_{I_{O_2}}$ until the Pa_{O_2} is above 70 mm of mercury on room air, then gradually reduce the tidal volume to 7 cc per kilogram and prepare to wean the patient from the ventilator as soon as possible.

14. If the Pa_{O_2} is below 150 to 250 mm of mercury, increase tidal volume gradually to 15 cc per kilogram; check blood gases frequently. If it is found that the Pa_{O_2} is not rising, then it may be necessary to add continuous positive-pressure or positive end-expiratory pressure ventilation (CPPV or PEEP). The compliance curves will indicate the optimum tidal volume to be used.[13]

15. If positive end-expiratory pressure is used, begin at 5 cm and gradually increase to 15 cm if necessary.[39,41] Great care must be taken in hypovolemic patients because of the danger of decreasing cardiac output and in patients with increased intracranial pressure with low cerebral compliance.[3,15,22,23]

16. Fluid balance must be very carefully followed and overhydration avoided. Multiple transfusions must be carefully filtered. The patient being mechanically ventilated may receive 500 cc distilled water from the humidifier through his lungs and cannot lose water via the lungs as he does normally. Further, the ventilator and positive end-expiratory pressure stimulate antidiuretic hormone secretion, and hyponatremia and a positive water balance may occur. Parenteral fluids, including nutriment, must be carefully monitored and kept below 2000 cc per day if possible and less if necessary. Diuretics such as Lasix may be needed in addition.

Serial measurements of lung compliance, careful charting of intake and output and serum and urinary electrolyte levels and osmolarities, daily weighing of the patient, serial radiological examination, and maintenance of normal serum albumin are necessary to avoid pulmonary edema.

17. When repeated x-rays, blood gas determinations, compliance measurements, and shunt estimates indicate a return of lung function toward normal, positive end-expiratory pressure is reduced to 5 cm of water, and then inspired oxygen concentration is reduced to 30 per cent, or room air. Tidal volume is then gradually reduced to 7 cc per kilogram. *At this stage the patient's radiograph should be clear, the compliance should be normal, and arterial oxygen tension should be 70 mm of mercury on room air and 450 mm of mercury on 100 per cent oxygen for 15 minutes.* The patient is then ready to be weaned from the ventilator.[62]

18. Correct hypocapnia by increasing inspired carbon dioxide concentration or dead space, or by using intermittent mandatory ventilation (IMV). Owing to the lag of cerebrospinal fluid acid-base adjustment, at least four hours in which Pa_{CO_2} is above 40 mm of mercury are needed before the ventilatory drive will be adequate.

In the unconscious or semiconscious patient encountered so often in the neurosurgical intensive care unit, the use of intermittent mandatory ventilation is preferred to conventional T-tube weaning. The frequency of ventilator-supported breaths is gradually reduced while adequate tidal volumes and sighs are provided as needed.

Weaning is a period of trial and error, and necessitates close monitoring at all times.

19. Throughout treatment, the patient must be turned hourly if possible.

20. Antibiotics are not used except to treat bacteriologically proved and clinically evident infections.[29]

21. Fiberoptic bronchoscopy is useful in clearing secretions.

Representative Case

1. A 43-year-old man aspirated gastric contents after an auto accident in which he received a closed head injury. He became acutely dyspneic, and a diffuse infiltrate showed on the chest roentgenogram.

Laboratory findings:

Hemoglobin (Hb) = 10 gm
Inspired oxygen concentration (F_{IO_2}) = 0.4
pH = 7.36
Pa_{O_2} = 84 mm of mercury; saturation of arterial blood (Sa_{O_2}) = 94 per cent
Pa_{CO_2} = 30 mm of mercury
$P\bar{v}_{O_2}$ = 38 mm of mercury; saturation of mixed venous blood (Sv_{O_2}) = 70 per cent
Barometric pressure = 727 mm of mercury
Respiratory quotient (R) assumed to be 0.8

a. Calculate alveolar oxygen tension (PA_{O_2}).
b. Calculate alveolar-arterial gradient ($\Delta A - a$).
c. Calculate arterial-alveolar ratio (a/A).
d. Calculate arterial oxygen content (Ca_{O_2}).
e. Calculate mixed venous oxygen content ($C\bar{v}_{O_2}$).
f. Calculate coefficient of oxygen delivery (COD).

2. The inspired oxygen concentration is increased to 100 per cent because of deterioration.

Laboratory findings:

P_B = 727 mm of mercury
Pa_{CO_2} = 30 mm of mercury
Pa_{O_2} = 60 mm of mercury; Sa_{O_2} = 90 per cent
$P\bar{v}_{O_2}$ = 30 mm of mercury; $S\bar{v}_{O_2}$ = 60 per cent

a. Calculate shunt and coefficient of oxygen delivery (COD)

3. PEEP is begun at 15 cm of water. These values are obtained: On 100 per cent oxygen

P_B = 727 mm of mercury
Pa_{CO_2} = 30 mm of mercury
Pa_{O_2} = 80 mm of mercury; Sa_{O_2} = 95 per cent

$P\bar{v}_{O_2}$ = 28 mm of mercury; $S\bar{v}_{O_2}$ = 59 per cent
Hb = 10 gm

a. Calculate arterial oxygen content (Ca_{O_2}).
b. Calculate mixed venous oxygen content ($C\bar{v}_{O_2}$).
c. Calculate shunt.
d. Calculate coefficient of oxygen delivery.
e. What would you do with PEEP (increase, decrease, or keep the same)?

4. The patient deteriorates and a static and dynamic pressure-volume curve is done. The static compliance curve on the left and dynamic characteristics curves shown in Figure 27–11 were performed before acute deterioration. The values from the latest pressure-volume curves with corrected tidal volume (TV), static pressure (SP), and peak pressure (PP) are as follows:

TV (liter)	*SP* (cm H_2O)	*PP* (cm H_2O)
.3	32	35
.4	36	39
.5	40	47
.6	49	57

Plot the new pressure-volume curves on a pressure-volume plot. What is your differential diagnosis for these changes?

Answers

1. a. $PA_{O_2} = F_{IO_2}(P_B - 47) - \dfrac{Pa_{CO_2}}{0.8}$
$= .4(727) - 47) - 37.5$
$= 272 - 37.5$
$= 234.5$ mm of mercury

b. $\Delta A - a = PA_{O_2} - Pa_{O_2}$
$= 234.5 - 84$
$= 150$ mm of mercury

c. $a/A = \dfrac{Pa_{O_2}}{PA_{O_2}}$
$= \dfrac{84}{234.5}$
$= .36$

d. $Ca_{O_2} = .003\ Pa_{O_2} + 1.39\ (Hb)\ (Sa_{O_2})$
$= .003\ (84) + 1.39\ (10)\ (.94)$
$= .252 + 13.06$
$= 13.3$ ml per 100 ml.

e. $C\bar{v}_{O_2} = .003\ P\bar{v}_{O_2} + 1.39\ (Hb)\ (S\bar{v}_{O_2})$
$= .003\ (38) + 1.39\ (10)\ (.70)$
$= .114 + 9.73$
$= 9.84$ ml per 100 ml.

f. $COD = \dfrac{Ca_{O_2}}{Ca_{O_2} - C\bar{v}_{O_2}}$
$= \dfrac{13.3}{13.3 - 9.8}$
$= 3.8$

2. a. $\dfrac{\dot{Q}s}{\dot{Q}t} = \dfrac{(.003)(P_{A_{O_2}} - P_{a_{O_2}}) + Hb(1.39)(DS_{a_{O_2}})^*}{(.003)(P_{A_{O_2}} - P_{a_{O_2}}) + Hb(1.39)(DS_{a_{O_2}} + C_{a_{O_2}} - C\bar{v}_{O_2}} \times 100$

$P_{A_{O_2}} = 1(727 - 47) - 30$
$\quad = 650$ mm of mercury

$C_{a_{O_2}} = (.003)(60) + (1.39)(10)(.9)$
$\quad = .18 + 12.51$
$\quad = 12.69$ mm of mercury

$C\bar{v}_{O_2} = (.003)(30) + (.139)(10)(.6)$
$\quad = .09 + 8.34$
$\quad = 8.43$ mm of mercury

$\dfrac{\dot{Q}s}{\dot{Q}t} = \dfrac{.003(650 - 60) + 10(1.39)(.10)}{.003(650 - 60) + 10(1.39)(.10) + 12.69 - 8.43}$

$\quad = \dfrac{1.77 + 1.39}{1.77 + 1.39 + (12.69 - 8.43)}$

$\quad = \dfrac{3.16}{7.42}$

$\quad = 43$ per cent

$COD = \dfrac{C_{a_{O_2}}}{C_{a_{O_2}} - C\bar{v}_{O_2}}$

$\quad = \dfrac{12.69}{12.69 - 8.43}$

$COD = 2.98$

---

* $DS_{a_{O_2}}$ = Desaturation of arterial blood.

3. a. $C_{a_{O_2}} = (.003)(80) + 1.39(10)(.95)$
$\quad = .24 + 13.21$
$\quad = 13.45 (13.5)$

b. $C\bar{v}_{O_2} = (.003)(28) + 1.39(10)(.59)$
$\quad = .08 + 8.20$
$\quad = 8.28 (8.3)$

c. $\quad P_{A_{O_2}} = 1(727 - 47) - 30$
$\quad\quad = 650$

$\dfrac{Qs}{QT} = \dfrac{.003(650 - 80) + 10(1.39)(0.05)}{.003(650 - 80) + 10(1.39)(0.05) + (13.45 - 8.28)} = 32$ per cent

d. $COD = \dfrac{13.5}{13.5 - 8.3}$
$\quad = 2.60$

e. Although the arterial oxygen tension increases with PEEP, the cardiac output is decreased and tissue oxygen delivery as reflected by the coefficient of oxygen delivery and mixed venous oxygen has deteriorated. Since we are concerned with tissue oxygen, we either must decrease PEEP despite the fact that it is associated with improved arterial oxygen tension or administer volume or pharmacological agents to increase cardiac output.

4. Since both static and dynamic pressure-volume curves are right-shifted, the differential diagnosis includes causes of respiratory distress that are associated with loss of lung volume or parenchymal lung disease. These include: (1) atelectasis, (2) displacement of endotracheal tube into main stem bronchus, (3) pulmonary edema, (4) pneumonia, and (5) pneumothorax.

If the right-shifted dynamic characteristics curve had largely exceeded the right-shifted static compliance curve, conditions associated with airway disease such as bronchoconstriction and mucous plugging would be considered as diagnostic entities.

The aim of treatment is anticipation, prevention, vigorous prompt treatment, and termination of treatment as soon as possible to prevent complications.

Complications

The major short-term complications are barotrauma and infection; the long-term complication is fibrosis.[34] Intubation carries the risk of tracheal tears, erosion, stenosis, and infection. Pressure ventilation may cause barotrauma in the form of alveolar rupture and pneumothorax. Pressure ventilation may also depress cardiac output.

The most important complication is infection. It is introduced first with gastric aspiration and is gram-negative in origin, so infection appearing in the first 48 hours is gram-negative. From the second to the eighth day, infections are usually due to *Staphylococcus* and are due to comtamination associated with intubation, suction and catheter technique, dressings, and cross contamination by doctors, nurses, patients, and equipment. Infection should be documented by clinical signs, specific cultures, and sensitivity studies before antibiotic therapy is given.[29] As soon as signs of clinical infection have cleared, the antibiotic should be stopped in an effort to reduce superinfection by resistant organisms, fungi, and viruses.

REFERENCES

1. Airway closure. Editorial. Brit. J. Anaesth., *44*, No. 7, July, 1972.
2. Abrams, J. S., Deane, R. S., and Davis, J. H.: Pulmonary function in patients with multiple trauma and associated severe head injury. J. Trauma, *16*:543–549, 1976.
3. Apuzzo, M. L. J., Weiss, M. H., Petersons, V., et al.: Effect of positive end expiratory pressure

ventilation on intracranial pressure in man. J. Neurosurg., 46:227–232, 1977.

4. Bellamy, R., Pitts, F. W., and Stauffer, E. S.: Respiratory complications in traumatic quadriplegia. J. Neurosurg., 39:596–600, 1973.

5. Berger, A. J., Mitchell, R. A., and Severinghaus, J. W.: Regulation of respiration. Part 1. New Eng. J. Med., 297:92–97, 1977.

6. Berger, A. J., Mitchell, R. A., and Severinghaus, J. W.: Regulation of respiration. Part 2. New Eng. J. Med., 297:138–143, 1977.

7. Berger, A. J., Mitchell, R. A., and Severinghaus, J. W.: Regulation of respiration. Part 3. New Eng. J. Med., 297:194–201, 1977.

8. Bergren, D. R., and Beckman, D. L.: Pulmonary surface tension and head injury. J. Trauma, 15:336–338, 1975.

9. Berk, J. L., Hagen, J. F., Tong, R. K., et al.: The role of adrenergic stimulation in the pathogenesis of pulmonary insufficiency. Surgery, 82:366–372, 1977.

10. Blaisdell, F. W.: Pathophysiology of the respiratory distress syndrome. Arch. Surg., 108:44–49, 1974.

11. Blaisdell, F. W., and Schlobohn, R. M.: The respiratory distress syndrome: A review. Surgery, 74:251–262, 1973.

12. Bone, R. C.: Compliance and dynamic characteristics curves in acute respiratory failure. Crit. Care Med., 4:173–179, 1976.

13. Bone, R. C.: Thoracic pressure-volume curves in respiratory failure. Crit. Care Med., 4:148–149, 1976.

14. Brackett, C. E.: Respiratory complications of head injury. In Proceedings: International Symposium on Head Injuries, Edinburgh and Madrid, April 2 to 10, 1970. Edinburgh and London, Churchill Livingstone, 1971.

15. Brown, A. S.: Intermittent positive pressure ventilation in the management of severe head injuries. In Proceedings: International Symposium on Head Injuries, Edinburgh and Madrid, April 2 to 10, 1970. Edinburgh and London, Churchill Livingstone, 1971.

16. Cameron, J. L., and Zuidema, G. D.: Aspiration pneumonia. J.A.M.A., 219:1194–1196, 1972.

17. Cameron, J. L., Reynolds, J., and Zuidema, G. D.: Aspiration in patients with tracheostomies. Surg. Gynec. Obstet., 136:68–70, 1973.

18. Clark, K.: Pre- and postoperative care of the neurosurgical patient. Adv. Neurol., 15:235–250, 1976.

19. Comroe, J. H., Forster, R. E., Dubois, A. B., et al.: The Lung, Clinical Physiology and Pulmonary Function Tests. Chicago, Year Book Medical Publishers, Inc., 1962.

20. Devereaux, M. W., Keane, J. R., and Davis, R. L.: Automatic respiratory failure associated with infarction of the medulla. Arch. Neurol., 29:46–52, 1973.

21. Douglas, M. E., Downs, J. B., Dannemiller, F. J., et al.: Acute respiratory failure and intravascular coagulation. Surg. Gynec. Obstet., 143:555–560, 1976.

22. Downs, J. B., Klein, E. F., and Modell, J. H.: The effect of incremental PEEP on PaO$_2$ in patients with respiratory failure. Anesth. Analg., 52:210–215, 1973.

23. Ducker, T. B., and Redding, J. S.: Pulmonary complications in neurosurgery. Clin. Neurosurg., 23:483–493, 1976.

24. Eaton, R. J., Senior, R. M., and Pierce, J. A.: Aspects of respiratory care pertinent to the radiologist. Radiol. Clin. N. Amer., 11:93–107, 1973.

25. Fairley, H. B.: Airway closure. Anesthesiology, 36:529–532, 1972.

26. Fishman, A. P.: Pulmonary edema: The water-exchanging function of the lung. Circulation, 46:390–408, 1972.

27. Fulton, R. L., and Jones, C. E.: The cause of post-traumatic pulmonary insufficiency in man. Surg. Gynec. Obstet., 140:179–186, 1975.

28. Fung, Y. C., and Sabin, S. S.: Theory of sheet flow in lung alveoli. J. Appl. Physiol., 26:472–488, 1969.

29. Goodpasture, H. C., Romig, D. A., Voth, D. W., et al.: A prospective study of tracheobronchial bacterial flora in acutely brain-injured patients with and without antibiotic prophylaxis. J. Neurosurg., 47:228–235, 1977.

30. Katz, J. D., Cronau, L. H., Barash, P. G., et al.: Pulmonary artery flow-guided catheters in the perioperative period. J.A.M.A., 237:2832–2834, 1977.

31. Krieger, A. J., and Rosomoff, H. L.: Sleep induced apnea. Part 1: A respiratory and autonomic dysfunction syndrome following bilateral percutaneous cervical cordotomy. J. Neurosurg., 39:168–180, 1974.

32. Krieger, A. J., and Rosomoff, H. L.: Sleep-induced apnea. Part 2: Respiratory failure after anterior spinal surgery. J. Neurosurg., 39:181–185, 1974.

33. Kumar, A., Falke, K. J., Geffin, B., et al.: Continuous positive-pressure ventilation in acute respiratory failure. Effects on hemodynamics and lung function. New Eng. J. Med., 283:1430–1436, 1970.

34. Lakshminarayan, S., Stanford, R. E., and Petty, T. L.: Prognosis after recovery from adult respiratory distress syndrome. Amer. Rev. Resp. Dis., 113:7–16, 1976.

35. Lamy, M., Fallat, R. J., Koeniger, E., et al.: Pathologic features and mechanisms of hypoxemia in adult respiratory distress syndrome. Amer. Rev. Resp. Dis., 114:267–284, 1976.

36. Laver, M. B.: Acute respiratory failure: More questions, fewer answers. Anesthesiology, 43:611–613, 1975.

37. Laver, M. B., and Lowenstein, E.: Lung function following trauma in man. Clin. Neurosurg., 19:133–175, 1971.

38. Lensen, I.: Regulation of cerebrospinal fluid composition with reference to breathing. Physiol. Rev., 52:1–56, 1972.

39. Levine, M., Gilbert, R., and Auchincloss, J. W.: A comparison of the effects of sighs, large tidal volumes, and positive end expiratory pressure in assisted ventilation. Scand. J. Resp. Dis., 53:101–108, 1972.

40. Lowe, R. J., and Moss, G. S.: Pulmonary failure after trauma. Surg. Annu., 8:63–89, 1976.

41. Lutch, J. S., and Murray, J. F.: Continuous positive-pressure ventilation: Effects on systemic oxygen transport and tissue oxygenation. Ann. Intern. Med., 76:193–202, 1972.

42. Markello, R., Winter, P., and Olszowka, A.: Assessment of ventilation-perfusion inequalities by arterial-alveolar nitrogen differences in intensive care patients. Anesthesiology, *37*:4–15, 1972.

43. Moore, F. D., Lyons, J. H., Pierce, E. C., et al.: Post-Traumatic Pulmonary Insufficiency. Philadelphia, W. B. Saunders Co., 1969.

44. Murray, J. F.: The adult respiratory distress syndrome (may it rest in peace). Amer. Rev. Resp. Dis., *111*:716–718, 1975.

45. North, J. B., and Jennett, S.: Abnormal breathing patterns associated with acute brain damage. Arch. Neurol., *31*:338–344, 1974.

46. Nunn, J. F.: Applied Respiratory Physiology. London, Butterworth & Co., Ltd., 1971.

47. Peters, R. M.: The Mechanical Basis of Respiration. Boston, Little, Brown & Co., 1969.

48. Pierce, A. K., and Robertson, J.: Pulmonary complications of general surgery. Ann. Rev. Med., 28:211–221, 1977.

49. Plum, F.: Hyperpnea, hyperventilation, and brain dysfunction. Ann. Intern. Med., *76*:328, 1972.

50. Plum, F., and Posner, J.: The Diagnosis of Stupor and Coma. 2nd Ed. Philadelphia, F. A. Davis Co., 1972.

51. Pontoppidan, H.: The black box illuminated. Anesthesiology, *37*:1–3, 1972.

52. Pontoppidan, H., Geffin, B., and Lowenstein, E.: Acute respiratory failure in the adult. Part 1. New Eng. J. Med., 287:690–698, 1972.

53. Pontoppidan, H., Geffin, B., and Lowenstein, E.: Acute respiratory failure in the adult. Part 2. New Eng. J. Med., *287*:743–752, 1972.

54. Pontoppidan, H., Geffin, B., and Lowenstein, E.: Acute respiratory failure in the adult. Part 3. New Eng. J. Med., *287*:799–806, 1972.

55. Porter, R., ed.: Hering-Breuer Centenary Symposium. Ciba Foundation Symposium. London, J. & A. Churchill, 1970.

56. Prys-Roberts, C.: Respiratory problems of the seriously injured patient. Injury, *5*:67–78, 1973.

57. Rie, M. A., and Pontoppidan, H.: Ventilatory Complications: Prevention and Treatment. *In* American College of Surgeons: Manual of Surgical Intensive Care. Philadelphia, W. B. Saunders Co., 1977, pp. 219–250.

58. Robin, E. D., Cross, C. E., and Zelis, R.: Pulmonary edema. Part 1. New Eng. J. Med., *288*: 239–246, 1973.

59. Robin, E. D., Cross, C. E., and Zelis, R.: Pulmonary edema. Part 2. New Eng. J. Med., *288*: 292–304, 1973.

60. Rosen, A. J.: Shock lung: Fact or fancy? Surg. Clin. N. Amer., *55*:613–626, 1975.

61. Rossi, N. P., and Graf, C. J.: Physiological and pathological effects of neurologic disturbances and increased intracranial pressure on the lung. A review. Surg. Neurol., *5*:366–372, 1976.

62. Sahn, S. A., Lakshminarayan, S., and Petty, T. L.: Weaning from mechanical ventilation. J.A.M.A., *235*:2206–2212, 1976.

63. Shapiro, A. R., and Peters, R. M.: A nomogram for planning respiratory therapy. Chest, *72*:197–200, 1977.

64. Theodore, J., and Robin, E. D.: Pathogenesis of neurogenic pulmonary edema. Lancet, *2*:749–751, 1975.

65. Theodore, J., and Robin, E. D.: Speculations on neurogenic pulmonary edema (NPE). Amer. Rev. Resp. Dis., *113*:405–411, 1976.

66. Webb, W. R.: Pulmonary complications of non-thoracic trauma: Summary of the national research council conference. J. Trauma, *9*:700–711, 1969.

67. Webb, W. R.: Adult respiratory distress syndrome. Conn. Med., *40*:1–4, 1976.

68. Weibel, E. R.: Morphometry of the Human Lung. New York, Academic Press, 1963.

69. West, J. B.: Respiratory Physiology. Baltimore, Williams & Wilkins Co., 1974.

28

UROLOGICAL PROBLEMS ASSOCIATED WITH CENTRAL NERVOUS SYSTEM DISEASE

Malfunction of the urinary bladder due to disease of the central and peripheral nervous systems is a major clinical, social, and economic problem that has been documented by several authors.[14,56] Bradley and co-workers estimated there were over one and a quarter million people in the United States suffering from neurological dysfunction of the urinary bladder.[19] Neurogenic bladder with its resultant urinary incontinence and malfunction is not only a psychological and social nuisance and embarrassment; its long-term effects on renal function and general health are often marked and occasionally lethal.

Ruch has emphasized that, although the neural control of the urinary bladder is of great clinical importance to neurologists and urologists, and although the urinary bladder provides unique opportunities for basic physiological study, the clinical and basic disciplines have influenced each other relatively little.[107] Because of the lack of interplay between the disciplines and the complexities of the nervous system controlling normal micturition, significant advances in therapy for neurological dysfunction of the urinary bladder have been few. Even though the basic voiding difficulty may be reasonably well understood, translation of basic knowledge into effective therapeutic measures has been difficult. A case in point is the attempt to produce effective micturition by electronically stimulating the detrusor muscle.[19] Despite 10 years of extensive research, routine clinical application of a system that worked reasonably well in the laboratory has been frustrated by the inability to couple electrical energy effectively to stimulate contraction of the detrusor smooth muscle cells.

ANATOMY AND PHYSIOLOGY

Central Pathways Involved With Micturition

The area of the cerebral cortex that has been most directly linked to micturition reflexes is the anteromedial part of the frontal lobes at the level of the genu of the corpus callosum and including the anterior portion of the cingulate gyrus (Fig. 28–1).[3] Lesions in this area lead to frequency, urgency incontinence, and inability to suppress the micturition reflex.

A second region above the brain stem, the hypothalamus, is involved in the micturition reflex. Anterior and medial hypothalamic regions influence the tone and motility of the vesical walls.[122] Selective stimulation in this area will produce detrusor contractions, as seen on cystometry.[69] A relationship between the area in the superior frontal gyrus and anterior ventral hypothalamus has been proposed, i.e., the frontal area normally excites, inhibits, and controls the anterior hypothalamus as well as adjacent basilar areas.[4] Lesions of either area produce the same urinary symptoms. The hypothalamus does receive afferent connections from various portions of the frontal lobes, including the cingulate gyrus. Basilar areas and the hypothalamus have

G. L. ROCKSWOLD AND S. N. CHOU

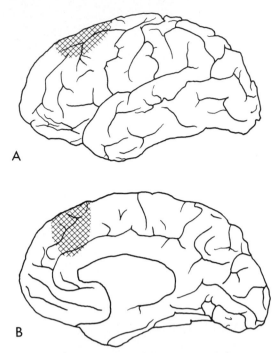

Figure 28–1 Cerebral area in frontal lobes at the level of the corpus callosum concerned with micturition reflexes. *A.* Lateral view. *B.* Medial view. (From Andrew, J., and Nathan, P. W.: Lesions of the anterior frontal lobes and disturbances of micturition and defaecation. Brain, *87*:233–262, 1964. Reprinted by permission.)

diffuse descending multisynaptic connections that project to the reticular formation of the brain stem.[31,124]

The second important series of connections is between the brain stem reticular formation centers for micturition and their connections with the parasympathetic motor neurons located in the sacral cord. A substantial body of knowledge appears to indicate that micturition is a brain stem reflex rather than one organized at the sacral level.[7,15,16,37] Barrington, in a classic series of experiments on the nervous mechanisms of micturition in cats, determined the level in the central nervous system of the origin of the motor tone of the bladder.[7] He found that section of the cord or medulla caused the bladder to lose tone, to dilate, and to lose spontaneous contractions. If the section was made at the midbrain level, the tone of the bladder increased and the capacity decreased. He concluded that the motor tone was arising in the rostral portion of the pons.

In later experiments, Barrington at-

tempted to identify more specifically the site of a micturition center from which the detrusor reflex arose.[8] Using Clarke and Horsley's stereotaxic device, he found that destroying a small part of the dorsal lateral part of the rostral pons at the level of the middle of the motor nucleus of cranial nerve V produced a permanent inability to void if the lesion was bilateral, but not if it was unilateral (Fig. 28–2). Subsequent experiments have confirmed this as the location of a very active detrusor motor center.[15,76]

DeGroat and Ryall have studied the reflexes of the sacral parasympathetic neurons by stimulating pelvic nerves and recording both intracellularly and extracellularly in the parasympathetic neurons.[37] They found that because the loop reflexes went to the brain stem, long-latency (150–250 msec) responses predominated in the cat with an intact spinal cord. Immediately following cord section, no activity could be recorded in response to either bladder filling or pelvic

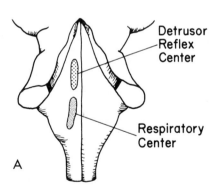

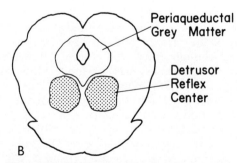

Figure 28–2 Diagram of micturition center for the detrusor reflex located in pontine reticular formation at the level of the motor nucleus of fifth cranial nerve. *A.* Posterior view. *B.* Cross-sectional view. (From Bradley, W. E., Timm, G. W., and Scott, F. B.: Innervation of the detrusor muscle and urethra. Urol. Clin. N. Amer., *1*:3–27, 1974. Reprinted by permission.)

Figure 28–3 Location of the efferent pathways to the urinary bladder in the lateral columns of the spinal cord. *A.* Cat. *B* and *C.* Human. *D.* Rhesus monkey. (*A* from Barrington, F. J. F.: The localization of the paths subserving micturition in the spinal cord of the cat. Brain, *56:*126–148, 1933. *B* from McMichael, J.: Spinal tracts subserving micturition in a case of Erb's spinal paralysis. Brain, *68:* 162–164, 1945. *C* from Nathan, P. W., and Smith, M. C.: The centrifugal pathway for micturition within the spinal cord. *J. Neurol. Neurosurg. Psychiat. 21:*177–189, 1958. *D* from Kerr, F. W. L., and Alexander, S.: Descending autonomic pathways in the spinal cord. Arch. Neurol., *10:*249–261, 1964. Reprinted by permission.)

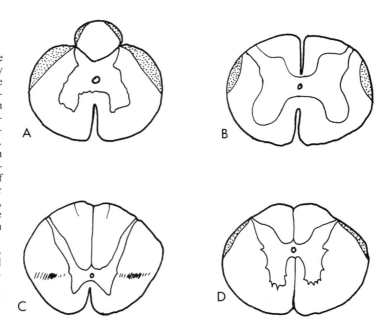

nerve stimulation. After 7 to 28 days, weak short-latency responses could be recorded that corresponded well to the establishment of reflex bladder function.

Several investigators have studied the course of the autonomic pathways to the urinary bladder in the spinal cord.[10,69,110] Experiments have been performed primarily in cats, but a few in Rhesus monkeys showed similar findings. It was determined that these pathways lie in the dorsal aspect of the lateral columns (Fig. 28–3). It was also determined that there was extensive crossover of the autonomic pathways in the lower thoracic and upper lumbar area. Because of this extensive crossover of the fiber tracts innervating the urinary bladder, bilateral spinal cord lesions were required to produce lasting urinary bladder dysfunction. Nathan and Smith determined that the principal afferent and efferent pathways for micturition in the spinal cord in man were also within the lateral columns (see Fig. 28–3).[91,92] They based this conclusion on careful correlation of a clinical evaluation of the patient with a postmortem histological examination of the spinal cord. They also concluded that unilateral lesions of the spinal cord pathways did not significantly interfere with voiding. McMichael found the posterior aspect of the lateral columns to be degenerated in a patient with isolated symptoms of abnormal micturition (see Fig.

28–3).[85] Findings are thus consistent with the experimental investigations in animals.

The supraspinal pathways of the striated muscle of the external anal and periurethral sphincters arise in the motor cortex and descend through the pyramidal tracts.[20] These descending pathways impinge on the pudendal nerve anterior horn cells in the sacral cord. Intact supraspinal control of the sphincters allows one to contract the sphincter at will during a micturition or defecation reflex. There are also reflex connections between detrusor sensory fibers that synapse on the anterior horn cells of the pudendal nerve nuclei, giving synaptic connections between the detrusor muscle and the external urethral and external anal sphincters.[17,40,49]

Peripheral Innervation of the Urinary Bladder and Sphincters

Peripheral innervation of the urinary bladder and sphincters in humans has been studied primarily by the dissection of cadavers and investigations in experimental animals.[58,71,93,109,125] Additional information has been obtained by studying the effect of sacral nerve blocks on the function of the urinary bladder in humans and by direct stimulation of ventral roots during rhizotomies to improve bladder function or to improve muscular spasticity.[60,89,99,100,115]

These studies indicate that the innervation to the urinary bladder arises primarily in the S3 and S4 sacral segments and to a lesser extent in the S2 sacral segment. It is parasympathetic in origin and passes over the ventral roots entering the pelvic plexuses and pelvic nerves to innervate the detrusor muscle. This parasympathetic innervation is essential for normal micturition; its interruption results in paralysis of the detrusor muscle. It also carries essential afferent impulses for the micturition reflex. Recently acquired experimental evidence in primates (Rhesus monkeys and chimpanzees) indicates that certain rootlets and fascicles within the sacral roots conduct impulses primarily to the urinary bladder and that others conduct impulses to the anal and urethral sphincters. Therefore, segregation, or a localized fascicular pattern, of nervous innervation of these structures is present within the sacral spinal roots.[97]

The sympathetic innervation of the bladder arises from the intermediolateral cell column of T10 to L2 and travels via the ventral roots and splanchnic nerves to the preaortic plexuses.[82] The fibers pass inferiorly and form a fine plexus between the iliac arteries that is termed the inferior hypogastric plexus. These nerves continue inferiorly over the sacral promontory and join the pelvic plexus and parasympathetic fibers to innervate the urinary bladder. The area of the trigone and bladder neck has been found to be particularly heavily innervated by sympathetic fibers.[44,45] Stimulation of the presacral or hypogastric nerves in experimental animals and man produces closure of the bladder neck.[51,72,82] The same effect can be produced with alpha-adrenergic stimulating agents such as epinephrine, ephedrine sulfate, or metaraminol bitartrate (Aramine).[42,72,82] Blockade of this effect and actual relaxation of the internal urinary sphincter can be produced with alpha-adrenergic blocking agents such as phenoxybenzamine (Diabenzyline) and phentolamine (Regitine).[51,72,118]

There is experimental evidence in cats that sympathetic pathways to the bladder exert a significant regulatory influence on micturition.[36,38,39,43] Stimulation of the bladder afferents in the pelvic nerves by electric pulses or vesical distention produced reflex firing in the hypogastric nerve, which produced an inhibition of bladder smooth muscle and transmission in vesical ganglia that allowed the bladder to accommodate larger volumes. Increased firing in the sympathetic fibers to the bladder neck increased outlet resistance and was thus complementary. With the onset of micturition and micturition pressures above a critical level, these reflexes are markedly inhibited, allowing micturition to proceed.

The pudendal nerve arises from the anterior primary rami of S2, S3, and S4.[52] The nerve terminates by dividing into three branches, the inferior hemorrhoidal, the perineal, and the dorsal nerve of the penis. The inferior hemorrhoidal nerve supplies the external anal sphincter as well as the adjacent skin. The perineal nerve, which has a deeper branch, innervates the striated muscle surrounding the membranous urethra as well as other perineal musculature. Normally, under resting conditions, continence is achieved at the bladder neck and proximal urethra.[5,26,77,78,113] The anatomical relationship between the proximal urethra and bladder base is critical in allowing the smooth muscle fibers that form the internal urinary sphincter to exert sphincteric resistance in a passive manner. When this anatomical relationship between the proximal urethra and bladder base is altered by detrusor contraction and perineal floor relaxation, the bladder neck opens and voiding occurs. Dye in the bladder does not extend into the urethra even under spinal anesthesia.[26] Bilateral pudendal nerve blocks or striated muscle relaxants do not result in urinary incontinence.[78] Under normal circumstances the external sphincter is used to maintain continence during sudden or marked increases in intravesical pressure and to interrupt urinary flow voluntarily.[42,72]

Summary of Events Occurring During Normal Micturition

The complex reflexes involved with micturition and their interreaction are not well understood. Based upon a synopsis of the evidence for the events occurring in micturition, however, the sequence may be as follows. There is very little increase in bladder wall tension as the volume of urine in the bladder gradually increases. The internal urinary sphincter passively maintains continence. At low resting pressures, the afferent discharge is insufficient to elicit the micturition reflex.[37] As urine volume increases, however, a certain critical pressure is reached, and the afferent discharge is of sufficient intensity to reach consciousness. Cerebral inhibition of the brain stem micturition center is released, allowing distention of the bladder to result in detrusor contraction via a brain stem reflex. Contraction of the bladder also leads to opening of the bladder neck by mechanical means.[62,63] There is also simultaneous relaxation of the external urethral sphincter via reflex connections between the pelvic and pudendal nerves.[40,49] Passage of the urine through the urethra reinforces excitation of the parasympathetic neurons via a long-routed brain stem reflex.[9] These combined actions produce a self-perpetuating reflex mechanism that continues until the bladder is empty. With the bladder empty, the external urethral sphincter again resumes its tone, and with bladder wall tension relieved, the reflexes become inoperable.

DIAGNOSTIC METHODS

Gas Cystometry

The basic neurourological diagnostic procedure is cystometry.[102] This procedure consists of retrograde filling of the urinary bladder through an indwelling catheter with either gas or liquid while intravesical pressure is recorded continuously. Carbon dioxide is preferred over saline because filling times are much faster and there is less artifact, owing to the lesser viscosity of the gas.[21] At the intravesical pressures recorded, there is no more than a 10 per cent decrease in volumes due to the compressibility of carbon dioxide as compared with saline.[30]

The principal observation that has been made from the cystometrogram is the presence or absence of a detrusor reflex. The reflex stimulus was passive distention of the bladder and the response was a contraction of the detrusor muscle producing an intravesical pressure rise. If a detrusor reflex was evoked the patient was asked to suppress the reflex as a test of detrusor reflex volitional control. Inability to suppress the reflex is an event frequently termed an uninhibited detrusor reflex (Fig. 28–4). Since

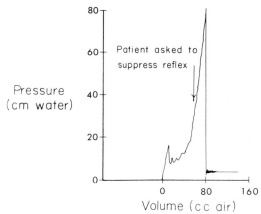

Figure 28–4 Cystometrogram demonstrating uninhibited detrusor hyperreflexia.

this situation often occurs with a low-volume reflex threshold it has been termed detrusor hyperreflexia. Clinically, these cystometrographic findings are associated with the sensation of urgency and frequent precipitate voiding with little voluntary control. In the case of complete absence of a detrusor reflex on cystometry (areflexia), the patient usually had difficulty in initiating effective voiding and in emptying the bladder. Cystometry should be routinely performed with the patient in the supine, sitting, and standing positions, as well as walking in place. Not infrequently detrusor hyperreflexia can be induced in one position but not another.[2]

Sphincter Electromyography

There are two basic methods of electromyography of the sphincters.[18,22] One involves the insertion of recording wires into the sphincters, which allows precise anatomical placement of the recording electrodes and is important for studying denervation potentials and evidence of muscle injury. This technique also has the advantage of simultaneously recording intravesical pressures and urinary flow rates. Its disadvantages are that only a small localized sample of muscle activity is obtained and there is discomfort for the patient associated with the insertion and reinsertion of the recording electrodes. The second major method makes use of externally mounted bipolar electrodes on an hourglass plug when the anal sphincter is being examined and external electrodes mounted on a catheter inserted into the urethra when the external urethral sphincter is being studied. These electrodes lie adjacent to the respective sphincter muscles and record the net electrical output of the sphincter (see Fig. 28–10). This type of recording obviates the discomfort and inconvenience of the insertion and reinsertion of needle electrodes.

Traditionally, electromyographic studies of the external anal and external urethral sphincters have been considered parallel because of the identical embryological origin of the structures, namely the cloaca.[13] Therefore, the more readily accessible external anal sphincter has frequently been evaluated electrically as representative of both sphincters. There is some evidence, however, to indicate that the various muscles of the pelvic floor do not act in concert in some pathological conditions.[119]

Patients should be routinely asked to contract the sphincters volitionally to determine if supraspinal innervation is intact.[102] Also, it is important to perform cystometry and electromyography of the sphincters simultaneously in order to study the interaction of the two essential elements of voiding, detrusor contraction and sphincter function. Combining these studies gives a dynamic picture of the peripheral events involved in micturition. Various abnormalities in detrusor or sphincter function can be determined that would not be readily apparent if the tests were not done simultaneously.

Evoked Response Technique

Contraction of either the external anal or external urethral sphincters can be produced by stimulation of the mucosa of the bladder or urethra (Fig. 28–5).[23,103] The pathway for this induced reflex is via the pelvic nerves and cauda equina to the sacral spinal cord. There the pudendal nerve nucleus is activated, producing contraction of the sphincters. The latency for this reflex evoked response has been determined to be approximately 50 to 80 msec (Fig. 28–6). Anesthetizing the mucosa of the bladder with local anesthetic obliterates the response, indicating that the response is not due to local stimulus spread. Caudal block also obliterates the response, indicating that the evoked response must pass through the sacral spinal cord.

This technique appears to be a useful clinical tool to determine the anatomical integrity of pathways from the bladder and urethra to the sacral spinal cord, including the pelvic nerves, cauda equina, and conus

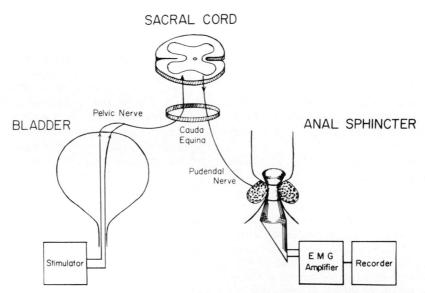

Figure 28–5   Diagram of neural pathways involved with evoked electromyographic technique. (From Rockswold, G. L., Bradley, W. E., Timm, G. W., and Chou, S. N.: Electrophysiological technique for evaluating lesions of the conus medullaris and cauda equina. J. Neurosurg., *45*:321–326, 1976. Reprinted by permission.)

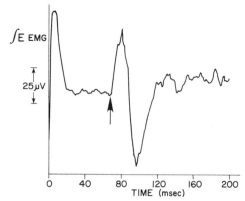

Figure 28–6 Evoked electromyographic response in the anal sphincter produced by stimulation of the urethra in a normal volunteer.

medullaris as well as the pudendal nerves. Various lesions have been shown to produce increased latencies and depressed responses or complete loss of response, depending on the extent of the lesion (Fig. 28–7).

Urethral Pressure Profiles

Urethral pressure profilometry is the measurement of the intrinsic pressures of the various segments of the urethra. Two basic techniques are in use for determining urethral pressure profiles. The most commonly used method is the mechanical withdrawal of a fluid- or gas-filled catheter

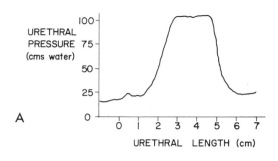

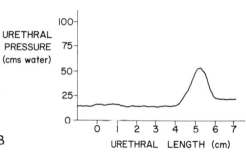

Figure 28–8 Urethral pressure profiles of patient whose intermittent urinary stream and retention were relieved by internal sphincterotomy. *A.* Before internal sphincterotomy. *B.* Post–internal sphincterotomy.

through the urethra while simultaneously measuring the critical escape pressure of the gas or fluid (Fig. 28–8).[24,59] Second, miniature transducers mounted on the tip of finely caliberated catheters that traverse the urethra have also been used.[22] These transducers are fragile and expensive.

It has been determined that the contribution of the striated muscles of the external sphincter to the urethral pressure profile is very small unless active contraction is performed.[42] The urethral pressure profile is largely determined by the tonus of adrenergically innervated smooth muscle. Therefore, when coupled with electromyography of the external sphincter and cystometry, urethral pressure profiles can be especially valuable in determining whether the amount of outlet urethral resistance is appropriate during bladder filling and voiding.

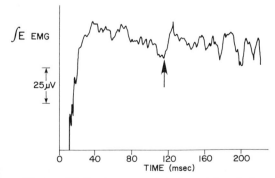

Figure 28–7 An example of a delayed fragmented electromyographic response in a patient with a sacral chordoma. (From Rockswold, G. L., Bradley, W. E., Timm, G. W., and Chou, S. N.: Electrophysiological technique for evaluating lesions of the conus medullaris and cauda equina. J. Neurosurg., *45*:321–326, 1976. Reprinted by permission.)

Urinary Flow Rates

Uroflowmetry is a good measure of the effectiveness of detrusor contraction and sphincter relaxation.[29,111] When coupled with intravesical pressure measurements, it

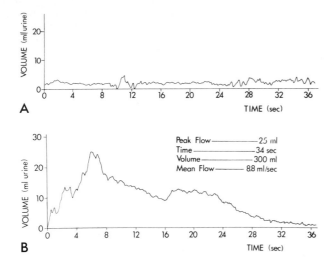

Figure 28–9 Urinary flow rate in a patient with detrusor-sphincter dyssynergia. *A.* Prior to sacral nerve block. *B.* After sacral nerve block.

can aid in defining anatomical obstruction of the urethra. Measurements of urinary flow can be determined from (1) variations produced in a constant magnetic field by electrolytes in the urine, (2) the energy imparted to a rotating disk by the urinary stream, (3) measurement of the weight of a column of urine, and (4) measurement of the cooling effect of urine on a hot wire.[22] Monitoring the weight of urine has proved to be an efficient and accurate method of measuring urine flow (Fig. 28–9).[121] It has been determined by Susset and associates that the total volume of urine in the bladder is the most important determinant of the flow rate in the normal situation.[111] As the volume in the bladder increases, the urinary flow rate increases proportionally. Flow rate is also related to the caliber of the urethra, which is wider in females, giving them on the average greater flow rates. The maximum urinary flow rate is the value most often noted. Maximum flow rates of less than 15 ml per second are usually abnormal and indicate ineffective detrusor contraction or outlet obstruction.

Denervation Suprasensitivity Test

Lapides and associates developed a test intended to diagnose lower motor neuron lesions of the urinary bladder and based on the fact that a denervated organ becomes suprasensitive to its neurohumeral transmitter.[81] The test consists of filling the bladder with water or gas and observing the in-travesical pressure at 100 cc of volume. After several control runs the patient is given 2.5 mg of bethanechol (Urecholine) and the cystometrogram is repeated at 10, 20, and 30 minutes following administration of the drug. A positive result indicative of denervation is an elevation of pressure greater than 15 to 20 cm above control value at 100 cc of volume.

Voiding Cystourethrogram and Intravenous Pyelography

A voiding cystourethrogram and an intravenous pyelogram should be a routine part of the evaluation of patients with neurological bladder dysfunction. The voiding cystourethrogram detects urethral pathological changes such as diverticulae and fistulae as well as urethral strictures or other evidence of obstruction. Bladder size and configuration are determined as well as the presence of trabeculation and vesical-urethral reflux. Excretory urography is the best means of screening the upper urinary tract. It is essential to rule out evidence of hydronephrosis, hypoplastic kidney, ureteral reflux, and other abnormalities that are uncommon but occasionally associated with chronic neurogenic bladder disease.

Urological Consultation

In the evaluation of neurological bladder disease, close cooperation with a urologist who is familiar with and interested in this problem is obviously very beneficial and at times essential. Treatment of upper urinary tract complications including calculosis, hydronephrosis, pyelonephritis, ureteral reflux, and lower urinary tract obstruction all falls within the domain of the urologist.

CLINICAL AND LABORATORY FINDINGS

Detrusor Reflex Dysfunction

Hyperreflexia

The cystometrogram is used to distinguish two abnormalities of detrusor reflex function that are very important in defining treatment.[102] The first is detrusor hyperreflexia, which is defined as detrusor reflex contraction that cannot be voluntarily suppressed by the patient (see Fig. 28–4). This reflex can occur at either very low volumes of gas or fluid, in which case it is termed a low-threshold detrusor hyperreflexia, or at higher volumes. Detrusor hyperreflexia has been referred to by many names, among them spastic bladder, uninhibited bladder, and hyperactive or hypertonic bladder. The urinary symptoms associated with detrusor hyperreflexia usually consist of frequency and urgency leading to incontinence if sphincter function is impaired. The incontinence is caused by inability to suppress the hyperactive detrusor reflex voluntarily.

Detrusor hyperreflexia can result from injury to or interruption of the pathways from the cerebral cortex to the brain stem and also from injury of the reflex arc between the brain stem centers and the sacral cord. Various neurological diseases occurring in the cerebrum that would interrupt these pathways would include head injury, brain tumors, cerebral vascular disease, hydrocephalus, and various degenerative diseases such as the dementias and multiple sclerosis.

Lesions involving the spinal cord would include trauma, arachnoiditis, degenerative diseases such as multiple sclerosis, tumors, herniated intervertebral discs, congenital deformities, and subdural and epidural hemorrhage or abscess. These lesions can produce either an incomplete or complete transverse myelitis. Following a complete transverse spinal cord lesion above the conus medullaris, detrusor hyperreflexia develops secondary to increased reflex activity in the isolated distal spinal cord.

Areflexia

Detrusor areflexia is the second major abnormality of detrusor reflex function (Fig. 28–10). Patients with the syndrome of an absent detrusor reflex most frequently relate a history of difficulty initiating voiding and not infrequently of complete retention. If voiding does occur, the flow rate is frequently decreased, the flow is intermittent, and significant residual urine remains. If there is uninhibited sphincter relaxation associated with the detrusor areflexia, incontinence may result. Incontinence may

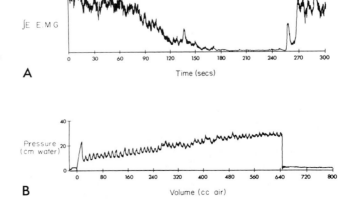

Figure 28–10 Uninhibited sphincter relaxation associated with detrusor areflexia and increasing bladder distention. *A.* Anal sphincter electromyogram. *B.* Cystometrogram.

also result from overflow and distention of the bladder.

The diagnosis of areflexia can be made only with caution, as voluntary suppression of reflex activity can result from the embarrassment or discomfort of the examination environment. Areflexia can also result from various nonneurological causes such as chronic infection, overdistention, or long-term catheter drainage of the urinary bladder. Various drugs can also produce areflexia. These include the phenothiazines and belladonna derivatives as well as various ganglionic blocking agents used for treatment of hypertension.

Various disease processes affecting the nervous system can also produce detrusor areflexia. These processes would include injury to the cauda equina or conus medullaris; spinal shock following injury to the supranuclear portion of the spinal cord; centrally located herniated lumbar discs; arachnoiditis of the cauda equina following myelography or herniated disc operations; spinal cord birth defects, most prominently myelomeningocele; tumors of the conus medullaris or cauda equina; and diabetes mellitus producing an autonomic neuropathy. It is important to rule out the presence of obstruction in the lower urinary tract in cases of areflexia. The evoked response technique described earlier can be used to determine whether there is denervation of the bladder from the various lesions listed.

Urinary Sphincter Dysfunction

Under normal conditions, a minimal tonic activity can always be recorded in the perineal muscles even when the bladder is empty and the patient is in a relaxed supine position. When the patient moves to a standing position there is usually a slight increase in activity. Cough or other Valsalva maneuvers produce an abrupt increase in the activity of the perineal muscles. There is a corresponding increase in intraurethral and intravesical pressure. During filling of the bladder an increase in electromyographic activity occurs in the periurethral striated muscle. As intravesical pressure rises, there is a simultaneous yet more marked rise in intraurethral pressure. During voiding the electrical activity of all the perineal muscles disappears. This cessation

of activity occurs almost simultaneously with the increase in intravesical pressure. There has been some controversy over whether the sphincters become silent just before or just after the intravesical pressure rise.[29,87,112,119] During voiding, intraurethral pressure is much less than intravesical pressure. As intravesical pressure begins to decline, the electrical activity of the sphincters gradually returns and intraurethral pressure increases correspondingly.

Spastic Sphincter

By the same mechanism that skeletal muscles of the lower extremities can become spastic and subject to hyperactive reflex activity, the urinary sphincter can be so affected. Rather than the usual reflex relaxation of the external urinary sphincter during detrusor contraction, there is enhanced sphincter contraction (Fig. 28–11). Sphincter electromyography demonstrates increased rather than decreased activity during detrusor contraction. This condition has been termed detrusor sphincter dysenergia.[18] It produces obstruction to the flow of urine, and bladder emptying may be inefficient and urinary stream poor. This syndrome is frequently associated with evi-

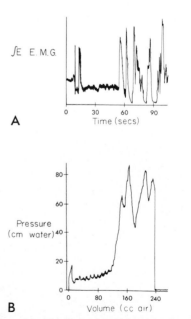

Figure 28–11 Detrusor-sphincter dyssynergia associated with detrusor hyperreflexia. *A.* Anal sphincter electromyogram. *B.* Cystometrogram.

dence of pyramidal tract impairment such as extensor plantar responses and spasticity in the skeletal muscles of the extremities. The patient is unable to relax or contract the sphincter satisfactorily on command. This type of sphincter dysfunction is most frequently seen with detrusor hyperreflexia but has been noted in detrusor areflexias as well. Various cerebral lesions producing pyramidal deficit such as a demyelinating process or brain tumor as well as various spinal cord lesions can cause this sphincter abnormality.

Another abnormal sphincter syndrome resulting from upper motor neuron lesions is a reflex relaxation of the urinary sphincter occurring during bladder filling or detrusor contraction.[18] This syndrome has been termed uninhibited urinary sphincter relaxation. It is associated with increased tone in the anal sphincter and impairment of the patient's ability to contract or relax the anal sphincter on command. At a critical intravesical pressure, reflex relaxation of the urinary sphincter occurs with associated sudden incontinence without prior sensation (see Fig. 28–10). The abnormal feature of this syndrome is the inability of the patient to suppress the relaxation of the sphincters voluntarily at a critical bladder pressure.

Atonic Sphincter

Denervation of the urinary sphincter secondary to injury or damage to the sacral cord, cauda equina, or pudendal nerves innervating the sphincter results in a patulous, ineffective sphincter with continuous urinary incontinence. Various degrees of denervation of the sphincter can occur, resulting in varying severity of the incontinence. Lesions causing this syndrome would be similar to those listed that produce areflexia of the detrusor muscle.

TREATMENT

Detrusor Reflex Dysfunction

Hyperreflexia

The goal of treating detrusor hyperreflexia is to reduce the hyperactivity of the detrusor muscle so that the bladder will accommodate a larger volume of urine without the symptoms of frequency and urgency. At the same time, effective voiding without the accumulation of significant residual urine should be maintained.

Drugs

A trial of drug therapy is indicated in patients suffering from detrusor hyperreflexia. Methantheline bromide (Banthine) is perhaps the initial drug of choice. Methantheline is a synthetic anticholinergic compound that, at the dosages usually used, blocks the postganglionic synapses.[65] Mode of action is assumed to be a simple competitive blockade of acetycholine. The usual dose is 50 to 100 mg four times daily. A closely related compound, propantheline bromide (Pro-Banthine), can also be used in doses of approximately 15 mg four times daily. Various antiganglionic agents (e.g., mecamylamine hydrochloride—Inversine) that produce autonomic ganglionic blockade can also be used in the treatment of detrusor hyperreflexia.[120] A significant problem with these agents has been the hypotension they cause. All the drug agents have a tendency to produce an increase in residual urine as well as side effects resulting from blocking the autonomic system at unwanted sites. These side effects would include constipation and blurring of vision.

These agents appear to be worth an initial trial in the case of detrusor hyperreflexia. The main difficulties are the close proximity of the therapeutic dose to doses producing unacceptable side effects, ineffective voiding, and increased residual urine.

Sacral Nerve Blocks

Selective sacral nerve blocks can be performed to determine which of the sacral nerves is operative in detrusor reflex activity.[60,98,100,117] By sequentially blocking several of the sacral nerves with local anesthetics and using cystometric control, the detrusor reflex can be abolished and bladder capacity significantly increased (Fig. 28–12). In essence this method determines the functional innervation of the detrusor muscle by determining which sacral nerves are primarily operative in detrusor reflex function. In a series of 50 patients so studied, the authors determined that the detrusor reflex could be abolished with unilateral sacral block in approximately 50 per cent.[100] Anesthesizing only two sacral nerves ipsi-

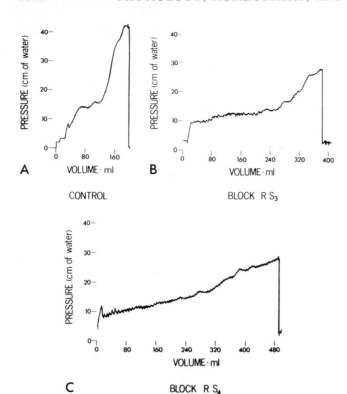

Figure 28–12 Cystometric response following sacral nerve blocks. *A*. Control cystometrogram showing low-threshold detrusor hyperreflexia. *B*. Cystometrogram following a unilateral S3 block showing little change. *C*. Cystometrogram following unilateral S3 and S4 blocks showing abolition of the detrusor reflex response.

laterally produced this effect in 17 patients. In this situation one can then consider either more permanent sacral blocks with phenol or a percutaneous radiofrequency lesion.[98] (The latter provides the opportunity for stimulation of the nerve root to determine the accuracy of the needle placement, and in addition, a graded ablation can be performed with cystometric control.) Sacral nerve lesions of this type will provide relief of symptoms for 3 to 12 months. Possible complications include a painful neuritis resulting from the intraneural injection of the phenol. Advantages include the avoidance of an operative procedure and the ease with which a block can be repeated in the case of recurrent symptoms.

Sacral Rhizotomy

If detrusor hyperreflexia can be reduced and bladder capacity increased by anesthesizing two or three sacral nerves, the patient can be considered a candidate for selective differential sacral rhizotomy.[99,101,115,116] Under the operating microscope, the individual fascicles of the selected sacral roots can be in turn stimulated and anesthetized to identify fibers

that innervate the bladder only. These fibers can be sectioned and the remainder of the nerve left intact. More physiological voiding can thus be restored for the patient by preserving the detrusor reflex and sphincter function and at the same time increasing bladder capacity (Fig. 28–13). The patients treated in this manner have had no postoperative difficulty with disturbance in sexual function. A tendency to recurrent symptoms has been observed over a period of long-term follow-up. In a group of 13 patients so treated, 5 developed recurrent symptoms within six months, while 6 remained symptomatically improved for over two years. There were no morbidity and no deaths in this group of patients.

End-Organ Denervation

Detrusor hyperreflexia has been effectively treated by denervation of the urinary bladder by section of the inferior hypogastric plexus transvaginally either unilaterally or bilaterally. Preoperative blocks of the pelvic nerves are performed to determine the effect of the block on clinical symptoms and the residual urine before the nerves are sectioned. In a series of 66 patients treated

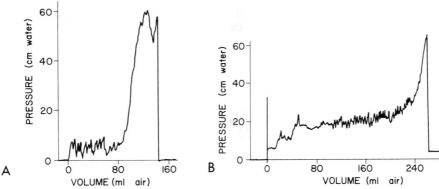

Figure 28–13 Cystometrograms before, *A*, and after, *B*, partial section of S3 and S4 ipsilaterally. Bladder capacity was significantly increased postoperatively, while the detrusor reflex was preserved. (From Rockswold, G. L., Bradley, W. E., and Chou, S. N.: Differential sacral rhizotomy in the treatment of neurogenic bladder dysfunction. Preliminary report of six cases. J. Neurosurg., *38*:748–754, 1973. Reprinted by permission.)

with unilateral or bilateral pelvic nerve section, there was primary failure in 4 patients and development of recurrent symptoms in 7 patients two months to five years after the procedure.[64] This technique has the obvious advantage of specific end-organ denervation. The completeness of the denervation would appear variable, however, especially in inexperienced hands.

Urinary Diversion

The indications for urinary diversion are infrequent in neurogenic bladder disease.[1,13,34,104] The major indication would be progressive renal failure due to obstruction or intractable infection that is unresponsive to conservative means of treatment. The most satisfactory diversion procedure is the ileal loop. Other procedures include suprapubic tube cystostomy, cutaneous vesicostomy, ureterostomy, anteversion of the urethra, and nephrostomy. All of them, however, have significant early and late complications. Renal deterioration may continue even after urinary diversion. All reasonable methods of conservative management should be performed prior to a permanent urinary diversion procedure.

Areflexia

Drugs

Treatment of patients with detrusor areflexia should be directed toward achieving satisfactory emptying of the urinary bladder with retention of minimal residual urine. Drugs again are worth an initial trial in the management of this problem. Bethanechol chloride (Urecholine) is probably the most frequently used and most useful drug for this purpose. Bethanechol is an analogue of acetylcholine that has a reasonably selective action on the gastrointestinal tract and urinary bladder.[73] The side effects include increased salivation, sweating, intestinal cramps, and diarrhea. Neostigmine (Prostigmin) is a synthetic anticholinesterase drug. It is sometimes useful when bethanechol is not effective, but in general it is not used as commonly. It is absorbed rather poorly from the gastrointestinal tract.[73]

Intermittent Catheterization

Intermittent catheterization can be an effective way of treating detrusor areflexia and secondary inability to empty the urinary bladder. It has been most extensively used in paraplegic and quadriplegic patients during the period of spinal "shock" to aid in emptying the bladder and to restore automatic or reflex bladder emptying. Guttman introduced the technique of intermittent catheterization for paraplegics following the second World War.[54,55] His reports clearly document its value in rendering the patient catheter-free and in significantly decreasing the incidence of infected urine. The complications of the indwelling Foley catheter, which include hydronephrosis, vesical-ureteral reflux, renal or vesical calculi, fistulae, prostatitis, seminal vesiculitis, and epididymitis, are decreased. It has only been with considerable delay and apparent reluctance that physicians in the United States have begun to accept the value of this technique.[12,55] More recently, however, several authors have again clearly demonstrated the value of intermittent catheterization following spinal cord injury.[12,47,83,95]

Ideally, intermittent catheterization should begin shortly after the injury so that an indwelling Foley catheter is never inserted. Numerous authors have shown, however, that intermittent catheterization may start several weeks or even months later and be of value in rendering the patient catheter-free and clearing up infection. The patient is catheterized by means of aseptic techniques approximately every four to six hours initially. Prior to catheterization, attempts are made to promote reflex emptying of the bladder by stroking the inner thigh, manipulating the anal sphincter, or squeezing the glans. As bladder function begins and some emptying of urine occurs, the catheterizations are spaced from the initial 4 hours to 6, 8, 12, and 24 hours, according to the amount of residual urine. Thereafter catheterization is done every 48 to 72 hours or once weekly, depending on bladder function, before it is abandoned completely. Urecholine in doses of 5 to 10 mg four times daily is effective in inducing the return of bladder tone and efficient detrusor contraction. The routine use of methenamine mandelate (Mandelamine) 1 gm and asorbic acid 1 gm four times daily is recommended to suppress urinary infection.

As noted, the use of intermittent catheterization can make patients catheter-free following spinal cord injury. This is because bladder filling provides the physiological stimulus for micturition by setting up appropriate afferent impulses to the spinal cord. Although there is no direct neurophysiological proof for this concept, it is known that continuous bladder drainage reduces the excitability of the detrusor and its ability to contract effectively to artificial stimulation in animals.[50] In addition the continuous distention of the external urethral sphincter by the cannula provides another source of unbalanced reflex activity between the detrusor muscle and the pelvic floor muscles. The absence of infec-

tion would also contribute to the earlier return of bladder reflex function.

Using this technique, the vast majority of patients can be rendered catheter-free. In one controlled prospective study two groups of 50 patients each were compared.[83] They had follow-up studies of up to five years in each group. One group was treated by the traditional method of an indwelling Foley catheter removed for trials of voiding, and the second group was treated by intermittent catheterization. Only 18 of 50 patients became catheter-free using the traditional techniques of an indwelling Foley catheter removed on several occasions for trials of voiding. All the patients treated with intermittent catheterization became catheter-free from one to six months after injury, the average time being three months. Intermittent catheterization was carried out for a period of 2 to 70 days, with an average of 11 days. The incidence of urinary infection, urinary calculi, and deterioration of renal function clearly showed intermittent catheterization treatment to be superior. It would appear to be conclusive that intermittent catheterization is the treatment of choice for patients with detrusor areflexia following spinal cord injury.

Intermittent catheterization is also useful in other diseases producing detrusor areflexia. Patients who have undergone laminectomy for various intraspinal lesions followed by a period of prolonged postoperative detrusor areflexia can be treated with intermittent catheterization. Recovery of spontaneous voiding is enhanced. If detrusor areflexia persists, the patient can be taught the technique of intermittent self-catheterization.[79,80,94,123] Patients have found this technique quite satisfactory over a long period of time. Objections to the possible introduction of an infection may be raised. It has, however, been shown that indwelling urinary catheters are perhaps the greatest source of infection.[35] The bladder has an inherent resistance to infection in the absence of a foreign body, but in the presence of an indwelling Foley catheter, virtually all patients with neurological bladder problems become infected within a few days. Patients using clean intermittent self-catheterization appear to have fewer problems with infection than those with chronic indwelling catheters. Also the various other complications of the indwelling catheter mentioned previously are avoided.

Detrusor Stimulation

Considerable effort has been put into developing a method of electronically stimulating the detrusor muscle in order to achieve effective urinary bladder evacuation.[19] Difficulty has, however, been encountered in rendering this a consistently effective technique. The single most important problem has been the inability to couple electrical energy effectively to stimulate contraction of the smooth muscle cells of the detrusor muscle. The cellular arrangement for spread of excitation in the detrusor muscle is such that two thirds to three fourths of the surface area of the detrusor muscle must be directly activated by electrical stimulation to produce effective evacuation. In addition the electrodes that cover such a large surface area must be sufficiently flexible to maintain contact with the bladder wall during the contour changes that occur during the course of bladder emptying. At the present time detrusor stimulation would appear to be an experimental technique that holds promise and should continue to be studied at certain centers.

Sacral Cord Stimulation

Evacuation of the bladder contents has been produced by placing permanent stimulating electrodes in the sacral spinal cord of patients with spinal cord injury.[53,67,68,90] This procedure has been performed only in patients who are completely paraplegic and in whom efforts to train a reflex bladder have been unsuccessful. The primary problem with this technique has been to obtain selective stimulation of the detrusor muscle only. Stimulation of the intermediolateral cell columns at the S1 and S2 levels has produced contraction of the external urethral sphincter via the pudendal nerve, causing outflow obstruction. In several patients, the obstruction has been relieved with a sphincterotomy. In addition, stimulation of other autonomic pathways produces erection, defecation, and hypotension. The authors reporting on this technique state that these side effects can be reduced by improving control of the stimulus.

Grimes and Nashhold reported a series of 10 patients, 6 of whom rely completely upon the bladder stimulator to induce micturition.[53] All these patients have remained totally continent of urine and maintain residual urine of less than 10 ml. Their infections have been markedly reduced. This technique appears to be promising. The indications for spinal cord stimulation would appear to be limited at the present time to complete spinal cord lesions with complete paraplegia and limited to those few patients in whom adequate reflex bladder function cannot be obtained with intermittent catheterization and other rehabilitative measures.

Urinary Sphincter Dysfunction

Spastic Sphincter

Treatment of the spastic sphincter syndrome is essentially the reduction of urinary outflow resistance by various means. Resistance can be increased at one or both of two points, namely, the bladder neck, or so-called internal urinary sphincter, and the periurethral striated muscle, or external urethral sphincter, located at the midurethra.

Drugs

As previously discussed, internal urinary sphincter resistance can be reduced by alpha-adrenergic blocking agents. The drug that has been used most extensively has been phenoxybenzamine (Dibenzyline).[74,75,86] This drug has been used in doses ranging from 10 to 30 mg daily. The only serious side effect has been orthostatic hypotension, which can usually be satisfactorily treated with elastic stockings. In cases of documented increased urethral resistance by urethral pressure profile during detrusor contraction, results have been very satisfactory.

Dantrolene sodium (Dantrium) has been used with benefit in carefully selected patients with external sphincter spasm.[88] Residual urine decreased to less than 100 ml in three patients and to less than 50 ml in another three patients treated with 200 to 250 mg per day. The one serious drawback to dantrolene sodium is its potential severe liver toxicity.

Sphincterotomy

Transurethral resection of the bladder neck or internal sphincter has been satisfactorily performed to reduce outlet resistance since Emmett first performed this type of intervention in 1937 (see Fig. 28–8).[46] It has been used most extensively in patients with traumatic cord lesions.[6,11,25,33] The frequency with which transurethral resection has been performed in this group of patients varies from 10 to 20 per cent. The procedure has also been performed in nontraumatic paraplegia.[66] A transurethral resection should be considered after six months of intermittent catheterization and a trial of alpha-adrenergic blockers has failed to establish satisfactory bladder emptying.

If electromyography and urethral pressure profiles reveal that the inappropriate outlet resistance is arising at the level of the external sphincter, transurethral external sphincterotomy may also be appropriate if conservative measures have failed.[61] Good results can be expected in a high percentage of patients if those patients are carefully selected.[61,105]

Pudendal Nerve Section

Bilateral section of the pudendal nerves is required to effectively relax the pelvic floor muscles. After arousing some initial enthusiasm this procedure is now seldom performed because of interference with or abolishment of erection in over 50 per cent of patients.[13,88]

Sacral Nerve Blocks

Marked improvement in urinary flow rates have followed sacral nerve blocks in patients with detrusor-sphincter dysenergia (see Fig. 28–9). Bilateral sacral nerve blocks are usually required, however, and they pose the same problems with erection as bilateral pudendal nerve section.

Atonic Sphincter

Treatment of the atonic or flaccid urinary sphincter with secondary incontinence consists of various measures to increase urethral outlet resistance. Treatment can be directed at either the internal or external urinary sphincters.

Drugs

Drugs causing alpha-adrenergic stimulation (ephedrine, phenylephrine, or imipramine) have been used to increase tone in the bladder neck and urethra by smooth muscle contraction.[32,41,70,84,96] The increased tone has improved symptoms of various types of urinary incontinence such as enuresis, stress and postprostatectomy incontinence, and uninhibited sphincter relaxation related to decreased urethral resistance. Ephedrine sulfate in doses of 50 to 150 mg daily gives good results in selected patients with reduced urethral pressure profiles.

Long-Term Stimulation of Urinary Sphincter

Urinary incontinence has been treated with long-term stimulation of the external urethral sphincter.[27,28,106] An implantable receiver, which is energized by an external electronic unit, is placed in the abdominal wall. Stimulating electrodes are inserted into the external urethral sphincter and connected to the implant. Continence is achieved by stimulation and secondary contraction of the sphincter; voiding is achieved by discontinuing the stimulating current. There must be functioning periurethral striated muscle for this technique to be successful. Severe denervation and atrophy will render the stimulation ineffective. A significant number of failures have occurred because of infection in the perineal wound, electrode protrusion, and inability to achieve satisfactory stimulation even during a relatively short follow-up period. This technique would be applicable only when all conservative methods had failed.

Artificial Prosthetic Urinary Sphincter

The use of an occlusive cuff around the urethra for the treatment of urinary incontinence was first advocated by Foley in 1947.[48] More recently Timm and co-workers developed an implantable prosthetic urinary sphincter that has now had significant clinical application.[57,108,114] This sili-

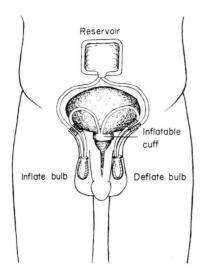

Figure 28-14 Diagram of prosthetic urinary sphincter consisting of four principal parts: reservoir, inflatable cuff, and inflating and deflating pumping mechanisms. (From Scott, F. B., Bradley, W. E., and Timm, G. W.: Treatment of urinary incontinence by an implantable prosthetic urinary sphincter. J. Urol., *112*:75–80, 1974. Reprinted by permission.)

cone rubber prosthetic urinary sphincter comprises four principal parts: a fluid reservoir, an inflatable occlusive cuff, an inflating mechanism, and a deflating pumping mechanism (Fig. 28–14). The cuff encircles the urethra in such a manner that when completely inflated it occludes the urethra. The reservoir contains a radiopaque fluid, sodium diatrizoate, which is utilized to inflate the cuff. The pumping mechanism is activated by squeezing a bulb that is placed subcutaneously in the labia or scrotum. The pumping mechanism contains valves that control the maximum pressure that can be exerted inside the cuff, preventing possible overinflation. Activation of the deflating pumping mechanism by squeezing another subcutaneous bulb opens the urethral cuff by returning fluid from the urethral cuff to the reservoir. With the cuff open, unimpeded voiding occurs.

This artificial sphincter has been used for neurogenic incontinence as well as post-prostatectomy and stress incontinence. The former has presented more difficulties in preoperative selection and postoperative management. Mechanical failures and infection secondary to the implanted foreign body have continued to cause failures. It is, however, a promising technique in the early phases of development and should be of benefit to carefully selected patients.

SUMMARY

Neurologic urinary bladder dysfunction is not a single disease entity. There are a multiplicity of causes and effects. Some problems are fairly easily diagnosed and treated, and others remain difficult and occasionally baffling. A complete neurourological investigation employing modern methods of assessment including high flow rate gas cystometry, integrated sphincter electromyography, and electrophysiological techniques to assess bladder innervation is necessary to delineate the voiding problem properly. Only then can appropriate therapy be initiated.

REFERENCES

1. Abramson, A. S.: Management of the neurogenic bladder in perspective. Arch. Phys. Med. Rehabil., *57*:197–201, 1976.
2. Andersen, J. T., and Bradley, W. E.: Postural detrusor hyperreflexia. J. Urol., *116*:228–230, 1976.
3. Andrew, J., and Nathan, P. W.: Lesions of the anterior frontal lobes and disturbances of micturition and defaecation. Brain, *87*:233–262, 1964.
4. Andrew, J., Nathan, P. W., and Spanos, N. D.: Disturbances of micturition and defaecation due to aneurysms of anterior communicating or anterior cerebral arteries. J. Neurosurg., *24*:1–10, 1966.
5. Ardran, G. M., Cope, V., Essenhigh, D. M., and Tuckey, M.: The primary vesical sphincter. Brit. J. Urol., *39*:329–333, 1967.
6. Band, D.: Urological management during the initial phase of traumatic paraplegia. Brit. J. Urol., *33*:361–369, 1961.
7. Barrington, F. J. F.: The relation of the hindbrain to micturition. Brain, *44*:23–52, 1921.
8. Barrington, F. J. F.: The effect of lesions of the hind and midbrain on micturition in the cat. Quart. J. Exp. Physiol., *15*:81–102, 1925.
9. Barrington, F. J. F.: The component reflex of micturition in the cat, I and II. Brain, *54*:177–188, 1931.
10. Barrington, F. J. F.: The localization of the paths subserving micturition in the spinal cord of the cat. Brain, *56*:126–148, 1933.
11. Bors, E.: Neurogenic bladder. Urol. Survey, *7*:177–250, 1957.
12. Bors, E.: Intermittent catheterization in paraplegic patients. Urol. Int., *22*:236–249, 1967.
13. Bors, E., and Comarr, A. E.: Neurological Urology. Baltimore, University Park Press, 1971.
14. Boyarsky, S.: Neurogenic Bladder. Baltimore, Williams & Wilkins Co., 1967.
15. Bradley, W. E., and Conway, C. J.: Bladder representation in the pontine-mesencephalic reticular formation. Exp. Neurol., *16*:237–249, 1966.
16. Bradley, W. E., and Teague, C. T.: Spinal cord

organization of micturition reflex afferents. Exp. Neurol., 22:504–516, 1968.

17. Bradley, W. E., and Teague, C. T.: Electrophysiology of the pelvic and pudendal nerves in the cat. Exp. Neurol., 35:378–393, 1972.

18. Bradley, W. E., Scott, F. B., and Timm, G. W.: Sphincter electromyography. Urol. Clin. N. Amer., 1:69–80, 1974.

19. Bradley, W. E., Timm, G. W., and Chou, S. N.: A decade of experience with electronic stimulation of the micturition reflex. Urol. Int., 26:283–303, 1971.

20. Bradley, W. E., Timm, G. W., and Scott, F. B.: Innervation of the detrusor muscle and urethra. Urol. Clin. N. Amer., 1:3–27, 1974.

21. Bradley, W. E., Clarren, S., Shapiro, R., et al.: Air cystometry. J. Urol., 100:451–455, 1968.

22. Bradley, W. E., Rockswold, G. L., Timm, G. W., and Scott, F. B.: Neurology of micturition. J. Urol. 115:481–486, 1976.

23. Bradley, W. E., Timm, G. W., Rockswold, G. L., and Scott, F. B.: Detrusor and urethral electromyelography. J. Urol., 114:891–894, 1975.

24. Brown, M., and Wickham, J. E. A.: The urethral pressure profile. Brit. J. Urol., 41:211–217, 1969.

25. Bunts, R. C.: Management of urological complications in 1,000 paraplegics. J. Urol., 79:733–741, 1958.

26. Caine, M., and Edwards, D.: The peripheral control of micturition: A cine-radiographic study. Brit. J. Urol., 30:34–42, 1958.

27. Caldwell, K. P. S.: The electrical control of sphincter incompetence. Lancet, 2:174–175, 1963.

28. Caldwell, K. P. S., Cook, P. J., Flack, F. C., and James, D.: Treatment of post-prostatectomy incontinence by electronic implant. Brit. J. Urol., 40:183–186, 1968.

29. Cardus, D., Quesada, E. M., and Scott, F. B.: Studies on the dynamics of the bladder. J. Urol., 90:425–433, 1963.

30. Cass, A. S., Ward, B. D., and Markland, C.: Comparison of slow and rapid fill cystometry using liquid and air. J. Urol. 104:104–106, 1970.

31. Cheatham, M. L., and Matske, H. A.: Descending hypothalamic medullary pathways in the cat. J. Comp. Neurol., 127:369–380, 1966.

32. Christopherson, J. B., and Broadbent, M.: Ephedrine and pseudo-ephedrine in asthma, bronchial asthma, and enuresis. Brit. Med. J., 1:978–979, 1934.

33. Comarr, A. E.: The practical urological management of the patient with spinal cord injury. Brit. J. Urol., 31:–46, 1959.

34. Comarr, A. E.: Management of the traumatic cord bladder today. Urol. Int., 20:1–11, 1965.

35. Cox, C. E., and Hinman, F.: Retention catheterization and the bladder defense mechanism. J.A.M.A., 191:105–108, 1965.

36. DeGroat, W. C., and Lalley, P. M.: Reflex firing in the lumbar sympathetic outflow to activation of vesical afferent fibers. J. Physiol., 226:289–309, 1972.

37. DeGroat, W. C., and Ryall, R. W.: Reflexes to sacral parasympathetic neurons concerned with micturition in the cat. J. Physiol., 200:87–108, 1969.

38. DeGroat, W. C., and Saum, W. R.: Sympathetic inhibition of the urinary bladder and of pelvic ganglionic transmission in the cat. J. Physiol., 220:297–314, 1972.

39. DeGroat, W. C., and Theobald, R. J.: Reflex activation of sympathetic pathways to vesical smooth muscle and parasympathetic ganglia by electrical stimulation of vesical afferents. J. Physiol., 259:223–237, 1976.

40. Denny-Brown, D., and Robertson, E.: On the physiology of micturition. Brain, 56:149–191, 1933.

41. Diokno, A. C., and Taub, M.: Ephedrine in treatment of urinary incontinence. Urology, 5:624–625, 1975.

42. Donker, P. J., Invanovici, F., and Noach, E. L.: Analysis of the urethral pressure profile by means of electromyography and the administration of drugs. Brit. J. Urol., 44:180–193, 1972.

43. Edvardsen, P.: Nervous control of urinary bladder in cats. I. The collecting phase. Acta Physiol. Scand., 72:157–171, 1968.

44. Edvardsen, P., and Setekliev, J.: Distribution of adrenergic receptors in the urinary bladder of cats, rabbits, and guinea pigs. Acta Pharmacol., 26:437–445, 1968.

45. El-Badawi, A., and Schenk, E. A.: Dual innervation of the mammalian urinary bladder. A histochemical study of the distribution of cholinergic and adrenergic nerves. Amer. J. Anat., 119:405–427, 1966.

46. Emmett, J. L.: Transurethral resection in treatment of true and pseudo cord bladder. J. Urol., 53:545–564, 1945.

47. Firlit, C. B., Canning, J. R., Lloyd, F. A., Cross, R. R., and Brewer, R.: Experience with intermittent catheterization in chronic spinal cord injury patients. J. Urol., 114:234–236, 1975.

48. Foley, F. E. B.: An artificial sphincter: A new device and operation for control of enuresis and urinary incontinence. J. Urol., 58:250–259, 1947.

49. Garry, R. C., Roberts, T. D. M., and Todd, J. K.: Reflexes involving the external urethral sphincter in the cat. J. Physiol., 149:653–665, 1959.

50. Geise, A., Bradley, W., Chou, S., and French, L.: Effect of indwelling catheter on electrical excitability of the bladder. Surg. Forum, 14:493–494, 1963.

51. Graber, P., and Tanagho, E. A.: Urethral responses to autonomic nerve stimulation. Urology, 6:52–58, 1975.

52. Gray, H.: The peripheral nervous system. In Goss, C. M., ed.: Gray's Anatomy of the Human Body. Philadelphia, Lea & Febiger, 1973.

53. Grimes, J. H., and Nashold, B. S.: Clinical application of electronic bladder stimulation in paraplegics. Brit. J. Urol., 46:653–657, 1974.

54. Guttman, L.: Statistical survey on one thousand paraplegics and initial treatment of traumatic paraplegia. Proc. Roy Soc. Med., 47:1099–1109, 1954.

55. Guttman, L., and Frankel, H.: The value of intermittent catheterization in the early management of traumatic paraplegia and tetraplegia. Paraplegia, 5:63–84, 1968.

56. Hald, T.: Neurogenic dysfunction of the urinary

bladder: An experimental and clinical study with special reference to the ability of electrical stimulation to establish voluntary micturition. Danish Med. Bull., *16*:Suppl. V:1–156, 1969.

57. Hald, T., Byrstom, J., and Alfthan, O.: Treatment of urinary incontinence by the Scott-Bradley-Timm artificial sphincter. Urol. Res., *3*:133–137, 1975.

58. Harmon, N. B.: The pelvic splanchnic nerves: An examination into their range and character. J. Anat., *33*:386–399, 1899.

59. Harrison, M. B., and Constable, A. R.: Urethral pressure measurement: A modified technique. Brit. J. Urol., *42*:229–233, 1970.

60. Heimburger, R. F., Freeman, L. W., and Wilde, N. J.: Sacral nerve innervation of the human bladder. J. Neurosurg., *5*:154–164, 1948.

61. Herr, H. W., Engelman, E. R., and Martin, D. C.: External sphincteromy in traumatic and nontraumatic neurogenic bladder dysfunction. J. Urol. *113*:32–34, 1975.

62. Hutch, J.: A new theory on the anatomy of the internal urinary sphincter and the physiology of micturition. Invest. Urol, *3*:36–58, 1965.

63. Hutch, J.: The internal urinary sphincter: A double-loop system. J. Urol., *105*:375–383, 1971.

64. Ingelman-Sundberg, A.: Urge incontinence in women. Acta Obstet. Gynec. Scand., *54*:153–156, 1975.

65. Innes, I. R., and Nickerson, M.: Atropine, scopolamine, and related antimuscarinic drugs. *In* Goodman, L. L., and Gilman, A., eds.: The Pharmacological Basis of Therapeutics. New York, Macmillan Co., 1975.

66. Jacobsen, B. E., Pedersen, E., and Grynderup. V.: Resection of the bladder neck in nontraumatic paraplegia. Acta Neurol. Scand., Suppl. 20, *42*:121–131, 1966.

67. Jonas, U., and Tanagho, E. A.: Studies on the feasibility of urinary bladder evacuation by direct spinal cord stimulation. II. Poststimulus voiding: A way to overcome outflow resistance. Invest. Urol., *13*:151–153, 1975.

68. Jonas, U., Heine, J. P., and Tanagho, E. A.: Studies on the feasibility of urinary bladder evacuation by direct spinal cord stimulation. I. Parameters of most effective stimulation. Invest. Urol., *13*:142–150, 1975.

69. Kerr, F. W. L., and Alexander, S.: Descending autonomic pathways in the spinal cord. Arch. Neurol., *10*:249–261, 1964.

70. Khanna, O. P.: Disorders of micturition. Neuropharmacologic basis and results of drug therapy. Urology, *8*:316–328, 1976.

71. Kimmel, D. L., and McCrae, L. E.: The development of the pelvic plexuses and the distribution of the pelvic splanchnic nerves in the human embryo and fetus. J. Comp. Neurol., *110*:271–298, 1958.

72. Kleeman, F. J.: The physiology of the internal urinary sphincter. J. Urol., *104*:549–554, 1970.

73. Koelle, G. B.: Parasympathomimetic agents. *In* Goodman, L. L., and Gilman, A., eds.: The Pharmacological Basis of Therapeutics. New York, Macmillan Co., 1975.

74. Krane, R. J., and Olsson, C. A.: Phenoxybenzamine in neurogenic bladder dysfunction. I. A theory of micturition. J. Urol., *110*:650–652, 1973.

75. Krane, R. J., and Olsson, C. A.: Phenoxybenzamine in neurogenic bladder dysfunction. II. Clinical considerations. J. Urol., *110*:653–656, 1973.

76. Kuru, M., Kurati, T., and Koyama, Y.: The bulbar vesico-constrictor center and the bulbosacral connections arising from it. A study of the function of the lateral reticulo-spinal tract. J. Comp. Neurol., *113*:365–388, 1959.

77. Lapides, J.: Structure and function of the internal vesical sphincter. J. Urol, *80*:341–353, 1958.

78. Lapides, J., Sweet, R. B., and Lewis, L. W.: Role of striated muscle in urination. J. Urol., *77*:247–250, 1957.

79. Lapides, J., Diokno, A. C., Gould F. R., and Lowe, B. S.: Further observations on self-catheterization. J. Urol., *116*:169–171, 1976.

80. Lapides, J., Diokno, A. C., Silber, S. J., and Lowe, B. S.: Clean intermittent self-catheterization in the treatment of urinary tract disease. Trans. Amer. Ass. Genitourin. Surg., *63*:92–95, 1971.

81. Lapides, J., Friend, C. R., Ajemian, E. P., and Reus, W. C.: Denervation supersensitivity as a test for neurogenic bladder. Surg. Gynec. Obstet., *114*:241–244, 1962.

82. Learmouth, J. R.: A contribution to the neurophysiology of the urinary bladder in man. Brain, *54*:147–176, 1931.

83. Lindan, R., and Bellomy, V.: Effect of delayed intermittent catheterization on kidney function in spinal cord injury patients; a long-term follow-up study. Paraplegia, *13*:49–55, 1975.

84. Mahony, D. T., Laferte, R. O., and Mahoney, J. E.: Part VI. Observations on sphincter-augmenting effect of imipramine in children with urinary incontinence. Urology, *1*:317–323, 1973.

85. McMichael, J.: Spinal tracts subserving micturition in a case of Erb's spinal paralysis. Brain, *68*:162–164, 1945.

86. McQuire, E. J., Wagner, F. M., and Weiss, R. M.: Treatment of autonomic dysreflexia with phenoxybenzamine. J. Urol., *115*:53–55, 1976.

87. Mueliner, S. R.: The voluntary control of micturition in man. J. Urol., *80*:473–478, 1958.

88. Murdock, M. M., Sax, D., and Krane, R. J.: Use of dantrolene sodium in external sphincter spasm. Urology, *8*:133–137, 1976.

89. Nagib, A., Leal, J., and Voris, H. C.: Successful control of selective anterior sacral rhizotomy for treatment of spastic bladder and ureteric reflux in paraplegics. Med. Serv. J. Canada, *22*:576–581, 1965.

90. Nashold, B. S., Friedman, H., Glenn, J. F., Grimes, J. H., Barry, W. F., and Every, R.: Electromicturition in paraplegia. Arch. Surg., *104*:195–202, 1972.

91. Nathan, P. W., and Smith, M. D.: The centripetal pathway from the bladder and urethra within the spinal cord. J. Neurol. Neurosurg. Psychiat., *14*:262–280, 1951.

92. Nathan, P. W., and Smith, M. C.: The centrifugal pathway for micturition within the spinal cord. J. Neurol. Neurosurg. Psychiat., *21*:177–189, 1958.

93. Oliver, J. E., Bradley, W. E., and Fletcher, T. J.: Spinal cord representation of the micturition reflex. J. Comp. Neurol., *137*:329–346, 1969.

94. Orikasa, S., Koyanagi, T., Motomura, M.,

Kudo, T., Togashi, M., and Tsuji, I.: Experience with non-sterile intermittent self-catheterization. J. Urol., *115*:141–142, 1976.

95. Perkash, I.: Intermittent catheterization and bladder rehabilitation in spinal cord injury patients. J. Urol. *144*:230–233, 1975.

96. Rashbaum, M., and Mandelbaum, C. C.: Nonoperative treatment of urinary incontinence in women. Amer. J. Obstet. Gynec., *56*:777–780, 1948.

97. Rockswold, G. L.: Innervation of the urinary bladder in higher primates and in man. Ph.D. thesis, University of Minnesota, June, 1976.

98. Rockswold, G. L., and Bradley, W. E.: The use of sacral nerve blocks in the evaluation and treatment of neurologic bladder disease. J. Urol., *118*:415–417, 1977.

99. Rockswold, G. L., Bradley, W. E., and Chou, S. N.: Differential sacral rhizotomy in the treatment of neurogenic bladder dysfunction. Preliminary report of six cases. J. Neurosurg., *38*: 748–754, 1973.

100. Rockswold, G. L., Bradley, W. E., and Chou, S. N.: Effect of sacral nerve blocks on the function of the urinary bladder in humans. J. Neurosurg., *40*:83–89, 1974.

101. Rockswold, G. L., Bradley, W. E., and Chou, S. N.: Differential sacral rhizotomy. Minn. Med. *57*:586, 1974.

102. Rockswold, G. L., Bradley, W. E., Timm, G. W., and Chou, S. N.: Neurologic bladder dysfunction; evaluation and treatment at the University of Minnesota. Minn. Med. *59*:687–691, 1975.

103. Rockswold, G. L., Bradley, W. E., Timm, G. W., and Chou, S. N.: Electrophysiological technique for evaluating lesions of the conus medullaris and cauda equina. J. Neurosurg., *45*:321–326, 1976.

104. Ross, J. C.: Diversion of the urine in the neurogenic bladder. Brit. J. Urol., *39*:708–711, 1967.

105. Ross, J. C., Gibbon, N. O. K., and Damanski, M.: Further experiences with division of the external urethral sphincter in the paraplegic. J. Urol., *89*:692–695, 1963.

106. Rowan, D., and Alexander, S.: Experience with electronic devices in management of incontinence and retention of urine. Proc. Roy. Soc. Med., *61*:705, 1968.

107. Ruch, T. C.: Central control of the bladder. *In* Handbook of Physiology, Vol II, Sec 1: Neurophysiology. Washington, D. C., American Physiological Society, 1960, pp. 1207–1224.

108. Scott, F. B., Bradley, W. E., and Timm, G. W.: Treatment of urinary incontinence by an implantable prosthetic urinary sphincter. J. Urol., *112*:75–80, 1974.

109. Sheehan, D.: Spinal autonomic outflows in man and monkey. J. Comp. Neurol., *75*:341–370, 1941.

110. Stewart, C. C.: On the course of impulses to and from the cat's bladder. Amer. J. Physiol., *2*:182–202, 1899.

111. Susset, J. G., Picker, P., Kretz, M., and Jorest, R.: Critical evaluation of uroflowmeters and analysis of normal curves. J. Urol., *109*:874–878, 1973.

112. Tanagho, E. A., Miller, E. R., Meyers, F. H., and Corbett, R. K.: Observations on the dynamics of the bladder neck. Brit. J. Urol., *38*:72–84, 1966.

113. Tanagho, E. A., and Smith, D. R.: Mechanism of urinary continence. I. Embryologic, anatomic and pathologic considerations. J. Urol, *100*:640–646, 1968.

114. Timm, G. W., Bradley, W. E., and Scott, F. B.: Experimental evaluation of an implantable externally controllable urinary sphincter. Invest. Urol., *11*:326–330, 1973.

115. Toczek, S. W., McCullough, D. C., Gargour, G. W., et al.: Selective sacral rootlet rhizotomy for hypertonic neurogenic bladder. J. Neurosurg., *42*:567–574, 1975.

116. Torrens, M. J., and Griffith, H. B.: Management of the uninhibited bladder by selective sacral neurectomy. J. Neurosurg., *44*:176–185, 1976.

117. Torrens, M. J.: Urodynamic analysis of differential sacral nerve blocks and sacral neurectomy. Urol. Int., *30*:85–91, 1975.

118. Tulloch, A. G. S.: Sympathetic activity of internal urethral sphincter. In empty and partially filled bladder. Urology, *5*:353–355, 1975.

119. Vereecken, R. L., and Verduyn, H.: The electrical activity of the periurethral and perineal muscles in normal and pathological conditions. Brit. J. Urol., *42*:457–463, 1970.

120. Volle, R. L., and Koelle, G. B.: Ganglionic stimulating and blocking agents. *In* Goodman, L. L., and Gilman, A., eds.: The Pharmacological Basis of Therapeutics. New York, Macmillan Co, 1975.

121. Von Garrelts, B.: Analysis of micturition: A new method of recording and voiding of the bladder. Acta Chir. Scand., *112*:326, 1956.

122. Wang, S. C., and Ranson, S. W.: Descending pathways from hypothalamus to medulla and spinal cord: Observations on blood pressure and bladder responses. J. Comp. Neurol., *71*:457–472, 1939.

123. Whitfield, H. N., and Mayo, M. E.: Intermittent non-sterile catheterization. Brit. J. Surg., *63*:330–332, 1976.

124. Wolf, G., and Sutin, J.: Fiber degeneration after lateral hypothalamic lesions in the rat. J. Comp. Neurol., *127*:137–156, 1966.

125. Woolard, H. H., and Norrish, R. E.: The anatomy of the peripheral sympathetic nervous system. Brit. J. Surg., *21*:83–103, 1933.

29

PREOPERATIVE EVALUATION; COMPLICATIONS, THEIR PREVENTION AND TREATMENT

PREOPERATIVE EVALUATION AND PREPARATION OF THE PATIENT

The surgeon's personal supervision of the preoperative evaluation and preparation of the neurosurgical patient is a sine qua non for the realization of the optimum in surgical care. The responsible surgeon may not personally conduct all aspects of the preoperative evaluation, but it is essential that he be in the role of captain of the team and, more specifically, participate personally in a comprehensive review of all steps in the evaluation so that he may make an informed judgment of what is best for the patient. He will find it necessary to examine the patient personally, and he must not permit the one-to-one surgeon-patient relationship to be blocked by the interposition of too many team members or excessive laboratory exercises. The patient must come to know the surgeon responsible for his care through actions and words.

The Medical System Review

A history, physical examination, and laboratory assessment are required for every patient being evaluated for a neurosurgical procedure. The comprehensiveness of this assessment will be determined by the complexity of the problem and by the degree of urgency that governs its surgical management; the following sections emphasize those aspects that assume importance in a neurosurgical practice.

The Acute Emergency

From a life-saving emergency procedure such as tracheostomy for respiratory obstruction to the surgical management of a strictly elective condition, there is a spectrum of urgency that will influence the amount of time that can safely be spent in obtaining a satisfactory history, executing a physical examination, and conducting a laboratory analysis. At the one extreme, no history is needed, the physical examination is made at a glance, and the operative procedure is executed with dispatch without laboratory testing. The patient who has passed into coma with an acute epidural hematoma may require management only slightly less prompt to save his life. But even under these stringent circumstances, the documentation of injury, the confirmation of important physical signs, and the collection of blood specimens usually can be effected. In the elective case, at the other end of the spectrum, one could not accept the history that reads, "The patient states he has hemorrhoids," followed by a physical examination that states, "He has."

The emergency problem requires the simultaneous collection of important historical facts, the execution of a properly tailored physical examination, and a laboratory assessment in keeping with the probable needs of the patient. The history may have to be obtained from other persons. A rapid, on-the-spot survey of the patient, who is often unable to communicate directly, is necessary, and in the case of the injured patient, injuries in all parts of the

W. E. STERN

body must be considered. The patient must be completely undressed and examined from head to toe. All pertinent observations must be charted; a flow sheet of vital signs, medications, supportive fluids, and urinary output should be included. All wounds must be examined, aseptic precautions being observed; a rapid but accurate neurological examination should note the level of consciousness, the function of special senses, other cranial nerve function, motor function, and of less importance, sensation and reflex activity; all orifices should be examined; special attention should be given to the scalp, the skull, the spine, and the obvious areas of injury. Simultaneously with the physical and neurological examinations, blood and urine samples should be obtained, and an intravenous infusion route should be established. The blood should be examined for standard data, including typing and cross-matching, in preparation for transfusion therapy. The urine should be examined for blood and glucose content. In cases of injury, a blood lipase and a urine fat examination may be profitable. The preferred intravenous fluid, which may be administered after the baseline body fluids have been sampled, is 5 per cent glucose in 0.445 per cent sodium chloride. In the cases of patients with severe or multiple injuries, a balanced electrolyte solution (extracellular fluid "mimic") may be preferable.

Less Urgent or Elective Problems

The following sections consider aspects of the preoperative evaluation that are likely to be necessary and possible in the nonemergency situation. They may not be sufficient alone, and in the case of the unresponsive or uncooperative patient, certain items clearly have to be sacrificed and other indirect means of assessment substituted.

General Nutritional Status

Weight Loss or Gain

Whether brought about by disease such as cancer, by specific neural processes involving the hypothalamic pituitary axis, or by imposed diet regimens or other kinds of starvation, weight loss may indicate exhaustion of glycogen stores and breakdown of body protein, a state of catabolism that may be associated with hypovolemia or, at least, with intolerance to further losses

such as blood loss at the time of operation. Furthermore, deficiencies, specifically hypoproteinemia or vitamin C deficiency accompanying a more general depletion, quite apart from their diagnostic import, may lead to poor wound healing following an elective surgical procedure. Intracranial disease with associated nausea and vomiting may have produced a state of acute malnutrition and weight loss, for example, in patients suffering from hypothalamic tumors with a failure to thrive and those with tumors of the hindbrain that produce recurrent vomiting and fluid loss, interfering with normal alimentation. Inadequate alimentation may also have resulted from other causes. Adult patients whose estimated caloric intake has been under 1500 calories per day may be suspected of being chronically deficient, and those receiving less than 1000 calories a day will be losing protein. Especially is this so in the severely injured patient. With inadequate general alimentation or with specific dietary restriction, vitamin C deficiency may be suspected. A laboratory determination of plasma proteins will detect the presence of severe protein depletion. Severe nitrogen depletion may be encountered in cases of metastatic disease involving the central nervous tissue, or in the chronically debilitated patient with pain.

Weight gain may be a matter of fluid retention and may be indicative of cardiac, renal, or other disease. A weight chart, a calculation of surface area on the basis of weight and height, and a calculation of expected blood volume should be in hand. This may be verified by a blood volume determination by one of several techniques (it must be remembered that a 10 per cent experimental error is to be expected in such determinations). Obesity may be a problem of surgical importance insofar as it can interfere with adequate ventilatory exchange and place an extra load on already marginal cardiac function. Rarely a local problem for surgical procedures on the cranium, it may be important in procedures on the spine or extremities. It may also influence the physician's judgment in selecting elective surgical therapy as the appropriate treatment. Excessive obesity may influence the optimal position on the operating table and determine the posture that will provide the best ventilatory exchange.

The malnourished, protein-depleted, or

vitamin-depleted patient should go to the operating room following a period of replacement or restorative therapy if the risk of the delay entailed balances favorably against the danger of the disease process. Oral therapy is preferred for a patient who can absorb from the gastrointestinal tract. An adequate diet with emphasis upon protein and carbohydrate content should be provided. The success of the regimen will, of course, be tempered by the tolerance of the patient. Parenteral hyperalimentation with protein (amino acids), glucose, and fat may be required, but rarely in the neurosurgical patient. A near-normal serum albumin concentration, as determined by laboratory examination, is the goal. Vitamin C should be administered to the depleted patient in doses of 1000 mg per day. Vitamin B complex may also be administered without danger of intoxication.[67]

Fluid and Electrolyte Status

Fluid and electrolyte deficiencies that require attention before operation may be encountered in patients who have diabetes insipidus from local hypothalamic-pituitary disease, in those who have had prolonged impairment of consciousness that interferes with adequate fluid and electrolyte maintenance, and in those whose central nervous system disease interferes with the normal thirst mechanisms that otherwise would govern fluid intake. Large solute loads of whatever origin, whether from nasogastric feedings or intravenous administration (glucose, osmotically active substances) or bleeding within the gastrointestinal tract, require an obligatory renal fluid loss and can produce deficiencies. An osmotic diuretic agent such as mannitol tends to cause less loss of urinary sodium and potassium than does furosemide. Clinically significant electrolyte deficiencies may, however, accompany the dehydration with recurrent dosage. Severe paroxysms of major trigeminal neuralgia may interfere with fluid and electrolyte maintenance. The patient who is febrile may have additional fluid loss in the form of sweat, and if he has been sweating overtly he will have lost relatively salt-free water. Diuretics may produce deficiencies; an example is the occurrence of hypokalemia following thiazide diuretic therapy. Hyperthyroidism, the presence of a tracheostomy, and a hot environment will increase

fluid loss, and the effect of large physical size is also self-evident. Cerebrospinal fluid losses by way of fistulae or external drainage apparatus may contribute to fluid and electrolyte loss, which, while tolerated in the adult, may cause a clinically significant deficiency in the infant or small child.

By contrast, obesity, old age, hypothyroidism, conditions that expand the extracellular fluid compartment, and pre-existing trauma or infection reduce the baseline requirements.

The bedside and laboratory assessments are most important. Patients who have lost water in excess of electrolyte (diabetes insipidus) will be thirsty, irritable, and restless, and may become disoriented; and in the late stages, they may become lethargic and comatose. They have dry mucous membranes, are febrile, and usually show tachycardia. In the laboratory assessment their serum water to solute ratio is low. (The serum osmolality is elevated.) The serum sodium and potassium levels and the hematocrit are elevated. The urine volume is large if the condition is due to diabetes insipidus, and it will show a low specific gravity (below 1.010).

When electrolyte loss exceeds water loss, as may be encountered in adrenal insufficiency, the clinical picture of weakness, lassitude, apathy, faintness, dizziness, and, in the late stages, lethargy and coma may be encountered. The patient may complain of muscle cramps, hypotension will be observed, and flaccidity of musculature and a decrease in skin turgor can be noted. The serum water to solute ratio is increased (serum osmolality is low); the serum sodium is decreased; the blood urea nitrogen, hematocrit, and protein values are increased. The laboratory examination should, therefore, include measurement of serum electrolytes, blood urea nitrogen, and serum osmolality and a hematocrit determination. A measure of 24-hour urinary sodium and potassium output may be necessary. The suspected mechanism of fluid or electrolyte loss, the clinical state of the patient, and the laboratory assessment will provide guides for replacement therapy in the depleted patient.

In the infant or small child, needed parenteral therapy should be provided in at least two doses spaced 12 hours apart and occupying, perhaps, four hours in each 12-hour period for the administration. The more practical method of filling the needs by continuous parenteral therapy will be especially applicable to the newborn and tiny infant. Such therapy is designed to send the patient to the operating room with a normal electrolyte pattern and a normal serum osmolality. The derangements may return postoperatively, but insofar as possible the patient should be in balance at the time of operation. For example, an antidiuretic hormone deficiency can be corrected by the administration of vasopressin tannate in oil or a synthetic analogue of vasopressin, 1-desamino-8-d-arginine vasopressin (DDAVP).[80] Excessive sodium loss resulting from adrenocortical secretion deficiency may be corrected by the administration of steroids.

Fortunately, preoperative derangements in fluid and electrolyte balance are rarely of such acute and fulminating nature as to jeopardize the welfare of the patient. By contrast, those encountered in the immediate postoperative period may place the patient's survival squarely in the hands of the surgeon. This is especially true in the case of the infant and young child.

Cardiovascular System

A history of prior heart failure and chest pain that could be of cardiac origin are essential points to note. A change in pattern of a symptom complex of presumed cardiac origin (e.g., anginal pain) requires attention. The patient's exertional tolerance in practical day-to-day activities and to more athletic physical exercise should be ascertained. His use of any cardioactive drugs, particularly digitalis or its equivalent, and drugs that counteract anginal attacks should be noted. Patients who have had myocardial infarcts in the recent past (less than six months) may present a risk that should preclude any elective surgical procedure that can be delayed without threatening life or risking significant neural deficit.[99]

Blood pressure should be recorded in the recumbent, sitting, and standing postures in the older patient, in the one in whom a borderline cardiac function is suspected, or in the one whose peripheral and especially cerebrovascular circulatory deficiencies might render him intolerant to the upright posture. This test may reveal perfusion lability in the hypovolemic individual or the one who has a borderline deficiency in total circulating fluid volume. The status of peripheral pulses in the carotid, brachial, radial, abdominal, femoral, tibial, and pedal loci should be assessed. Cardiac arrhythmias must be noted. The capacity of the venous system to empty with appropriate posturing is a useful test of adequacy of venous return. The chest examination findings are important to note as well as the presence of edema about the trunk or in the extremities.

In the absence of specific historical or physical findings suggestive of cardiac disease that would require a more comprehensive assessment of cardiac function by an internist-cardiologist, the screening laboratory tests to be obtained are posteroanterior and lateral roentgenograms of the chest and an electrocardiogram. A two-hour postprandial blood glucose determination may also be helpful in overall assessment of risk.

The foregoing appraisal will suggest necessary prophylaxis or therapy. This will include the treatment of incipient cardiac failure, the electrocardiographic revelation of electrolyte disturbances, particularly correctible hyperkalemia or hypokalemia; it will help in selection of the appropriate anesthetic agent, and will call attention to precautions that should be observed in loading the cardiovascular system with fluid. It will indicate the prophylactic or therapeutic administration of cardioactive drugs. The presence of atrial fibrillation will require that a decision be made whether this dysrhythmia should be converted. The presence of ventricular tachycardia requires investigation and correction of its cause, which may be of extracardiac origin. Complete heart block may occur without symptoms and requires the most careful monitoring. A cardiologist should be consulted in the management of these problems.

Respiratory System

Just as cardiac function is important in guaranteeing adequate cerebral perfusion as well as for body welfare in general, so also is there a very close relationship between adequacy of the respiratory system and cerebral function and the maintenance of normal mass dynamics within the intracranial chamber.

A history of chronic lung or cardiopulmonary disease, asthma, emphysema, and bronchiectasis will require further investigation. Heavy smoking may also demand further evaluation, as will a history of wheezing, shortness of breath, or productive cough.

Severe obesity, wheezing, rales, signs of fluid collections, cyanosis and clubbing of the fingertips, and an increased anterior-posterior diameter of the thorax are warning signs of impending respiratory problems.

Posteroanterior and lateral chest roentgenograms are essential. In the absence of historical or physical examination findings that suggest difficulty with the respiratory system, the chest roentgenogram is the only screening examination that is needed. Otherwise, pulmonary function evaluations and perhaps expert consultation may be indicated. In the screening evaluation, testing should include a measurement of vital capacity, timed vital capacity (forced expiratory volume, or FEV_1), and maximal breathing capacity (MBC, or maximal voluntary ventilation, MVV). The vital capacity accurately reflects the presence of any restrictive disease. The timed vital capacity is related to air flow resistance in the lung. The maximal breathing capacity is an overall assessment of the patient's ability to sustain a good ventilatory effort. A patient who expels less than 0.6 liter per second and whose maximal breathing capacity is less than 50 per cent of the predicted value will require preoperative corrective respiratory therapy or support. Other danger signs are a vital capacity of less than 1 liter in an adult or a forced expiratory flow (FEF, or maximum expiratory flow rate, MEFR) of less than 100 liters per minute. Patients with such findings can be poor operative risks and require preoperative therapy. A maximal breathing capacity of less than 40 liters per minute in adults again has the same ominous significance. As a supplemental test, arterial blood gas values may be needed.[23,26,50,82]

In the presence of pleural effusions, vital capacity should be improved by thoracentesis. All patients who are able to cooperate should be encouraged to cough effectively and aerate their lungs deeply during the days before operation; this is particularly appropriate to the bedridden patient and the one who may be operated on in the prone position. For patients with compromised respiratory function, deep breathing exercises, coughing protocols, postural drainage, and air humidification can be helpful. When intelligently prescribed and monitored, devices such as blow-bottles and incentive spirometers also may be helpful. Reliance should not be placed on artificial ventilatory machines except in paresis of function. Unless respiratory disease is dominant, the positive-pressure breathing apparatus should be avoided when patients are suffering from increased intracranial pressure or intracranial mass lesions because of the reversal of the venous pressure gradient during the obligatory positive-pressure phase of the machine-induced cycle. Cigarette smoking should be stopped at least one week preoperatively. Almost every patient who is to be operated on under general anesthesia should be coached preoperatively in the mechanics of deep, full inspiratory ventilation. This coaching helps to obtain a more adequate ventilation postoperatively and minimizes complications.

Gastrointestinal System

A history of recent and persistent vomiting requires a determination of its cause, especially if it is due to other than the intracranial disease. The minimal requirements are to assess the patient's water and electrolyte balance and to correct deficiencies. In view of the risk posed if steroid therapy is needed, a history of peptic ulcer is important. A history of jaundice or alcoholism should alert the surgeon to the possibility of hepatitis and metabolic liver disease. In the latter case, the known influence on drug metabolism and coagulation processes can dictate appropriate therapy and prophylaxis. Recent constipation or gastrointestinal bleeding warrants further investigation. For example, ulcerative colitis may be exacerbated postoperatively, and the presence of esophageal varices poses an obvious threat.

The findings of jaundice or hepatic enlargement indicate the need for more extensive investigation of the hepatobiliary system. A rectal examination should exclude the presence of impaction or other impediment to normal defecation.

In the absence of other indicators of liver dysfunction, the recommended screening tests are the prothrombin test, a hepatitis B surface antigen determination, and total serum bilirubin and serum glutamic oxalo-acetic transaminase measurements. Patients with a history of peptic ulceration may deserve measurement of gastric acidity and serum gastrin if sufficient time exists before the operation.[27,105]

Acute distension—in particular, acute gastric distention—requires prompt decompression, usually by nasogastric suction, with the appropriate monitoring and replacement of fluid and electrolyte loss. Patients with peptic ulceration, distention, or documented hyperacidity should receive antacid therapy or, possibly, one of the newer hydrogen molecule blocking agents.

Endocrine System

In addition to the special problems of the patient who suffers specific disease of or direct secondary effects upon the neurohypophyseal system and who requires a detailed investigation, as discussed in Chapter 25, there are elements in this system that require emphasis and pertain to the proper preparation and management of any patient who is anticipating major surgical stress.

A family or personal history of diabetes mellitus, excessive fluid intake or output, impaired sexual function (including the menstrual cycle), asthenia, intolerance to previous operative procedures or anesthetics, and a history of prior medication with adrenocortical steroids all necessitate further assessment.

The signs of endocrinopathy should be noted, especially the state of primary and secondary sexual characteristics, adipose tissue distribution, body habitus, hair distribution and texture, and skin character and color.

In the absence of significant indicators of endocrine deficiency from the history or physical examination, the screening laboratory testing may be limited to a routine urine examination, a determination of serum electrolytes and osmolality, and, as the best screening test for diabetes mellitus, a two-hour postprandial blood glucose value. If the results of the latter fall between the normal and flagrantly abnormal values (110 to 180 mg per 100 ml), a glucose tolerance test should be performed.[1] It should be noted that patients who have not been eating, have been vomiting, or have been taking a low-carbohydrate diet may show abnormal glucose tolerance tests and

require the usual three-day preparation on a fixed carbohydrate intake prior to the testing. With major spinal or intracranial disease, serum thyroxine and calcium determinations may also be used as a routine screening step prior to operation.

Diabetes Mellitus

The patient with diabetes mellitus (particularly one with chronic disease difficult to control) suffers from an increased risk of cardiovascular complications. His fluid, electrolyte, nutritional, and general metabolic management must be tightly controlled. When possible the patient should be stabilized in the hospital prior to a major operation. The internist and surgeon should work as a team to correct the metabolic imbalance, to correct any acidosis, and to assess cardiac, hepatic, and renal functions. The patient whose disease is not well controlled is best managed by administering regular insulin, usually in three or four divided doses per day. Examination of freshly secreted urine for glucose content and repeated determination of blood glucose values offer the guides to appropriate insulin and glucose therapy. Diagnostic and operative procedures to be undertaken with the patient in the fasting state should be scheduled, when possible, as the first procedure of the day. A baseline fasting blood glucose specimen should be drawn before the procedure, and the results should be known prior to initiating the anesthesia. An intravenous route for the administration of either 5 per cent dextrose in half-normal saline or other appropriate solution should be started.[30,59]

Prior Steroid Therapy

Many patients have received local steroid therapy (i.e., for painful bursae or joints); such local injections do not make prophylactic steroid therapy necessary under the stress of an operative procedure, nor does a history of a prior short-term course of steroid therapy that has been completed over a matter of a few days. The patient who has received steroids for a longer period *within a year's time* of the anticipated operative procedure, however, should be treated as though he may still have the residue of adrenocortical suppression; in the face of the added stress of diagnositc studies and operative procedures, he should be given supportive steroid therapy. If time permits, the adequacy of the adrenal responses may be tested (see Chapter 25). Patients who are receiving maintenance doses of cortisone or its equivalent must have these doses supplemented to meet the added stress of the surgical procedure.

Acute Adrenal Insufficiency

Acute adrenal insufficiency is rarely found in the preoperative period of evaluation in neurosurgical problems, but it may follow the abrupt withdrawal of corticosteroids administered incident to the assessment of endocrine function during the preoperative examination. In hypothalamic-pituitary disease, it may be precipitated by the stress of diagnostic procedures, and the risk is even greater during the definitive surgical procedure itself. In the acute deprival situation, intravenous fluids in the form of sodium chloride in an iso-osmotic solution should be administered and 100 mg of a soluble form of adrenocortical steroid should be administered rapidly by the same route.

Prophylaxis for Possible Steroid Deficiency

In preparing the patient to undergo various stressful diagnostic tests when a reasonable question of overt or latent adrenal insufficiency exists and, most certainly, in the presence of known hypothalamic-pituitary disease, prophylactic therapy is indicated.[45] On the morning of the procedure 50 to 100 mg of hydrocortisone or its equivalent may be given intramuscularly, or 50 to 100 mg of hydrocortisone or its equivalent may be given orally. In the event that the procedure is to be prolonged, this medication may be supplemented by the intravenous administration of soluble steroid at the rate of approximately 10 mg per hour. It should be noted that although oral cortisone is about equal in rapidity of absorption and availability to intramuscular hydrocortisone, it is superior in these respects to intramuscularly administered cortisone. For the equivalent milligram dosage of the various glucocorticoids available today one would do well to consult current pharmacological sources.

A word of caution: The administration of thyroid replacement therapy in the face of panhypopituitarism without associated adrenocortical replacement therapy may produce an acute collapse. During the preoperative evaluation and study of pituitary-hypothalamic deficiency states, thyroid replacement is usually unnecessary unless the patient is obviously myxedematous.

Hematological System

An adequate history is, perhaps, the most important part of the assessment of the adequacy of the coagulation process. Suggestions of the defects derived from the history should lead to further consultation with a specialist. An inquiry concerning consanguinity and other familial indices of bleeding diatheses should be made. A history of the patient's previous operations, including tooth extractions, and attendant bleeding problems should be elicited. Bleeding episodes such as prolonged oozing from skin wounds, subcutaneous bleeding, and bleeding from mucous membranes and other exposed areas are important symptoms. The occurrence of spontaneous petechial rashes or purpura, epistaxis, confluent ecchymoses, bleeding into joints, menorrhagia, hematuria, or cerebral hemorrhage should be noted. A history of severe liver disease or jaundice should be recorded. A history of prior medications, including vitamin K and anticoagulant therapy in any form, and the presence of drug sensitivities or alcoholism are essential to record. The prior use of aspirin within a week of operation should alert the surgeon to its effects upon platelet function and the need for further investigation.

The objective physical evidence of any of those items suggested under History should be noted as well as the appearance of anemia.

A complete blood count including hemoglobin and hematocrit determinations should be a seldom-violated routine. A serological test for syphilis also is indicated. From the peripheral blood smear, an estimate of platelet adequacy can be obtained; this should be requested. The prothrombin time and partial thromboplastin time are two further screening tests that give an adequate assessment of the hematologically important proteins of the blood (protein deficiencies are not identified by the history). One may consider the thrombin time (as a measure of the third stage of clotting) as an additional screening test.[90] For a more detailed analysis of a suspected platelet deficiency, a *template* (controlled incisions with standardized venous pressure) and a platelet count are recommended. A detailed analysis of platelet deficiency must consider the number of platelets and their functional adequacy. A decrease in numbers to as few as 50,000 per milliliter may be tolerated at operation. It is essential to make a functional assessment by clot retraction test and platelet aggregation studies.

In the presence of biliary obstruction or extrahepatic biliary disease, the oral administration of vitamin K_1 with bile salts is desirable. If oral administration is not possible, parenteral vitamin K in the form of menadione sodium bisulfite (Hykinone), 10 mg per day, is recommended. It the patient has been receiving dicumarol or allied drugs, these, of course, should be discontinued before the operative procedure for as long as possible, preferably several days. For the more immediate reversal of drug-induced hypoprothrombinemia the parenteral administration of vitamin K_1 (Mephyton), given slowly, intravenously, in a dose of 25 to 50 mg at rates not to exceed 5 mg per minute, is to be recommended. The adequacy of prothrombin levels should be checked repeatedly as a monitor of adequate preparation of the patient. The effect of an initial dose of vitamin K_1 administered parenterally may be transient, and repetitive doses at four- to six-hour intervals may be required until the prothrombin concentration is stabilized. (It is worth mention that routine prophylactic administration of vitamin K_1 to the newborn infant is recommended in a dose of 0.5 to 1 mg parenterally.) It should be noted that the water-soluble vitamin K analogs are not effective in correcting the coagulation defect produced by these drugs.[35]

To counteract heparin therapy (as detected by the Lee-White coagulation test or the partial thromboplastin time), protamine sulfate is the drug of choice. The usual dose is 1 to 1.5 mg to antagonize each 1 mg of heparin. The material should be given in a 1 per cent intravenous solution no more rapidly than 50 mg over a 10-minute period.

For the preoperative correction of hypo-volemia due to acute blood loss, whole blood transfusions may be necessary. Preparation of a patient with severe anemia of more chronic form is better accomplished by administering red cell suspensions to restore the desired hematocrit level (circa 30 per cent or above). This latter technique is especially applicable not only for the elderly but for any patient with a poor vascular tree and in borderline cardiac decompensation.[66,79] Chronic blood loss together with weight loss must be treated by a similar program of parenteral replacement, since long-term nutritional therapy by diet and iron supplement is rarely possible as a preoperative regimen in the neurosurgical case.

For elective surgical procedures in which transfusion of whole blood is anticipated, preoperative phlebotomy can be recommended so that the patient's own blood will be available, intraoperatively, thereby avoiding the high risk of transfusion-mediated hepatitis.

Genitourinary System

In the standard urological system review it is important to note any history of obstructive uropathy or previous inflammatory disease that may relate to the frequently encountered need for placement of an indwelling urethral catheter prior to an operative procedure, as discussed later.

No specific items are required other than the standard physical examination, including a rectal and pelvic examination.

A standard urinalysis and blood urea nitrogen and creatinine values should be obtained. If screening reveals predisposing factors or overtly defective renal function, a more detailed examination is indicated. This includes a urine culture and tests of renal function such as concentration and dilution tests, the endogenous creatinine clearance test, and an excretory urogram, which will assess anatomy as well as function.

Urethral Catheters

Because the genitourinary tract remains an important portal for gram-negative septicemia, it is necessary that significant obstructive uropathy be overcome and active infection be treated. Routine urethral catheterization is to be avoided, but a catheter should be placed in patients with obstructive uropathy or with specific neural deficit that interferes with adequate drainage. Catheterization will also be needed for a prolonged operative procedure, one performed under hypothermia, one associated with high risk of hypovolemia, or one during which the administration of hyperosmolar diuretic agents (urea or mannitol) will be needed.

Irrespective of the reason for using a catheter, one of the smallest size compatible with adequate drainage should be utilized. It must be placed under aseptic conditions by the no-touch technique after thorough preparation of the urethral meatus. Medicated ointment is used as a lubricant at the time of catheterization. A closed gravity drainage system is recommended such that the catheter drains into a sterile bag from which specimens may be collected and in which urinary volume may be measured without the necessity of disconnecting the catheter from the collecting device. During transportation the catheter should be firmly connected to the drainage bag. In male patients catheters that are to be in place for prolonged periods should be taped to the lower abdomen to prevent meatal and urethral pressure and erosion, especially when the tissues are anesthetic. When a catheter is removed, even in the absence of clinical signs of infection, a culture of the terminal urine should be obtained and the results examined before the genitourinary system is considered rehabilitated.

Peripheral Vascular System

A history of heart disease, prior major phlebitis, pulmonary embolism, extremity ulceration, or painful claudication is of significance.

Particular note should be made of obesity, the adequacy of the peripheral pulses, and the presence of stasis ulceration or other areas indicative of ischemia. Examination should be made of suitable areas for parenteral fluid administration.

No specialized tests are indicated in the absence of clinical evidence of insufficiency. A complete blood count and hematocrit determination will disclose the presence of polycythemia or erythrocytosis, either one of which is a predisposing factor to thrombosis. Specific assessment of intracranial circulatory dynamics requires separate consideration.[94]

The serious complication of deep vein thrombosis deserves preoperative prophylactic consideration. The risk factors include: age over 45, past history of thrombophlebitis or pulmonary embolism, varicose veins or ulcers, prior myocardial infarction, cardiac arrhythmias, congestive heart failure, extremity paralysis, serious infection, malignant disease, and prominent obesity. Whereas it is valuable to urge that all preoperative patients (when they are able) be as active as possible to prevent postural stasis, it is especially important for those who are in the high-risk categories listed. These patients should be as mobile as their condition permits from the day they are admitted to the hospital. Because of the clear indication that properly constructed elastic stockings will assist in venous flow, it is strongly recommended that all patients in the high-risk categories be fitted with individually tailored, graded-pressure stockings with maximum pressure distally and decreasing pressure into the thigh. Such stockings should be fitted and worn preoperatively.[47,54,64] A recent study strongly suggests that intermittent external pneumatic compression of the calves by inflatable boots is an effective measure to prevent deep vein thrombosis in neurosurgical patients. This method deserves careful consideration.[88a]

Neurosurgeons should be aware that the evidence is irrefutable that the prophylactic use of heparin in small doses can reduce the incidence of deep vein thrombosis. The landmark work of Kakkar and colleagues has now established that small doses of heparin (utilized prophylactically) can also reduce the incidence of fatal pulmonary embolism and augment the effectiveness of normal blood anticoagulants. Once thrombin forms, then much more heparin is needed. In low dosage, heparin does not change any of the coagulation factors as measured, nor did it, in Kakkar's series, increase the occurrence of serious postoperative hemorrhage in patients whose operations were not neurosurgical. The disturbing aspect of considering low-dosage heparin for many neurosurgical procedures is that the incidence of wound hematomas is greater in the heparin-treated group than in the controls. The use of prophylactic heparin in low dosage may be considered for those patients in the high-risk group and whose operative procedure is such that a wound hematoma could be tolerated. Heparin is administered, 5,000 units subcutaneously, 2 hours preoperatively and every 8 to 12 hours thereafter for seven days or until the patient is ambulatory, whichever is the longer.[48] The safety of such low-dosage, prophylactic heparin protocols in a wide spectrum of neurosurgical patients has received recent support.[7a,102a]

Additional Historical Review

Prior therapy that may dictate special prophylactic management or assessment is worthy of recapitulation: *steroids, anticoagulants, aspirin, antihypertensive agents, antidiabetic medications, thiazide diuretics, anticonvulsants, and vasoactive drugs.*

The surgeon should note the presence of any of the following: an allergic history; sensitivity to any topically applied, ingested, or systematically administered material; prior transfusions and the patient's tolerance to them; and any history of previous operative procedures or administration of anesthetics and the patient's tolerance to them.

Preparation for the Specific Operative Procedure

Evaluation of the Operative Site

The surgeon must examine the site of operation, ascertain the state of nutrition of the skin, note the presence of any localized manifestation of a generalized disease or any specifically localized skin disease (infection) that may require therapy in advance of the operative procedure. The presence of acne, folliculitis, furunculosis, or other localized infection should be noted, and when needed, cultures of the lesions should be obtained and local measures directed toward eradication of the process. The state of the skin hygiene should be observed, and if the proposed incision is in proximity to contaminated or dirty areas, plans should be made to exclude the latter from the field.

Prior exposure to ionizing irradiation, especially if the dosage has been canceroci-dal, may interfere with wound healing. Poi-kiloderma with a loss of skin appendages, the lack of elasticity, the presence of a cica-trix, or the presence of telangiectasia may indicate a poor blood supply and decreased healing potential. Incisions should be planned to avoid such areas, but when they must be violated, planning to permit wide mobilization of tissue to accommodate excision and possible grafting may be profitable, as may consultation with a plastic surgeon.

The presence of previous operative scars must be taken into account in planning the incision, recognizing the relationship between such scars and a possible compromise of blood supply, for example, to a scalp flap.

If donor sites will be needed for bone or other grafts, these should be inspected. Potential venotomy and arteriotomy sites should also be selected.

Discussion with Patient and Family

Direct personal communication between the surgeon and the patient and the responsible members of the family is an essential step in the preparation for the operative procedure. Not only must the patient and the family develop confidence in the surgeon, but the surgeon must be able, through his personal contact, to mobilize all psychological and emotional resources in support of his patient. With few exceptions, competent anesthesiologists will consult with the patient prior to operation, and the surgeon may assist this relationship.

The surgeon must, whenever possible, present to the patient and to the members of the family his recommended plan of treatment. His words with the family are best limited to one or two of the most responsible members, who may then convey them to the other relatives. It is a disservice to frighten the patient, but it is important that the patient, commensurate with his level of intelligence, emotional stability, and neurological integrity, have his questions answered and receive a rational explanation of the reasons for the operation, what is to be expected, something of the risks that are being undertaken, and the alternatives available. The responsible member of the family must be apprised also of the major aspects of the proposed therapy, the reasons behind it, the alternatives that have been considered, and the major risks that are faced. Except under emergency, life-threatening conditions or under circumstances in which time does not permit a geographically distant relative to arrive, it is poor practice for a surgeon to undertake

COMPLICATIONS AND TREATMENT

a major surgical procedure upon a patient without having first met, face to face, with the nearest of kin. Only through appropriate communication can a truly informed consent exist, irrespective of whatever documents may be signed.

Systematic Checklist

The surgeon and his team should systematically check each step of preoperative evaluation. Together, they should note the presence of deficiencies or abnormalities that have been uncovered and what measures have been or need to be taken to correct these, thereby providing prophylaxis against identifiably possible complications. A written note in the hospital record indicating that such a systematic survey has been made, as well as the results of the discussion with the patient's family in respect to the consent for operation, is recommended.

Antibiotics

The presence of an infection with a known etiological agent should lead to the institution of culture-dictated antibiotic therapy in full therapeutic dosage. The urgency of the basic neurosurgical condition will determine whether an established infection may be eradicated prior to the operation or whether the latter must proceed in the face of a known infection. Indeed, it may be the case that the surgical procedure itself is directed primarily toward eradicating the primary cause of the infectious process.

The indiscriminate use of antibiotic medication is to be deplored. If administered before bacterial contamination occurs, however, antimicrobial agents used as a supplement to the host's defenses can be of great value in the prevention of infection. Controlled studies have shown that their use after bacteria have been in the wound for about three hours has little antibiotic effect. Preventive antibiotics are indicated in patients with wounds contaminated with dirt or other foreign bodies, in those with wounds associated with devitalized tissue or ischemia, and in those whose host defenses are impaired by immunosuppression, low blood volume, anemia, reduced pulmonary function, and the like. Also, antibiotics are indicated if the surgeon anticipates entering a previously noncommuni-cating contaminated zone or site of frank infection. A greatly prolonged operation may justify their use. When possible, the medication should be available at the operative site via the systemic circulation prior to the incision and should be continued throughout the procedure and for several hours thereafter.[2,57] Preventive use of antibiotics may be desirable in cerebrospinal fluid shunting procedures.[84]

Local Operative Site Preparation

When the site of the proposed operative procedure is known, preliminary cleansing of the area at home or during the preoperative in-hospital stay should be undertaken in the absence of any shaving. This will take the form of regular shampoos or showers using hexachlorophene-medicated soaps or their equivalent. Special attention must be given to eliminating crusts and to other areas of skin blemish that may be hiding loci for bacteria. Operations planned on the distal part of the extremities require a program of hygiene for nails, fingers, or toes. The patient may be given a nail brush and directed to carry out a careful surgical toilet.

For operations involving the thoracic and lower spine or the extremities, preliminary shaving may be done on the evening before operation if the procedure is scheduled as the first case. Otherwise it is better to perform the nonsterile surgical preparation of the operative site on the morning of operation. For the elective craniotomy or posterior cervical procedure, all hair clipping should be done on the ward; in the case of the urgent problem that leads to the patient's coming to the operating suite unprepared, the preparation should be in a room separate from the operating theater. The reasons for postponing head clipping and shaving until the day of operation are: The patient has a warm scalp, appears more normal to his family, and rests more easily that night; the shave is close and fresh when done immediately prior to operation; and abrasions made during the preparation are relatively clean and do not act as culture sites for bacteria.

Preparation of the Operative Team and Equipment

When an operating team has worked closely together over a period of months, there will be little need for elaborate preliminary planning of the basic and routine details of managing a modern neurosurgical operating room. Major variations in the operative procedure, special problems, changes in personnel, and the development of new techniques and instrumentation suggest the need for special preoperative planning. The wise surgeon may find it important to carry out his operative procedure in the dissection room in advance of operation, especially if it is a procedure with which he is not fully familiar. Particularly is this true when a new procedure or a major modification of an old one is contemplated or if a procedure is planned upon a part of the body in which the anatomical features bear review (such as extremities or cervical triangles).

If special instruments are required, a check should be made on their availability and their condition (aneurysm therapy instruments, for example), and the members of the staff should be familiar with their complexities. The mechanical features of the operating table and its attachments should be mastered so that adjustments during the operation can be made with dispatch. When a new operating position for the patient or complicated new equipment is to be utilized, a preliminary "dry run" in the operating room with members of the team on hand to become acquainted with positioning and equipment is a wise undertaking.

The need for venotomies (cut-downs), central venous catheters, or pulmonary artery catheters should be anticipated and provided for on the day before operation. These measures will take advantage of the help of catheterization laboratories in the case of the last two procedures and will contribute to safety and the saving of operating room time.

If special lighting arrangements, stimulators, radiofrequency generators, crysurgical units, microscopes, special equipment for monitoring arterial blood pressure, pulmonary or blood gases, blood flow, venous or cerebrospinal fluid pressure, electrocardiogram, or temperature are needed, the members of the team should be familiar with their safe and effective use. Consultation with the anesthesiology and laboratory staffs about the value and technical operation of such devices is important. Attention must be given to the safe grounding of all electrical equipment. New devices that pass electrically produced energy through human tissue should have been animal tested and their safety established. The possible influence of electrical instrumentation upon implanted systems such as cardiac pacemakers should lead to protective measures.[70,95]

If prosthetic items are to be utilized, their availability should be ascertained, and if prior sterilization is needed, this should be accomplished with adequate time afterward for "breathing" of such materials as plastics if these require gas sterilization.

Special medications that may be needed during the operative procedure, such as hypotensive agents, antivasoactive medications, antibiotics, or steroids, should be arranged for in advance of the actual operation.

The responsible surgeon and anesthesiologist should discuss the general plans and anesthetic requirements of the operative procedure on the day before operation whenever possible, but in any case in advance of inducing anesthesia.

It should be the responsibility of a designated member of the surgical team to insure that all important and useful diagnostic data are available at the time of operation. These include radiological studies and results of clinical laboratory determinations that will affect management. If special laboratory aids are to be requested during the operative procedure, arrangements for these must be made.

Advance preparation of adequate amounts of blood of the appropriate type or of other vascular supporting fluids should be made. If, for hematological reasons, the need for fresh blood or platelets or other special blood products is anticipated, arrangements with the blood bank should be made.

THE OPERATIVE PROCEDURE

Prophylactic Measures During the Operation

Medications

Preanesthetic Medications

Agents that significantly increase intracranial pressure, depress respiratory function, contribute to vasospasm, produce prolonged postanesthetic obtundation, or have an excessive vagotonic effect are, all else being equal, undesirable agents to employ for major intracranial procedures. To counteract the vagotonic effects of certain anesthetic agents and the adverse neural bombardment, which might set the stage for cardiac arrest, atropine-like drugs usually are indicated in the preanesthetic medication protocol. Since an intravenous route is readily available in the operating room, the atropine or atropine-like medication may be administered to an adult patient intravenously and need not contribute to the patient's discomfort by premature administration. The medication is, however, best administered prior to an infant's arrival in the operating room.[89]

Steroids

When treating a patient with steroid deficiency or suspected deficiency or when it is anticipated that the operation will render the patient deficient, the surgeon should insure that the patient arrives in the operating room having received a "loading" dosage of steroids as described in the section on the preoperative evaluation of the endocrine system. For his continued prophylactic or replacement needs of adrenocortical steroids, intravenous administration of approximately 10 mg of a soluble solution such as hydrocortisone sodium succinate should begin at the time of anesthetic induction and be administered in the dosage of 10 mg per hour throughout the operative procedure. Patients who are receiving glucocorticoids for the control of central nervous system edema (e.g., dexamethasone) should continue to receive such medication intraoperatively. If the operative manipulation is likely to initiate an edematous process with the resulting significant neurological deficit, a "loading" dose of dexamethasone (10 mg) should be administered intraoperatively.

Diuretic Agents

The intravenous infusion of hyperosmotic agents is of great value for decreasing brain and spinal fluid bulk with a consequent decrease in intracranial and cerebrospinal fluid pressures. The two solutions recommended are urea in 10 per cent invert sugar, administered in a 30 per cent solution in a dosage of 1 to 1.5 gm per kilogram of body weight, and mannitol administered in a 20 per cent solution in distilled water in doses of 1 to 3 gm per kilogram of body weight. (If a higher concentration of mannitol is to be used, e.g., 25 per cent, the solution may require warming to prevent crystallization.) The 30 per cent urea solution must be mixed immediately before administration; this is aided by convenient commercial packaging. The author prefers urea since a smaller total volume of fluid need be administered to deliver the desired dose and it has greater short-term efficiency. These intravenous solutions should be started at the beginning of the operative incision and the rate of administration judged so that the infusion will be completed at about the time that the dura mater is to be opened for the definitive intracranial manipulation. Precautions must be observed to insure that the intravenous administration is entirely intravascular; the extravasation of such hypertonic solutions is severely irritating and can cause soft-tissue damage. The use of intravenous furosemide in a dosage of 1 mg per kilogram body weight as a diuretic to cause decrease in brain bulk has been encouraging. It does give a greater electrolyte loss than do osmotically active agents. In practice, however, this objection may not be serious.[9] The degree of diuresis produced by these agents requires the presence of an indwelling catheter and free external drainage not only for bladder decompression but for measurement of the amount of fluid loss.[46,112,115]

Antibiotics

If a suppurative or other infectious focus is identified at operation, a sample of the area should be promptly examined by Gram stain and appropriate cultures should be initiated. Antibiotic administration should be based upon the configuration and staining characteristics of any organism that is identified. A high blood level of the antibiotic agent should be obtained by prompt intravenous administration intraoperatively. For most infectious or frankly suppurative foci, if they are contained and walled off from the free cerebrospinal fluid spaces or normal brain tissues, the antibiotic mixture of polymyxin 0.1 per cent, neomycin 1.0

per cent, and bacitracin 500 units per milliliter may be used for local instillation or irrigation. This solution should be freshly prepared, but may last several days if refrigerated. This same medication may be utilized to swab areas of potential contamination such as exposed mucous membranes of the accessory nasal sinuses. Known specific infections such as tuberculosis dictate the use of other agents topically.

Positioning

One general admonition may be helpful here. If the surgeon studies his patient after the latter has been finally positioned for operation and considers how he himself might feel after assuming that position for several hours, he may immediately recognize defects and areas of possible pressure, stretch, or angulation that require correction.

Headrests of the conventional bolster type, used in the prone and sitting positions, may produce abrasions and decubiti or areas of folliculitis, particularly on the vulnerable areas of the chin, forehead, and malar eminences. Permanent blindness from pressure on the globe for long periods has been reported.[44] In the case of the infant or small child, frequent (every 15 minutes) adjustment of the patient's head upon the headrest is important to prevent the development of decubiti. The head-piece should be designed in the form of a soft doughnut to keep pressure off the external ear and distribute weight over as broad an area as is compatible with the surgical exposure. The adult patient who undergoes an operation of several hours' duration also deserves precautionary adjustment of the head periodically to preclude serious scalp decubiti or epilation. The utilization of pin-fixation headrests avoids such pressure areas but introduces the local injury produced by the pin itself. On balance, the pin units are to be preferred, but are not applicable in the case of the soft or thin cranium.

The sitting position often puts disproportionate pressure upon the iliac tuberosities and buttock region, which therefore require special padding. One should insure that the patient's spine is neither compressed nor stretched between a rigid head fixation device and the unyielding seat of the operating table.

The prone position makes vulnerable the anterior thoracic cage, the anterior pelvis, the patellar regions, and the feet. Special bolstering of the anterior shoulder region is often needed to provide free chest expansion. For operations on the lumbar and lumbosacral areas, the positioning should be so arranged that there is minimal pressure upon the anterior abdominal wall. The bolsters should be placed anterior to the pelvis rather than across the abdomen itself and should be sufficiently soft that they do not compress the lateral femoral cutaneous nerves. The acute "jackknife" posture, by ignoring compression of the abdomen, will not only increase the venous bulk and pressure within the operative site but will place the more vulnerable retroperitoneal and other intra-abdominal anatomical structures closely against the vertebral column and may cause significant femoral vascular compression.

The indifferent electrode plates of electrical devices introduce firm, hard surfaces that should be kept away from bony prominences. Furthermore, a broad surface of skin contact will help prevent burns by the plate.

The positioning of extremities must take into account those areas vulnerable to neural pressure and postures that can produce neural stretch. This is especially important when the upper extremity is hyperabducted in the prone position. Axillary padding for the patient lying in the lateral decubitus position is usually needed, as is protection of the upper leg in the vicinity of the fibular neck. No extremity should be allowed to hang in a dependent position.

Cervical Manipulation and Positioning

The anesthesiologist should bear in mind the condition of cervical spondylosis or other disease or injury of the cervical spine. Hyperextension or hyperflexion often will not be well tolerated by the patient during endotracheal intubation, and intubation may be performed better with the patient awake. For example, when the neck is fractured, the surgeon can maintain correct alignment and traction during the intubation of the awake patient. With the utilization of neuromuscular blocking agents the protective effect of the envelope of muscles about the cervical spine is lost. The anesthesiologist and the surgeon must be alert to the fact that, in giving them an ideal position for operative exposure, the increased ease provided by the paralyzing agents may also permit them to exceed the safe limits of manipulation of the spine, with potential hazard to the underlying spinal cord. When the vertebral canal is compromised, the surgeon must resist the temptation to flex the cervical spine acutely to improve the ease of his exposure. It may be necessary to perform the procedure with the cervical spine and head in a neutral position to maintain optimal alignment of the spinal column vis-à-vis the underlying neural tissue.

Acute rotation of the adult head and neck is likewise to be avoided. This problem arises particularly when the patient is undergoing a laterally oriented craniotomy. The head and neck must not be acutely rotated while at the same time the patient is allowed to remain in the supine position. Rather the entire trunk should be rotated so that prolonged maintenance of the position will not produce cervical vascular occlusion, cervical cord insult, or severe discomfort in the postoperative period.

Special Problems of the Sitting Posture

There are two problems almost unique to the sitting posture that require special mention: maintenance of antigravity peripheral circulatory support and the danger of air embolization. A third danger that may accompany the sitting position is the formation of a hematoma following ventricular collapse. When adequate precautions are taken to meet these problems, the position has great surgical advantage.

The patient is anesthetized in the recumbent position and placed in the sitting position gradually. Monitoring of his blood pressure during the time of his gradual elevation into the sitting position is a necessary measure and preferably is performed with an intra-arterial monitor. At times some form of peripheral vasoconstrictor or beta-receptor stimulator, such as the noncatecholamine mephentermine or ephedrine, may be needed. Mechanical circulatory support must be provided at the minimum by snug wrapping with elastic stockings from the toes to the groin and by broadly distributed, gentle but firm pressure upon the freely hanging abdomen. A more efficient method is the utilization of the pneumatic or antigravity suit that may be inflated to distribute pressure evenly. The lower extremities should be not completely dependent, but aligned more or less horizontally with the knees slightly flexed. It is important that the patient's weight be equally distributed upon the buttocks and that a posturally sound spinal curvature be maintained to avoid postoperative backache.

A catheter placed in the right atrium is needed to aid in detecting and treating air embolism (the technique has been described by Michenfelder and co-workers).[65] In patients in whom severe blood loss and fluid replacement judgments may be difficult, the author has initiated the use of a double-lumen Swan-Ganz catheter with one lumen floating in the pulmonary artery and the other in the atrium. It provides the added advantage of detecting increases in pulmonary artery pressure, which are one sign of embolization of air.

Meticulous attention must be paid to occluding vascular channels in the wound. Since, on the venous side at least, they may not be full or readily visible as blood-containing structures, the surgeon must be alert to occlude these channels as he proceeds through his operative exposure. In the soft-tissue approach it is better practice to obliterate the channel before it is opened. During the bony exposure the emissary apertures must be promptly filled with bone wax; tiny openings may be occluded with the cutting current of the electrosurgical unit. When bone is cut the edges must be promptly waxed, and the wound must be generously irrigated with a physiological saline solution throughout the exposure so that open channels may be filled with solution rather than air. At the completion of the bony exposure, attention should be given to all parts of the exposure to insure that portals of entry for air have been shut.

Continuous monitoring of the pulse and electrocardiographic tracing is required; continuous monitoring of the blood pressure is also strongly recommended if not mandatory. The work of Bethune and Brechner indicates the great value of monitoring exhaled carbon dioxide and central venous pressure.[10] The ultrasonic appliance utilizing the Doppler principle introduced by Maroon and co-workers is the most sensitive noninvasive detection apparatus available and is highly recommended.[62]

Preparation of the Sterile Operative Site

A general principle to observe is that the patient's skin deserves as much attention as the surgeon's hands in the preparation of the operative field. Solutions should not be allowed to flow into the eyes or into the external ear canal. They should not be allowed to puddle or pool about the site or in the drapes so that they are in long-term contact with the exposed skin during the operative procedure with the threat of a local reaction or burn. Adjacent areas of contamination such as the anus or other sites of drainage should be excluded from the operative site by a boundary of adherent plastic film.

Not only must the surgeon give attention to the preparation of the primary operative site; he should also insure that his anesthesiologist gives equal attention to skin preparation and aseptic technique during the placement of intravenous catheters or intra-arterial monitors.

Instrument Use

The indifferent electrode of the electrosurgical unit must have sufficient contact over a broad surface of skin and with an appropriate coupling jelly to decrease resistance and to prevent burns. The active electrode should be housed in an insulated container on the operating table so that inadvertent activation of the tip will not cause a burn (through moistened drapes or by contact with instruments that penetrate to the patient's skin).

Power cutting instruments, apart from requiring familiarity and practice prior to their utilization at the operating table, require continuous cooling irrigation at the cutting site and safeguards in handling to avoid dural lacerations.

The operating loupe and the operating microscope provide most useful magnification for selected procedures. Their use changes the surgeon's perspective; his depth of focus is changed, his movements are magnified; he has a more limited field within which to operate. It is important that he realize that during magnification the scope of his cognizance of what is going on in the rest of the wound is reduced, and he must be alert to the development of complications that may require him to discard the magnifying instrument. Magnifying devices also enhance the problem of wound contamination. These disadvantages with their attendant potential complications may be reduced with laboratory practice.

Parenteral Fluid Administration

For major surgical procedures two separate well-placed intravenous routes are preferable. Whereas needles are followed by fewer complications of postinfusion phlebitis, the convenience of the flexibility of catheters usually leads to their preferential use during the operative procedure. Operations upon small persons usually require a venotomy prior to the start of the procedure. Parenteral fluids that are to be administered rapidly should be at room temperature or, if large volumes are to be given, raised to body temperature prior to their administration to avoid triggering cardiac dysrhythmias or arrest. Warming coils are available for cold blood that must be administered promptly after arrival from the blood bank.

The basic, noncolloid fluid for administration is a solution of 5 per cent glucose in 0.445 per cent saline.

Intraoperatively, the urinary output will provide a guide for the volume of crystalloid solution needed and, except when dehydration effects are wanted, may be matched milliliter for milliliter. Other measurable loss should also be matched by replacement. Prolonged operations should be accompanied by administration of that portion of the day's 24-hour fluid requirement (calculated on a surface area basis) accounted for by the duration of the procedure. The serum osmolality is an excellent guide in judging the adequacy of hydration. Severe dehydration or overhydration is to be avoided. The goal is a serum that is iso-osmolar or slightly above (295 to 300 mOsm per liter). The influence of osmotic diuretic agents and glucose-containing solutions on the osmotic pressure must be taken into account when interpreting results of laboratory determinations. In an air-conditioned operating room and under conditions in which anesthetic gases are moistened, insensible loss may be relatively small. In circumstances of a hot ambient environment, heavy surgical drapes, and the administration of dry anesthetic gases, such loss may be substantial and requires replacement.

Whereas the healthy adult patient will tolerate loss equivalent to one whole-blood transfusion from an operative procedure without the need for replacement, blood loss in excess of this should be matched as it is lost. In the case of an infant or a debilitated or anemic patient, all blood should be replaced as lost. Preparation for such an exigency by having the patient's own blood available for administration will sharply reduce the risks of whole-blood transfusion. In the elderly individual and in one with compromised cardiac or pulmonary function, the administration of red cell mass may be preferable to whole blood. Central venous or, preferably, pulmonary wedge pressures can offer guidance to the fluid loading of the cardiovascular system. Blood is preferably administered from collapsible bags rather than from rigid containers to preclude the threat of air embolization, especially if it is pumped to hasten its delivery. If the blood is discolored or has a foul odor, it should be rejected. The banking of blood with citrate-phosphate-dextrose rather than acid-citrate-dextrose may decrease the problem of acidosis from the administration of large amounts of blood and its depressant effect on serum calcium. Electrocardiographic monitoring will detect citrate intoxication by revealing an increase in the QT interval.[63] Cardiac arrhythmias require symptomatic treatment, but the administration of alkali probably should be discouraged. The same may be said of calcium until more information is available. It is possible that when blood is administered very rapidly, the ionized calcium may be influenced in such a way as to justify calcium administration. If hyperkalemia is a problem, it is desirable to administer blood that is less than 10 days old. The operating room staff carries great responsibility in insuring that the wrong blood is not administered to the patient.

Control of Body Temperature

In infants and small children, conserving and maintaining body temperature in a normal range is the goal and can usually be accomplished by using thermostatically controlled blankets (tested to insure they will not produce burns) placed beneath the patient. Thermostatically controlled and tested heat lamps may also be used. Monitoring of rectal or esophageal temperatures should be a routine procedure for such patients.[81] Severe hyperthermic episodes may occur intraoperatively, e.g., as a sequel to existing (perhaps unsuspected) infection. Malignant hyperthermia is encountered as a rare but dangerous response to certain pharmacological agents, e.g., succinyl choline or inhalation agents or both. Such experiences offer additional support to the recommendation that temperature monitoring be part of every major procedure.

Core temperature monitoring (preferably with esophageal thermometers) is also an essential accompaniment to inducing hypothermia. The vulnerable appendages of the body (external genitalia, fingers, and toes) should be wrapped and protected from the refrigeration medium. Hypothermia to 29° to 30° C is readily induced in all but the very obese patient by a combination of a blanket with a variable temperature control beneath the patient (for ease of rewarming) and chipped ice applied to cover the exposed trunk and extremities. The ice is easily removed as the desired level of temperature is approached. Shivering must be controlled by neuromuscular blocking agents. Continuous electrocardiographic monitoring is mandatory, and the occurrence of cardiac arrhythmias requires a prompt reversal of the cooling process. The prophylactic use of certain drugs (propranolol) will protect against dysrhythmias of the cold heart. A word of caution is offered about the elective combination of hypothermia and arterial hypotension: The patient who is rendered hypothermic has his autoregulatory mechanisms depressed and is more sensitive to hypotensive drugs, and the blood pressure may be more difficult to maintain at the desired level.

Major complications attendant upon the utilization of hypothermia include cardiac arrest, myocardial infarction, gastric ulceration, and respiratory infections.[11,83]

Control of Blood Pressure

Techniques for the reduction of arterial pressure as a tool in the management of certain intracranial disease processes, especially aneurysms, include deepening of anesthesia, changing of the patient's posture, and the administration of ganglionic blocking agents such as trimethaphan (Arfonad) and sodium nitroprusside. The former may be preferred in the control of hypertensive episodes, and the latter for inducing hypotension. It is essential that the monitoring of blood pressure be accurate, reliable, and continuous; this can be provided by utilizing an intra-arterial catheter.[102] Under general anesthesia, the sitting position will produce a differentially lower blood pressure in the intracranial vessels than in the brachial or radial arteries. These differences in pressure must be remembered if manipulation of systemic arterial pressure by pharmacological agents is contemplated. Similarly, the impairment of autoregulatory mechanisms produced by hypothermia must be taken into account because it increases the sensitivity of the patient to hypotensive agents. This increased sensitivity may make it difficult to maintain the desired blood pressure. Hypothermia alone will induce some hypotension, and hypotension alone may decrease body temperature.[27,81]

Deliberate intraoperative pharmacological support to counteract hypotension for protection against cerebrovascular insufficiency in the sitting position may be achieved by the use of phenylephrine.

Intraoperative Complications

Low Perfusion States

The diagnosis of acute blood loss as a cause for low perfusion will usually be obvious to the surgeon and anesthesiologist except in the situation of a patient with multiple injuries who is losing blood in areas remote from the operative field. The estimate of the volume of blood lost may be more difficult. A mild hypotension (70 to 90 mm of mercury) and a moderate tachycardia (110 to 130) suggest a loss of about 25 per cent of the patient's original blood volume. A severe hypotension (0 to 50 mm of mercury) means a 50 per cent or greater volume loss. In the small child and infant the actual amount of blood lost may seem small to the surgeon but be sufficient to produce a low perfusion state in the tiny body. In an infant of 5 kg weight, the loss of 100 ml of blood represents 20 to 25 per cent of its blood volume (8 to 8.5 per cent of body weight) and is serious. Acute intraoperative blood loss

may also result from bleeding in injured parts of the body remote from the operative field or from gastrointestinal hemorrhage due to an acute stress ulcerative state. Acute adrenocortical steroid insufficiency, myocardial infarction, a severe reaction to blood transfusion, massive pulmonary embolization, massive atelectasis or respiratory obstruction, overwhelming gram-negative intoxication and drug excess all may produce an inadequate perfusion syndrome.

The correction for a low perfusion state due to acute blood loss is the replacement of blood. This must be effected rapidly, and the monitoring guides to administration are the arterial pressure and the central venous and pulmonary wedge pressures. The goal is to restore the prehemorrhage blood volume. The measurement of actual loss or the indirect calculation of percentage of normal blood volume that has been lost will dictate immediate volume replacement. A loss of 10 per cent or less of blood volume may be met by the administration of 2 liters of an extracellular fluid "mimic" in the adult. Blood loss of greater volume requires the use of blood as well. The prehypovolemic blood pressure serves as a baseline for comparison in monitoring blood pressure and its return to what is normal for that particular patient. The precautions in the administration of whole blood noted earlier should be observed. Signs of pulmonary edema should be watched for by the anesthesiologist as blood replacement proceeds. A dynamic response of central venous or pulmonary wedge pressure may offer more valuable guidance than absolute values. It should be remembered that arterial hypotension secondary to pulmonary embolism (air or clot) should not be treated with volume replacement but rather with pressor agents.

If the clinical state does not respond to appropriate blood administration, and if ventilatory problems (atelectasis, pneumothorax, or obstruction) have been excluded, primary cardiac causes should be suspected. Electrocardiographic data will be helpful. Serum transaminase values should be obtained, and a blood culture should be initiated for possible gram-negative septicemia. A sample of freshly drawn blood should be returned to the blood bank with the blood bag and pilot tube for investigation of possible blood incompatibility (discussed later under Transfusion Reaction). Drug excess should be excluded. Adrenal insufficiency should be prophylactically excluded by the intravenous administration of hydrocortisone (100 mg immediately and repeated after a period of observation). Monitoring of urinary outflow is desirable. Patients in the sitting position will not long tolerate acute blood loss sufficient to produce a low perfusion state and should be placed in the recumbent posture as promptly as possible.

Bleeding Diatheses

Surgeons with limited experience may incorrectly ascribe to a bleeding diathesis blood loss that, in truth, is the bleeding that should be expected from multiple open vascular channels. As an illustration, the broad surface of dura mater adjacent to a major dural sinus is a field from which large amounts of blood may be seen to ooze from a myriad of sites. Such loss must be recognized as resulting from the surgeon's manipulation and not from any obscure defect in blood coagulation. The same is true in areas that have previously been operated upon and in which large planes of scar tissue are exposed.

Bleeding at the time of operation that does not respond to the usual hemostatic measures of the surgeon requires prompt investigation for a hemolytic reaction to blood transfusion. A prothrombin time and a clotting time will detect preceding anticoagulant therapy. Previous heparin therapy may be counteracted with protamine sulfate; if a warfarin anticoagulant has been used, vitamin K_1 should be administered intravenously. If multiple transfusions have been used and if the blood is not fresh, then platelet abnormalities may be the most important of considerations and require fresh blood or platelet transfusions. The previously noted caution in respect to calcium use should be observed. Platelet administration is both costly and risky, since each unit carries the same threat of hepatitis transmission as does one unit of whole blood. Platelet administration is therefore best offered after consultation with a hematologist.

A severe spate of bleeding that is not due to mechanical factors or the surgical technique itself requires a careful hematological screening on an emergency basis for the identification of deficiency states, as already discussed in preoperative evaluation. A platelet count, a fibrinogen determination, a template bleeding time (controlled incisions with standardized venous pressure), a prolonged one-stage prothrombin time, a partial thromboplastin time, and a clot retraction test should be ordered. Studies of platelet aggregation under various conditions, if available, may be useful in detecting platelet functional disorders such as occur in many hematological diseases. The majority of patients who bleed excessively will not have any demonstrable coagulation deficiency.

Consumption coagulopathy or disseminated intravascular coagulation (DIC) may be responsible for intraoperative and postoperative bleeding. It is to be feared at the time of extensive surgical tissue destruction, other massive trauma with shock, septicemia with shock, hemolytic transfusion reactions, and conditions requiring the use of large volumes of old banked blood. It manifests itself intraoperatively by uncontrolled bleeding, yet is accompanied by macrothromboembolism and microthromboembolism, especially in the lungs and kidneys. The bleeding diathesis is, in part, due to the consumption of the clotting factors by disseminated intravascular clot formation, which aggravates the usual hypercoagulability accompanying operative procedures. Thrombin is formed, which in turn activates plasmin, and fibrinolysis develops. A basic phenomenon is that breakdown products of fibrin and fibrinogen act as anticoagulation agents. The administration of banked blood may further dilute some factors. Expert emergency hematological assessment is called for, in addition to the surgeon's harboring a clinical suspicion. The diagnosis will be aided by the laboratory revelation of thrombocytopenia, low fibrinogen and plasminogen levels, prolonged one-stage prothrombin time, a prolonged partial prothrombin time, and an assay of fibrin and fibrinogen split products in the serum (thrombin time and diluted thrombin time). The key diagnostic item is determining soluble fibrin monomer via the protamine sulfate test. The death rate is high, and the danger period extends into the postoperative phase with pulmonary and renal failure, continued bleeding, and sepsis. The correct intraoperative therapy is still controversial. Whether to use heparin or to replace consumed platelets and other coagulants depends on the individual circumstances. If the patient is bleeding, replacement rather than heparinization would appear to be wise.[14,22]

Epsilon-aminocaproic acid may be administered in an adult in the dose of 20 gm in 500 ml of saline or 5 per cent dextrose in half-normal saline over a 30-minute period. This material may be useful in combating fibrinolytic states, particularly in genitourinary tract bleeding, and has been recommended by Cliffton for controlling hemorrhage not due to specific factor deficiencies.[20] The danger of inducing thrombotic manifestations by its use must be recognized.

Operative procedures for patients with hemophilia should be conducted in centers where the full resources of hematological consultation and laboratory assessment are available. The advent of concentrates of factor VIII and mixed concentrates of factors VIII and IX from human plasma permits successful correction of the basic deficiency of these ingredients. Factor VIII assay or partial thromboplastin time determinations must be easily available to assess the degree of deficiency and the course of therapy preoperatively and postoperatively. For major intracranial procedures the factor VIII levels must be 35 per cent or more to realize adequate hemostasis. Either glycine-precipitated factor VIII or cryoglobulin concentrate may be used. The former is predictable in its potency and may be preferred, but the greater availability of the latter and its ease of preparation may dictate its use. The two agents may be used together. Dosage depends upon the degree of deficiency.[70,106]

In the case of platelet deficiencies, platelet concentrates may be used to combat thrombocytopenia and are indicated with platelet counts below 100,000.

Transfusion Reaction

Urticarial reactions are usually well treated by stopping the blood and using antihistamines. The possibility of pyrogenic reactions further emphasizes the value of monitoring body temperature. The occurrence of a more severe intraoperative transfusion reaction may be heralded by increased bleeding in the form of diffuse oozing throughout the operative field. A temperature rise may be noted. Hypotension may be observed, and hemoglobin may appear in the urine. If any reaction is suspected, administration of blood should be stopped promptly. With the exception of urticarial reactions, which do not require laboratory analysis, a fresh blood specimen (clot), taken from a different vein and avoiding any hemolysis, plus the old blood and its pilot tubes should be sent to the blood bank promptly for examination of plasma hemoglobin, direct Coombs test, antibody screen, and retype and cross match. The next obtainable urine specimen should also be submitted for analysis for hemoglobin. A second blood specimen obtained four to six hours later should be submitted for bilirubin analysis. A catheter should be placed in the bladder, and the urinary output should be monitored. The output of urine should be maintained at a level of approximately 1 ml per kilogram of body weight per hour or more. Urinary output may be stimulated by the rapid administration of an infusion of saline or mannitol or the use of furosemide, especially if fluid overload is possible. The value of the intravenous infusion of 5 to 6 gm of either sodium bicarbonate or sodium lactate (1 m lactate solution) is in question; it may be desirable provided the acid-base balance of the patient is monitored. The continuous or repetitive administration of these agents is not recommended.[4,63,103]

Air Embolism

The surgeon who operates on a patient in the sitting position should be constantly alert to the possibility of air embolization. It falls, however, to the anesthesiologist to report the first signs; it is to be hoped that these will be detected before the catastrophic changes in cardiac functions cause irreversible changes and death. A continuous monitor of cardiac signs should be available to the anesthesiologist. An intra-arterial pressure monitor is recommended, and an esophageal stethoscope is needed. In the hierarchy of detection methods, ultrasonic scanning utilizing the Doppler principle stands at the top of the list. Carbon dioxide determination at the end of the respiratory cycle (end-tidal) is next in order of efficiency and is followed in usefulness by alterations in central venous pressure, air aspiration, electrocardiographic changes, hypotension, and esophageal stethoscope sounds.[12] Irrespective of the monitoring technique that is used, therapeutic considerations strongly recommend the availability of a catheter in the atrium of the heart for air aspiration. Aspiration of the air can be accomplished via a central venous catheter or by having access to the lumen of a Swan-Ganz catheter that is in the atrium. The other lumen of the Swan-Ganz catheter may be located in the pulmonary artery, where the pulmonary artery pressure may be monitored and will be noted to rise in air embolization.[68] The risk of using the Swan-Ganz catheter is overshadowed by the value of the information obtained about seriously ill patients, particularly those in whom considerable blood loss is likely.

The surgeon should be alert to the presence of gas bubbles in the vascular tree. The occurrence of hypotension and peripheral circulatory failure indicates the process is far advanced.

At the first sign of air embolization, the wound should be thoroughly irrigated with saline solution and carefully inspected for sites of air ingress; these should be promptly occluded. Simultaneously with the surgeon's manipulation, the anesthesiologist should raise the venous pressure intracranially by cervical occlusion or increasing intrathoracic pressure. Re-examination of the wound for sites of bleeding after the venous pressure is raised may permit effective closure of the site of the air ingress. Aspiration through the atrial catheter by the anesthesiologist may recover frothy blood and bubbles of air. Compromise of cardiovascular function requires that the patient be placed in the recumbent position rapidly. An approrpiate pressor agent (phenylephrine) is used. If cardiac function ceases, cardiac resuscitory measures similar to those for cardiac arrest should be applied.

Acute Brain Swelling

Massive swelling as an intraoperative complication may prevent the completion of the elected operative procedure. It may preclude obtaining satisfactory exposure of the desired portion of the intracranial space. It may cause fracturing of the brain tissue against the margins of the craniotomy, it may cause internal dislocations and herniations with potential lethal effects, and it may prevent the satisfactory closure of the protective coverings over the brain. The differing causes of the problem suggest the appropriate management.

The primary disease process that brings the patient to operative treatment may be associated with high intracranial pressure manifested at the time the dura mater is about to be opened. This disease process may have produced acute cerebrospinal fluid system obstruction, one of the various brain edemas, hemorrhage, or venous obstruction. Whereas the management of this problem is the management of the primary disease, per se, the problem of the acutely swollen brain may be alleviated by the methods to be described.

Any process that produces acute engorgement of the venous system of the intracranial chamber may result in an acutely swollen brain, and any process that raises the intrathoracic venous pressure will predispose to the problem. Difficulties with intubation that produce straining, breath holding, coughing, or "bucking" will contribute to the same process, as will a lightening of the level of anesthesia that permits the patient to engage in voluntary respiratory efforts in competition with the anesthetic cycle. Acute respiratory obstruction due to twisting or kinking of the anesthetic conduits will produce the same change and, in addition, rob the patient of oxygen. A gradual accumulation of excess carbon dioxide will produce venous engorgement. It is these complications, related to the respiratory system and anesthetic, that are second in frequency only to the primary disease as the cause of acute brain swelling intraoperatively.[41,95]

By his operative manipulation of brain tissue the surgeon can induce acute brain swelling. Faulty retraction causes intraparenchymatous hemorrhage, and the disengagement of critical veins may produce major venous engorgement or infarction. Manipulation may cause tissue dislocation with resulting obstruction to venous or cerebrospinal fluid outflow. Prolonged exposure of the brain, brain drying, strangulation of brain substance along sharp tissue edges, or the use of hypo-osmolar solutions for topical irrigation will contribute to swelling.

The intravenous administration of excessive amounts of water (hypo-osmolar solutions such as 5 per cent glucose in water) may initiate and certainly will aggravate brain swelling.

An operation planned on a brain known to be swollen requires that every reasonable adjunct in prophylaxis be applied to assist the surgeon in accomplishing his procedure. The patient should arrive in the operating room prepared with anti-edema doses of steroids (dexamethasone 10 mg loading dose followed by 4 mg every six hours for an adult). This protocol should be continued intraoperatively. The choice of the anesthetic agents should be made with a knowledge of their affect upon intracranial pressure and cerebral perfusion pressure.[86,96] The intraoperative use of a controlled respiratory cycle that can provide a ventilatory pattern to reduce the arterial P_{CO_2} to 25 to 30 mm of mercury (hyperventilation) is desirable. An osmotic (preferred) or tubular diuretic agent should be administered, and under especially severe circumstances, the addition of modest hyperthermia (30° C) will offer the best opportunity to deal successfully with the problem. The respiratory and anesthetic-related causes are often first noticed by the surgeon, but the corrective measures are in the hands of the anesthesiologist. It the anesthetic is so light as to permit the patient to react against his endotracheal tube or otherwise resist smooth respiratory cycling, the addition of a neuromuscular blocking agent to the point of paralysis is needed. The machine that controls the ventilatory cycle should be capable of effecting a negative pressure whereby the breathing cycle returns to zero baseline or slightly below to enhance venous return to the heart. Such use of mild hyperventilation with the addition of a negative phase to the respiratory cycle will help overcome most respiratory-induced acute brain swelling. *Mild* hyperventilation can, within the limits of autoregulatory competency, decrease cerebral bulk by decreasing cerebral blood flow. Most general anesthetic agents used in neurosurgery decrease the brain's metabolic needs for oxygen and offer, thereby, protection against the dangers of hypoxia due to the hyperventilation. These same maneuvers will correct for carbon dioxide retention, but the anesthesiologist must ascertain that his carbon dioxide absorbing techniques are efficient and that no obstruction exists within the system.[41,95]

The unexpected intraoperative occurrence of acute brain swelling requires prompt appraisal by surgeon and anesthesiologist. Easy communication between the two is essential and often requires preoperative consultation. The steps in management of the swelling are those just reviewed, and the surgeon will need to exercise patience while these measures take effect. A hematoma, an area of badly contused brain, or ventricular obstruction may be responsible for or contribute to the swelling, and, if present, clearly requires resection or evacuation. The successful treatment of the primary disease, as by tumor mass excision or cyst evacuation, will often offer the best therapy for the acutely swollen brain, and this goal must not be lost sight of during the preoccupation with secondary effects. A generous internal decompression in the case of a large infiltrative glioma is an example in point.

Although positioning the patient in the sitting posture usually assists in preventing acute brain engorgement, acute herniation of tissue may occur during operative manipulation in the posterior fossa. This may result from the development of an acute epidural or subdural hematoma in a hydrocephalic state secondary to the collapse of the ventricular system, which can follow ventricular puncture or the release of an obstruction in the sitting posture.[18] For this reason, ventricular drainage should be deliberate and gradual and should be effected just before the dura mater is to be opened and not earlier unless there are compelling reasons to do so. It is preferable to decompress the ventricular system intermittently as needed rather than to permit continuous drainage throughout the procedure.

Cardiac Dysrhythmias and Irregularities

Cardiac arrhythmias can result from myocardial hypoxia, which, in turn, may follow laryngospasm, bronchospasm, and other intrapulmonary causes. They may be induced by drugs with vasoactive or cardioactive properties. Epinephrine in association with infiltration anesthetic agents is an example; the author rarely uses epinephrine in this role. Alterations in the pH and ionic balance in the body may be responsible. Citrate-containing blood anticoagulant-preservatives may lower the pH and depress the serum calcium. The surgeon and anesthesiologist should be aware of the arrhythmogenic potential of either of these changes. Especially are these likely when multiple transfusions of whole blood are administered. Vigorous administration of alkali or calcium is, in the light of our current knowledge, probably not indicated.

The vagotonic effects of certain anesthetic agents and excessive vagal stimuli incident to procedures such as intubation or suctioning may also produce cardiac arrhythmias.[75] These neurogenic mechanisms may be protected against by administering atropine and atropine-like substances. The administration of large volumes of cold intravenous solutions causes trouble, as can the infusion of large quantities of old blood with a high potassium content. Blood should be warmed before it is administered, and if a potassium load is a problem, blood should be sought that is less than 10 days old. The sitting position with its threat of air embolization introduces another possible cause for cardiac dysrhythmias, as does the placement of catheters intravascularly adjacent to or into the atrium. Surgical manipulation of the floor of the fourth ventricle and medulla may produce vagotonic effects upon cardiac function and will deserve prompt prophylaxis or treatment with atropine.

It is recommended that continuous electrocardiographic monitoring be a routine procedure in major neurosurgical operations. The audible monitor will alert not only the anesthesiologist but also the surgeon to the initial stages of dysrhythmia. The monitoring of blood gases and pH will detect hypoxic or metabolic mechanisms. Here again, possible causes suggest the prophylactic and therapeutic management, and the relationship of dysrhythmias to cardiac arrest should be obvious. Atropine is helpful in treating atrial dysrhythmias or heart blocks. Lidocaine is the drug of choice for ventricular arrhythmias.

Cardiac Arrest

Although the surgeon may note a change in color of the operative field and a cessation of the normal tissue movement that is synchronous with the arterial pulse, the anesthesiologist is usually the first to be aware of cardiac arrest. Electrocardiographic monitoring may provide the first indication of the problem, but can be deceptive and indicate cardiac action in the absence of an effective contraction. The disappearance of measurable blood pressure or of major arterial pulsations is sufficient to make the diagnosis of cardiac arrest. The absence of femoral, aortic, or carotid pulse is verified, and the following protocol is promptly initiated.

The patient is placed supine on the operating table. The surgeon places himself in an advantageous position and initiates closed chest cardiac compression with the heel of his hand over the lower end of the sternum. He exerts a downward force such that there is a 3 to 5 cm excursion of the sternum toward the vertebral column. The rate of compression will vary but should minimally be 60 times per minute; the hand is then released fully to permit cardiac refilling; the efficacy of the massage can be observed by the reappearance of a palpable pulse in a large vessel. The surgeon directs the anesthesiologist to stop all anesthetic agents and administer 100 per cent oxygen with appropriate insufflation of the lungs for adequate aeration and oxygenation. If not already provided, an intravenous route is prepared immediately for administration of fluid. The external defibrillator is called for, electrocardiographic monitoring is initiated, and a variety of drugs are prepared in the event of their need. The primary team of surgeon and anesthesiologist offers the first and most important line of therapy, namely, the maintenance of adequate tissue perfusion with well-oxygenated blood. A relief surgeon should be available to continue the cardiac massage in an unbroken rhythm.

Irrespective of the state of cardiac function electrically, the first procedure is to provide adequate perfusion of tissue (particularly the myocardium) to overcome hypoxia. The correction of any hypovolemia also should be of high priority. If electrocardiographic tracings demonstrate that cardiac contractions are occurring in a fairly normal pattern but are of weak effort, resulting in significant hypotension, an alpha agent such as dopamine or norepinephrine may be required. Dopamine is preferred because of its inotropic effect and lessened dysrhythmogenic possibility. If the electrocardiographic tracing demonstrates that ventricular fibrillation has occurred, external defibrillation is indicated immediately. The heart should be shocked to a standstill, and massage should be continued thereafter. If the cardiac contraction returns, but is weak and unresponsive to an intravenous alpha agent, 1 ml of a

10 per cent solution of calcium chloride may be administered intraventricularly by needle through the closed chest. If the electrocardiogram demonstrates that complete asystole exists, cardiac standstill is observed, and there is no response to massage, 0.5 ml of 1:1000 epinephrine or 4 ml of 1:20,000 epinephrine may be administered by needle through the closed chest into the right ventricle. Digitalis may have to be administered. Cardiac massage may be continued over several hours, although within the first hour the vast majority of patients will show evidence if there is to be spontaneous resumption of cardiac function. If it is ascertained that the closed technique is not providing a satisfactory peripheral pulse in spite of the efficiency of the massage (which should not contuse the liver or fracture ribs), then open cardiac massage performed via a thoracotomy through the left fourth intercostal space may be required.

When reasonable myocardial contractions have been restored and a peripheral pulse can be maintained without massage, a second phase of management is instituted: this involves guaranteeing the adequacy of oxygenation (measured by blood Po_2 and Pco_2 determinations) through effective ventilatory cycling, if necessary, by means of an endotracheal tube or cuffed tracheostomy tube and machine-driven ventilation. Restoration and preservation of normal circulatory volume of appropriate composition are mandatory. Dopamine is the agent of choice if pharmacological agents are needed to maintain blood pressure. Correction of acidosis (measured by pH determination) by the use of intravenously administered sodium bicarbonate may be necessary.[39]

Wound-Related Intraoperative Complications

The Incision

Unless there are medical indications to the contrary, incisions should be placed for the best cosmetic effect. The violation of this principle causes a complication that is frequently irrevocable. Incisions that cross visible furrows or flexion creases (forehead, high anterior cervical areas, and extremities) represent complications in their own right. Incisions about the scalp should, when possible, be hidden behind the hairline. Anterior and anterolateral cervical incisions should be placed in the circumferential lines of the neck, following the normal creases. A correctly placed longer incision will be less conspicuous than a shorter incision that crosses skin folds of scalp, neck, or extremities.

Procedures that do not preserve at least one major supply of blood to scalp flaps may be associated with ischemia, necrosis, and sloughing. An incision that isolates an island of scalp between a pre-existing scar and the new incision leaves that area of isolation vulnerable to ischemic necrosis. When there is a conflict between a cosmetically desirable incision and one that insures the adequate blood supply of the scalp, the latter consideration takes priority. Spring scalp clips for hemostasis are a frequent cause of varying depths of scalp margin injury, and the risk is higher when the scalp is thin or has a borderline blood supply. Subcutaneously placed prostheses or foreign bodies that will produce a tumefaction should be located so as not to lie beneath a cutaneous suture line. Prolonged angulation of the scalp after it has been reflected such as to occlude its arterial supply will cause ischemia. Incisions through tissues that have been previously irradiated may pose problems in healing, especially if the skin is atrophic and hypovascular.

For anterior exposures the Souttar, or modified coronal, incision will avoid the cosmetic disadvantages of incisions in front of the hairline.

Injury to branches of the facial nerve supplying the occipitofrontalis muscle (corrugation of the forehead) is a complication of incisions in the frontal region. Anterior scalp flaps should be reflected so that the plane of dissection hugs the periosteum to preserve the nerve supply to this muscle.

Incisions that sweep low in the temporal area to the level of the zygomatic arch risk injury to branches of the facial nerve destined to the orbicularis oculi muscle. Incisions that extend into the preauricular region must be placed posteriorly enough or high enough above the zygomatic arch to avoid these filaments. Layer-by-layer development of the incision, good lighting, and a deliberate search for neural structures (electrical stimulation of suspected facial nerve branches may be helpful) usually can prevent such a complication.

Suboccipital incisions that overlie the external occipital protuberance will be vulnerable to local decubital pressure. Incisions should avoid the course of the greater occipital nerve.

In the lumbosacral region, if cosmetic appearances are a consideration, a transverse skin incision may be preferable to a vertical one. The threat of wound contamination from the proximity of a low lumbosacral incision to the anal orifice also may be a determinant in favor of a transverse incision.

Disadvantageous and often unacceptable scarring and contracture result when incisions cross the major flexor creases of the joints. They should, therefore, be so designed as to not violate the flexor creases and, at the same time, to provide adequate exposure. This is accomplished through the development of skin-flap techniques for peripheral nerve operations. Cognizance of the location of important nerves in extremity exposures will repay the surgeon for refreshing his memory of anatomy. An example in point is the avoidance of the major cutaneous nerves of the forearm in incisions about the elbow for transposition of the ulnar nerve.

The cosmetic considerations involved in placing new incisions on old sites have been noted. In general, when the old site is to be utilized again, the old scar should be excised lest defects in wound healing, further cicatrization, and abnormal scar formation occur.

Bone Exposure, Removal, and Replacement

Violation of Cosmetic Considerations

CRANIAL DEFECTS.   Bone defects that lie anterior to the hairline and are wider than a few millimeters should be filled or covered, for they will produce scalp dimpling or worse. The twist drill hole opening is not cosmetically objectionable, but the standard burr opening certainly is. Bone defects of the cranium can be painful as a sensitive scalp angulates over the bony margin. Defects the size of a 25-cent piece or larger anywhere over the vault and when unprotected by muscle bulk (temporal or occipital musculature) should be repaired by cranioplasty techniques.

FLAP RECESSION.   Bone flaps that are allowed to "ride" freely, unsecured to the host bone, may become dislodged or recessed and are cosmetically unacceptable, especially in adults. In contrast, in children with growing skulls, the endosteal role of the dura mater can be expected to repair the defects, and growth to mold the skull. A well-beveled design of the flap edges, careful wire fixation of the bone flap, and, if necessary, the covering of gaping areas when these lie outside the hairline give acceptable results. Power cutting instruments produce a wider kerf with greater recession than the thin Gigli saws, which may, as an added advantage, be manipulated to produce helpful locking notches in the cut.

Nasal Sinus Entry

CEREBROSPINAL FLUID LEAK.   Cerebrospinal fluid leakage through the ostia of the accessory nasal sinuses can be expected if the mucous membrane of the sinus is violated and free communication with the cerebrospinal fluid pathways is allowed to remain. Such postoperative leakage may be prevented by folding the mucous membrane into the sinus and packing the open cavity with muscle stamps or a cellulose sponge (soaked in triple antibiotic mixture), or by suturing a flap of dura mater or periosteum across the opening of the sinus. Transsphenoidal procedures through the nasopharynx can be associated with a high incidence of leakage, and leakage is also a complication of exenterating the sella turcica via the intracranial approach. In any case, it is prevented or treated by closing the barrier, utilizing muscle, cellulose, fat, or a prosthesis.

Entry into the mucous membrane–lined cavity of an accessory nasal sinus or into the mastoid cells runs the risk of inoculating or spreading infection into the craniotomy site. Large mastoid cells are best plugged with the materials mentioned. If the mucous membrane of the accessory nasal sinuses is entered, the sinus may be collapsed upon itself or fully exenterated and stripped of its mucous membranes and managed as described for a cerebrospinal fluid leak.

In temporal exposures, mastoid air cells may extend in front of the external auditory canal. Their opening may set the stage for cerebrospinal fluid passage into the middle ear, eustachian canal, and nasopharynx. Whenever mastoid cells are opened, they should be plugged.

INFECTION. Plain radiological study of the site of proposed operation should be a routine step in the preoperative evaluation. If it is noted that the accessory nasal sinus site or the mastoid air cell site is one where infection has been established, and if the operative procedure requires violation of these areas, the utilization of antibiotics before, during, and after the operation is recommended.

Bone Necrosis

"Free" bone flaps or other bone that is separated from its periosteum is in danger of necrosis of an aseptic type due to loss of blood supply. To prevent aseptic necrosis of a "free" bone flap, the scalp flap should be turned "full thickness," with the periosteum remaining attached to the scalp. When the periosteum is left attached to the bone, the osteoplastic bone flap technique should be employed to preserve the blood supply of the periosteum.

Dural Sinus Exposure

HEMORRHAGE. Hemorrhage from exposure of the major dural venous sinuses, particularly the longitudinal and the transverse, may be of such volume as to require that the operative procedure be discontinued and completed at a second stage. This is especially true in the case of an underlying neoplasm attached to a vascular pedicle adjacent to or involving the sinus.

THROMBOSIS. Acute occlusion of a major dural sinus, in particular the longitudinal sinus, if located anterior to the major rolandic draining veins, may be tolerated, but the threat of hemorrhagic venous infarction still exists. Acute occlusion behind the entrance of the major rolandic veins poses a high risk of catastrophic hemispheric swelling, paralysis, or death. The major pattern of venous drainage should be ascertained before operation by angiographic studies, and the operation should be planned to accommodate the circumstances. The surgeon should recall that an incomplete removal of the offending lesion with the preservation of a patent dural sinus may be better therapy than total removal that forces occlusion of a previously patent sinus.[43,49] Freeze-killing of fragments of residual neoplasm by use of a cryoprobe may be a helpful adjunct in this and similar problems.

EMBOLIZATION. Air embolization from the opening of a major dural venous sinus is a threat when positive-negative ventilatory cycling is being utilized or when the patient is in the sitting position. Openings in the sinus should be closed promptly, and when embolization is threatened, the wound should be kept moist with irrigating fluid while the aperture is repaired.

Bone Instability

CRANIUM. Bone flaps of the osteoplastic design that are not securely fastened to the host tissue may become dislodged, or may click or produce other annoying sounds. Correct design of the flap, the use of beveling and notching, and appropriate means for securing the flap at the time of closure can prevent this type of instability.

SPINE. Spinal instability may result from progression of the primary disease (neoplasm, infection, or trauma) whereby the weight-bearing elements no longer are competent, or from the operative treatment itself, which interferes with elements such as pedicles and facets. The dislodgment or necrosis of grafts (anterior cervical area) may permit malalignment. Extensive bone removal in the growing spine of a child may be followed by deformity. In the management of the disease, if sacrifice of facets, pedicles, or vertebral bodies is required, postoperative bracing becomes a necessity until such time as radiological and clinical evidence indicates sufficient healing to permit weight bearing unsupported by external means. Local back or radicular pain, local gibbus formation, limitation of pre-existing spine movement, and the occurrence of neurological deficit that has not previously been observed are clinical signs of trouble. Radiological studies including carefully supervised flexion and extension posture and laminagraphic studies will provide an assessment of the integrity of the weight-bearing mechanism of the spine and suggest whether supportive measures are needed.[98]

When grafts are utilized to stabilize the spine, extrusion of the graft, failure of fusion, and collapse of the graft with angulation of the column are complications that may require therapy to re-establish appropriate continuity. If firm fusion takes place in association with angulation and if the latter is not a concern clinically, the x-ray deformity, per se, need not be treated.

Extradural Exposures

Because the surgeon can avoid brain manipulation and contamination of the subarachnoid space with blood, there is less morbidity from an extradural exposure than from an intradural one. The complications that follow extradural exposures and that are related to the exposure, per se, usually result from the stripping of the dura mater from the inner table of the skull and the floors of the various fossae. In gaining operative exposure through this maneuver, a space is produced into which postoperative bleeding may occur.

Subfrontal and Subtemporal Areas

The bony anatomy of the floor of the two fossae should be studied radiologically and by examination of a skull prior to the exposure. It is well to have a dried skull available in the operating room so that the surgeon may follow landmarks and avoid losing orientation. The extradural subfrontal exposure carries the risk of laceration of the dura mater, which in the aged may be especially thin and readily torn. If the dura mater is stripped to expose the cribriform plate, multiple dural lacerations may occur even with meticulous technique, in which event the stage is set for the development of cerebrospinal fluid leakage. Dural lacerations in these areas require watertight closure, at times via an intradural route.

The temporal fossa is vulnerable to hematoma formation in any dead space. Not only are the branches of the middle meningeal artery closer to their vessel of origin, but the apertures in the floor of the middle fossa are vascular, and a hematoma in this locale may, with smaller bulk than in other loci, produce brain stem compression and distortion.

Extradural dead space should be obliterated by intradural inflation or instillation techniques and by careful suturing of the dura mater to cranial tissues. Following temporal fossa extradural exposures, blood or cerebrospinal fluid may collect behind the tympanic membrane, which may rupture and produce an external leak.

Defects in the floor of the middle fossa, particularly overlying the course of the facial nerve, may permit damage to the nerve through either direct trauma or the application of the electrosurgical unit, which is grounded via an indifferent electrode. Stripping of the dura mater from the anterior surface of the petrous pyramid may interrupt function of the greater superficial petrosal nerve, resulting in an absence of tearing homolaterally. Delayed hemorrhage from an incompletely or inadequately occluded middle meningeal artery, either at its foramen in the floor of the middle fossa or from the dura mater, may be a complication of this exposure. Third or sixth nerve palsies may result from dissections carried too far mesially and anteriorly in the epidural space along the floor of the middle fossa. The subfrontal extradural exposure usually made through a formal osteoplastic craniotomy is best drained with a closed vacuum-assisted self-contained plastic assembly.

The syndrome of local brain compression followed by signs of brain stem compression and distortion must, in the postoperative course of an epidural exposure, be attributed to hematoma formation and should not be explained on the basis of cerebral swelling or other mechanisms of intradural origin. Prompt re-exploration of the wound is indicated.

Spinal Canal

Epidural exposures below the termination of the spinal cord and exposures of nerve roots produce complications primarily because of the misidentification of anatomical structures and the obscuring of vision when the expected bleeding from the generous venous plexus found in the epidural space cannot be controlled. Injury to major dura-enveloped nerve roots is most often produced by attempts to expose the nerve root without first delineating the dural sac itself or, in the case of re-explorations, by the failure to expose more normal or virginal tissue from which the dissection into the diseased area is then developed. Injuries to vascular structures anterior and anterolateral to the vertebral canal and injuries to the abdominal contents result from close application of these vulnerable structures to the vertebral body when the abdomen is compressed anteriorly. These injuries also stem from the failure to recognize the depth of exposure and the fact that tactile signals may not always be available to the surgeon as he passes his instruments through a diseased intervertebral disc.

Spinal epidural hematomas may occur when large venous channels are opened and are not obliterated by reducing spinal flexion (thereby reducing abdominal pressure) in combination with gentle packing, ample irrigation, strategic but accurate coagulation, and patience.

Epidural exposures of the spinal cord, per se, run the risk of instrumental contusion of nerve roots or of the cord itself (witness the high incidence of aggravation of spinal cord functional deficits following the epidural exposure of centrally herniated thoracic intervertebral discs). Employment of narrow-lipped instruments and the gentlest technique, best initiated at the lateral boundaries of the laminae, with minimal displacement of the dura mater during bone exposure will reduce the severity and frequency of this complication.

Intradural Exposures

Brain and Parenchyma

Surface retraction of brain tissue must be done with flat, broad instruments; it must be gradually and gently accomplished and maintained, preferably without movement, by bone-anchored holders whenever possible. The surface of the brain should be protected with a nonadherent film; the edge of the retractor should not angulate or cut the brain surface, and its tip should be in view at all times. Retractors should not be placed over a bleeding surface; the bleeding will often continue behind the retractor and aggravate the existing contusion. Vigorous and massive retraction may dislocate tissue from one major intracranial compartment into another and cause incarceration with all the adverse effects of such herniations. A more basal bony exposure, as in the frontotemporal region, can provide access with less brain retraction than an exposure that requires the surgeon to work over a ledge of bone.

The disengagement of strategic veins may be followed by hemorrhagic venous infarction, which, if of sufficient magnitude, will require resection of the infarcted area lest severe swelling compromise the patient's course postoperatively. This is especially true in frontal lobe exposures and particularly so if bilateral frontal lobe retraction from the falx cerebri is to be under-

taken. Occlusion of the rolandic, thalamic, or internal cerebral veins may be followed by severe neurological deficit. The angiographic anatomy of the venous drainage pattern should be studied prior to operation.

Incisions in the parenchyma of the brain must take into account the direction of the major projection pathways of the cerebrum so that they may be split rather than transected.

Probing of the brain parenchyma for whatever reason utilizes a variety of instruments, depending upon the goal. Probing for lesions or for ventricular fluid is best carried out with a bluntly pointed cannula that separates rather than cuts. Coring of the brain for biopsy runs a significant risk of hemorrhage because of the cutting effects of the open-ended biopsy needle. All probing tracts should be promptly irrigated and observed to note bleeding. If it is troublesome, a transcortical incision of more formal nature may be needed to cope with the problem. Electrode placement into the depths of the brain for stimulation or recording and for long-term implantation should utilize small-caliber, blunt instruments 1 to 1.5 mm in diameter. The incidence of deep hemorrhage at the site of an electrode implant in the basal ganglia is in the neighborhood of 0.5 per cent. Sharp-ended needles such as lumbar puncture needles and larger-caliber cutting probes should be avoided except for biopsy.

Blood spilled into the subarachnoid spaces is followed by head pain, fever, impairment of consciousness, and signs of meningeal inflammation that may involve the entire neuraxis and may be responsible for a communicating hydrocephalic state.[33] Protection from heavy blood contamination of the free cerebrospinal fluid spaces should be provided for during the exposure by gentle packing. Firm clots should be prevented by irrigation; if they occur, they should be lifted out of the wound and the spaces should be thoroughly rinsed prior to closure to eliminate as much of the irritating materials of blood origin as possible.

Retraction of the walls of the ventricle, particularly the caudate nucleus, must be gentle lest it produce contusion and impairment of consciousness postoperatively. The major venous draining channels of the lateral ventricle should be left undisturbed to avoid major venous infarction. Foreign material, particularly blood, cyst contents (e.g., keratins), or particles from cottonoid patties, evokes a ventriculitis. The risk of aqueductal block from blood obstructing the third ventricle must be recognized. If the choroid plexus requires excision or coagulation, absolute hemostasis must be obtained to prevent delayed bleeding in the nontamponaded chamber. Procedures that expose large areas of the choroid plexus to a fluid-filled cavity not in ready communication with the cerebrospinal fluid pathways should include resection of the choroid plexus to prevent the formation of loculated collections of fluid. Intraventricular exposures may be followed by the delayed formation of porencephalic dilatation.

Paresis of function after handling of cranial nerves may be anticipated. The surgeon should visually ascertain the integrity of the nerve at the time of closure in order to predict future function. Operations along the free edge of the tentorium may injure the fourth cranial nerve, and exposures in the mesial temporal fossa may injure the third, fifth, or sixth cranial nerves. Manipulation of the ninth and tenth cranial nerves in the posterior fossa may produce either transient arterial hypertension or irregularities of cardiac function. These effects may be damped by the application of a patty soaked in a topical anesthetic agent. Manipulation of the branches of the trigeminal nerve or of the ganglion may be followed postoperatively by the development of herpes simplex (*Herpesvirus hominis*) eruptions in the cutaneous distribution of the disturbed branch.

Spinal Cord and Nerves

Spinal nerve root manipulation may be followed by paresthesias or dysesthesias, and if the manipulation has been severe, a chronic pain syndrome combined with motor deficit may result.

The diseased cord does not tolerate operative retraction without risk of aggravation of functional deficit. The comments on extradural spinal canal exposures are pertinent here. Cord manipulation is better tolerated if the dentate ligaments are detached and the ligaments themselves handled directly rather than via retractors applied against cord tissue. Dissections are best made in a direction away from the spinal cord so as not to aggravate an already displaced cord in the removal of mass lesions. Some protection against spinal cord edema may be afforded by the use of steroids as in cerebral edema.

Comments relative to spinal nerve root manipulation apply here. The cauda equina responds to both chemical and physical irritants with paresthesias and dysesthesias. All irritating materials should be irrigated from the subarachnoid space that contains the roots of the cauda equina. Manipulation of the spinal cord or the cauda equina may be associated with temporary interference with urinary vesical function postoperatively. The dura mater should be closed over the roots of the cauda equina, or where this is not possible, a nonreactive prosthesis such as a freeze-dried homologous dural graft may be utilized. If the arachnoid has not been opened, the dura mater may be left open, if necessary, for decompression. A dural closure of some sort should be fashioned if the arachnoid barrier has been opened, irrespective of where the operative site is located along the spinal canal.

Decompressions, Resections, and Dead Spaces

A dead space that remains after an internal decompression or resection may be the site of fluid loculation that does not communicate with the subarachnoid space or the ventricular system. Such a fluid mass may grow and require subsequent drainage. Postoperative hematomas may also develop in relaxed decompression sites. Such intradurally evacuated spaces should be filled with physiological saline solution. Displacement and expression of the fluid remaining in the dead space by the expanding brain in the postoperative state may require 24-hour external drainage. The placement of internal radiopaque markers (metallic clips or other opaque substances) can provide a visual monitor of postoperative tissue displacement, which may indicate the development of a postoperative fluid collection that will require evacuation. Such a step is likewise helpful in following the subsequent course of a primary disease process that has not been totally eradicated, as in the case of continued tumor growth. The availability of computer scanning offers a superior method of detecting these events.

Manipulation of Intracranial Vessels

Manipulation of intracranial vessels, particularly those at the base of the brain, can be associated with a localized or a propagating form of spasm.[3,52,109] Mechanical trauma to the wall of a vessel by puncturing, stretching, severe pinching, the application of vascular occlusive techniques close to the origin of a vessel that itself is not intended for occlusion, vigorous stripping of adjacent arachnoid, manipulation about a pre-existing atherosclerotic plaque, and envelopment of a vessel with freshly spilled whole blood may, in each instance, contribute to acute spasm. Local trauma and subarachnoid bleeding are the main offenders; delayed onset of arterial spasm is the most troublesome, however. Fortunately, this spasm rarely occurs except secondary to the rupture of vascular lesions such as aneurysms. Locally induced spasm at the time of operation may be kept at a minimum by recognizing and avoiding the traumatic mechanisms of its production and by irrigating and lifting blood away from the major vessels. Local application of pharmacologically vasoactive substances such as 3 per cent papaverine may be useful in reversing the acute local spasm.

Prostheses

Problems arise with cranioplasty plates, which, unless well seated and anchored to the bone, become dislodged and can produce both an unsatisfactory cosmetic result and an area of pressure necrosis of the scalp. Extrusion and secondary infection are encountered most often in the case of sharp-edged metallic prostheses (tantalum and stainless steel). For the covering of cosmetically important burr openings, the author prefers small discs of stainless steel wire mesh. Some of the commercially available plastic covers have caused inflammatory reactions and required removal. Wires utilized for anchoring a bone flap, if not properly recessed, may produce painful nodulations or may erode a thin scalp, as can shunt apparatus. Synthetic dural substitutes may require removal because of the sterile inflammatory process they evoke. Rarely is this necessary after the use of freeze-dried homologous dural grafts. The complications related to the implantation of radiofrequency stimulation devices are treated in other sections.

Stereotaxic Procedures

The neurological complications peculiar to the various intracerebral stereotaxic procedures depend upon the anatomical site of the target. The multiplicity of syndromes that may be produced by stereotaxic procedures must be considered individually for each procedure. The following complications have been encountered in those directed toward the globus pallidus and thalamic nuclei (nucleus ventralis thalami) and utilizing a variety of techniques in the management of patients with dyskinesias. Alterations in mental function have included confusion, somnolence, lethargy, personality changes, depression, negativistic responses, and suicide attempts. Other neurological functional disturbances that have been seen include hemipareses, akinetic mutism, visual field defects, and seizures. The occurrence of transient arterial hypertension during lesion-making alerts the surgeon to the possibility of bleeding. Prophylactic use of pharmacological measures to prevent abrupt rises in arterial pressure during these procedures may be advisable. Intraparenchymatous hemorrhage may occur, as may thalamic abscess, meningitis, and more superficial wound infections or the migration of permanently implanted flexible cannulae. Infection, hemorrhage, and the migration of implanted devices are generic complications common to any stereotaxic procedure. The other complications are more specifically related to the site of the target and the technique of lesion production.

Spinal stereotaxic procedures, notably percutaneous cordotomy, are associated with few complications that are not related to the specific technique. Any stereotaxic technique in which electric current is employed is associated with the complications caused by defects in the equipment and its use. These include surges of current exceeding safe levels and the formation of gas pockets with subsequent explosion and tissue destruction. Such complications can be avoided by careful selection and preliminary animal testing of the equipment prior to its adoption, as discussed in the section on preparation of electrical equipment.

Trans-sphenoidal procedures have included surgical removal of tissue, implantation of radioactive elements, or the utilization of cryoprobes to remove or destroy either normal or abnormal intrasellar tissue. The complications vary somewhat with the technique employed, but cerebrospinal fluid rhinorrhea, meningitis, extraocular muscle palsies, visual field defects, and the complications incident to ablation of hormonal production lead the list. The incidence of cerebrospinal fluid rhinorrhea has been reduced by the utilization of plugging techniques; when it does occur, it requires the administration preoperatively, intraoperatively, and postoperatively of antibiotic medication.[38,76,78,111]

Skeletal Traction

In the child, when the skull is firm enough for the application of skeletal traction, techniques should be utilized that penetrate the full thickness of the skull rather than those that involve the use of tongs, which penetrate only into the diploic spaces and from which continuous bleeding may be troublesome. The apparatus designed to penetrate both tables of the skull and to be anchored beyond the equator of the globular configuration of the skull will be less likely to fall out than the "ice tong" grasping unit that is introduced between the two tables of the skull (Crutchfield style).

In the adult, if the biting tongs of the Crutchfield design are to be used, a set of tongs should be provided that can be opened to at least 11 cm between points and are equipped with adjusting devices for control of the angle of the tines.[25] A single member of the surgical team should be responsible for checking the firmness of the grip of the tongs daily. Penetration of a tine is usually signaled by unilateral cranial pain in the distribution of the first division of the fifth nerve. The occurrence of such head pain requires replacement of the tongs, as does the disengagement of the tongs, under which circumstances replacement at a new site is recommended. Repetitive cleansing of the scalp wounds should insure external drainage of the inevitable secretions. More serious infection requires removal of the tongs. These complications and their management are independent of the details of traction, which are beyond the scope of this discussion, but it is well to remember that malalignment and distraction may be avoided by repeated radiological documentation of the effects of therapy —as often as several times per day if necessary.

Special Wound Problems

The complications encountered in the management of contaminated wounds, irrespective of their location, result from infection and healing defects arising from incomplete elimination of contaminating foreign material and inadequate removal of devitalized, necrotic, and avascular tissue. The management is the conversion of the contaminated wound into a clean one by thorough wound excision (debridement) so that the wound site is transformed into one of well-vascularized tissue. It is usually not desirable, except in the case of badly contaminated extremity wounds akin to those of warfare, to delay wound closure for secondary, staged operations unless inflammation is present. In spite of pre-existing contamination, if a dural defect exists, dural closure is a first principle. A dural substitute or graft may be required to accomplish this, and if an avascular substitute is needed, adequate soft-tissue covering is essential.

Intraoperative complications in association with re-explorations, particularly of wounds that have healed completely, may result from trauma incurred when structures are difficult to identify. Such complications may be minimized by designing the operative approach to expose previously unexposed or virginal tissue planes to permit the safer development of the dissection. Skin scars are best excised during the re-explorations. The use of the least amount of buried, nonabsorbable foreign material (suture material) that is compatible with wound integrity is to be recommended.

Most purulent processes are contained within their naturally defined limits. If they are located in the depths of brain tissue, they may have to be probed. Probing techniques should avoid transfixing the purulent collection with the exploring and evacuating needle to avoid the inoculation of surrounding, noninfected tissue. A preoperative identification of the offending organism will permit the preoperative and intraoperative administration of systemic antibiotics. Purulent processes that are discovered for the first time intraoperatively should be examined by Gram stain, and antibiotic medication therapy should be instituted systemically and, often, locally (see earlier section of this chapter on antibiotics). If external drainage is the technique of management elected, the procedure must provide wide drainage and, if possible, saucerization of the wound. Completely loculated and walled purulent processes that simulate tumors within the brain substance should be excised.

Wound Dressing and Support

The complications resulting from dressings, splinting, bracing, and casting usually are related to inadequacy of padding, the application of dressings that are too tight and that constrict vascular supply, or the fixation of extremities at too extreme an angle. Areas of necrosis of the scalp, painful compression and necrosis of the external ear, local wound compression with suture line ischemia, compression of a thin scalp over bony or prosthetic prominences, neural compression, bony prominence decubiti formation over the trunk and extremities are all preventable complications that still occur.

POSTOPERATIVE COMPLICATIONS

Major Complications Directly Involving the Wound

The incidence of wound complications that require special attention on the part of the surgical staff either in the form of special dressings and ward procedures or in the form of more formal operative management is approximately 6 per cent on a major surgical service. Leading the list are wound hematomas and wound infections. Next in frequency is the occurrence of areas of skin (scalp) necrosis, wound separation or frank dehiscence, and cerebrospinal fluid leakage. Wound infections are responsible for over half of the significant complications of the wound itself.[6]

Skin Margins

Skin overlap and skin separation, which may set the stage for infection or cosmetic complications, can be avoided by proper attention to suture placement and the avoidance of excessive suture-line tension. The latter may be prevented by generous undermining of skin flaps and the occasional use of relaxing incisions. Irrespective of whether a one- or two-layer suture-line closure technique is used, it is essential that the tension-bearing fascial plane (galea aponeurotica in the case of the scalp) be included in the closure. If a single-layer closure is used, the sutures should be allowed to remain in place for 10 to 14 days. The best cosmetic effects are obtained by using a line of buried sutures plus fine dermal sutures, either intradermal or transdermal, with special attention to accurate approximation of the epidermis.

The most common cause of scalp edge necrosis has been the utilization of scalp clips of the spring type. The second most common cause is interference with the blood supply from the base of the scalp flap either by angulation or by defective flap design. The third cause is denuding of the under surface of the scalp of its blood supply. The use of the superficial temporal artery for anastomoses has posed such problems. A fourth cause is suture strangulation. Pressure dressing necrosis has also been observed. The more gentle clip of the malleable type with less spring (the Michel and Adson designs) or the Boston Children's Hospital spring clip may be preferable to the more efficient, but harsher, tighter spring clip of the Raney design. Use of the latter should be avoided on thin scalp edges and edges of flaps with compromised blood supply. The necrosis produced by the clips is usually superficial. A crust or eschar will form and slough. During this process meticulous attention to wound dressings and wound pressure is important. If the necrosis involves the full thickness of the scalp, excision and secondary closure are recommended.

Wound Dehiscence and Disruption

General factors such as vitamin C and B-complex deficiencies, anemia, protein depletion, and diabetes mellitus must be recognized. Local factors such as infection, wound closure under excessive tension, powerful muscle action applied to an unhealed incision, necrosis of wound margins from whatever cause, or an expanding process in the sound depths (e.g., cerebrospinal fluid collection, hematoma, abscess) are all inimical to sound healing. The diagnosis of wound separation is obvious from examination; any moisture on a dressing should lead to immediate, aseptic examination of the wound.

Major dehiscences require prompt correction in the operating room. The underlying cause of the separation must be corrected, e.g., if a fluid collection exists, this should be evacuated. A wound culture should be obtained. Wound closure must be meticulous, and the wound must be properly supported. Wounds that are particularly vulnerable for dehiscence are those located in the interscapular area where the action of muscles of the shoulder girdle and upper extremities places tension upon the wound. This problem is best avoided by careful layer-by-layer closure with nonabsorbable suture material and reinforcement of the wound with a padded figure-of-eight shoulder support. The surgeon must be aware of the patient's deficiencies in wound healing capacity and correct these by providing therapy as required. Wound dehiscences are often followed by secondary infection of the wound, the management of which is discussed later in this chapter.

Wound Hematoma

Wound hematomas may compromise neural function and may be responsible for intracranial tissue dislocations, herniations, and lethal compression-producing syndromes. They may produce irreversible changes in spinal cord function, they may be the nidus for subsequent infection, they may compromise the healing of the wound and be associated with wound dehiscence, they may be of sufficient magnitude to embarrass the quality and, at times, the quantity of circulating blood. Significant wound hematomas are encountered in approximately 1 to 1.5 per cent of all surgical procedures on a large neurosurgical service. Their diagnosis, when they are located in the depths of the wound, is through indirect

evidence. The wound hematoma may be only one of several factors responsible for a syndrome of deterioration, yet because of its confluence and because it occupies space, it may be the one factor amenable to correction by its elimination. It may be either in its own right of sufficient volume to cause trouble or of minor consequence until it is associated with one or more additional processes.

Superficial Hematoma

Suture-line hematomas that result from inadequate hemostasis of the scalp margins can usually be gently expressed at the time of wound dressing. A scalp vessel that continues to bleed may be controlled by a strategically placed suture as a ward procedure under aseptic precautions.

The commonest limited hematoma is the subgaleal hematoma that manifests itself while the wound is still fresh. It consists of liquefied blood, often with an admixture of other tissue fluid (cerebrospinal fluid), causing a tumefaction beneath the flap. (A useful prophylactic maneuver at the time of the primary operation is placement of a suture that approximates the galea on the one hand and the pericranium on the other in the midportion of the scalp flap.) The diagnosis is obvious from examination of the wound. Its presence may be responsible for fever and headache or local cranial discomfort in the postoperative state. Its management is usually by evacuation of the fluid collection through an 18-gauge needle. Puncture is made through an anesthetized portion of a surgically cleaned area of scalp that is not compromised by the pressure of the hematoma. The indications for aspiration are: tension upon the suture line, pressure-thinning of the scalp, fever, local pain, or the clinical suspicion that the area is infected. Small collections that are not tense, do not threaten the suture line, or are unassociated with a systemic response may be left alone and will resolve. Sufficient bleeding may occur into the subgaleal space of an infant to require replacement or iron therapy or both. In the infant, such a hematoma as may follow craniectomy for craniosynostosis may require evacuation. Rarely is open drainage needed in an adult. A single evacuation followed by gentle compression of the wound by a pressure dressing is usually sufficient. Head dressings should not be so tightly placed as to prevent normal tissue drainage within craniocervical planes. The material removed should be submitted for culture in every instance. The patient may be nursed in a posture that raises the head and guarantees adequate drainage. Spontaneous evacuation of a subgaleal hematoma into the dressing should be followed by meticulous wound cleansing (shaving if necessary) and an occlusive sterile dressing after culture material has been taken from the site of evacuation.

Deep Hematomas: the Brain Compression-Dislocation Syndromes

When a surgically significant wound hematoma (beneath the bony integument) develops above the tentorium, the following *cardinal changes are of the greatest clinical importance:* (1) development or worsening of local cranial pain and headache; (2) progressive worsening or development of previously nonexistent signs of neurological deficit corresponding to the local site of the operative procedure; (3) progressive alteration and deterioration in the patient's level of consciousness; (4) development of signs of herniation and brain stem dislocation and distortion, including pupillary signs of unilateral or bilateral thrid cranial nerve or diencephalic or midbrain compression, changes in respiratory functional patterns, extraocular muscle palsies, impairment of vestibulo-ocular reflexes, homolateral corticospinal dysfunction, decorticate and decerebrate posturing, appearance of other false localizing signs such as contradictory hemianopic visual field defects, and blood pressure and pulse changes that are usually in the direction of a widening pulse pressure and a rising blood pressure with a fall in pulse rate. The clinical picture is usually that of a progressive, unremitting deterioration, but some fluctuation in the course may be anticipated. *The change in the level of consciousness is perhaps the most important of all the observations.*

AIDS IN DIAGNOSIS. Local wound findings usually are not helpful, nor will a search for signs of increased intracranial pressure by ophthalmoscopy or other mensuration be of value. Although they do not reveal the precise mechanism of the dislocation, if internal radiopaque markers are available for comparison with films taken immediately after operation, radiographs may indicate progressive dislocation of intracranial structures. The presence of a bulky head dressing and the usual postoperative edema of the scalp militate against the practical application of serial echoencephalography, which is otherwise useful in determining shifts of the midline structures. Lumbar punctures are best avoided; even if performed, they give information of questionable value in leading to the correct diagnosis. Improved techniques for the continuous monitoring of intracranial pressure may provide an early warning system to detect ominous dynamic changes in the intracranial contents, of which hematoma formation is but one. Computed tomography is the most effective and least disturbing technique available for accurate diagnosis of the problem. Postoperative cerebral angiography may give clear evidence of displacement of vascular structures from beneath the bone flap suggestive of either an epidural or subdural collection; its use may be valuable in distinguishing diffuse swelling of the brain tissue from a localized mass such as would be produced by hematoma formation. In the temporal fossa, where hematomas are particularly dangerous, the angiographic differentiation between temporal lobe swelling and hematoma may not be sufficiently reliable to base management upon it.

MANAGEMENT. The presence of a growing hematoma, whether in the space outside the dura mater, beneath the dura mater, or within the parenchyma, or, as is often the case, a combination of these, is a surgical emergency when any part of the clinical picture previously described presents itself. The lesion is life threatening and the tempo of the process is often rapid. Management consists of prompt re-exploration of the operative wound. All adjuncts to control increased intracranial pressure and cerebral edema may be necessary so that the full extent of the wound may be explored to uncover hematomas lying in the deep recesses of the wound.

Surgeons cannot rely upon drains to prevent the development of hematomas beneath the bony integument nor can they rely upon catheters or puncture techniques for their evacuation in the face of the acute syndromes of deterioration. An exception to this may be the occurrence of a hematoma at the site of a stereotaxic procedure that is, generally speaking, inaccessible to operative attack. In this circumstance an approach to the hematoma by the introduction of a hollow cannula for its evacuation may be a justifiable maneuver.

Posterior Fossa Hematoma

Hematomas occurring in wounds below the tentorium may, when located in the soft tissues of the neck, transmit their pressure upon central nervous tissue in a way not encountered in wounds above the tentorium where osteoplastic craniotomy procedures interpose a bony barrier. By contrast, craniectomy and myoplastic closure are the surgical techniques usually employed in the posterior fossa. This sets the stage for soft-tissue pressures outside the dura mater to be transmitted to the underlying neural tissue. Balanced against this feature of the posterior exposure is the advantage that in the absence of a watertight dural closure, tissue fluid (including blood) that collects in the spaces deep to the dura mater may be decompressed into the soft tissues of the neck, thereby preventing serious brain stem and other central nervous tissue compression. The clinical signs differ only slightly from those described earlier. Aggravation of neurological deficit noted preoperatively is of the same importance. Headache may be prominent; deterioration in the level of consciousness remains of critical importance. Disturbances in extraocular muscle coordination and function again may be observed. Alterations in vital signs are more prominent under the circumstances of posterior fossa hematomas; in particular, the respiratory pattern is altered (a decrease in rate, a change of rhythm, the appearance of irregularities in the cycle, and a net decrease in the adequacy of ventilatory exchange). Sighs and hiccoughs may be ominous signs. Alterations in muscle tone and in posturing of the extremities may be more frequently encountered. The progressive, although slightly fluctuating and occasionally intermittent, nature of the clinical picture requires exploration of the wound. There are no reliable diagnostic tests that will exclude with sufficient clini-cal certainty the presence of a hematoma with the possible exception of the computed tomographic scan. Even this excellent technique may be "blind" to low-lying posterior fossa hematomas unless the instruments are specially adaptable. The diagnosis as well as the treatment is effected by operative exploration.

A word of caution is in order in the management of patients with wide suboccipital craniectomies. The nursing of these patients must recognize the need for maintaining the head, cervical area, and upper trunk in a neutral, unangulated position. Postoperatively, compression of underlying brain tissue may be aggravated by placing bolsters under the neck or by acute hyperextension of the neck (with the infolding of dressings and soft tissue upon the brain), leading to prompt apnea. Both have been encountered with catastrophic results. For example, the posture utilized for the performance of a tracheostomy may trigger this mechanism of posterior fossa tissue compression.

Hematoma Following Ventricular Collapse

In the patient with hydrocephalus, the recognized incidence of supratentorial, subdural, or, occasionally, extradural hematomas must lead to a suspicion of this complication postoperatively. Particularly is this true if the patient has been operated on in the sitting position or has had a very large ventricular system evacuated abruptly or, indeed, has collapsed or, after ventricular tapping, has undergone head manipulation that may have shaken the relaxed brain from its surrounding integument and initiated bleeding. Ventricular evacuation, whenever it is performed, should be done gradually.[18]

Intraspinal Hematoma

Hematomas in intraspinal wounds manifest themselves primarily by the rapid development of or worsening of pre-existing neural deficit corresponding to the level of the operative wound and by the onset of local pain or the aggravation of pre-existing operative site pain. The management is immediate operative exploration of the wound and evacuation of the hematoma.[61]

Cerebrospinal Fluid Leak and Pseudomeningoceles

Soft-tissue closure of an operative wound within which the dura mater has been left open may permit spillage of cerebrospinal fluid because of inadequate suture placement. Whereas the problem is usually that of an inadequate layer-by-layer closure of the wound at deeper levels, occasionally a strategically placed skin suture is all that is required. This should be followed by elevation of the wound to relieve it of the hydrostatic pressure of the cerebrospinal fluid system.

The demonstration of blood or cerebrospinal fluid behind the tympanic membrane, rupture of the membrane, or the presence of rhinorrhea requires the administration of antibiotic medications active against the gram-positive cocci in full therapeutic doses. An intact tympanic membrane should be left undisturbed. Blood or cerebrospinal fluid in the external ear canal should be allowed to drain freely; the canal should not be packed or irrigated. Nasal decongestants may be helpful in guaranteeing nasal drainage in the case of rhinorrhea. Forceful nose-blowing is to be discouraged. The patient may be nursed in a semi-sitting position. Drainage will usually cease in a matter of 24 to 48 hours. Antibiotics should be continued for three days after drainage has stopped. Although a source of complaints of stuffiness or fullness in the ear, dry blood in the canal should be left undisturbed for approximately six weeks and then removed with care. Most cerebrospinal fluid leakage, other than that through the normal orifices of the head, is through wounds of the posterior fossa dura mater and spinal theca.

The basic management of external cerebrospinal fluid wound leakage is posturing to decrease the hydrodynamic pressure on the site of leakage; the utilization of antibiotic chemotherapeutic agents in full therapeutic dosage; reinforcement of the wound either by dressings, by suture, or by more formal closure; and correction of the underlying mechanism responsible for the persistence of a head of pressure that seeks decompression through external drainage. If possible, the patient should be nursed so that the site of drainage is not in a dependent position. When the site of drainage is remote from the lumbar and lumbosacral region, repetitive lumbar punctures or closed lumbar drainage may be effective. The key to the control of most cerebrospinal fluid leakage is in the appropriate care of the wound itself. It must further be recognized that if the leak is based upon a need for decompression of the cerebrospinal fluid pathways, the patient may develop signs of increasing intracranial pressure due to the stoppage of the decompressive flow following repair. Treatment must then be directed toward the more basic process.

Pseudomeningoceles most commonly form in wounds that have been inadequately closed, and they are especially frequent at posterior fossa wound sites in which the myoplastic muscle closure has been incomplete. Increased pressure within the wound from whatever cause will aggravate the process whereby cerebrospinal fluid leaks into a closed space and distends it by its hydrostatic and pulsatile force. The site of greatest vulnerability in the posterior fossa is at the apex of the wound, the area where muscle closure in the midline over the craniectomy site is most deficient.

In managing a fresh wound in the posterior fossa where muscle approximation appears to be deficient, the muscle may be anchored to multiple drill holes placed along the superior margin of the craniectomy site, thereby mobilizing the deep layers of tissue for adequate wound support. If the underlying disease process has been corrected and cerebrospinal fluid circulation re-established or at least accommodated by appropriate shunting mechanisms, any pseudomeningocele that may have formed will, over a period of months, usually decrease in bulk and be reasonably well tolerated. In its early phases it may be tender and its tenseness may threaten the integrity of the overlying skin incision and require wound revision. Decompression of the area by indirect methods such as lumbar puncture or continuous drainage with a closed system may be effective if combined with gentle wound support, but the full, tense sac usually reflects a temporary, if not permanent, change in the normal cerebrospinal fluid pressure toward a higher resting pressure due to interference with absorption. Shunting of the cerebrospinal fluid into the peritoneum is usually associated with a collapse of the mass. If a valve-like flap of tissue encourages the continued collection of cerebrospinal fluid into such a pseudocyst, operative treatment will be the proper management. It is certainly the proper management in the case of the wound that has been inadequately or incompletely closed. For the long-standing pseudomeningocele, the shiny-walled sac must be excised and a careful layer-by-layer closure of the wound accomplished to prevent recurrence.

Infants who undergo repair of lumbar and lumbosacral meningoceles and myelomeningoceles should be nursed in a prone position on a Bradford frame or similar structure with the site of repair uppermost and the infant so restrained that all urine and feces drain away from the wound. When possible such operative wounds may be dressed with an adherent plastic film applied by spray, and the infant may be positioned so that the wound is visible and any contamination readily cleansed. This is preferable to a gauze dressing that can become saturated with excreta and act as a contaminated compress.

Small openings in the dura mater, particularly in the spinal theca and the sheaths of nerve roots, may be associated with an outpouching of intact arachnoid and the collection of fluid in the pouch, thereby producing a traumatic arachnoid cyst that acts as a compressing mechanism for irritation of the underlying nerve tissue. The development of such arachnoid cysts in the cranium may cause bone erosion and tumefaction beneath the scalp. In the spinal spaces this complication is more often seen following intervertebral disc operations in the lumbar-lumbosacral area. It is associated with the development of a radicular syndrome of pain postoperatively, which is aggravated by compression of the surgical wound. If persistent, the wound should be explored, the cyst evacuated, and the small rent in the dura mater repaired or, alternatively, more widely opened so that the cyst will decompress through its own ostium.

Parenchymal (Brain) Fungus

This complication may develop following the combination of a defect in closure of the integument (dura mater, skull, or scalp) with any of the several forms of brain swelling or edema. It is seen with massive cerebral contusions, extensive intracranial neoplasia (usually of the glial series), and widespread cerebritis. The brain forces its way through the dural opening and, if the more superficial layers of closure are inadequate, may be found beneath the galea or extruding through the scalp incision. Its occurrence is one of the major disadvantages of the marsupialization technique in the management of brain abscess and a compelling reason to avoid external decompression techniques for malignant tumors. Management consists of wide operative exposure, amputation of the necrotic and herniating brain tissue, watertight dural closure, and layer-by-layer closure of the overlying tissues.

Foreign Body Rejection

Foreign body rejection usually manifests itself by the local signature of an inflammatory response (cellulitis), wound drainage, or both. In its initial stages the response is a sterile reaction, but if the wound should drain, this may then be followed by secondary infection. The materials that have evoked reactions have been the synthetic compounds (rubber items, metallic implants) and, rarely, substances of biological origin that are usually inert (freeze-dried tissues). When the foreign substance lies in contact with the subarachnoid space or the ventricular system, it may provoke a leptomeningeal response, a sterile meningitis. The author has also encountered a sterile cerebritis with wound drainage that continued until all gelatin sponge was removed from the tumor bed.

In addition to causing an inflammatory reaction, foreign material may act as a mechanical barrier that interferes with vascularization of neighboring tissue or it may be the cause of wound decubitus or wound separation. The occurrence of an inflammatory response, with or without wound suppuration, or the exposure of a prosthesis requires that the foreign substance be removed. Successful replacement of the prosthesis must await complete wound healing. The utilization of prosthetic devices in performing shunts for the diversion of cerebrospinal fluid has been associated with a high incidence of infection. The occurrence of septicemia, ventriculitis, or local sepsis may be obvious, but nonspecific complaints such as nausea, vomiting, and malaise require attention. Fever is usually common to all shunt infections. Therapy requires removal of the shunt assembly and either immediate replacement of a fresh assembly or closed external drainage, the administration of antibiotic medication, and delayed replacement of the shunt apparatus.[34,73,84]

Tissue Necrosis

Aseptic necrosis is a phenomenon that may involve the scalp, bone flaps that are denuded of their periosteum, or bone grafts that have been transposed to a new bed. The wound response to necrosis may give rise to tumefaction from fluid collection and eventual external drainage, which, although initially sterile, is associated with the ever-present danger of contamination and secondary infection. In the presence of either of these complications the devitalized sequestrum must be removed. Bone necrosis that is followed by a cosmetically unacceptable or hazardous bony defect will require correction by cranioplasty. If at the time of removal it can be ascertained that no infection exists, cranioplasty may be combined with removal, but the safer course is to defer cranioplasty to a time 6 to 12 months thereafter.

Wound Infections

General factors that increase the patient's susceptibility to a wound infection include obesity, old age, prolonged hospitalization, uncontrolled diabetes mellitus, infections elsewhere in the body, and steroid or immunosuppressive therapy. Local factors that contribute are the nature of the wound (if traumatic), the length of the operative procedure, the occurrence of scalp margin necrosis, wound dehiscence, cerebrospinal fluid leakage, and the presence of a foreign body, dirt, devitalized tissue, or hematoma. Re-explorations, the utilization of wound drains in excess of 48 hours, faulty dressing technique, or secondary wound inoculation (i.e., via the patient's fingers) also increase the risk. The possibility of a deliberate, factitial mechanism should not be ignored. The existence of these local factors focuses attention on the need for meticulous technique in the management of wounds. The threat of dissemination of the local infection into the cerebrospinal fluid pathways is a real one, but is usually encountered only in the presence of a cerebrospinal fluid leak of fistula.

In the absence of either a leak or the direct implantation of infection into the cerebrospinal fluid compartments at the time of the operative procedure, wound infections usually remain contained within the confines of the operative site. Soft-tissue infection alone or soft-tissue infection in combination with osteomyelitis (in a ratio of 2 : 1) is the common picture. Postoperative epidural, subdural, and cerebral abscess or septicemia rarely occurs.[6] The severe morbidity and mortality figure of about 20 per cent from intradural sepsis compares unfavorably with the figure of approximately 4 per cent in the case of extradural infections.[55]

Stitch abscesses lie superficial to the first plane of tissue strength, i.e., the galea or superficial fascia, but they can be precursors to major wound infections. The stitch should be removed; cultures should be taken; the scalp should be shaved, if necessary, and thoroughly cleansed. The local site of abscess formation is permitted to evacuate to the exterior and heal, which it usually will with little more than meticulous dressing technique. Systemic antibiotics are not indicated, and local antibiotics are usually not required. The condition must be thoroughly healed before the patient is permitted abroad without a proper occlusive head dressing.

Although a wound infection may develop clinical manifestations at any time in the first months following operation, it rarely manifests itself before the second postoperative day, and the majority of infections will become evident within the first weeks. The clinical tempo of the process will depend upon the site of the infection, the pathogenic agent, the number of organisms in the inoculum, the general and local factors encountered, and, importantly, whether antibiotics that would mask the clinical development of the syndrome have been administered. There may be an associated systemic response. The early metabolic response to an operative procedure will be associated with ½° to 1° C of fever in the first and second days, but after that and in the absence of other mechanisms that could evoke a febrile response, the fever should abate rapidly. Wound pain, which may be prominent initially, should likewise steadily decrease in intensity. Tissue edema in the wound should resolve after the first two to three days, and, as the wound fluid redistributes, the tissues immediately in the vicinity of the incision should become flat and reactionless and appear without inflammation to the inspecting eye and nontender to the gently palpating gloved finger. Quite apart from the systemic response of fever, malaise, leukocytosis, tachycardia, or elevated sedimentation rate, any or all of which may be absent, the local manifestations of wound infection may be those of fullness in the wound, redness, edema, suture stretch, pigskin appearance of the epidermis, tenderness, or, indeed, fluctuation if the process is superficial. Drainage sites may show discoloration, give rise to odor, or be associated with a neighboring adenopathic response.

If the local indications point to the presence of infection, the wound should be opened. If there is significant doubt that the wound is the site of trouble and if the wound is fresh, a blunt-nosed hemostat may be gently inserted into its depths. This is a reasonable approach *only* for the purposes of excluding the presence of suppuration and liquefaction in the wound. A wound culture of such a probed tract should be made. If, after this maneuver, there is clear evidence of infection, the patient should be taken to the operating room and the wound should be opened to expose the full reaches of the infection. If it is reasonably certain that wound suppuration exists in the absence of external drainage, probing is to be avoided and the patient should be taken to the operating room where the wound may be opened under optimal conditions. The principle underlying management is the exposure of all parts of the wound occupied by the liquefied, necrotic tissue. Sealed tissue planes should be left intact, but pockets or septae that enclose loci of infection should be gently broken down so that the wound may drain freely to the saucerized center. Infected bone or a foreign body requires removal. If the infection involves any part of the bone flap, the entire flap should be removed. Where undetached host bone is infected, all dead (nonbleeding) bone should be rongeured back to healthy-looking, bleeding bone. The dural barrier should be left intact. If the infection lies deep to the dura, the local area of cerebritis should be excised and the dura reconstituted.

In major craniotomy infections, after the bone flap has been removed and cultures have been taken and the wound has been irrigated with antibiotic solution, it should be gently packed with fine mesh gauze. Catheters may be incorporated for the subsequent introduction of local antibiotic medications (polymyxin 0.1 per cent, neomycin 1.0 per cent, and bacitracin 500 units per milliliter). Other noninjurious solutions may be preferred. The scalp edges are loosely approximated with stainless steel sutures (protected by bolsters) to prevent severe retraction. The scalp should be sufficiently relaxed that dressings can readily be changed in the depths of the wound. The fine mesh gauze is removed and replaced at one- to three-day intervals, and the wound is permitted to close from its base and to obliterate all pockets through the healing of the scalp flap to the underlying tissue. Subsequent wound margin revision may be necessary to obtain a cosmetically acceptable closure. Cranioplasty, if required, should be deferred for 12 months following such a purulent infection.

In the management of laminectomy infections the same general principles should be observed: saucerization of the wound, evacuation of all recesses of infection, and open packing. Devitalized tissue must be trimmed away in the course of wound toilet. Once a healthy bed of granulation tissue covers all exposed bone, the wound may be secondarily closed.

Meticulous adherence to wound dressing technique, patient isolation, or wound occlusion and isolation must be observed whatever the site of the infection.

Depending upon the organism responsible for the infection, systemic antibiotics should be administered and continued until serial wound cultures for the pathogens are negative, at which time it is reasonable to perform secondary closure and to discontinue isolation techniques. Although the basic principle of adequate operative evacuation of a purulent collection still pertains, the management of infections of closed fluid spaces involving the ventricular cavity or loculations thereof may require the local instillation of antibiotics in preference to external evacuation. Most examples of postoperative leptomeningitis can be treated by systemically administered antibiotic therapy.

It is the surgeon's responsibility to attend his wound and manage it until it is in a safe state before delegating this task to others.

Complications Related But Not Limited to the Wound

Tissue Edemas

One of the primary challenges of the surgical management of disease involving central nervous tissue in its confines within the skeleton is that of tissue swelling, which may accompany disease preoperatively, intraoperatively, and in the postoperative phase.[5] The intraoperative aspects of this problem have already been discussed.

Certain of the edemas are caused by direct physical trauma and cell membrane rupture, the physical injury of radiation, the local effect of certain toxic chemical agents, and by inflammation-inducing agents such as bacteria, the deprivation of tissue of needed nutriment including oxygen, and the creation of severe osmotic gradients across cell membranes. Other mechanisms that contribute to an increase in brain bulk include swelling of the vascular compartment of the intracranial chamber (frequently on the venous side, rarely on the arterial side), obstruction to the normal passage of cerebrospinal fluid, the presence or creation of a foreign mass of tissue, or any combination. Although no one of these mechanisms, alone, may be responsible for the clinical difficulties, correction of a single factor may be sufficient to tip the scales favorably. Conversely, to ignore a single factor may do the opposite. Operative procedures confined to the epidural space with minimal or no manipulation of central nervous tissue are associated with minimal morbidity insofar as the serious tissue edemas are concerned. The tissue edemas that occur outside the confines of the bony integument incident to operations upon the head, spine, and peripheral nerves rarely pose a problem in the absence of hemorrhage or infection. Ischemic necrosis with attendant tissue edema can be seen under these circumstances; this has been discussed under the complications of wound management.

The edema that is due to direct operative trauma begins immediately, reaches its peak usually on the second postoperative day and subsides steadily thereafter. If the primary disease process is associated with edema, the latter will be aggravated by operative manipulation, even though the goal of operation is to so treat the disease that the balance is favorable for recovery.

Edemas due to such mechanisms as fluid and electrolyte imbalance (water intoxication) can come about at any time in the course of the disease when the environment is changed, but most critically at the time the edema of trauma is maximal. Should infection intervene, the tempo of the edema process will coincide with the inflammatory process and may summate with other mechanisms. One such mechanism that must not be forgotten is cerebral fat embolization, especially in the patient who has suffered extensive and multiple wounds.[8,100]

If respiratory obstruction occurs, this likewise will interfere with a smooth course by contributing to the adverse effects of any one of the tissue edemas.

Whereas any of the processes, irrespective of their timing, may be of sufficient severity to influence the postoperative course adversely, it is the combination of effects coinciding with maximal tissue edema from operative trauma that poses that most common problem, and this will be encountered from the time of operation through the first few postoperative days. Rigid limits upon the danger period cannot be set, but the first three postoperative days are the most critical.

The diagnosis of significant tissue edemas depends upon an awareness of the possible mechanisms and the probable tempo to be expected according to their differing causes, especially noting the timing of the response to operative manipulation. A series of observations of the patient's neurological status in the immediate postanesthetic recovery period, with special attention to the level of consciousness, will provide a baseline for comparison and determination of subsequent deterioration. The appearance of or the worsening of preexisting neurological deficit corresponding to the site of operation will be the commonest clinical manifestation of a wound-related cerebral edema. Blunting and deterioration of the level of consciousness represent a more severe response and a manifestation of a more widespread effect including the occurrence of dislocations and incarcerations. It is important to recognize that the initial peak of edema with its associated aggravating factors may tip the scales in the direction of severe dislocation and herniation of brain tissue, which, once established, will result in irreparable and incapacitating neural damage, if not death, regardless of the subsidence of the initiating process.

Cerebral angiography may give a useful clue and demonstrate the picture of diffuse edema in contrast to a focal hemorrhage. Angiography may also reveal the presence of widespread vasospasm as a possible underlying contributor to the swollen state of the tissues, but it must be remembered that the edema process itself may secondarily compress the vascular tree. The advent of computed tomography provides an effective diagnostic tool for the identification of the edema and its discrimination from other space-occupying processes of surgical importance.

If, on clinical and other grounds of assessment, it is not possible to separate the tissue edemas from a possible hematoma or other evacuable mass lesion (fluid loculation), the wound should be explored promptly.

The nonoperative management of the cerebral edemas requires attention to each of the mechanisms that can cause aggravation of the increased tissue mass. Respiratory exchange must be adequate to maintain the P_{CO_2} in normal or low range. The patient is nursed to enhance venous drainage and respiratory exchange, rectal elimination is made easy to avoid straining, troublesome coughing and hiccoughing are controlled. Respiratory depressant drugs are avoided. Cerebral venous drainage must be unobstructed, and cerebral vascular bulk may be reduced by mild hyperventilation techniques.

If artificial ventilatory apparatus is employed to replace spontaneous respirations or to provide hyperventilation, the automatic cycle should have a small negative phase to avoid the deleterious effects of an exclusively positive-pressured, artificial inflation and to replace the negative intrathoracic pressure of inspiration, which normally aids in venous return from the cranium. A time-cycled, volume-limited respirator is the machine of choice. The serum should be maintained at least iso-osmolar by avoiding hypo-osmolar fluid ad-

ministration. For maintenance fluid, the author prefers 5 per cent dextrose in a 0.445 per cent sodium chloride solution. Instead of restricting fluid severely, the serum osmolality is checked frequently and the fluid is given in amounts required for basic needs.

Osmotic diuretics (urea, mannitol, or glycerol) or, less optimally, furosemide are useful and should be employed when the process is expected to be self-limited and reversible. The agents should be administered in time to blunt the approaching peak of the edema process or to reverse an acute rise in intracranial pressure as detected by monitoring techniques. Administration of hypo-osmotic solutions, either intravenously or orally, should be limited to avoid severe dehydration and hyperosmolality. Other corrective measures may sustain the beneficial effects of the short courses of therapy. The long-term administration of dehydrating and hyperosmolar agents may precipitate a hyperosmolar state, which has signs that mimic those of edema. The hyperosmolar state may result from unsuspected diabetes mellitus producing a nonketotic coma. The gluconeogenic effects of steroids may aggravate the process (see section on preoperative fluid and electrolyte status and intraoperative administration of osmotically active agents).

Adrenocorticosteroids of the group devoid of appreciable sodium-retaining activity are helpful in preventing and controlling certain forms of cerebral edema. Dexamethasone is the current drug of choice and is administered parenterally or by mouth. For an adult patient the usual loading dose is 10 to 16 mg followed by a maintenance dose of 4 to 6 mg every six hours during the acute phase. A protocol of rapidly tapering dosage can then complete the course in a total of five to seven days. Oral medication should replace the parenteral medication as soon as the patient is able to accept it. Oral antacid therapy is recommended for all patients receiving such steroid therapy. If prolonged steroid therapy is needed it is usually well tolerated at a lower dosage of 1 to 2 mg every six hours by mouth.

For the patient who is seriously ill from cerebral edema following operation for neoplasm, trauma, infection, or vascular disease, the challenge is great. Each of the adjuncts just reviewed is mobilized. Respiratory adequacy of oxygenation is assured by endotracheal intubation (or tracheostomy after 48 hours if the process is going to be prolonged). The arterial partial pressure of carbon dioxide is maintained at 26 to 30 mm of mercury. Maintenance fluids and steroids are administered as described. The patient's core body temperature is reduced to 30°C by external cooling measures, and shivering as detected clinically or by electrocardiographic monitor is controlled with chlorpromazine. Arterial blood pressure monitoring is instituted to allow control of severe hypotension or of hypertensive overshoot with nitroprusside. Anticonvulsants are administered to protect against seizure activity, and antibiotics are used according to principles that were outlined previously. Clinical and manometric monitoring of behavior and intracranial pressure permits the intermittent administration of osmotic diuretics to control the acute pressure plateau waves. The recent reports of the adjunctive use of barbiturates in control of acutely raised intracranial pressure in such cases deserves attention.[87] This protocol of management may tide the patient over his acute process until the abnormal pressure is naturally reversed or until corrective operative measures can be applied. When they are accessible, operative resections of hemorrhagically infarcted or contused areas that "feed" the edema-producing process have been helpful. These resections also provide decompression. Massive decompressive craniectomies have not been utilized by the author. Excellent reviews of this subject have been published by Shapiro and co-workers and Stullken and Sokoll.[86,87,96]

The management of the edemas that involve the spinal cord follows closely the pattern of management outlined earlier.

Vasospasm

The section on the tissue edemas is pertinent to this discussion, and it is difficult to say whether vasospasm, when associated with cerebral swelling, is secondary to mechanisms independent of those responsible for the edema or whether the mechanism causing the vasospasm is primary and responsible in turn for cerebral ischemia and secondary edema. Most evidence supports the former concept. Angiographic studies clarify the presence and the extent of vasospasm. Postoperatively, the surgeon must be concerned about the delayed-onset, prolonged vasospasm that is almost always associated with intracranial vascular disease (usually an aneurysm) and subarachnoid bleeding. Whether the spasm observed angiographically is only fortuitously associated with the adverse neural function or whether it is an epiphenomenon, a bellwether of other derangement, or the etiological agent of the neural deficit is not clear. The management is essentially the same as for brain edema, but the dilemma is obvious.[60] If the process is one of vasospasm and severe tissue swelling, the introduction of any greater volume of blood bulk into the intracranial chamber may be deleterious. What is wanted is a decrease of bulk of other tissues and an increase in adequate perfusion of tissue. Decreased tissue bulk is usually associated with improved cerebral perfusion; for example, increased cerebral blood flow accompanies the administration of a hyperosmotic agent such as urea. If the process is one of cerebral ischemia such as may attend vascular occlusive procedures in the management of intracranial vascular disease, the following steps may be considered to improve cerebral circulation: Maintenance of arterial oxygenation within the normal range (avoidance of hyperventilation or hypoventilation), control of cerebral edema, reduction in cerebrospinal fluid pressure (including removal of cerebrospinal fluid if safely possible), and attention to extracranial factors that influence cardiac output and cerebral perfusion. In view of the effects upon brain bulk, the risks of shunting blood away from the ischemic region, the transformation of an ischemic infarct into a hemorrhagic one, and the existence of impairment in autoregulation, neither arterial hypertension nor hypotension should be permitted. A normotensive milieu should be preserved. The nice balance that the surgeon wishes to maintain is adequate perfusion without increasing intracranial vascular bulk to a dangerous extent.

Although the principles just enuciated are sound, neurosurgeons should be familiar with the reported value of supporting circulatory load and prescribing vasoactive substances to raise systemic arterial blood pressure, decrease cerebrovascular resistance, and combat vasospasm. The utilization of colloid-induced hypervolemia with or without pharmacological vasoconstriction, to raise the systemic blood pressure 40 to 60 mm of mercury constitutes one pattern of therapy.[51a] The administration of a peripheral vasoconstrictor, e.g., phenylephrine, with simultaneous administration of nitroprusside, as an alternative pattern, is based upon the vasodilatory effect of nitroprusside on cerebral vessels.[3a] Comprehensive monitoring of arterial blood pressure by means of intra-arterial techniques, urinary output, cardiac rhythm, and central venous or pulmonary artery wedge pressures is requisite in such management plans.

To prevent vascular sludging and platelet aggregation, low molecular weight dextran or aspirin or both are rational considerations.[60] Clinical application of the intravenous infusion of isoproterenol and aminophylline is based upon experimental data suggesting the value of preventing the degradation of cyclic adenosine monophosphate. Trials of this method deserve scrutiny.[31]

Bleeding

The cause of bleeding beyond the confines of the operative wound is usually related to specific bleeding diatheses. The spread of blood from the operative site into the tissue planes and fluid spaces such as the ventricular cavities and the subarachnoid channels may evoke symptoms of a ventriculitis, ventricular obstruction, interference with cerebrospinal fluid absorption, hydrocephalus, increased intracranial pressure, and painful meningeal reactions involving the head, spine, and distribution of the nerve roots.[33]

Complications Not Related to the Wound

Local Complications

With the exception of the phlebitis that may follow intravenous therapy, which is discussed in a later section, certain local complications that do not involve the operative site bear note. The list itself suggests the prophylaxis and treatment needed: decubitus ulcerations, corneal abrasions, burns from hypothermia techniques or electrical apparatus, burns from chemicals used for skin preparation, adhesive tape reactions and excoriations, and friction burns from sliding or other handling of the patient. The abrasions, decubiti, and areas of folliculitis that may result from headrest use have been noted earlier. These complications require prompt local therapy and, like a first- or second-degree burn, will, with protection against secondary infection, heal kindly. If the full thickness of the skin or scalp is involved, an eschar may require surgical debridement, excision, or grafting. The occurrence of local *Staphylococcus aureus* suppuration and septicemia from infected intra-arterial monitoring emphasizes the need for attention to aseptic technique whenever the skin is violated and especially when a monitoring device is to be left in situ postoperatively.

Respiratory System Complications

Immediate—Recovery Room

Any facility in which the postoperative neurosurgical patient is cared for should be equipped with a bag, valve, mask unit (BVMU), endotracheal intubation tray, and sterile tracheostomy tray with varying sizes of tubes and cuff attachments. An electrocardiographic monitor and an external defibrillator should be accessible, and all members of the staff should be instructed as to their location and use. Mechanical respirators and ventilatory equipment should be readily at hand or promptly available upon emergency call. Solutions and medications for emergency use should be stocked on the nursing unit and in the recovery room.

OBSTRUCTION. With the exception of severe laryngeal stridor or spasm, most causes of respiratory obstruction, be it improper positioning of the unconscious patient, aspiration, mucus plugs, or the like, usually can be diagnosed promptly and corrected by improved positioning plus nasopharyngeal and upper respiratory tract toilet. A nasopharyngeal airway may be required and tolerated better than an oropharyngeal airway. An endotracheal tube may be required (a low-pressure, soft-cuff tube should be employed). Endotracheal intubation or immediate tracheostomy will be needed for severe stridor or laryngeal spasm. In the prophylaxis against recurrent respiratory obstruction, if it is anticipated that the process will be reversible, the endotracheal tube may be left in situ for 48 or more hours. If the process is not expected to reverse itself in this time, it is preferable to perform a tracheostomy. The caution previously mentioned relative to persistent tracheal suctioning is pertinent here, and if any cardiac irritability has been demonstrated intraoperatively, the maneuver should be accompanied by continued electrocardiographic monitoring and the administration of oxygen before and during suctioning.

HYPOVENTILATION. Some degree of underventilation may be a fairly regular postoperative accompaniment of otherwise uncomplicated anesthesia. A patient may be especially susceptible to severe ventilatory deficiency if he has had preoperative respiratory system deficiencies, has had underventilation intraoperatively, or has had an operative procedure or a primary disease process that has involved neural control of respiration and has produced depression. As an example of this last, operations performed in the posterior fossa, on and around the brain stem, and those performed on the upper spinal cord (as discussed in the section on percutaneous cordotomy) may produce a degree of neural paresis of function that might be tolerated alone, but may require assisted ventilation when combined with the effects of the pharmacological agents used for the operation. This form of hypoventilation may show a delayed onset as a sequel to tissue edema in strategic neural centers and may require assisted ventilation over several days. The action of neuromuscular blocking agents during anesthesia may carry over into the recovery room. This and other forms of pharmacological depression of respiration may be at the basis of the hypoventilation observed. The administration of antidotes to counteract drug-induced depression is indicated, as is mechanical respiratory assistance.

Although the respiratory signs of hypoventilation may be obvious, such signs may be absent in the early postoperative period. A recovery-room check on arterial blood gases should probably be routine after almost *all* major operations. The patient may demonstrate mild arterial hypertension, tachycardia, and restlessness. These signs must not be misinterpreted as due only to pain, for the treatment of the latter could compound the former problem. Confirmatory and critical laboratory measurement is a determination of arterial P_{CO_2} and P_{O_2} values. Unless the patient has chronic pulmonary disease, an arterial P_{CO_2} above 42 to 45 mm of mercury suggests a state of hypoventilation and yet can be acceptable if the patient's progress is satisfactory in the circumstances of recovery of respiratory function. Hypoxia may be combated by the administration of oxygen by catheter or mask, but hypercarbia must be overcome by mechanical ventilatory assistance. When ventilatory assistance is required, in contradistinction to the management of tracheobronchial secretions, cuffed tubes are needed. They must be intermittently deflated and adjusted to prevent tracheal necrosis or subsequent cicatrix.[15,82,116]

Tracheostomy-Related Complications

Unmanageable obstruction, the inability to place an endotracheal tube (or of the wakeful patient to tolerate one), the presence of local laryngeal obstruction, or a neurological deficit interfering with the adequate neural control of respiration may require tracheostomy with a cuffed tube. Inflation of the cuff will permit mechanical respiration and also protect the tracheobronchial tree during any administration of fluid by way of the alimentary tract. Tracheostomy-related complications include bleeding at the site of tracheostomy, major mediastinal artery erosion, mediastinal emphysema, tracheitis, tracheomalacia, tracheal perforation, delayed cicatrix, and posttracheostomy pneumothorax (either unilateral or bilateral). To prevent introducing an infection into the respiratory tree through the tracheostomy portal requires meticulous attention to technique. The inspired air should be moistened by using a nebulizer or by administering sterile saline solution topically directly into the tracheostomy.

Atelectasis

Atelectasis is second only to pulmonic infection as the most frequent complication of the respiratory system encountered immediately postoperatively. Some reports place it first. The diagnosis rests upon an awareness that it is so frequent and that the stage is set for its occurrence by hypoventilation, aspiration, or neural paresis. Apprehension or obvious respiratory distress, an acute rise in temperature, an increase in pulse rate, deviation of the trachea, decreased chest expansion, flatness to percussion, and decreased breath sounds on auscultation are familiar signs of extensive atelectasis. Less flagrant degrees should be suspected on the basis of the clinical course. The differential diagnostic considerations include tension penumothorax, acute pulmonary edema, pleural effusion, and pulmonary embolization. Bedside radiological examination of the chest will be helpful. Microatelectasis probably occurs after all major operations. It may be associated with a low arterial Po_2 and a normal chest roentgenogram. Management must be prompt, direct, and vigorous. The approach is mechanical and takes the form of opening up the collapsed alveoli by stimulating cough and deep inspirations. Also indicated is the humidification of respired air (ultrasonic nebulization may be helpful), suctioning of secretions that cannot be raised by cough, and the judicious use of intermittent respiratory assistance or other techniques such as the incentive spirometer for lung inflation to two to three times the tidal volume. Pulmonary physical therapy in the form of chest percussion and a regimen to insure the continued maintenance of the cleansed respiratory tract after the atelectatic area has been opened up are recommended. It should be noted that underhydrated patients may be more vulnerable to atelectasis as a result of being unable to mobilize inspissated plugs of mucus.

The administration of 100 per cent oxygen for 15 minutes or 75 per cent oxygen for 30 minutes as a trial period while monitoring the arterial Pco_2 and Po_2 will give an indication of the severity of the problem and the adequacy of therapy. If assisted respirations are used or if artificial cycling is employed, the cycling pattern of one third inspiration to two thirds expiration with a tidal volume of 10 to 12 ml per kilogram represents a reasonable guide. The blood pH should be maintained at 7.3 or above.[15,53]

Bronchospasm

Bronchospasm may be a manifestation of an asthmatic attack or of obstructive lung disease. It may be precipitated by suctioning and it may accompany an allergic reaction. Its management is by the administration of oxygen, the use of bronchodilators, humidification of the inspired air, and the early administration of large doses of corticosteroids for two to three days followed by abrupt discontinuation. Any associated acidosis should be reversed, and antibiotics may be indicated on occasion.

Pneumonia

Inflammation and infection of the substance of the lung has been, in the author's experience, the single most important postoperative complication involving the respiratory system; the term as used here encompasses bronchopneumonia, pneumonitis, and lobar pneumonia. One of the major mechanisms responsible in the neurosurgical patient is aspiration. One patient in four in the author's group developed the infection incident to aspiration. The aspiratory event may occur quite obviously as with vomiting, or it may occur repeatedly but silently as in the presence of a tracheostomy tube that alters the mechanics of swallowing. The management requires antibacterial and mechanical measures. Careful cultures by the laboratory are needed to identify the organisms responsible so that the correct choice of antibiotics may be made. Mechanical therapy invokes those measures necessary to guarantee an environment both oxygen-rich and humid. It insures the elimination of any irritants in the inspired air, the provision for adequate tracheobronchial suction, the encouragement of coughing, or other appropriate combinations of mechanical techniques to clear the tracheobronchial tree of secretions. Adrenocorticosteroids are indicated early in acute chemical aspiration but not under the circumstances of aspiration of particulate matter such as vomitus and not in the later phases of the process in any case. Serial chest roentgenograms will assist in following the patient's course. The patient must be turned regularly; deep respiration must be encouraged; a pulmonary physical therapist, if available, should assist the patient in voluntary deep ventilatory maneuvers. Oxygen poisoning (with its central nervous system effects consisting of muscular twitching, nausea, mood changes, paresthesias, impairment of consciousness, and seizures) may be encountered if a tight-fitting, occlusive mask is utilized with high concentrations of oxygen (80 per cent at one atmosphere) or if the ventilatory unit is connected to an endotracheal or tracheostomy tube and the concentration and pressure of oxygen are very high. Under these conditions oxygen metering is advisable.

The danger of the development of sepsis by way of contaminated nebulizers speaks for itself; they should be sterilized daily. The same is true of the indiscriminate interchanging of nasal, oral, and tracheal catheters in the toilet of secretions. Sterile catheters and gloves should be utilized during each suctioning.

Patients who have vocal cord weakness or paralysis should be given nothing orally until return of function guarantees protection of the tracheobronchial tree. The combination of tracheostomy and upper gastrointestinal tract feeding exposes the patient to soiling of the tracheobronchial tree. The respiratory passages are easily contaminated if liquid administered through a nasal gastric tube ascends along the outside of the tube. Wherever possible the tracheostomy should be removed prior to the institution of nasogastric tube feedings. When the two techniques must be used together, a tracheostomy cuff is inflated during the time of nasogastric feeding and for approximately 30 minutes thereafter. During this time the patient's head should be elevated, and it is preferable during this period that no tracheal suctioning be carried out. For long-term alimentation in combination with tracheostomy, consideration should be given to gastrostomy.

Pulmonary Edema

Pulmonary edema may be produced experimentally by bilateral cervical vagotomy or by lesions in the medulla or hypothalamus, which reminds us of the occasional primary neural causes of pulmonary edema. The more common causes, however, are the precipitation of left ventricular heart failure (overloading the circulation with too much parenteral fluid) and obstruction in the respiratory tree. In the elderly patient, especially sensitive to overloading of the vascular system, the monitoring of central venous pressure is to be recommended.[56] A rising central venous pressure usually indicates that the volume in the circulatory tree is being sustained and, if previously deficient, is now re-paired. A pressure in excess of 10 to 12 cm of water indicates that fluid volume is, at least, adequate and further fluid should be administered only with caution. A cause and effect relationship between abnormally high intracranial pressure and pulmonary edema may be assumed if the two occur together, and therapy must be directed toward reducing the pressure to normal. Acute pulmonary edema is combated further by rotating tourniquets on the extremities, phlebotomy, the administration of oxygen, and rapid digitalization if cardiac failure is imminent or supervenes. Intermittent positive-pressure breathing impedes the venous return to the thorax and is effective (although it may also aggravate intracranial vascular congestion), and the seriousness of the problem usually dictates its use. Rapidly acting diuretic agents such as ethacrynic acid may aid therapy. Central venous pressure monitoring is required, electrocardiographic monitoring is recommended, and blood gas determinations may be useful adjuncts in the laboratory documentation of progress.

Pneumothorax

Tension pneumothorax requires prompt insertion of a large-bored needle or trochar to equalize the pressure, followed by closed water-seal drainage with suction to accelerate re-expansion of the lungs. If the pneumothorax is small and the tension feature is absent, it may be left alone. The breathing of oxygen speeds the absorption of the retained air.

Pulmonary Embolization

Pulmonary embolization is fourth in frequency (after pneumonia, atelectasis, and obstruction) as a cause of respiratory distress postoperatively on a neurosurgical service. Patients who are at particularly high risk are those with heart disease, obesity, or polycythemia, a previous history of thrombophlebitis, or embolization. Patients who have had a protracted illness at bed rest are also at special risk. The danger of relying on soft-tissue tamponade to control bleeding intracranially or intraspinally has deterred us from recommending that such high-risk patients receive anticoagulant drugs postoperatively on a prophylactic basis.[29] (See also Peripheral Vascular System in the earlier discussion of preoperative evaluation.) The clinical manifestations are protean, and pre-existing phlebothrombosis as a warning state may be difficult to identify.

The diagnosis of pulmonary embolization may be quite challenging but is to be suspected in the presence of substernal chest pain, hypotension, tachycardia, sweating, and hyperpnea. There may be fever, cough, hemoptysis, pleuritic pain, pulmonary consolidation, friction rub, or pleural effusion. Electrocardiographic and plain roentgenographic studies and arterial blood gas determinations should be obtained for assistance in the differential diagnosis. Pulmonary radionuclide scanning (including both ventilation and perfusion scans) provides a high degree of accuracy in diagnosis. If the ventilation and perfusion scans are positive, the diagnosis approaches 95 per cent accuracy, but pulmonary angiography is the ultimate diagnostic step and is recommended prior to the institution of long-term anticoagulation or specific operative procedures.

The postoperative patient who has a nonfatal pulmonary embolism should receive immediate anticoagulant therapy in the form of heparin. If warfarin is to be used subsequently, adequate prothrombin deficiency should be effected prior to the discontinuation of the heparin. If anticoagulant therapy is contraindicated (the primary disease process is a hemorrhagic one and not satisfactorily controlled), if the patient has sustained embolization in the presence of correct anticoagulant therapy, or if a long-term process is anticipated, then vena caval interruption should be considered.[51] The author has permitted the use of therapeutic heparinization after an arbitrary period of five postoperative days in craniotomy or laminectomy cases without other contraindications. If treatment is mandatory at an earlier stage or in the face of contraindications to anticoagulation, one of the various intravascular devices can be used.

Cardiac Complications

Cardiac Arrest

Most cases of cardiac arrest are encountered intraoperatively. In the postoperative state, conditions that have been interpreted as cardiac arrest have been found in association with laryngeal or other respiratory obstruction, high increased intracranial pressure, pneumonia, and convulsive seizure activity. Arrest may be incorrectly diagnosed as the primary pathophysiological process when, in fact, it is a secondary accompaniment to the more basic mechanism of medullary failure in which respiratory failure precedes the cardiac collapse. Therapy directed toward "cardiac arrest" when the primary problem is medullary failure with respiratory paralysis will not be effective unless the primary process giving rise to the respiratory failure can be reversed. The postoperative monitoring of vital functions can assist the attending nursing and surgical staff in separating the mechanisms and identifying cases of primary cardiac arrest for which therapy can be profitably offered. The protocol of management is set forth earlier in this chapter.

Dysrhythmias

In the absence of pre-existing dysrhythmias, the only dysrhythmia encountered afresh in the postoperative state, in the author's experience, has been that of supraventricular tachycardia. In this situation, consideration should be given to the prescribing of digitalis or quinidine or both under the supvervision of a cardiologist. The primary cardiac dysrhythmias to be feared are ventricular tachycardia and ventricular fibrillation, and the latter requires the same management as cardiac arrest. The prompt use of lidocaine, the best drug for ventricular dysrhythmias, is recommended. The presence of complete heart block renders the patient vulnerable to cardiac arrest. For the management of persistent dysrhythmias and the application of conversion techniques, a cardiologist should be consulted. The placement of catheters for central venous pressure determinations requires that electrocardiographic monitoring be available so that the tip of the catheter does not precipitate cardiac irregularities. The role of potassium intoxication and possibly also of low calcium values as sequelae to multiple blood transfusions deserve note and have been commented upon earlier in this chapter.

Myocardial Infarction

Myocardial infarction must be considered in the differential diagnosis of the major pulmonary complications, particularly severe pulmonary embolization or infarction. Electrocardiographic abnormalities may be seen in patients suffering from subarachnoid hemorrhage, and the possibility that such processes can cause structural changes in the myocardium alerts the surgeon to the need for monitoring and the correction of dysrhythmias, if indeed they are correctable, to prevent myocardial injury. (See the section on preoperative evaluation of the cardiovascular system.)

Congestive Heart Failure

Congestive heart failure may be precipitated through fluid overload and is a precursor and accompaniment of pulmonary edema. The sudden development of arterial hypertension from whatever cause may unmask incipient failure postoperatively. Its management by the application of rotating tourniquets, phlebotomy, adequate oxygenation, rapid digitalization, and the utilization of diuretics is best conducted under the supervision of a cardiologist.

Complications Related to Fluid, Electrolyte, and Hormonal Needs

Hypovolemia and Hypotension

The commonest cause of postoperative hypovolemia is inadequate replacement of fluid that is lost intraoperatively. One exception to this is the infant who may lose sufficient blood into the subgaleal or intracranial spaces to produce postoperative hypovolemia. Another exception is fluid loss by involvement of other systems in the patient with multiple injuries.

The patient may present with cool extremities, a faint peripheral pulse, a narrow pulse pressure, decreased urinary output, and a low normal or subnormal brachial cuff blood pressure (below 90 mm of mercury in a normotensive individual or 40 to 50 mm of mercury below the preoperative control values in the hypertensive individual). The patient may become restless and thirsty, and a low central venous or pulmonary artery pressure will be recorded. The occurrence of hypovolemia and hypotension in the elderly patient, however, may result in myocardial damage and exist in the face of an elevated central venous pressure. The clinical signs of venous distention may also accompany the cardiovascular abnormalities associated with pulmonary embolism, right heart failure, cardiac tamponade, or congestive atelectasis. Certain of the signs accompanying hypovolemia may accompany any of the major cardiopulmonary complications previously considered. Hypotension is one of the cardinal signs also associated with atelectasis, pneumothorax, pulmonary embolization, and myocardial infarction. Endocrinological deficiency in patients with primary disease involving the hypothalamic-pituitary region or in those for whom pituitary destruction is undertaken may explain the hypotension. Sepsis as the result of a gram-negative organism may be accompanied by hypotension. The patient with endotoxic causes for signs of circulatory deficiency may present the picture of so-called "warm shock" because of arteriocapillary-venous dilatation. Acute gastric distention may produce hypotension, and we cannot forget that hypotension may accompany transfusion reactions.[7]

Hypotension may also accompany the administration of certain pharmacological agents (particularly opiates). Patients with central nervous system disease may not tolerate central nervous system depressants without some effect upon the cardiovascular system. Even small doses of codeine may offend. Patients who are still under the effect of the drugs of anesthesia and those with compromised brain stem function may respond adversely with hypotension to changes in position. Such a sensitivity to motion also occurs in the hypovolemic state. This latter state will usually rectify itself if the patient is permitted to remain recumbent and undisturbed.

The recognition of hypovolemia in the immediate postoperative state or at any time throughout the postoperative course requires prompt restoration of circulating blood volume.

The patient should be nursed in the recumbent posture with the lower extremities elevated. A central venous catheter or pulmonary artery catheter can provide monitoring data that are useful in diagnosis and as a guide in therapy. A urinary catheter should be available to measure the hourly output of urine. The administration of a well-balanced electrolyte solution (extra-cellular fluid "mimic"), red cell mass, or whole blood, or all three is indicated. A blood loss of 10 per cent or less usually requires, in the adult, 2 liters of a solution such as Hartman's; if the loss is greater, then blood is needed as well. In the absence of specific contraindications this fluid may be administered rapidly as long as the central venous pressure remains below 10 cm of water or thereabouts. A *rising* central venous pressure, irrespective of the absolute value, usually indicates that replacement is approaching the desirable level. Urinary output should attain approximately 0.5 ml per kilogram of body weight per hour for the adult. For the infant, urinary output will need to be much higher. The same precautions as described for intraoperative blood administration should be observed. The patient who is hypotensive as a result of hypovolemia and who has received fluid estimated to produce an adequate circulating volume as determined by central venous pressure but who does not show a satisfactory return of blood pressure to normal levels may respond to vasoactive drugs (beta-mimetic agents and alpha- and beta-adrenergic blocking agents).[21,37,56,97]

In the first 12 to 24 hours the use of the hematocrit as a guide may cause one to underestimate blood loss, since hemodilution will not be complete and a normal hematocrit may merely indicate that plasma and red cells were lost in equal proportion. If the patient can sustain the hypovolemic state until readjustment occurs after 24 hours postoperatively, he will then present with a reduced hematocrit and a reduced hemoglobin level, his total circulating volume having been made up by the mobilization of fluid from extravascular spaces. Once hypovolemia has been corrected it is the quality of the circulating blood that becomes important; anemia may be the factor that requires combating. In the first few hours postoperatively, therefore, replacement and re-establishment of adequate volume are recommended. By the end of the first 24 hours the hematocrit should reflect the hemodilution that has occurred, and an estimate may be made of the red cell mass that is necessary to restore oxygen-carrying capacity to normal levels, assuming that total volume is normal. When both volume and hematocrit are low, whole blood is preferred.

Anemia

When a normal blood volume exists, anemia is best counteracted by administering packed red cells. The hematocrit should probably be maintained above 30 per cent. The patient's red cell mass and the plasma volume may be measured, recognizing a 10 per cent margin of error incident upon such measurements. The formulae proposed by Moore may be useful guides in supplementing the clinical evaluation of the patient in determining the need for postoperative blood administration.[66]

The significant incidence of viral hepatitis subsequent to whole blood transfusion offers an important deterrent to the administration of whole blood in the absence of firm clinical indications. Postoperatively, if the patient's clinical progress is satisfactory, wound healing is progressing, and complications have not developed, then the mere presence of a mild to moderate anemia is not in itself an indication for transfusion. The relative risk is less if the patient continues oral iron therapy upon discharge.[93]

Under the circumstances of blood loss for which blood replacement has not restored hemoglobin and hematocrit to normal levels, medicinal iron may be prescribed (ferrous sulfate, 300 mg three times a day for a course of therapy to be extended over three to six months).

Dehydration

Postoperatively the patient may inherit a state of dehydration incident to changes that have occurred preoperatively and intraoperatively. The intraoperative causes of dehydration are discussed in previous sections. A state of dehydration initiated intraoperatively (the administration of osmotic diuretic agents or the advent of diabetes insipidus) may be inherited as a postoperative problem. It may be aggravated by drainage from the operative site, sweating, or adrenocortical deficiency. A large solute load secondary to high protein or high caloric nasogastric feedings will also demand of the kidneys an obligatory fluid loss.

The commonest pattern of dehydration encountered in the postoperative neurosurgical patient is that of water loss in excess of electrolyte loss (hypertonic dehydration), as described in the section on preoperative assessment of fluid and electrolyte

**TABLE 29-1 DAILY WATER LOSSES
OF VARIOUS AGE GROUPS***

AGE	INSENSIBLE LOSS PER M² BODY SURFACE (ml)	URINARY OUTPUT NEEDS PER M² BODY SURFACE (ml)
Newborn	800	900
2 mo–2 yr	1150	900
3–8 yr	950	600
Over 8 yr	750	600

* Adapted from Paulsen, E. P.: Amer. J. Surg., *107*:392, 1964.

balance. Such hypertonic dehydration is corrected by administering 5 per cent dextrose in half-normal sodium chloride solution. If renal function is impaired, 5 per cent glucose in water is a preferable solution; however, an excess of this hypo-osmolar solution will contribute to cerebral edema. In the infant or small child, the decreased concentrating capacity of the kidney requires more water per unit of surface area, and in addition to that needed to replace urinary loss, fluid must be administered to take into account the uncompensated water loss from insensible sources. The differences between the water losses of varying age groups are noted by Paulsen (Table 29–1).[72]

It must be noted that insensible loss may be reduced significantly by nursing the patient in an Isolette with a moist environment, but overhydration is a complication of the humid or moist ambience. If the mechanism of hypertonic dehydration is diabetes insipidus and fluid replacement cannot keep up with loss, the administration of antidiuretic hormone, as outlined earlier, is recommended (see section on diabetes insipidus).

Electrolyte loss in excess of water may bring about hypotonic dehydration. This situation is encountered in adrenocortical insufficiency, as described in the section on preoperative assessment. The correction of this problem is by the immediate administration of a balanced electrolyte solution.

Serial serum osmolality determinations should be made and will be a useful guide to the preservation of an iso-osmotic environment (285 to 295 milliosmoles per liter of serum).

The essential bedside clinical measurements necessary in the management of pa-

tients suspected of being either dehydrated or water intoxicated include daily body weights obtained under standard and reproducible conditions and a fluid intake and fluid output flow and balance sheet. These should be associated with hourly urinary output measurement, cumulative urinary output calculation, and urinary specific gravity determinations. Serum osmolality measurements should be regularly available, and the serum and urinary sodium concentrations should also be measured together with the measurement of the laboratory parameters noted in the section on preoperative assessment of the fluid and electrolyte balance.

In the wakeful patient who is able to take fluid by mouth, dehydration is usually corrected and prevented by the mechanism of thirst. If the patient is able to take fluids orally to keep up with or to repair his loss, he himself will maintain or correct a deranged internal milieu. Certain central nervous lesions, however, either because they impair consciousness enough to blunt or eliminate the thirst stimulus or because they interfere with the thirst mechanisms per se, may render the patient completely dependent upon careful external assessment and management by the physician.

A word of caution is in order: the physician himself may contribute to dangerous degrees of dehydration by withholding adequate maintenance fluids from the neurosurgical patient on the partially erroneous theory that a dehydrated state will help to avoid brain edema. The patient should receive adequate maintenance fluid in the postoperative period. The key to the matter is the administration of the proper kind of fluid (iso-osmolar) rather than the withholding of that fluid necessary to meet insensible losses, match an obligatory loss, and provide an adequate urinary output.

Water Intoxication and
the Syndrome of Inappropriate
Secretion of Antidiuretic Hormone

Water intoxication can be produced by obligatory administration of hypo-osmolar solutions such as 5 per cent dextrose in water, independent of clinical and other laboratory assessment. It may also occur in infants nursed in an incubator with a moistened gas environment. Patients who have been on low sodium diets or receiving diuretics that have lowered the body sodium stores are particularly susceptible to overhydration. The administration of exogenous antidiuretic hormone (ADH) or the "inappropriate" continuing internal secretion of the hormone incident to associated diseases, drugs, anesthesia, the operative procedure, the primary disease, dehydration, or some combination thereof, will produce a change in renal tubular pore size. The kidney retains water, urine volume decreases, and body water, including brain water, increases. The patient complains of headache, nausea, anorexia, and vomiting. Some irritability and restlessness or impairment of consciousness may be noted, as may drowsiness, confusion, or stupor. Nausea may supervene and motor incoordination may be present. Muscle cramps followed by seizures and coma signify a serious degree of water intoxication. The skin is moist, and sweating is increased. In the laboratory assessment serum sodium levels fall (usually below 120 MEq/per liter) and serum osmolality falls, as do potassium, blood urea nitrogen, and creatinine levels. Urinary volume decreases and urinary sodium increases, as does its osmolality. Serum antidiuretic hormone fails to return to expected baseline levels.

In the differential diagnosis, the syndrome of inappropriate secretion of antidiuretic hormone (SIADH) is distinguished from water intoxication by the decreased urinary sodium in the latter. A second condition from which it must be distinguished is adrenocortical insufficiency (pituitary insufficiency), which is identified by a serum cortisol assay and by the higher serum potassium, creatinine and blood urea nitrogen values.

The fundamental step in correcting inappropriate antidiuretic hormone levels is to withhold fluids until general homeostasis is reestablished through central nervous system and renal mechanisms. Monitoring of serum osmolality and sodium and urinary sodium is recommended. Severe cases may be treated with an osmotic diuretic (urea or mannitol) or a tubular diuretic (furosemide); with these drugs attention must be paid to replacement of sodium and potassium. Lithium carbonate has been employed.[108] It may be valuable on a short-term basis, but myocardial irritability, thyroid dysfunc-

tion, and other toxic side effects of lithium (drowsiness, tremors, and the like) discourage its use in neurosurgical patients. Demeclocycline, an antibacterial compound, induces a reversible decrease in urinary concentrating ability, and although its effects are delayed for several days, it may have use in chronic problems and is clearly superior to lithium.[25a,33a]

Diabetes Insipidus

Diabetes insipidus is a frequent accompaniment of operations in the vicinity of the tuberculum sellae, sella turcica, dorsum sellae, third ventricle, lamina terminalis, and hypothalamic region. In these circumstances it may be expected and anticipated as a postoperative accompaniment. For a day following operation the diuretic effects of osmotically active agents that have been used intraoperatively to decrease brain bulk and decrease intracranial brain pressure may still be responsible for abnormally high urinary output. Urinary output should be monitored as described in the section on dehydration. Especially is this important in the case of small persons, infants, and children, in whom, in the face of rapidly developing diabetes insipidus, dehydration may reach a dangerous level unless monitoring is frequent and correction is instituted promptly.

In addition to the fulminant immediate onset, there are three other patterns encountered: one may see an immediate but transient period of diabetes insipidus; there may be a delay in onset of a few days; or one may see a diabetic type of urinary output immediately after operation followed by an interval of relatively normal response (the maximum in the author's experience has been eight days), followed, then, by more flagrant diabetes insipidus. It is, therefore, important to look for the development of the complication over the course of the first eight days postoperatively. Irrespective of the timing of the process, diabetes insipidus is manifested by the obligatory loss of electrolyte-poor or very low specific gravity urine with low osmolality and by a rise in serum osmolality and a lack of the normal antidiuretic hormone release in response to this rise. The kind of dehydration that develops leaves plasma solutes and red cells retained. The serum water to solute ratio falls, and the serum sodium rises, as do the serum proteins and hematocrit.

Diabetes insipidus needs to be distinguished from primary polydipsia in which antidiuretic hormone secretion is reduced by continued hydration. One can readily distinguish between these two conditions by withholding water. Another technique for aiding diagnosis is noting any change in the rate of urinary flow following the injection of hypertonic sodium chloride solution. A decrease will be observed in the case of primary polydipsia, whereas the flow will be unimpaired or increased in the patient suffering from true diabetes insipidus. (The author has not encountered the problem of nephrogenic diabetes insipidus in which the kidney is incapable of reabsorbing water even under the influence of exogenously administered antidiuretic hormone.)

The goal of correct intraoperative fluid control is to bring the patient to the recovery room and to the intensive care unit iso-osmotic and in normal balance, with his blood loss replaced and his maintenance requirements met. If the patient is iso-osmotic (this may be confirmed by a determination of serum osmolality), the backbone of management of diabetes insipidus, if it develops, is the matching of urinary output with intake. The intake fluid of choice is a solution of 5 per cent dextrose in 0.445 per cent sodium chloride. Since urinary output is measured every hour, fluid administration for each hour is based upon the volume of urinary output the preceding hour. Urinary output should be maintained in excess of 0.5 ml per kilogram of body weight per hour in an adult. In an infant or young child this figure must be increased because of the decreased concentrating capacity of the kidneys and the infant's need for more water to handle the same solute load. As long as fluid can be administered to keep up with urinary output, the patient may be managed by such a balancing technique. The difficulties are twofold: (1) If the urinary output becomes unwieldy (for example, a 70-kg man might normally excrete 70 ml of urine per hour, but in diabetes insipidus he could excrete 1000 ml per hour), if there is any defect in the technique or adequacy of fluid administration, it is possible for rapid dehydration with circulatory collapse to occur in a short space of time. The small patient is even more vulnerable; the intravenous route becomes his lifeline. (2) The other difficulty is the distinct inconvenience of administering large amounts of fluid and the need to guarantee adequate bladder drainage. In an adult it is wise to administer exogenous antidiuretic hormone when urinary output reaches a volume of approximately six times the normal expected output over two successive hours. In the case of the small child or infant, a less voluminous outflow is an indication for the administration of the medication.

The medication of choice is vasopressin tannate by injection. This is a water-insoluble compound suspended in oil. Each milliliter contains 5 units. Details of injection technique are important: The vial should be warmed to approximately 40° C in a water bath and then vigorously shaken to insure that the suspension is well mixed. The injection must be intramuscular and well placed in a well-vascularized tissue; the site of injection must be vigorously massaged at the completion of administration. The starting dose is usually 0.4 ml (2 units). A response should be observed within an hour. In the absence of a response within the hour, or at the most, two hours, the dosage may be repeated—with a check on each of the details mentioned. A pharmacologically active dose of vasopressin tannate in oil will usually be sufficient for the succeeding 24 to 36 hours, at which time it may be expected that a second dose will be required. The action of aqueous vasopressin has been unpredictable and it is not recommended for the management of the usual postoperative case of diabetes insipidus. A synthetic analogue of vasopressin (DDAVP) is now available and appears to be excellent.[80] For long-term management, however, the utilization of lysine vasopressin (Diapid), inhaled for absorption by the nasal mucous membranes, may suffice in mild cases after the acute stage is stabilized. Additional adjunctive compounds are discussed in the excellent article by Shucart and Jackson.[88]

The primary danger associated with the administration of exogenous antidiuretic hormone is that the patient's fluid dosage will not be adjusted to his decreased need and that he will develop signs of water intoxication. In the first 48 hours in the management of an adult patient, urinary output may be matched milliliter for milliliter on a retrospective basis. Insensible fluid loss, if calculated to be normal, may be ignored during this period, since the water of oxidation will supply a part of this need. The patient will be mildly thirsty when his level of consciousness permits this stimulus to be active, and further fluids may be added gradually, beginning on the second postoperative day or thereafter.

When the patient's thirst mechanisms appear to be active and his level of consciousness is normal, and provided that his level of intelligence and age permit him to govern himself, he may then gauge his intake by himself and become independent of the medical staff. Instruction in the administration of the vasopressin, the measurement of urinary output, and the recording of its specific gravity should be provided before the patient is discharged, and it may be well that he wear on his person a medically identifying tag indicating his dependence upon the antidiuretic hormone should this be a semipermanent requirement.

Electrolyte Imbalance

HYPERNATREMIA. Most examples of hypernatremia are explicable on the basis of dehydration. Impaired renal tubular concentrating capacity as a result of renal disease, primary aldosteronism, the exogenous administration of mineralocorticoids, or diabetes insipidus can contribute to dehydration, as will the other recognized causes associated with increased respiratory activity, fever, vomiting, and diarrhea. Whether a true neurogenic hypernatremia exists—other than that due to mechanisms of diabetes insipidus or hypodipsia (impairment of thirst mechanisms) or gastrointestinal or renal disturbances—is unsettled. Nevertheless, certain patients, especially those who have undergone operations in the hypothalamic area, may, in the absence of overt dehydration, demonstrate a persistently increased serum sodium level.[74]

HYPONATREMIA. Most examples of hyponatremia are due to a dilutional mechanism based on excessive water intake. When such general medical conditions as renal disease, cirrhosis, or congestive heart failure are excluded, the primary difficulty is usually the result of the activity of antidiuretic hormone and the administration of exogenous water. It deserves emphasis that antidiuretic hormone may often be inappropriately released in patients with central nervous system disease or lung disease. This hormone release also may occur as a result of the operative manipulation, anesthetic and other drug administration, and similar factors. The administration of water in such a setting will contribute to dilutional hyponatremia. In measuring the serum sodium, it is to be remembered that one is measuring concentration rather than total body sodium. The latter may be normal and yet the serum sodium will measure low if extracellular fluid is expanded. The expansion of extracellular fluid by hypotonic solutions will decrease aldosterone secretion, and there will be an accompanying urinary sodium loss. These mechanisms give rise to the so-called but probably misnamed "salt-wasting" syndrome. Exogenous sodium will not help this state of affairs, *but fluid restriction usually will.* If a third factor, a "natriuretic hormone," exists, it is possible that urinary sodium loss in association with dilutional hyponatremia may be due to the release of this factor, which stimulates natriuresis. If this factor is elaborated in the brain, its release in combination with inappropriate antidiuretic hormone secretion could explain the rare examples of "cerebral salt wasting" that are not purely dilutional.[107,113,114]

Steroid Insufficiency

Steroid insufficiency is encountered in the circumstances of inadequate replacement of needs created by disease and operations on the hypothalamic-pituitary area and in the far less common circumstance of primary adrenal disease. Assessment techniques and prophylactic management have been presented earlier. Deficiency can cause a shock-like state, impairment of consciousness, a fall in blood pressure, tachycardia, fever, abdominal pain, nausea, vomiting, and reduced urinary outflow. Vascular collapse and death are the catastrophic manifestations of acute adrenal failure. The less fulminating picture may be manifested by weakness, general lassitude, decreased peristalsis, mild abdominal distention, anorexia, and nausea. Hyponatremia, hypoglycemia, hyperkalemia, and a low level or absence of plasma cortisol are the prominent laboratory findings. The treatment of acute insufficiency is by the parenteral administration of hydrocortisone sodium succinate or its equivalent in doses of 100 mg or more.

The author's usual protocol of management in the postoperative period is the administration of 200 mg of parenteral soluble cortisone preparation in divided doses during the first 24 hours. This dosage is tapered in decreasing decrements to the equivalent of 50 mg per diem by the sixth postoperative day. Further reduction is individualized to a discharge maintenance dose equivalent to 25 to 50 mg per diem in divided oral doses of cortisone.

Steroid deficiency often becomes a problem with the transfer of the neurosurgical patient to the care of physicians who are not aware of the degree of ablation of hypothalamic-pituitary stimulation of adrenal function and of the patient's dependence on exogenous cortisone. This may result in attempts to reduce steroid therapy to a point below that of maintenance levels (which in the average adult is in the neighborhood of 25 mg of cortisone or its equivalent per 24 hours). Patients who have had total ablation of the pituitary gland require 25 to 50 mg per 24 hours. The increased needs incident to stress, injury, and disease should be remembered. The patient's dependence upon exogenous steroid should be indicated on a medical identification tag that is worn at all times.

Genitourinary Tract Complications

Catheter-Related Problems

Infection in association with the use of catheters takes the form of urethritis, epididymitis, orchitis, cystitis, and a less well-defined family of infections generally entitled "genitourinary tract infection." Acute pyelonephritis has also been encountered. Trauma to the urethra incident to the placement of the catheter or to forced extraction of a balloon bag by a disoriented patient has occurred.

The diagnosis of middle and lower urinary tract infection is usually not too challenging a problem, but it is worth remembering that a catheter is also a route for the introduction of gram-negative organisms followed by gram-negative septicemia and endotoxemia. The steps in treatment for the commonly encountered postoperative catheter-related urinary tract infections are several. First, the adequacy of urinary drainage must be insured. The catheter cannot be removed until spontaneous mechanisms provide drainage and an adequate urinary flow. At such time it should be removed since its presence is inimical to maintaining a sterile system. Culture of the urine is mandatory. The therapeutic administration of antibiotic medication will depend upon the organism involved.

Neurally Induced Complications

The neural mechanisms that govern the genitourinary system and that may be deranged postoperatively are several and complex: Impairment in the level of consciousness may produce no more than incontinence with complete evacuation of clean urine. At other times urinary retention followed by retention overflow occurs. Lesions of the paracentral lobule, of the cingulum, and of downstream portions of the motor pathways may introduce a neuroparetic mechanism leading to defective bladder evacuation. The most frequent occurrence is in association with spinal cord lesions.

The circumstance of incontinence with the evacuation of clean urine is to be preferred to the placement of a catheter as long as bladder evacuation is complete. This can usually be determined by palpation and gauging the force of the urinary stream. In the male patient an external device affixed to the penis will provide a reservoir for drainage of urine. The problem is more difficult in the female, and if skin care deteriorates as a result of incontinence, an indwelling urethral catheter may be necessary.

In the management of urinary retention, pharmacological agents that may depress autonomic neural balance should be minimized. If there is no recognized neurological structural change and if the patient's level of consciousness is close to normal, he should be permitted to fill his bladder to a point at which he will have an appropriate stimulus to evacuation. The need for catheterization should, under these circumstances, not be tied to the clock. When the stimulus is present, it is reasonable to catheterize the patient if he is unable to void after a trial of the usual adjuncts. The patient should be catheterized as a single aseptic procedure, and a trial at normal voiding should be made thereafter upon refilling.

A trial of parasympathomimetic agent such as bethanechol chloride (Urecholine) may be given when it is ascertained that no organic obstruction exists. (Contraindications are asthma, myocardial ischemia, or coronary artery disease.) The oral dosage is 5 to 50 mg and the subcutaneous dosage is 2.5 to 5 mg (0.5 to 1.0 ml). An antidote of atropine sulfate and epinephrine should be available for administration.

For the management of the urinary tract of a patient who has sustained injury to the spine with neural involvement, the ideal approach is that of intermittent aseptic catheterization every 8 to 12 hours, conducted by a competently drilled medical staff. In the absence of the facilities and personnel for meticulous adherence to the rigid protocol of this approach, the utilization of the indwelling catheter with closed gravity drainage, as described in the section on preoperative evaluation of the genitourinary system, is the method of choice.

Oliguria and Anuria

Acute renal failure postoperatively may result from either renal ischemia or intravascular hemolysis. The latter can result from the transfusion of mismatched blood or the accidental infusion of distilled water or other hemolytic agents. If such hemolysis is suspected, prompt administration of a single dose of mannitol or furosemide is to be advised. The intravenous administration of 5 to 6 gm of an alkalizing solution of sodium bicarbonate or sodium lactate may be considered, although its value is questioned. Renal ischemia may exist as a postoperative complication in the absence of preexisting disease and is usually related to decreased renal perfusion intraoperatively. It is to be feared in patients with multisystem injuries, especially crush injuries. Urinary output will be diminished (oliguria) and if the insult is severe, urinary sodium will rise, urinary osmolality will become iso-osmolar with serum, and urinary specific gravity will fall (usually below 1.018). Oliguria has been defined as a urine output of 400 ml per 24 hours or less, which for a 70-kg patient would be 0.25 ml per kilogram body weight per hour or less. The primary therapeutic approach in the treatment of renal ischemia is the restoration of normal renal blood flow by providing normal circulating blood volume and promoting normal cardiac output. In restituting circulatory volume, fluid therapy must not overload the patient; monitoring of the central venous pressure is a useful adjunctive guide. Following the restitution of circulating blood volume, a test dose of mannitol may be given, but if oliguria persists, additional mannitol is contraindicated. The problems then are those of the management of the major complications of renal failure, the prevention of overhydration and the avoidance of potassium intoxication. The management of the persistently oliguric or anuric patient is to be accompanied by restriction of fluid intake, a low-potassium diet, frequent serum potassium determinations, and electrocardiographic determinations. Exchange resins may be given by mouth or by enema. Acidosis should be combated by administering either sodium bicarbonate or sodium lactate as mentioned. Renal dialysis may be required.[4,117]

Alimentary System Complications

Hiccough

Hiccough can be a symptom of impending medullary collapse, often in association with other respiratory irregularities, e.g., sighing. In the usual postoperative state, hiccough is less often a specific index of focal neurological disease. It may be seen with diaphragmatic irritation due to atelectasis, pneumonia, and pleuritis. It may also be a precursor to vomiting and can be controlled by suction through a nasogastric tube. If mild, it may be treated by placing a few drops of volatile oil (oil of eucalyptol or cloves) on the back of the tongue. Periodic inhalation of carbon dioxide in concentrations of 5 to 7.5 per cent to the point of creating hyperpnea may be helpful. Carbon dioxide therapy must be used with caution in patients who have disease that may have rendered the brain stem respiratory centers refractory to carbon dioxide stimulation. Added carbon dioxide under such conditions may contribute to carbon dioxide intoxication. Chlorpromazine hydrochloride in doses of 25 to 50 mg intramuscularly is effective and is probably the best pharmacological agent available for the control of hiccoughing. The author has never encountered hiccoughing so intractable as to require phrenic nerve blockade or section.

Vomiting

Vomiting is encountered in patients suffering from disease that secondarily dislocates and distorts or directly compresses the brain stem. The management under these circumstances is that of the primary disease process. In the postoperative phase of patient care the same mechanisms may be active, but if the primary disease has been adequately treated by removal or decompression, other causes for vomiting should be sought. One of the common causes is too early or too vigorous alimentation during the time the gastrointestinal tract's mobility is decreased, as discussed in the following section on abdominal distention. The pharmacological depression of vomiting is best brought about by use of the phenothiazine agents, particularly chlorpromazine hydrochloride or prochlorperazine maleate. (Chlorpromazine by intramuscular injection or by rectal suppository in doses of 25 mg by either route may be repeated; in the adult patient the larger suppository of 100 mg may be needed.)

Abdominal Distention

We are concerned here with a decrease in gastrointestinal motility in the postoperative period. Acute gastric distention, which can cause hypotension, is treated by prompt nasogastric tube decompression, and the latter may be needed if retention or aerophagia follows alimentation. Decreased motility of the small bowel is not so much a problem as decreased motility of stomach and large bowel, although there are particular circumstances in neurosurgical practice in which the entire bowel may be quiescent (paralytic ileus). These include injuries of the spinal column and its neural contents, operations upon lumbar and lumbosacral intervertebral disc spaces, and the presence of inflammatory or infectious disease processes involving either the vertebral bodies or the intervertebral disc spaces or both. In the multiply injured patient other specific causes for impaired gastrointestinal motility should be sought, and certain of the comments relative to hiccough and vomiting are pertinent here. The use of pulmonary therapeutic measures such as intermittent positive-pressure apparatus may contribute to abdominal distention by encouraging insufflation of air, which is slowly absorbed because of its high nitrogen content.

Prior to the initiation of alimentation, evidence of gastrointestinal motility should be in hand. Preferably the patient should be a bit hungry, bowel sounds should be heard, and the patient should be passing flatus. Feedings should be small in volume, beginning with 30 to 60 ml per hour (with aspiration prior to the next feeding to insure no retention if a nasogastric tube is in place). The protocol may then be rapidly accelerated as the patient tolerates it. The patient should be in a semi-Fowler or upright position to discourage regurgitation. All the psychological factors should be made optimal for retention of oral or nasogastric intake. The presence of a nasogastric tube, necessary at times, often contributes to aerophagia, and when possible the tube should be removed and the patient's gastrointestinal system allowed to remain undisturbed until spontaneous motility re-establishes itself. Esophagitis and stricture may develop following the presence of a nasogastric tube in place for 10 days or more in a supine patient. Therefore, it is recommended that patients be nursed with the head and trunk elevated if at all possible, particularly if the tube must be continued beyond 10 days.

Retained rectal gas may be deflated by the passage of a well-lubricated rectal tube, which should not be left in place more than 5 to 10 minutes at a time.[40]

Gastrointestinal Ulceration and Bleeding

Although disease of the nervous system is not the only cause for gastrointestinal hemorrhage as a phenomenon of stress, latent gastrointestinal disease and known pre-existing disease may become clinically manifest or aggravated after the stress of a neurosurgical operation or the insult of the primary neurological problem. Trauma, pre-existing arterial hypotension, and gram-negative endotoxemia predispose to ulceration. Whether steroid therapy in an otherwise healthy patient predisposes to ulceration is moot. Ulceration has been encountered in a severely complicated case of brain tumor with superimposed infection and as a result of nasogastric tube suctioning. Whereas any part of the gastrointestinal tract may be involved in the ulcerative or hemorrhagic manifestations, the stomach and duodenum lead the list. The usual manifestation of stress ulceration is bleeding. Daily stool checks for blood in patients at particular risk may offer early warning. Treatment is by correction of the predisposing conditions, the reduction or elimination of steroid therapy when this can be tolerated, the removal of nasogastric tubes if they are offending, and the treatment of bleeding disorders if they are present. For the patient at risk, prophylactic antacids should be administered, every two hours if the patient cannot eat or one to three hours after each meal if he can eat. Iced antacids may also be of value. In other than mild cases, the patient should be prepared for operation, blood should be made ready, and the opinion of a general surgical colleague should be sought. Gastric icewater lavage may be helpful in mild cases. If the bleeding persists and cannot be readily controlled, operative therapy may be the only recourse.[19,24,32,105,110]

Parotiditis

Salivary gland infection may cause fever and discomfort postoperatively. It is usually found in the debilitated, aged, or dehydrated patient. It may be prevented by good nursing care in maintaining excellent oral hygiene. The use of a lemon and glycerin mixture or other stringent solution to encourage salivary flow is recommended. Lemon curd is palatable to children. The use of chewing gum carries the risk of aspiration. Adequate hydration is an important part of both prophylaxis and therapy. In the presence of parotiditis (which will be accompanied by pain, fever, and leukocytosis) secretions from the excretory ducts should be cultured and antibiotic therapy instituted.

Jaundice, Hepatitis, Liver Necrosis

A single episode of hemolysis from whatever cause may produce jaundice within 24 hours. Hemolysis may result from the normal destruction of transfused blood cells, particularly old blood, or from a transfusion reaction. Hemolytic transfusion reactions can occur in the absence of incompatibility, but the latter is the major cause for the serious responses. The resolution of a large hematoma may likewise be associated with hyperbilirubinemia and jaundice, and postoperative septicemia may produce hemolysis and jaundice. The possibility of the occurrence of jaundice in patients who have had pre-existing liver disease is obvious. The stress of anesthesia and the operative procedure, particularly in the alcoholic patient, may precipitate hepatic decompensation. Certain drugs such as the phenothiazine derivatives may induce jaundice, and the rare occurrence of this complication following halothane anesthesia is known to all. Hepatocellular disease as a result of drug use will give rise to fever and elevated serum bilirubin and serum glutamic oxaloacetic transaminase (SGOT) levels. Subsequent exposures to the suspected drug should be avoided whenever possible. The possibility of malaria transmitted through blood transfusions should not be overlooked. Hepatitis more frequently results from viral transmission by blood administration. Although transfusion-transmitted hepatitis, both symptomatic and asymptomatic, varies depending upon the source of the blood, it nevertheless occurs in approximately 10 per cent of patients receiving an average load of five transfusions. Approximately a third of these patients are symptomatic, showing evidence of jaundice. Hepatitis associated with transfusion may become evident in from 14 to 180 days following transfusion.[63] The occurrence of an anicteric form of hepatitis may explain an adverse turn in the patient's convalescence characterized by exhaustion, anorexia, nausea, weight loss, and abdominal discomfort. Liver enzyme and serum bilirubin analyses may provide the clue to diagnosis.

Fecal Impaction

Postoperative fecal impaction not only may be responsible for fever, local pain, abdominal discomfort, and anorexia, but at the time the impaction is corrected it is locally most distressing. Prevention is the best approach. "Bowel rounds" should be included in the thinking of the attending surgical staff on the night of the third postoperative day. Most patients who have undergone major operative procedures, unless there is some specific contraindication to it, should receive a mild laxative at that time. The following morning if, after a warm breakfast, there has been no spontaneous bowel evacuation, an enema should be administered. In the absence of satisfactory results from the enema, a rectal examination should be performed, and if impaction is present, gentle manipulation may initiate the evacuation. Local instillation of glycerin suppositories and mineral oil will assist in softening the stool so that, spontaneously or by manual extraction, the impaction may be overcome.

Hematological and Transfusion-Related Complications

A protocol for the bedside administration of blood is worthy of adoption. A nurse should be present for the first 15 minutes of the transfusion and should visit every 15 minutes thereafter; vital signs should be recorded every 30 minutes. For the first half hour, blood should be given slowly, either at a "keep open" rate or at approximately 50 drops a minute. Thereafter the rate may be accelerated to 60 to 80 drops per minute.

Allergenic reactions are most commonly associated with urticaria but may be accompanied by muscle pain, joint pain, asthmatic symptoms, pulmonary edema, and edema of the face and larynx. If any of these occur, the transfusion should be stopped. Antihistamines should be administered for simple urticarial reactions; intravenous epinephrine may be indicated for bronchospasm, hypotension, or severe urticaria. A laboratory analysis is usually not indicated in such cases.

Pyrogenic reactions are frequently caused by leukocyte antibodies, but may also result from chemical or bacterial contamination. When such reactions appear, the transfusion should be stopped immediately. If repetitive transfusions are required, leukocyte-poor blood such as washed blood (in contrast to packed cells) or frozen blood should be used.

The administration of incompatible blood generates the most serious reactions, which are accompanied by hemolysis and cause such symptoms as fever, pain in the chest or back or legs, and a drop in blood pressure.

When any reaction other than the simple urticarial-allergenic type occurs, the remaining blood of the transfusion and its pilot tubes should be submitted to the laboratory. A specimen of the patient's blood, freshly drawn from a separate vein with precautions against hemolysis, should be sent to the laboratory for examination of plasma hemoglobin, a direct Coombs test,

an antibody screen, and retyping and crossmatching. The first available urine specimen should be submitted for analysis for hemoglobin. A second blood specimen obtained four to six hours later should be submitted for examination for bilirubin. In the case of a pyrogenic reaction, the transfused blood specimen should be cultured and the possible transmission of other diseases (malaria) should be recognized.

In the management of severe reactions, the maintenance of urinary flow is essential. A catheter should be placed in the bladder, and urine flow should be stimulated to a rate of 1 ml per kilogram per hour or better in the adult. Such urine flow stimulation may be assisted by utilizing mannitol or furosemide, the latter being preferred in circumstances in which circulatory overload is a concern. Oligemic shock must be corrected, and if additional blood is needed, fresh compatible blood, washed blood, or frozen blood may be elected. Alkalinization of the urine may be indicated if severe acidosis occurs, but audit of the patient's acid-base status is the best guide to such therapy. Steroid therapy may also be indicated. The primary concern, however, is maintenance of an adequate urinary flow.

If the patient is normovolemic or hypervolemic but requires improved oxygen-carrying capacity, packed cells or washed cells should be administered in preference to whole blood. Circulatory overload may be recognized by a distended venous bed, pulmonary edema, tachypnea, and on occasion, hypertension, facial flushing, and cardiac enlargement. The fluid administration should be stopped, rotating tourniquets on the extremities should be instituted promptly, and phlebotomy may be required. Prompt monitoring of the central venous pressure may be necessary.[63,104]

Venous Thromboses and Inflammation

Phlebitis secondary to intravenous therapy is a common complication, especially when indwelling catheters are utilized. This complication and the mechanisms behind it offer an explanation for some examples of postoperative fever and occasionally of gram-negative sepsis. The local signs are pain, redness, swelling, tenderness, fever, and leukocytosis, and it is significant that the inflammatory response may be at some distance from the site of introduction of the catheter. Such an inflammatory response requires removal of the catheter. The extremity should be elevated, and warm moist packs should be applied. Venous thrombosis as a result of the process may deny the surgeon access to this particular route for therapy. The author has made it a rule to avoid, whenever feasible, the administration of intravenous fluids into the lower extremities. Catheter placement should be made after surgical preparation of the skin and the application of local antibiotic at the site of introduction. The catheter should not be allowed to remain in place more than 48 hours. When possible and with a cooperative patient who will permit the extremity to remain undisturbed, the scalp needle technique should replace the catheter technique. For prolonged intravenous therapy, subclavian puncture for the introduction of fluid by way of a caval catheter may be preferred.[58]

For the more serious forms of deep vein thrombosis, the risk factors include: age over 45, past history of thrombophlebitis or pulmonary embolism, varicose veins or ulcers, prior myocardial infarction, cardiac arrhythmias, congestive heart failure, extremity paralysis, infection, malignant disease, and prominent obesity. The incidence of postoperative deep vein thrombosis on the author's service is approximately 0.6 per cent and does not differ from other neurosurgical services in this regard.[85] All patients in the high-risk categories should continue to wear the properly constructed elastic stockings described in the preoperative preparation section of this chapter. They should also be encouraged in repetitive lower extremity exercises against resistance (footboard) from the moment of wakefulness. They should be mobilized as soon as possible. External evidence of inflammation may be minimal, but pain is a common symptom. An inappropriate increase in pulse rate may be noted. An increase in the circumference of the extremity and pain in the calf upon acute dorsiflexion of the ankle and foot are useful signs if present. Tenderness along the course of the venous structures may be identified, or the more obvious evidences of inflammation, heat, redness, and fever, may occur. The patient who complains of stiffness or aching in his calves, particularly after the beginning of ambulation, or one who develops a limp (the significance of which may be clouded by neurological deficit) must be ob-

served with care for other signs of phlebothrombosis. The combination of a mild pulse increase and temperature rise should lead the physician to measure calf circumference, examine the venous drainage, and determine the presence of a positive Homans' sign. Exclusive reliance upon clinical indications, will, however, result in missed diagnoses, and the first sign of trouble may be in the form of a pulmonary embolus. More reliable methods for detecting deep vein thrombosis include ultrasonic scanning utilizing the Doppler principle, impedence plethysmography, venography, and the use of iodine-125-tagged fibrinogen. Because of the significant risk attendant upon therapeutic anticoagulation, particularly in the neurosurgical patient, confirmation of the diagnosis by venography or isotopic studies can be justified in doubtful cases.

At the first indication of deep vein thrombosis, and in the absence of pulmonary embolization, the patient should be placed at bed rest with the extremities elevated without creasing or acute flexion of either the thigh or the knee. Properly constructed graded-pressure elastic stockings, as previously noted, should be prescribed. Heat may be applied. If the diagnosis is confirmed, therapy should be specific and vigorous. If the diagnosis is made within the first few postoperative days or if other relative contraindications to anticoagulation exist (bleeding ulcer, urinary tract bleeding), venacaval interruption should be seriously considered. If, on the contrary, the process is detected after the initial four to five days, it is probably safe to initiate anticoagulation. Such may be the case earlier in the postoperative period in patients whose disease and operative procedure do not involve intracranial and intraspinal manipulation.

Anticoagulation can be offered according to a subcutaneous, intermittent intravenous, or continuous intravenous protocol. If the facilities are available, continuous intravenous heparin at a rate of 1000 units per hour is initiated following a loading dose of 10,000 units. Monitoring of the partial thromboplastin time (activated PTT) and its maintenance at between two and three times the normal is essential. It must be remembered that the dosage of heparin will vary with the individual patient's response, and repeated monitoring to obtain a level approaching three times the normal activated partial thromboplastin time is wanted. If the patient has a pulmonary embolus, the loading dose of heparin should be between 15,000 and 20,000 units. The patient should then be started on warfarin within a week. After anticoagulation levels are obtained with the latter medication, the heparin may be discontinued. The warfarin is continued for six weeks, and the elastic stockings are worn for six months to help prevent the postphlebitic state.

Diffusely Disseminated Infection

Bacterial meningitis has been encountered in several groups of patients: (1) those who have contamination of the meninges from an associated wound infection; (2) those with cerebrospinal fluid rhinorrhea; (3) those with cerebrospinal fluid fistulae following operative procedures on the dura mater, particularly over the spinal meninges; (4) those with operations that have violated the barriers between meninges and contaminated spaces such as the accessory nasal sinuses or the mastoid air cells (i.e., operations for pituitary tumors, eighth nerve tumors, orbital decompressions); and (5) those undergoing repair of meningoceles or myelomeningoceles. Ventriculitis has been seen most often when indwelling prosthetic devices or shunting techniques have been used and after prolonged intraventricular operative procedures, especially if associated with a chemical ventriculitis caused by blood or the spillage of cyst fluid. The *Staphylococcus,* pneumococcus, enterococcus, and *Pseudomonas* and *Klebsiella* bacilli are the organisms that have been most frequently encountered. Operations that can be expected to transgress the barrier between a known infected site and the intradural spaces should be planned so that antibiotic therapy is administered before, during, and after the procedure. Active sinusitis and mastoiditis are examples of such infected sites. "Prophylactic" therapy postoperatively is far less effective than the program just described, but is indicated if a frankly infected space has been entered or if the site, although clean, cannot be excluded from the field and remains a source of contamination. Established meningitis usually responds to systemically administered antibiotics, but ventricle infections may, if drainage is defective, require intraventricular medication as well as closed external ventricular drain-

age or ventricular perfusion. For long-term intraventricular therapy the Ommaya reservoir is a useful device.[77]

In addition to the other possible causes of bacteremia and septicemia, attention should be directed to the role of indwelling urethral catheters, indwelling intravenous infusion catheters, pressure monitoring devices, and mechanical respirators and nebulizing equipment as routes for the introduction of infection, particularly gram-negative infection. The presence of a prosthetic device, particularly a cerebrospinal fluid shunting apparatus, may play a role in the production of bacteremia and septicemia.[34,73]

"Sterile" Inflammatory Responses

Fever of "Unknown" Etiology

Some of the less frequent causes of postoperative fever that may be unsuspected but have been encountered in the management of the neurosurgical patient postoperatively include anemia, large subgaleal collections of fluid or other hematoma resolution, steroid deficiency, salivary gland inflammation, phlebitis in association with intravenous therapy, fecal impaction, and drugs. Most examples of fever of "unknown" origin can be traced to a specific cause as one expands the check list, which needs reviewing in the management of each postoperative problem.

Meningismus

Blood spilled into the subarachnoid space may be associated with an immediate febrile response (more often seen in infants and children) or a delayed response with a secondary rise in temperature following the first few postoperative days. In the mild form the temperature rise is slight (1° to 1.5°C), and the process may be associated with little more than pain at the operative site or, more commonly, in the spine, low back, and lower extremities. More severe reactions produce higher fever, prominent headache, neck guarding, back pain, and radicular pain (often sciatic in distribution). Their occurrence requires the performance of a lumbar puncture. The fluid is often grossly bloody, and the protein content is increased. Drainage of such fluid in the absence of any contraindication thereto is helpful, and repeated lumbar punctures are to be recommended. The patient's complaints will usually resolve over the course of a week. The problem may be aggravated by the coexistence of a subgaleal collection of blood that communicates with the subarachnoid space and provides a source of chronic contamination and perpetuation of the syndrome. Evacuation of the subgaleal collection plus lumbar puncture is helpful. Each fluid specimen should be cultured to insure that neither a primary nor a secondary infection develops in the spaces harboring the irritating fluid. Hydrocephalus may be a transient or semipermanent consequence of a large contamination of the cerebrospinal fluid pathways with blood. The spilled blood can overwhelm the absorptive capacities of the arachnoid villae; it can also contribute to the development of an obliterative meningeal inflammatory process, as can repeated widespread operative exposure of strategic meningeal cerebrospinal fluid pathways, especially those of the posterior fossa. Hydrocephalus may be the consequence.[91]

Exposing large areas of central nervous tissue to manipulation or the removal of large blocks of tissue with attendant tissue necrosis may produce a similar postoperative reaction. Fever may appear from the day of operation and remain elevated as long as four weeks (the more usual course is limited to the first two weeks). High fever (41° C) and tachycardia may be the only major findings, but local wound pain and some signs of meningeal irritation are usually associated. The latter complaints are more prominent the higher the blood content in the fluid, but sterile meningeal reactions do occur following the manipulation and excision of tissue in which necrosis is considered the more responsible mechanism rather than the spillage of blood. In the author's experience the cerebrospinal fluid response has varied from a few hundred to several thousand white cells per cubic millimeter. Early in the process the polymorphonuclear cells dominate over 90 per cent. As the days pass the mononuclear response becomes more prominent, and near the termination of the response (although fever may still be present) there appears to be a rapid reversal of pattern to a dominantly mononuclear cellular response with final clinical resolution. There is usually neither peripheral blood leukocytosis nor superimposed encephalopathy during the course of the sterile meningeal reaction, important

points in distinguishing it from bacterial infection. The cerebrospinal fluid protein is usually increased to more than 120 mg per 100 ml, and the figure may rise to 1000 mg per 100 ml. With protein content in excess of 200 to 300 mg per 100 ml clinical signs are usually present. The cerebrospinal fluid glucose determinations vary; they may be quite low (values as low as 24 mg per 100 ml have been encountered), but they may be in the normal range (60 to 70 per cent of blood glucose). A rare occurrence is the very late onset of such a sterile meningeal reaction (one example occurred seven weeks following a posterior fossa exploration).

The course of such an illness is about three weeks with complete resolution and no sequelae. The presence of any foreign body introduces the question of whether that item is the basis of the reaction. With rare exceptions, the pyrogenic reactions have resolved under symptomatic therapy. If clear evidence of wound inflammation, suppuration, or breakdown is present, the local indications for management dominate the picture and exclude these cases from the sterile reactions mentioned.[17]

Since antibiotics are used for a variety of other complications, the possibility that their use may mask a bacterial infection must be kept in mind. In the face of this possibility a patient's illness may be sufficiently fulminant that it is necessary to treat him as though he were suffering from a bacterial infection. It is worth noting, however, that the patients with sterile meningeal responses do not demonstrate the clouding of consciousness or other aggravation of neurological deficit expected with bacterial infection. Cultures are sterile, and there is no peripheral leukocytosis. Repeated inspection of the wound is needed. The serial cerebrospinal fluid cellular, protein, and culture data should be charted for ready comparison. Wound collections should be evacuated with the precautions mentioned under wound care. Fever is managed by the use of rectal or oral acetaminophen and external cooling. Dexamethasone has, in certain cases, produced dramatic improvement and may be recommended in dosage similar to that used in combating the cerebral edemas[16] The use of therapeutic ionizing radiation in the management of the patient in the postoperative stage may be associated with an aggravation of or precipitation of a reaction similar to those just described, introducing once again the role

PHYSIOLOGY, HOMEOSTASIS, AND GENERAL CARE

of destruction of tissue in the mechanism. Again, the management is conservative after excluding specific bacterial infection.

Patients who are operated on immediately following a myelogram may, in the immediate postoperative state, suffer from a reaction to the preoperative study. This may involve signs of meningeal irritation, headache, fever (39° C), leukocytosis in the cerebrospinal fluid as high as 9200 cells (of which the majority are polymorphonuclear), and an increase in the cerebrospinal fluid protein as high as 1000 mg per 100 ml followed by a rapid decrease. The possible role of the postmyelogram reaction must, therefore, not be forgotten in the differential diagnosis of the "sterile" meningitides.

Allergic Sensitivity Reactions

The possible reactions to drug administration or adhesive tape and other surface applications have been noted in earlier sections. The author has encountered rashes in association with morphine, codeine, anticonvulsant agents, and atropine. Such rashes may last for several days and, although troublesome to the patient, are usually not dangerous. They may be associated with an otherwise unexplained fever. In mild form they should be combated by antihistamine administration (diphenhydramine in a dosage that may need to be high enough to make the patient mildly drowsy) and cornstarch baths with tepid water. Triamcinolone-containing lotions may be applied, and steroids may be administered orally or parenterally. The primary problem is to avoid exacerbating the condition by applying something that is more irritating than the underlying process.

Hyperpyrexia (Hyperthermia)

Fever is a common sign accompanying many surgical complications. When so associated it is usually the result of the action of a pyrogen (of bacterial, leukocytic, or other origin) upon the hypothalamus. Primary "central" hyperthermia may occur with injury or disease of the hypothalamus itself, which then is rendered incapable of coordinating thermoregulatory responses from central and peripheral thermoreceptive structures. Patients are endangered by fevers in excess of 39° C, and efforts should be made to reverse febrile trends approaching that temperature; vigorous therapy is indicated if that temperature is exceeded. Treating the cause is fundamental, but symptomatic therapy is also indicated. The patient should be naked or covered by a loosely anchored sheet of light linen. Tepid water bathing with skin rubbing to the point of rubor followed by gentle alcohol rubbing will help. External ambient temperature control is needed; a propeller fan will aid surface evaporation, which, again, is enhanced by producing skin rubor. A hypothermic blanket may be placed beneath the patient (but not over him). The covering linen sheet may be sprinkled with alcohol while the fan plays upon it. Oral or rectally instilled acetaminophen is effective. Chlorpromazine will control shivering, and ice water enemas may be used if the response is inadequate. Severe, intractable hyperpyrexia demands formal hypothermia induction by external cooling (refrigeration blankets, ice) aided by the use of neuromuscular paralyzing agents of which pancuronium is the drug of choice (artificial ventilatory measures must be available).

Miscellaneous Complications

Seizures, Postictal Paresis

In the postoperative period, convulsive activity may produce a clinical state that mimics postoperative deterioration from other more serious causes, particularly if it causes impairment of consciousness of postictal paresis of neurological function. The possibility of its occurrence should be remembered in the management of the postoperative patient. The goal is to protect against any seizure activity that, even as a transient phenomenon, will aggravate brain metabolic needs or contribute to intracranial venous engorgement, which a generalized seizure will most surely do. Patients who have had seizures preoperatively should be placed on an adequate anticonvulsant regimen in the immediate postoperative period. Should seizure activity first appear in the early postoperative period, prompt anticonvulsant medication is indiciated. Diazepam, sodium phenobarbital, and sodium diphenylhydantoin are the most useful medications.

Confusion Unexplained by Site of Operation

Elderly patients or patients who have been moved from one environment to another may become confused, disoriented, and difficult to manage. Their dislocation to strange surroundings and their lack of rapid adaptation to changes made at a time during which their memory was impaired provide a partial explanation. This process may also be observed in the absence of any operative procedure involving central nervous tissue per se. It may be precipitated or aggravated by the inappropriate use of sedation. Surgeon and anesthesiologist must recognize how sensitive are patients, particularly elderly ones, to any central nervous depressants after procedures on the central nervous system. Thirty milligrams of codeine given hypodermically have been associated with impairment of the level of consciousness in an adult. Some anesthetic agents such as methoxyflurane (Penthrane) should be avoided in view of the prolonged sedation produced in the postoperative period.

Decubitus Ulceration

The aged patient, the debilitated patient, and the paralyzed or comatose patient are all vulnerable to skin breakdown. The risks are increased if urinary or fecal incontinence exists to macerate the skin. The autonomic paralysis accompanying paraplegia robs the patient of protective vascular reflexes, and ischemia develops rapidly. If there are no contraindications to frequent turning (bony instability, hypovolemia, serious diencephalic or brain stem disease), patients should be turned to expose all areas of the skin to room air every one to two hours. The skin should be dry (assisted by nonallergenic powders) and treated at least daily with a solution of 5 per cent tannic acid in 95 per cent isopropyl alcohol. Bony prominences may be additionally toughened with tincture of benzoin. Synthetic "sheepskin" padding is useful under the trunk and pelvis, and heel cradles can prevent breakdown in the Achilles area. Danger signs are persistently reddened areas or blanching of the skin without prompt reactive hyperemia. If decubital blisters or ulcers occur, the therapy is exposure and weightlessness. Excision of the core of devitalized tissue with plastic repair will be required in cases of deep ulceration. All comments relative to "surgical" nutrition and wound healing are also applicable here.

CONCLUDING COMMENT

Each complication requires as prompt recognition and management as possible. One complication is often superimposed upon another in a dangerous train leading to irreversible illness and death. Whatever the surgeon does to help his patient, he must recognize the attendant risks and possible complications. He must be prepared to meet these by a survey of the likely kind of complication that might be expected during the predictable phases of the patient's course or at the time of major changes in the patient's condition. He must anticipate the need for preventative methods or provide promptly the therapeutic measures once the complication develops. The responsible surgeon, himself, must accept the need for repetitive, personal involvement in the care of his patient. In the recent past the author has cared for a patient with the following complications occurring either simultaneously or sequentially: a postoperative wound hematoma, pneumonia, blood in the cerebrospinal fluid, wound pseudomeningocele, urinary retention, cystitis, epididymitis, salivary glandulitis, and electrocardiographic irregularities secondary to the administration of epinephrine in the management of laryngeal edema. This patient recovered, yet many of these complications might have been fatal. The surgeon, in effect, hand-carries his patient through his surgical management.

REFERENCES

1. Alexander, R. W.: Diabetes mellitus—current criteria for laboratory diagnosis. Calif. Med., *110*:107–113, 1969.
2. Alford, R. H.: Prevention of bacterial disease by oral and parenteral antimicrobial agents. Southern Med. J., *66*:32–39, 1973.
3. Allcock, J. M., and Drake, C. G.: Ruptured intracranial aneurysms—the role of arterial spasm. J. Neurosurg., *22*:21–29, 1965.
3a. Allen, G. S.: Cerebral arterial spasm. Part 8: The treatment of delayed cerebral arterial spasm in human beings Surg. Neural., *6*:71–80, 1976.
4. Austen, G.: Management of postoperative acute renal failure. Amer. J. Surg., *116*:346–361, 1968.
5. Bakay, L., and Lee, A. C.: Cerebral Edema. Springfield, Ill., Charles C Thomas, 1965.
6. Balch, R. E.: Wound infections complicating neurosurgical procedures. J. Neurosurg., *26*:41–45, 1967.
7. Barbour, C. M., and Little, D. M., Jr.: Postoper-

ative hypotension. J.A.M.A., *165*:1529–1532, 1957.

7a. Barnett, H. G., Clifford, J. R., and Llewellyn, R. C.: Safety of mini-dose heparin administration for neurosurgical patients. J. Neurosurg., *47*:27–30, 1977.

8. Bergentz, S. E.: Fat embolism. Progr. Surg., *6*:85–120, 1968.

9. Bergland, R. M., and Page, R. B.: Furosemide— a non-osmotic diuretic for neurosurgical use. A.A.N.S. Annual Meeting, April 6–10, 1975.

10. Bethune., R. W. M., and Brechner, V. L.: Recent advances in monitoring pulmonary air embolism. Anesth. Analg., *50*:255–261, 1971.

11. Boba, A.: Hypothermia, appraisal of risk in 110 consecutive patients. J. Neurosurg., *19*:924–933, 1962.

12. Buckland, R. W., and Manners, J. M.: Venous air embolism during neurosurgery. A comparison of various methods of detection in man. Anaesthesia, *31*:633–643, 1976.

13. Burke, J. F.: Preventive antibiotic management in surgery. Ann. Rev. Med., *24*:289–294, 1973.

14. Cafferata, H. T., Aggeler, P. M., Robinson, A. J., and Blaisdell, F. W.: Intravascular coagulation in the surgical patient. Its significance and diagnosis. Amer. J. Surg., *118*:281–291, 1969.

15. Cahill, J. M.: Respiratory problems in surgical patients. Amer. J. Surg., *116*:362–368, 1968.

16. Cantu, R. C., and Ojemann, R. G.: Glucosteroid treatment of keratin meningitis following removal of a fourth ventricle epidermoid tumor. J. Neurol. Neurosurg. Psychiat., *31*:73–75, 1968.

17. Cantu, R. C., Moses, J. M., Kjellberg, R. N., and Connelly, J. P.: An unusual cause of aseptic postoperative fever in a neurosurgical patient. Review of concepts of the pathogenesis of fever, hypoglycorrhachia, and inflammation. Clin. Pediat. (Phila.), *5*:747–754, 1966.

18. Chadduck, W. M., and Martinez-G, J. de D.: Epidural hematoma complicating ventricular decompression. Southern Med. J., *60*:755–761, 1967.

19. Clarke, J. S., Coulson, W. F., Guth, P. H., et al.: Gastroduodenal stress ulcers—Interdepartmental Conference, University of California, Los Angeles. Calif. Med., *116*:32–46, 1972.

20. Cliffton, E. E.: Prediction, diagnosis and treatment of excessive bleeding at surgery. *In* American College of Surgeons, Committee on Pre and Postoperative Care: Manual of Preoperative and Postoperative Care. Philadelphia, W. B. Saunders Co., 1967.

21. Committee on Trauma, American College of Surgeons: Early Care of the Injured Patient. 2nd Ed. Philadelphia, W. B. Saunders Co., 1976.

22. Corrigan, J. J., Jr., and Jordan, C. M.: Heparin therapy in septicemia with disseminated intravascular coagulation. New Eng. J. Med., *283*:778–782, 1970.

23. Cotes, J. E.: Lung Function: Assessment and Application in Medicine. 2nd Ed. Philadelphia, F. A. Davis Co., 1968.

24. Crawford, F. A., Hammon, J. W., Jr., and Shingleton, W. W.: The stress ulcer syndrome. Amer. J. Surg., *121*:644–649, 1971.

25. Crutchfield, W. G.: Redesigned Crutchfield skull tongs. Technical note describing the combined "squeeze" and "hook" principle. J. Neurosurg., *25*:656–657, 1966.

25a. DeTroyer, A., and Demanet, J. C.: Correction of antidiuresis by demeclocycline. New Eng. J. Med., *293*:915–918, 1975.

26. Diament, M. L., and Palmer, K. N.V.: Spirometry for preoperative assessment of airways resistance. Lancet, *1*:1251–1252, 1967.

27. Drake, C. G.: Further experience with surgical treatment of aneurysms of the basilar artery. J. Neurosurg., *29*:372–392, 1968.

28. Dykes, M. H. M., and Walzer, S. G.: Preoperative and postoperative hepatic dysfunction. Surg. Gynec. Obstet., *124*:747–751, 1967.

29. Eckmann, L., Girardin, R., Hochuli, R., Montigel, C., and Allgöwer, M.: Experience with preoperative and early postoperative application of hydroxy-coumarins in surgical patients. Progr. Surg., *5*:38–86, 1966.

30. Everson, E. C.: Management of diabetes. *In* American College of Surgeons, Committee on Pre and Postoperative Care: Manual of Preoperative and Postoperative Care. Philadelphia, W. B. Saunders Co., 1967.

31. Flamm, E. S., and Ransohoff, J.: Treatment of cerebral vasospasm by control of cyclic adenosine monophosphate. Surg. Neurol., *6*:223–226, 1976.

32. Fogelman, M. J., and Garvey, J. M.: Acute gastroduodenal ulceration incident to surgery and disease. Analysis and review of 88 cases. Amer. J. Surg., *112*:651–656, 1966.

33. Foltz, E. L., and Ward, A. A., Jr.: Communicating hydrocephalus from subarachnoid bleeding. J. Neurosurg., *13*:546–566, 1956.

33a. Forrest, J. N., Cox, M., Hong, C., et al.: Superiority of demeclocycline over lithium in the treatment of chronic syndrome of inappropriate secretion of antidiuretic hormone. New Eng. J. Med. *298*:4:173–177, 1978.

34. Forrest, D. M., and Cooper, D. G. W.: Complications of ventriculo-atrial shunts; a review of 455 cases. J. Neurosurg., *29*:506–512, 1968.

35. Goodman, L. S., and Gilman, A.: The Pharmacological Basis of Therapeutics. New York, Macmillan Co., 1965.

36. Gump, F. E.: Changes caused by injury. Cont. Surg., *9*:13–18, 1976.

37. Hardaway, R. M., James, P. M., Jr., Anderson, R. W., Bredenbert, C. E., and West, R. L.: Intensive study and treatment of shock in man. J.A.M.A., *199*:779–790, 1967.

38. Hardy, J. and Ziric, I. S.: Selective anterior hypophysectomy in the treatment of diabetic retinopathy. J.A.M.A., *203*:73–78, 1968.

39. Hardy, J. D.: Cardiac arrest. *In* American College of Surgeons, Committee on Pre and Postoperative Care: Manual of Preoperative and Postoperative Care. Philadelphia, W. B. Saunders Co., 1967.

40. Harrower, H. W.: Postoperative ileus. Amer. J. Surg., *116*:369–374, 1968.

41. Hayes, G. J., and Solcum, H. C.: The achievement of optimal brain relaxation by hyperventilation techniques of anesthesia. J. Neurosurg., *19*:65–70, 1962.

42. Hodgkin, J. E., Dines, D. E., and Didier, E. P.: Preoperative evaluation of the patient with pulmonary disease. Mayo Clin. Proc., *48*:114–118, 1973.

43. Hoessly, G. F., and Olivecrona, H.: Report on 280 cases of verified parasagittal meningioma. J. Neurosurg., *12*:614–626, 1955.

44. Hollenhorst, R. W., Svien, H. J., and Benoit, C. F.: Unilateral blindness occurring during anesthesia for neurosurgical operations. Arch. Ophthal. (Chicago), *52*:819–830, 1954.

45. Hume, D. M.: Adrenal insufficiency. *In* American College of Surgeons, Committee on Pre and Postoperative Care: Manual of Preoperative and Postoperative Care. Philadelphia, W. B. Saunders Co., 1967.

46. Javid, M., and Settlage, P.: Effect of urea on cerebrospinal fluid pressure in human subjects. Preliminary report. J.A.M.A., *160*:943–949, 1956.

47. Kakkar, V. V., et al.: Deep vein thrombosis of the leg. Is there a "high risk" group? Amer. J. Surg., *120*:527–530, 1970.

48. Kakkar, V. V., Corrigan, T. P., and Fossard, D. P.: Prevention of fatal postoperative pulmonary embolism by low doses of heparin. Lancet, *2*:45–51, 1975.

49. Kalbag, R. N., and Woolf, A. L.: Cerebral Venous Thrombosis with Special Reference to Primary Aseptic Thrombosis. London, Oxford University Press, 1967.

50. Kazemi, H.: Pulmonary-function tests. J.A.M.A., *206*:2302–2304, 1968.

51. Kirklin, J. W., and Nunn, S. L.: The cardiovascular system in care of the surgical patient. *In* American College of Surgeons, Committee on Pre and Postoperative Care: Manual of Preoperative and Postoperative Care. Philadelphia, W. B. Saunders Co., 1967.

51a. Kosnik, E. J., and Hunt, W. E.: Postoperative hypertension in the management of patients with intracranial arterial aneurysms. J. Neurosurg., *45*:148–154, 1976.

52. Landau, B., and Ransohoff, J.: Prolonged cerebral vasospasm in experimental subarachnoid hemorrhage. J. Neurol., *18*:1056–1065, 1968.

53. Laver, M. B., and Bendixen, H. H.: Atelectasis in the surgical patient: recent conceptual advances. Progr. Surg., *5*:1–37, 1966.

54. Lewis, C. E., et al.: Elastic comparison in the prevention of venous stasis. A critical reevaluation. Amer. J. Surg., *132*:739–743, 1976.

55. Lewis, R. L: A survey of possible etiologic agents in postoperative craniotomy infections. J. Neurosurg., *25*:125–132, 1966.

56. Longerbeam, J. K., Vannix, R., Wagner, W., and Joergenson, E.: Central venous pressure monitoring. A useful guide to fluid therapy during shock and other forms of cardiovascular stress. Amer. J. Surg., *110*:220–230, 1965.

57. Lowbury, E. J. L., et al.: Aseptic methods in the operating suite. A report to the medical research council by the sub-committee on aseptic methods in operating theatres of their committee on hospital infection. Lancet, *1*:705–709, 763–768, 831–839, 1968.

58. McCabe, W. R.: Antibiotics and their complications in surgery. Amer. J. Surg., *116*:327–332, 1968.

59. McKittrick, J. B.: Surgery in diabetes. *In* Cole, W. H., and Zollinger, R. M., eds.: Textbook of Surgery. 8th Ed. New York, Appleton-Century-Crofts, 1963.

60. McMurty, J. G., Pool, J. L., and Nova, H. R.: The use of rheomacrodex in the surgery of intracranial aneurysms. J. Neurosurg., *26*:218–222, 1967.

61. Markham, J. W., Lynge, H. N., and Stahlman, G. E. B.: The syndrome of spontaneous spinal epidural hematoma. Report of three cases. J. Neurosurg., *26*:334–342, 1967.

62. Maroon, J. C., Edmonds-Seal, J., and Campbell, R. L.: An ultrasonic method for detecting air embolism. J. Neurosurg., *31*:196–201, 1969.

63. Merritt, J. A.: Complications related to blood replacement. Amer. J. Surg., *117*:333–336, 1968.

64. Meyerowitz, B. R.: Venous thrombosis in surgical patients. Amer. J. Surg., *113*:521–524, 1967.

65. Michenfelder, J. D., Martin, J. T., Altenburg, B. M., and Rehder, K.: Air embolism during neurosurgery. J.A.M.A., *208*:1353–1358, 1969.

66. Moore, F. D.: Metabolic Care of the Surgical Patient. Philadelphia, W. B. Saunders Co., 1959.

67. Moore, F. D.: Surgical nutrition: parenteral and oral. *In* American College of Surgeons, Committee on Pre and Postoperative Care: Manual of Preoperative and Postoperative Care. Philadelphia, W. B. Saunders Co., 1967.

68. Munson, E. S., Paul, W. L., Perry, J. C., de Padua, C. B., and Rhoton, A. L.: Early detection of venous air embolism using a Swan-Ganz catheter. Anesthesiology, *42*:223–226, 1975.

69. Nishioka, H. Results of the treatment of intracranial aneurysms by occlusion of the carotid artery in the neck. J. Neurosurg., *25*:660–682, 1966.

70. Olsen, E. R.: Intracranial surgery in hemophiliacs. Report of a case and review of the literature. Arch. Neurol. (Chicago), *21*:401–412, 1969.

71. Parker, B.: Electrical testing for safety of the operating room and intensive care unit. Bull. Amer. Coll. Surg., *54*:187–189, 1969.

72. Paulsen, E. P.: Postoperative fluid, electrolyte, caloric requirements in children. Amer. J. Surg., *107*:390–395, 1964.

73. Perrin, J. C. S., and McLaurin, R. L.: Infected ventriculoatrial shunts, a method of treatment. J. Neurosurg., *27*:21–26, 1967.

74. Pleasure, D., and Goldberg, M.: Neurogenic hypernatremia. Arch. Neurol., *15*:78–87, 1966.

75. Porter, R. W., and French, J. D.: The physiologic basis of cardiac arrest during anesthesia. Amer. J. Surg., *100*:354–357, 1960.

76. Rand, R. W.: Cryosurgery of the pituitary in acromegaly: Reduced growth hormone levels following hypophysectomy in 13 cases. Ann. Surg., *164*:587–592, 1966.

77. Ratcheson, R. A., and Ommaya, A. K.: Experience with the subcutaneous cerebrospinal-fluid reservoir. Preliminary report of 60 cases. New Eng. J. Med., *279*:1025–1031, 1968.

78. Ray, B. S., Pazianos, A. G., Greenberg, E., Peretz, W. L., and McLean, J. M.: Pituitary ablation for diabetic retinopathy. II. Results of yttrium 90 implantation in the pituitary gland. J.A.M.A., *203*:85–87, 1968.

79. Rhoads, J. E.: Nutrition. *In* Moyer, C. A., Rhoads, J. E., Allen, J. G., and Harkins, H. N., eds.: Surgery: Principles and Practice. 3rd Ed. Philadelphia, J. B. Lippincott, 1965.

80. Robinson, A. G.: DDAVP in the treatment of

central diabetes insipidus. New Eng. J. Med., *294*:507–511, 1976.

81. Roe, C. F., Santulli, V., and Blair, C. S.: Heat loss in infants during general anesthesia and operations. J. Pediat. Surg., *1*:266–274, 1966.

82. Sackner, M. A.: Management of pulmonary insufficiency. Calif. Med., *110*:355–357, 1969.

83. Sahs, A. L.: Hypotension and hypothermia in the treatment of intracranial aneurysms (section VII part 2, report on the cooperative study of intracranial aneurysms and subarachnoid hemorrhage). J. Neurosurg., *25*:593–600, 1966.

84. Schoenbaum, S. C., Gardner, P., and Shillito, J.: Infections of cerebrospinal fluid shunts: Epidemiology, clinical manifestations and therapy. J. Infect. Dis., *131*:543–552, 1975.

85. Schulze, A.: Zum Problem der Thrombose und Embolie nach neurochirurgischen Operationen. Acta Neurochir. (Wien), *14*:278–286, 1966.

86. Shapiro, H. M.: Intracranial hypertension therapeutic and anesthetic considerations. Anesthesiology, *43*:445–471, 1975.

87. Shapiro, H. M., Wyte, S. R., and Loeser, J.: Barbiturate-augmented hypothermia for reduction of persistent intracranial hypertension. J. Neurosurg., *40*:90–100, 1974.

88. Shucart, W. A., and Jackson, I.: Management of diabetes insipidus in neurosurgical patients. J. Neurosurg., *44*:65–71, 1976.

88a. Skillman, J. J., Collins, R. E. C., Coe, N. P., et al: Prevention of deep vein thrombosis in neurosurgical patients: A controlled, randomized trial of external pneumatic compression boot. Surgery, *83*:354–358, 1978.

89. Smith, R. M.: Current issues in pediatric anesthesia. Amer. J. Surg., *107*:396–399, 1964.

90. Smith, W. W.: Bleeding diatheses in surgical patients, Monogr. Surg. Sci., *1*:3–57, 1964.

91. Stein, B. M., Tenner, M. S., and Fraser, R. A. R.: Hydrocephalus following removal of cerebellar astrocytomas in children. J. Neurosurg., *36*:763–768, 1972.

92. Stein, M., and Cassara, E. L.: Preoperative pulmonary evaluation and therapy for surgery patients. J.A.M.A., *211*:787–790, 1970.

93. Stern, W. E.: Preoperative preparation for neurosurgery with emphasis upon fluid, electrolyte and steroid use. Neurochirurgia (Stuttgart), *6*:176–187, 1963.

94. Stern, W. E.: Circulatory adequacy attendant upon carotid artery occlusion. Arch. Neurol. (Chicago), *21*:455–465, 1969.

95. Stern, W. E., and Bethune, R. W. M.: Application of adjunctive technics for the control of intracranial pressure with emphasis upon the surgical exposure of the pituitary fossa. Ann. Surg., *154*:662–673, 1961.

96. Stullken, E. H., Jr., and Sokoll, M. D.: Anesthesia and subarachnoid intracranial pressure. Anesth. Analg., *54*:494–500, 1975.

97. Symposium on Shock, Third (Boston Univ.) Surgical Service Eleventh Annual Seminar. Amer. J. Surg., *110*:293–354, 1965.

98. Tachdjian, M. O., and Matson, D. D.: Orthopedic aspects of intraspinal tumors in infants and children. J. Bone Joint Surg., *47-A*:223–248, 1965.

99. Tarhan, S., Moffitt, E. A., Taylor, W. F., and Giuliani, E. R.: Myocardial infarction after general anesthesia. J.A.M.A., *220*:1451–1454, 1972.

100. Thomas, J. E., and Ayyar, D. R.: Systemic fat embolism. A diagnostic profile in 24 patients. Arch. Neurol., *26*:517–523, 1972.

101. Van den Berg, J., and Van Manen, J.: Graded coagulation of brain tissue. Acta Physiol. Pharmacol. Neerl., *10*:353–377, 1962.

102. Vander Ark, G. D.: Cardiovascular monitoring in neurosurgery. Clin. Neurosurg., *22*:462–475, 1975.

102a. Van Dulken, H., and Thomeer, R. T. W. M.: Letter to the Editor. J. Neurosurg., *47*:974, 1977.

103. Walter, C. W.: Blood donors' blood and transfusions. *In* American College of Surgeons, Committee on Pre and Postoperative Care: Manual of Preoperative and Postoperative Care. Philadelphia, W. B. Saunders Co., 1967.

104. Walter, C. W.: Safe electric environment in the hospital. Bull. Amer. Coll. Surg., *54*:187–189, 1969.

105. Watts, C. C., and Clark, K.: Gastric acidity in the comatose patient. J. Neurosurg., *30*:107–109, 1969.

106. Wessler, S., and Avioli, L. V.: Changes in surgical management of hemophiliacs. Pseudotumor of the ilium. J.A.M.A., *206*:2292–2296, 1968.

107. Wessler, S., and Avioli, L. V.: Inappropriate secretion of antidiuretic hormone. J.A.M.A., *205*:349–352, 1968.

108. White, M. G., and Fetner, C. D.: Treatment of the syndrome of inappropriate secretion of antidiuretic hormone with lithium carbonate. New Eng. J. Med., *292*:390–392, 1975.

109. Wilkins, R. H., Alexander, J. A., and Odom, G. L.: Intracranial arterial spasm: A clinical analysis. J. Neurosurg., *29*:121–134, 1968.

110. Williams, L. F., Jr.: Gastrointestinal hemorrhage as a postoperative phenomenon. Amer. J. Surg., *116*:375–381, 1968.

111. Wilson, C. B., Winternitz, W. W., Bertan, Z., and Sizemore, G.: Stereotaxic cryosurgery in the pituitary gland and carcinoma of the breast and other disorders. J.A.M.A., *198*:587–590, 1966.

112. Wise, B. L.: Effects of infusion of hypertonic mannitol on electrolyte balance and on osmolality of serum and cerebrospinal fluid. J. Neurosurg., *20*:961–967, 1963.

113. Wise, B. L.: Fluid and electrolytes. *In* Neurological Surgery, Springfield, Ill., Charles C Thomas, 1965.

114. Wise, B. L.: The management of postoperative diabetes insipidus. J. Neurosurg., *25*:416–420, 1966.

115. Wise, B. L., and Chater, N.: The value of hypertonic mannitol solution in decreasing brain mass and lowering cerebrospinal fluid pressure. J. Neurosurg., *19*:1038–1043, 1962.

116. Wyte, S. R.: Ventilation of the neurosurgical patient. Clin. Neurosurg., *22*:444–461, 1975.

117. Zimmerman, B.: The diagnosis and management of acute renal failure. *In* American College of Surgeons, Committee on Pre and Postoperative Care: Manual of Preoperative and Postoperative Care. Philadelphia, W. B. Saunders Co., 1967.

V

ANESTHESIA AND OPERATIVE TECHNIQUE

30

ANESTHESIA

The anesthetic management of the neurosurgical patient should concern the neurological surgeon as well as the anesthesiologist. Probably in no other field can the skills of the anesthesiologist so profoundly affect the work of the surgeon. This is particularly true for intracranial operations, because all anesthetic agents and techniques may significantly alter normal cerebral physiology and, secondarily, intracranial dynamics. Intelligent management of the patient requires that the anesthesiologist fully understand the procedure planned by the surgeon and know the patient's preoperative neurological status. When he has this information, consultation with the neurosurgeon will permit selection of the proper anesthetic agents and techniques, and determination of possible need for special techniques and monitoring devices. The neurosurgeon should be aware of the major effects of anesthesia on cerebral physiology and should be familiar with both the cerebral and systemic effects of the various special techniques available to him.

GENERAL PRINCIPLES

Airway

Providing an adequate airway is vitally important in all phases of the care of patients with intracranial disease. This is so not only because of the undesirable effects of hypoxia and carbon dioxide accumulation but also because of the direct relationship of intracranial pressure to intrathoracic and intra-abdominal pressure. Any degree of airway obstruction may trigger the vicious circle of increased intracranial pressure, cerebral hypoxia, and irreversible edema. Managing the airway in the comatose patient requires careful evaluation of the depth of coma and the prognosis. In light coma the presence of adequate muscle tone, active protective reflexes, and adequate tidal volume and respiratory rate permits a "wait and watch" approach. Deeper coma associated with deterioration of any of these factors or the presence of excessive tracheobronchial secretions requires endotracheal intubation. In general, any patient who requires an oropharyngeal or nasopharyngeal airway should be intubated unless immediate improvement is anticipated. If the prognosis indicates a long-term problem, elective tracheostomy should be done after intubation. With use of modern soft plastic tubes and highly compliant cuffs, endotracheal intubation is usually safely tolerated for as long as seven days.

The use of armored endotracheal tubes during operations has solved most of the problems related to unusual operative positions or inaccessibility of the airway. Specific airway problems may be encountered in patients with fixed cervical spine, fracture of the cervical spine, limited mandibular motion, or head and neck trauma; these patients must have careful preoperative evaluation to determine the feasibility of intubation. If loss of the airway is likely when general anesthesia is induced, the patient should be intubated while awake. The introduction of the fiberoptic laryngoscope and bronchoscope has greatly simplified many of these previously difficult airway problems. Rarely, intubation is mechanically impossible or carries sufficient potential hazard to warrant an elective preoperative tracheostomy.

Postoperative airway problems may re-

J. D. MICHENFELDER, G. A. GRONERT, AND K. REHDER

sult from dysfunction of the ninth, tenth, or twelfth cranial nerve, usually caused by operative trauma during the removal of a tumor of the fourth ventricle.[4] Damage to the vagus nerve is most important to assess, since it may result in loss of protective airway reflexes and interfere with swallowing. The potential hazard of aspiration in these patients makes tracheostomy mandatory. Bilateral damage to the twelfth cranial nerve may also make tracheostomy necessary because of the resulting loss of motor function and inability to maintain an airway.

Premedication

As in all operative procedures, the purpose of premedication in neurosurgery is to ensure that the patient is in a suitable state for smooth induction of anesthesia, is protected from harmful reflexes, and is free of anxiety. In the patient with intracranial disease, there is often a narrow margin between inadequate medication, resulting in struggling or straining, and excessive medication, resulting in airway obstruction, hypoventilation, or circulatory depression. In general, excessive medication should be avoided by using narcotics or hypnotics minimally if at all in infants, in patients with increased intracranial pressure, and in comatose patients. Atropine is a useful drug in most patients; it reduces tracheobronchial secretions and, in sufficient dosage, will minimize vagal effects on the heart secondary to anesthetic drugs or operative manipulation. Such vagal reflexes may be expected during pneumoencephalography, carotid angiography, carotid operations, orbital exploration or decompression, trigeminal nerve procedures, and posterior fossa exploration. Antiemetics may be a useful addition to the premedications to prevent nausea and retching, which are particularly likely to occur during pneumoencephalography and ventriculography under regional anesthesia.

Local Anesthesia

Before World War II, regional anesthesia was often the anesthetic method of choice for intracranial operations, in part because of the deficiencies in techniques and personnel available for administering general anesthesia. In some respects local anesthesia is particularly well suited for operations on the brain: the brain itself is insensitive to pain, and with adequate infiltration of the extracranial tissues, operative pain is minimal; the patient's response to manipulation and retraction of the brain can be assessed accurately; and central nervous system depression by anesthetic agents is minimized. The disadvantages of local anesthesia are equally apparent: uncooperative patients may require sedation to the point of uncontrolled depression of the central nervous system; cooperative patients become increasingly uncomfortable from prolonged maintenance of a rigid position; any patient may experience nausea with retching, straining, and coughing; control of the airway is not always possible; and the maintenance of adequate ventilation is not assured. With the introduction of new agents and techniques and the increasing availability of trained personnel for the administration of general anesthesia, the desirability of regional anesthesia in most institutions has decreased to the point at which it now is reserved for only a few neurosurgical procedures. These generally include procedures that require continuous evaluation of the patient's neurological status, such as carotid ligation, percutaneous cordotomy, stereotaxic operations, and electrocorticography; or brief uncomplicated procedures such as pneumoencephalography, cerebral angiography, myelography, and drilling of burr holes for extracerebral hematomas, ventricular drainage, or ventriculography.

The *use of regional anesthesia in no way reduces the need for continuous monitoring and care of the patient.* Premedication for patients scheduled for operation under regional anesthesia should not be excessive; it is preferable to provide sedation intravenously as required during the procedure. Incremental doses of either diazepam or droperidol-fentanyl (Innovar) are usually highly effective. Selection of the proper local anesthetic for infiltration should be based primarily on the anticipated length of the procedure. For a craniotomy of several hours' duration, intermittent fortification of the initial anesthetic by infiltration is necessary. The addition of epinephrine to the local anesthetic is optional, but its use prolongs the anesthesia and significantly reduces loss of blood from the highly vascular tissues of the scalp.

It is a common misconception that "sick" or comatose patients will not tolerate general anesthesia and must, therefore, be operated upon under regional anesthesia. This may have been true in past years; however, current techniques of general anesthesia permit a significantly greater degree of control of the patient's vital functions than is possible with any regional technique. If regional anesthesia is selected for a comatose patient, an adequate airway must be provided, either by preoperative tracheal intubation or by tracheostomy.

Neuroleptanalgesia

In recent years, a new group of drugs has been introduced that is capable of producing a sedated but rousable patient with emotional detachment or psychic indifference.[37] Such a state is produced by the combination of a so-called neuroleptic drug such as droperidol or haloperidol and a narcotic, specifically phenoperidine or fentanyl. The latter drugs are in themselves emetics; the addition of a neuroleptic drug counteracts this effect and, in addition, provides a cataleptic state, diminishes sensitivity to epinephrine and norepinephrine, and may produce undesirable extrapyramidal effects. In the United States the available preparations are Innovar (a combination of droperidol and fentanyl in a 50:1 ratio), droperidol alone, and fentanyl alone. Operations not requiring muscular relaxation may be performed using these agents alone. Circulation is said to be stable, but drug antagonists may be needed on emergence. Properly administered, neuroleptanalgesia does not interfere with the patient's ability to cooperate; hence, it has been recommended for electrocorticography and for diagnostic neurosurgical procedures. Because these drugs may either induce or remove tremor, their use during thalamotomy is questionable. Supplemental nitrous oxide, relaxants, and controlled respiration produce satisfactory anesthesia for both adult and pediatric neurosurgical procedures. Recognition that this technique usually reduces and never increases intracranial pressure has caused it to become popular for anesthetizing patients with intracranial mass lesions.

General Anesthesia

The ideal agent for general anesthesia in neurosurgery should be potent, nonirritating, nonexplosive, stable, and nontoxic; should permit rapid, smooth induction and awakening (without coughing, retching, or vomiting); should abolish laryngeal and pharyngeal reflexes at light levels of anesthesia; and should be compatible with epinephrine. It should not increase intracranial pressure or unduly depress the cardiovascular or other organ systems of the body. No agent meets all these criteria; accordingly, individual preferences generally include the combination of two or more agents in an attempt to approach the ideal. Basic to most combinations is nitrous oxide. Variation exists primarily in the selection of supplementary agents. Recommended agents have in the recent past included halothane, ethyl ether, trichloroethylene, methoxyflurane, enflurane, and various intravenously administered drugs such as hydroxydione, narcotics, thiopental, muscle relaxants, and neuroleptanalgesics.

Nitrous oxide is generally administered in a 60 to 70 per cent concentration; the resultant limitation on the inspired oxygen concentration is the primary disadvantage to its use. Relative contraindications to nitrous oxide arise during and after air encephalography and in procedures in which air embolism is a possible complication.[41] In severely depressed semicomatose patients, supplementation with other agents may not be required, particularly if ventilation is controlled. Similarly, in alert patients, nitrous oxide may be used along with large doses of muscle relaxants and controlled ventilation; this combination provides adequate analgesia and amnesia for most neurosurgical procedures, although some recommend supplementation with an opiate. Nitrous oxide has been reported to cause modest increases in intracranial pressure.[19] This effect is probably of little clinical significance and can be totally blocked by combination with barbiturates, narcotics, and hyperventilation. Those who have abandoned volatile anesthetics for intracranial procedures rely upon such combinations with nitrous oxide to prevent elevations in intracranial pressure. The combination of nitrous oxide and a relaxant also may be used for electrocorticography because it rarely interferes with the observation of significant electrical patterns.[6]

Those who still use volatile anesthetics tend to prefer either halothane or enflurane. These agents remain popular with some because they provide a number of the ideal requirements for anesthesia. They are potent and nonexplosive; they reduce pharyngeal reflexes at light levels of anesthesia; and they are characterized by a smooth, rapid induction and emergence. Objections to their use relate primarily to the potential for an increase in intracranial pressure secondary to cerebral vasodilation.[42,59] In addition, halothane has been associated with the rare occurrence of hepatic necrosis, and enflurane, at high concentrations, may cause seizure activity, particularly in combination with hypocapnia.[31] For intracranial operations the major objection relates to the possible intracranial pressure effects. Clinical studies have demonstrated that, for halothane at least, elevations in intracranial pressure can be avoided by hyperventilation (to a Pa_{CO_2} of 25 to 30 mm of mercury) prior to the initiation of halothane.[1] Presumably this would be effective with all the volatile agents. Additionally, since the cerebral vasodilating effect of the volatile anesthetics is dose related, they should only be used in the lowest concentration compatible with adequate anesthetic depth. Volatile agents are particularly useful in those circumstances in which nitrous oxide may be contraindicated (following air contrast studies or in patients in whom venous air embolism is a significant risk) and in patients in whom careful control of blood pressure is mandatory (e.g., operations for aneurysm).

Until recently methoxyflurane was considered to be a satisfactory agent for many neurosurgical procedures. It is now, however, recognized that metabolic breakdown products (fluoride primarily) are potentially nephrotoxic and that this effect is directly time-dose related.[25] Thus, methoxyflurane should only be used for relatively short operations (less than four hours) and then only at the lowest possible concentrations. Another disadvantage of its use is the prolonged emergence from the depressive effects on the central nervous system. This is a crucial consideration after intracranial procedures because the anesthetic effects cannot be differentiated from the effects of cerebral edema, infarction, or hemorrhage. Delayed recognition of such complications will postpone corrective measures, possibly beyond reversibility. Ethyl ether is objectionable because of the prolonged emergence associated with its use and the hazard of explosion. Trichloroethylene was at one time frequently selected for neurosurgery. Its incompatibility with soda lime and the occurrence of tachypnea and ventricular arrhythmias associated with its use caused most anesthesiologists to abandon it after halothane was introduced.

When first introduced, the intravenous agent ketamine was thought to be an ideal general anesthetic (so-called dissociative anesthesia) for brief neurosurgical and neurodiagnostic procedures, particularly in children. It soon was recognized, however, that ketamine is a potent cerebral vasodilator, and thus its use in any patient with potentially increased intracranial pressure should be avoided.[10]

Regardless of the primary agent selected, there are certain requirements of every general anesthetic administered for intracranial operations. Induction should be as rapid and smooth as is possible; in adults this is best accomplished with intravenously administered barbiturates such as thiopental or methohexital. Endotracheal intubation should be attempted only when laryngeal reflexes are completely abolished or when total paralysis of the skeletal muscles has been produced. Intubation should be preceded by topical application of a local anesthetic, such as 4 per cent lidocaine, to the trachea and larynx. Considerations regarding techniques of ventilation are discussed elsewhere in this chapter.

The pediatric neurosurgical patient may be anesthetized with the same agents, with some modifications, as the adult. An induction technique using rectally administered thiopental, thioamylal, or methohexital, although generally smooth, is not well suited because of possible depression of vital centers and prolongation of postoperative recovery. Routine considerations include the monitoring and maintenance of body temperature and careful attention to blood loss and replacement. Special techniques such as deliberate hypotension and hypothermia are rarely, if ever, required in children, and control of intracranial pressure (assuming the existence of adequate ventilation) is seldom a problem.

Some neurosurgeons advocate the injection of epinephrine into and around the incision to produce local hemostasis. Epinephrine is compatible with most anesthetic agents under certain conditions, notably control of dosage and adequate ventilation. It is not generally recommended for use with halothane, as instances of ventricular fibrillation have been reported. Nonetheless, epinephrine has been used by some in combination with both halothane and methoxyflurane.

SPECIAL CONSIDERATIONS

Electrocorticography and Stereotaxis

Anesthesia for electrocorticography and stereotaxic procedures may present special problems that require significant alterations in the usual anesthetic techniques. These alterations are necessitated by the potential need for an "awake" electroencephalographic pattern or a rational response from the patient during the procedure. This has been accomplished by a variety of techniques, none entirely satisfactory. The objections to local anesthesia have been discussed. These can be partly remedied by inducing general endotracheal anesthesia after completing that part of the procedure that requires an awake patient; this can be technically difficult and hazardous because of the limitations imposed by the draped open head. The opposite approach has also been used: beginning with general endotracheal anesthesia and then, when needed, arousing the patient; then completing the operation using local infiltration or reinducing general anesthesia. This is an unpredictable method, frequently associated with coughing, which necessitates either urgent extubation of the patient or the use of muscle relaxants. The former may be hazardous, and the latter can be a frightening experience for the patient. The patient may not be immediately oriented or cooperative. Many of these hazards can be avoided by using drug combinations to produce

neuroleptanalgesia. This, when combined with local anesthesia, is possibly the most satisfactory method. Electrocorticography can also be satisfactorily accomplished in most patients under endotracheal nitrous oxide anesthesia combined with muscle relaxants and moderate hyperventilation. Nitrous oxide rarely interferes with significant electrical patterns; if necessary, it may be discontinued for periods of 10 to 15 minutes, during which time "awake" electroencephalographic patterns can be recorded without risk of subsequent patient recall of the event.

Posterior Fossa Procedures

The management of patients undergoing exploration of the posterior fossa may at times present unusual problems. If the patient is placed in the sitting position, the potential hazards of postural hypotension and air embolism are introduced in exchange for the advantages of improved operative exposure, reduced bleeding, and accessibility of the patient's airway. Both the incidence and severity of complications secondary to the sitting position can be minimized by appropriate prophylaxis; these are discussed in a later section of this chapter.

Proper monitoring of these patients is particularly important because of the need to recognize surgical proximity to the vital centers of the brain stem. Traditionally, the respiratory rate and rhythm of the patient have been carefully observed as a means of detecting untoward stimulation of the brain stem. With most types of general anesthesia, however, spontaneous respiration inevitably leads to carbon dioxide accumulation secondary to the depressive effects of anesthetics; this in turn may be associated with arterial and intracranial hypertension, cardiac arrhythmias, and increased bleeding. For these reasons, mechanical passive hyperventilation of the patient may be preferable. This technique necessitates the monitoring of cardiac rate and rhythm, which is best accomplished by oscilloscopic display of the electrocardiogram. Those experienced in electrocardiogram interpretation have found this to be an extremely sensitive means of detecting brain stem stimulation. In most instances, the arrhythmias produced by brain stem manipulation are immediately corrected by operative retreat. Antiarrhythmic drugs should generally be avoided since they may block subsequent recognition of brain stem stimulation. In a series of over 1400 posterior fossa explorations performed at the Mayo Clinic, the monitoring of cardiac rather than respiratory rate and rhythm has not been misleading.

Diagnostic Procedures

Neurodiagnostic procedures that may require the attendance of an anesthesiologist include cerebral angiography, pneumoencephalography, ventriculography, myelography, and computer tomography. The type of anesthesia indicated for these procedures is frequently debated; however, there are certain areas of broad agreement. For computer tomography, anesthesia is required only in the patient who is unable to remain physically quiet during the procedure. In this circumstance intravenous sedation alone may be adequate, but in a few patients general endotracheal anesthesia will be required. For the remaining diagnostic procedures, either general or local anesthesia may be used. In children and uncooperative adults, general anesthesia is the method of choice, and the requirements are, with few exceptions, identical to those discussed for neurosurgical procedures. For cooperative adults, the choice of anesthesia is probably not a critical consideration. All the standard neuroradiological procedures can be done with local anesthesia and appropriate sedation. An apparent advantage of local anesthesia is that it permits monitoring of the patient's level of consciousness, evaluation of his response to the examination, and the option to terminate a procedure before irreparable damage has occurred. Proponents of general anesthesia, particularly as regards cerebral angiography, believe that inhalational agents will protect the patient from possible untoward reactions.[17,50] Regardless of the technique selected, the patient should be monitored continuously by personnel trained in the disciplines of anesthesia, and if local anesthesia is used, all the standard equipment and drugs necessary for endotracheal intubation and the induction and maintenance of general anesthesia must be immediately available.

When general anesthesia is required either during or following air encephalography, it is important to avoid the use of nitrous oxide.[41] This is so because the solubility of nitrous oxide in blood is 30 times that of nitrogen, and it will, therefore, rapidly equilibrate with the intraventricular air space long before the nitrogen is eliminated. As a result, the intraventricular gas volume will tend to expand, producing a significant increase in intracranial pressure. This effect can be turned to advantage by using nitrous oxide as the exchange gas and maintaining nitrous oxide anesthesia throughout the examination.[14] Under these circumstances, stopping the anesthetic will be accompanied by a rapid decrease in the intraventricular gas volume.

SPECIAL ANESTHETIC TECHNIQUES

Hyperventilation

Passive hyperventilation combined with adequate oxygenation is considered by many anesthesiologists to be an effective means of producing a "relaxed" or "slack" brain. Evaluation of this effect in the anesthetized patient is a complex problem. There seems to be confusion about the definition of "controlled ventilation" and "hyperventilation." Controlled ventilation implies only control of rate and volume of ventilation. Not included in the definition is whether it is performed manually or by a mechanical ventilator, with or without muscle relaxants, with or without a negative expiratory phase, and whether the subject is anesthetized or conscious. Controlled ventilation can result, therefore, in hyperventilation, normoventilation, or hypoventilation. Hyperventilation implies an increased alveolar ventilation in relation to metabolic rate such that, under normal circumstances, an arterial P_{CO_2} of less than 40 mm of mercury is produced.

Conflicting reports concerning the effect of hyperventilation on intracranial pressure exist in the literature. Hyperventilation has been reported to reduce ventricular fluid pressure in man and in dogs.[18,54] The decrease may be relatively large when the initial ventricular fluid pressure or the initial arterial carbon dioxide tension is high. With increasing minute volumes, however, progressively lesser effects and even an increase in the pressure may be observed. At a constant level of hyperventilation, a gradual increase in ventricular fluid pressure with time has been reported, and a transient rise above baseline levels has been observed at the end of hyperventilation.[24,54] This has been attributed to an adaptation of the cerebral vasomotor system to the Pa_{CO_2}.

Hyperventilation may fail to produce the expected decrease in ventricular fluid pressure during arterial hypotension, possibly because the cerebral vessels lose their ability to react to changes in Pa_{CO_2}. In patients with reduced brain volume, e.g., in hydrocephalus, lesser changes in pressure may be expected. Poor synchronization with the respirator and inadequate muscle relaxation may result in increased ventricular fluid pressure. The adverse intracranial effects of coughing or straining or sustained elevation of Pa_{CO_2} may persist despite elimination of the causative factor and subsequent hyperventilation.[16]

A redistribution between blood and cerebrospinal fluid volumes with no net loss of fluid from the cranium has been demonstrated in anesthetized hyperventilated dogs by Rosomoff.[39] He found little or no change in cerebrospinal fluid pressure during hyperventilation when pH and Pa_{CO_2} were normal prior to the onset of hyperventilation. He believes that reduction of intracranial tension may be seen if hypercapnia rather than eucapnia is the starting point. Symbas and associates reported that the cerebrospinal fluid pressure in dogs remained unchanged or decreased when the dogs were ventilated with pressures of less than 20 cm of water and with a tidal volume less than 400 ml.[49]

Some authors report a beneficial effect from a negative expiratory phase; others see little or no change. This difference of opinion may be explained at least partially by the findings of Werkö, who observed that the relation of mask pressure to pleural pressure varied considerably in three patients he studied.[57] It is difficult to predict changes in pleural pressure from changes in endotracheal pressure without knowledge of pulmonary resistance (airway plus pulmonary tissue resistance), pulmonary compliance, and respiratory effort.

Potential harmful effects of hyperventilation are cerebral vasoconstriction with possible cerebral hypoxia, tetany, shift of the hemoglobin dissociation curve to the left (Bohr effect), decrease in cardiac output, increase in whole-body oxygen consumption, increase in fixed acids, and decrease in arterial oxygen tension. Some of these effects warrant further comment.

An abrupt decrease in Pa_{CO_2} results in an exponential decrease in P_{CO_2} of tissue and cerebrospinal fluid and a concomitant decrease in hydrogen ion in the cerebrospinal fluid. After a few hours of hyperventilation, a "normal" pH results from a decrease in bicarbonate ion of the cerebrospinal fluid that is proportional to the lowered P_{CO_2}. If hyperventilation ceases, the Pa_{CO_2} will rise initially, to be followed a few minutes later by the P_{CO_2} of the cerebrospinal fluid. The bicarbonate ion in the cerebrospinal fluid remains low, however. This produces an acidotic cerebrospinal fluid and stimulation of the central chemoreceptors; thus, a transient period of active hyperventilation may be observed despite normal chemical composition of the blood. It was recently suggested that the obligatory hypoventilation eventually necessary, after hyperventilation, to restore depleted supplies of body carbon dioxide, can last as long as an hour and may result in arterial hypoxia.[47]

Reported biochemical changes in the blood associated with hyperventilation vary and include a decrease in standard bicarbonate, a progressive decrease of buffer base and an increase of lactic acid, a decrease of bicarbonate with unchanged buffer base and only slightly elevated lactic acid levels, and a bicarbonate deficit with a rise in lactic and pyruvic acids. Recently, striking increases in brain and cerebrospinal fluid lactate, independent of blood levels, were found in anesthetized dogs hyperventilated for six hours.[34]

The reported effects of hyperventilation on cerebral function are inconsistent. Clutton-Brock found, in conscious volunteers, increased pain thresholds with active hyperventilation; he suggested that cerebral hypoxia may be produced by hyperventilation.[8] Robinson and Gray found similar responses in passively hyperventilated, conscious subjects, although increases of pH above 7.55 did not further raise the pain threshold.[38] Retinoscopy showed constricted retinal vessels. Contrary to the findings of Clutton-Brock, these authors did not find any change in pain response when they hyperventilated their patients with oxygen; they did not believe that the cerebral effects of passive hyperventilation were due to hypoxia. Barach and associates concluded that all degrees of hyperventilation at normal atmospheric pressure were detrimental to cerebral function.[5] Allen and Morris found a depression of the critical flicker-fusion test in 17 of 21 hyperventilated patients and concluded that hyperventilation in a patient under anesthesia can cause demonstrable cerebral malfunction, which is, however, minor in degree and duration.[3] Whitwam and associates, however, were unable to demonstrate any deterioration in cerebral function after passive hyperventilation in five volunteers, as measured by the critical flicker-fusion test.[58] Alteration of the blood-brain barrier after hyperventilation was recently described in cats, when Pa_{CO_2} was maintained below 20 mm of mercury for five hours. Cohen and associates were unable to demonstrate biochemical evidence for cerebral hypoxia during halothane anesthesia at a Pa_{CO_2} of 25 mm of mercury.[9] Alexander and co-workers observed, during nitrous oxide anesthesia with Pa_{CO_2} levels below 20 mm of mercury, an insignificant decrease in aerobic utilization of glucose accompanied by mild, readily reversible electroencephalographic changes consistent with mild hypoxia.[2] These authors concluded that only minimal hyperventilation should be used in patients with arterial hypotension or central nervous system disease, in the patient of advanced age, or in the febrile patient whose cerebral metabolic rate is increased. Sugioka and Davis found decreased cerebral oxygen tension in dogs during hyperventilation with room air, and an increase in cerebral oxygen tension when 5 per cent carbon dioxide was added to the inspired gas mixture.[46] These authors believed that cerebral hypoxia was produced by cerebral vasoconstriction caused by hypocapnia. The validity of their methods has been questioned.

Apparently, no generalizations regarding the consequences of passive hyperventilation can be made. Variability in the observed effects relates to the degree of hypocapnia, the duration of hyperventilation, the presence or absence of muscle relaxants, the presence or absence of a negative expiratory phase, the position of the patient, his condition, the nature of the operative procedure, and the interrelationship of respiratory rate, tidal volume, and airway pressure. On the basis of extensive clinical experience involving the use of passive hyperventilation, however, it is reasonable to conclude that this technique is hazardous only when used at the extremes of the previously mentioned variables. Its use in neurosurgery has virtually abolished the previously common complications related to inadequate ventilation and hypercapnia. It is likely that continuing investigations ultimately will resolve most of the existing controversies.

Deliberate Hypotension

The indications for induced hypotension in neurosurgery are not clearly defined. There is near general agreement regarding its value in operations for aneurysm; other indications may include highly vascular lesions such as meningiomas, hemangioendotheliomas, and arteriovenous anomalies. Its application for the sole purpose of reducing brain bulk has been condemned; such an effect has never been substantiated and, if it does occur, probably results from a reduction in cerebral blood flow only. The primary objections to hypotension in neurosurgery result from the uncertainties regarding the adequacy of cerebral blood flow, and the possible complications of "retractor anemia" or reactionary hemorrhage.

The effect of hypotension on cerebral blood flow is an important consideration. In normotensive supine persons a reduction in the mean arterial pressure to 60 mm of mercury is well tolerated. At pressures below this level, the variation in opinion and experience and results suggests, in at least some patients, ischemic damage may occur. The work reported by Eckenhoff and associates is an outstanding exception to this generalization.[12] In this study, use of a 24-degree head-up tilt and ganglionic blockade lowered the systolic pressure to 70 mm of mercury in 23 patients and to 50 mm of mercury in 6 patients; these pressures were maintained for average periods of 42 and 39 minutes, respectively. Oxygen tension of jugular blood was used as an index of cerebral blood flow, and in no patient did the Po$_2$ decrease below a level of 27 mm of mercury, well above the presumed critical level of 15 to 20 mm of mercury. Rosomoff has cautioned against a direct application of this work to neurosurgery, since these patients were not studied during craniotomy.[40] Furthermore, the demonstration of an "adequate" jugular blood oxygen tension does not guarantee that regional cerebral blood flow is adequate. The potential untoward effects of hypotension on the heart, kidneys, and liver are well known and need not be reviewed here.[21]

Techniques recommended for the induction and maintenance of hypotension for neurosurgery vary; familiarity with the method selected is probably the most important consideration. Prior to the time that sodium nitroprusside was made commercially available in 1974, most anesthesiologists preferred either ganglion-blocking agents or deep anesthesia with halothane, supplemented by positive-pressure ventilation and varying degrees of head-up tilt. Although both these techniques are associated with a decrease in cardiac output, there is some evidence that ganglionic blockade produces a less significant decrease and may, therefore, be preferred to deep anesthesia with halothane as the primary method. Of the several ganglion-blocking agents available, the most commonly used are hexamethonium (100 to 300 mg), pentolinium (3 to 20 mg), or trimethaphan given as 0.1 to 0.2 per cent solution by intravenous drip. Trimethaphan offers a distinct advantage because the rapid onset and brief duration of action permit momentary control in accordance with operative requirements. Disadvantages associated with its use include the common occurrence of tachyphylaxis and an unpredictable degree of sensitivity to vasopressors. If vasopressors are administered, subsequent induction of hypotension with trimethaphan is often difficult or impossible. The theoretical disadvantage of histamine release with this drug has not been demonstrated to provide a significant contraindication to its use in man.

Since 1974 sodium nitroprusside has rapidly gained in popularity as the agent of choice for inducing hypotension.[53] This drug is a direct vasodilator that is potent, evanescent in action, and rarely associated with either resistance or tachyphylaxis. Several studies have demonstrated either no change or an increase in both cardiac output and cerebral blood flow during modest levels of hypotension induced by sodium nitroprusside. Reversal of hypotension is rapid upon discontinuation of the drug, and a vasopressor is rarely required. Several deaths have been reported following administration of large doses of sodium nitroprusside and have been attributed to cyanide toxicity. Animal studies have clearly demonstrated that cyanide release from the nitroprusside molecule does occur and that at doses exceeding 1.5 mg per kilogram (administered rapidly during a one- to three-hour period) intoxication is manifested. Clinical experience indicates that such a dose is rarely required, and at doses less than 1.0 mg per kilogram intoxication does not occur.

Supplementation of drug-induced hypotension by increasing the mean airway pressure has been recommended by Enderby as a method of maintaining a stable level of hypotension.[15] The resultant increase in central venous pressure with this technique may be undesirable in neurosurgery, depending primarily on the degree of head-up tilt. The latter not only is an important consideration in providing adequate venous drainage but also is an obvious means of reducing intracranial arterial blood pressure. The proper degree of head-up tilt can be determined only in relation to the arterial pressure as measured in the arm, since for every inch of elevation of the head above the heart (assuming the arm cuff to be level with the heart), a decrease of 2 mm of mercury in intracranial arterial pressure occurs. Thus, the arbitrary placement of limits on the "safe" degree of head-up tilt has little significance; rather, this limit varies directly with the arterial pressure. It is equally apparent that for intracranial operations the judicious use of head-up tilt is an important supplement to induced hypotension, regardless of the primary method selected.

For most neurosurgical procedures, the duration of hypotension required is brief; hence, the selection of long-acting agents or methods that do not permit rapid reversal should be avoided. For the same reason, the combination of hypothermia with hypotension is rarely desirable. This method has been recommended as a theoretical means of reducing the possibility of ischemic damage to vital organs secondary to hypotension; that it does so has not been proved clinically. The combination converts a brief, relatively simple procedure into a prolonged, complicated one and probably introduces as many hazards as it is intended to overcome. Exceptions are the techniques described by Brown and Horton and Small and Stephenson, in which hypotension is produced intermittently by rapid intracardiac pacing of the heart, resulting in virtual arrest of the circulation; in these procedures, hypothermia is essential to provide sufficient time for surgical correction of an aneurysm.[7,43]

There can be no absolute contraindications to induced hypotension in neurosurgery, since at any time it may provide the only chance for a successful operative outcome. As an elective procedure, it should be restricted to patients without significant systemic disease. Its use in patients with increased intracranial pressure should be avoided until the dura has been incised and the brain decompressed. After the definitive operative procedure, the pressure must be returned to normal before the dura is closed and the operative field is lost to view. If ganglion-blocking agents are used the possibility of postoperative cycloplegia should be anticipated and not mistaken for evidence of an intracranial disaster.

Hypothermia

Hypothermia has been a controversial technique since first introduced in 1940 by Smith and Fay.[45] In neurosurgery the method enjoyed periods of great enthusiasm: in 1955, after the initial use of moderate hypothermia in the operative repair of aneurysms;[23] in 1957, after experimental evidence indicated its efficacy in the treatment of cerebral infarction and injury; and in 1960, after profound levels of hypothermia and circulatory arrest were utilized in the repair of aneurysms. In each instance, initial interest has been followed by disenchantment because of disappointing results and unexpected complications. The current status of hypothermia is difficult to evaluate, but a continuing interest in techniques that permit selective profound cooling of the brain or safe periods of circulatory arrest during moderate hypothermia suggests that a new wave of enthusiasm may be gathering.

Despite this continuing controversy, the therapeutic basis of hypothermia is well established. A reduction in body temperature is accompanied by a significant, predictable reduction in oxygen requirements of the whole body including the brain. Thus, if the brain can safely withstand 4 minutes without perfusion at 38° C, this period will be approximately doubled at 30° C, quadrupled at 22° C, and at 16° C more than 30 minutes of continuous circulatory arrest is tolerated. The promise of a bloodless operative field for the intricate repair of intracranial vascular lesions assures a continuing interest in hypothermic techniques.

Studies concerned with the systemic effects of induced hypothermia have not uncovered any significant deleterious effects within well-defined limits. Above 28° C, and in the absence of shivering, cardiac output is maintained in relation to oxygen requirements, and cardiac arrhythmias, although frequent, are rarely serious problems. Below 28° C, progressive impairment of myocardial function and increasing myocardial irritability necessitate support of the circulation by extracorporeal techniques. This significant alteration in technical requirements provides a convenient point for the separation of moderate and profound hypothermic techniques.

Acid-base alterations relate primarily to the temperature achieved rather than the technique used. Confusion on this subject results from an inability to define normal values at an abnormal temperature. A decrease in temperature is accompanied by an increase in solubility of carbon dioxide, an increase in carbon dioxide combining power, a decrease in buffer capacity, and an increase in pK. Correction factors are available for these changes, but interpretation of the resulting values is controversial. Significant alterations in the metabolic component of the acid-base profile have not been found in the immediate posthypothermia period so long as shivering, inadequate tissue perfusion, or prolonged periods of circulatory arrest were avoided. Apparent progressive respiratory alkalosis will accompany cooling if normothermic levels of ventilation are maintained. There is, however, evidence in poikilotherms that this is appropriate and normal at temperatures below 37° C.[36] The combined effect of decreasing temperature and increasing pH on the binding of oxygen by hemoglobin (leftward shift of the dissociation curve) has been considered a possible cause of tissue hypoxia. This is, in part, counteracted by the increased solubility of oxygen; nonetheless, some investigators have recommended either the addition of carbon dioxide to the inspired gases or the intravenous infusion of dilute solutions of hydrochloric acid during hypothermia.

Function of the kidneys, liver, and endocrine system is depressed during hypothermia but returns to normal within 24 hours after rewarming.[56] Disturbances of blood coagulation have been encountered after profound hypothermia.[55] This appears to be a multifaceted problem that may result from inadequate doses of heparin during cooling, inadequate reversal of heparin after cooling, release of fibrinolysins, or the destruction of platelets and other clotting factors secondary to either mechanical trauma or extreme temperatures.

Shivering, easily recognized on the electrocardiogram by the characteristic disturbance of the baseline, is common during cooling and rewarming. It must be corrected, either by increasing the depth of anesthesia or by administering muscle relaxants. The potential deleterious effects of shivering result from an increase of 50 to 200 per cent in oxygen requirements that may not be accompanied by an appropriate increase in cardiac output. In this situation, a vicious circle of increasing anaerobic metabolism, progressive metabolic acidosis, and further cardiac depression may result. If shivering occurs during cooling, the decrease in temperature may be halted or reversed. The practice of permitting a patient to rewarm by allowing him to shiver is potentially hazardous and may account for the syndrome of "rewarming shock."

The anesthetic requirements for hypothermia in neurosurgery are not importantly different from those already discussed for intracranial procedures. Premedication with the so-called lytic cocktail, consisting of large doses of promethazine, chlorpromazine, and meperidine, is not necessary and probably should be avoided because of the risk of severe respiratory and cardiovascular depression. Light premedication, induction with a short-acting barbiturate, and maintenance with inhalation agents will minimize the potential problem of delayed destruction and excretion of depressant drugs secondary to cooling of the liver and kidneys. Since cold itself is an anesthetic, the maintenance concentration of the selected agent can be diminished when the patient's temperature is below 30° to 32° C; below 18° to 22° C, probably no anesthetic is required. Monitoring of the patient ideally should include the use of the electrocardiogram, multiple temperature probes, and measurement of direct arterial pressure and central venous pressure. The temperatures monitored should, at a minimum, include the nasopharyngeal temperature (as an index of brain temperature) and the esophageal temperature (as an index of heart temperature).

Techniques for cooling differ. Moderate levels of hypothermia (28° to 30° C) are almost always accomplished by surface cooling methods, generally with blankets that permit the circulation of a cooling liquid, or by direct immersion in an ice bath. The latter, although more rapid, is less controllable and is associated with a significant downward drift in temperature because of the large surface-to-core gradients created. The production of profound whole-body levels of hypothermia requires an extracorporeal circuit and the open-chest technique of Drew and Anderson or, as is more common, the closed-chest technique, as described by Patterson and Ray and by Michenfelder and associates.[11, 27, 32] With these methods, large temperature gradients opposite to those encountered with surface cooling are commonly observed. For this reason, after induction of profound hypothermia an upward drift of core temperature is to be expected during the period of circulatory arrest. Selective cooling of the brain to profound levels of hypothermia is also possible and requires an extracorporeal system similar to that described by Kristiansen and co-workers.[20]

The primary indication for hypothermia in neurosurgery is for those procedures in which temporary cessation or significant reduction in part or all of the cerebral blood flow is contemplated. The level of hypothermia produced should be determined by the anticipated duration of reduced or absent blood flow required by the surgeon for repair of the lesion. This is, admittedly, a restricted indication and applies primarily, if not exclusively, to intracranial vascular lesions. Its use as a means of protecting the brain during the removal of large cerebral tumors, craniopharyngiomas, and tumors close to the vital centers is of questionable validity. Although a reduction in brain bulk occurs with hypothermia, hypothermia should not be used for this purpose alone, since simpler and safer techniques are available. Even its use in the repair of aneurysms has been questioned because of a failure to demonstrate an associated decrease in morbidity and mortality.

Monitoring

The success or failure of a number of the techniques and procedures previously discussed depends, in part, upon adequate monitoring of the patient. Standard monitoring techniques are not always satisfactory: Indirect measurement of blood pressure may be misleading, particularly during induced hypotension or hypothermia; palpation of the radial pulse or auscultation of the heart sounds will not always reveal cardiac arrhythmias or permit accurate diagnosis; and respiratory rate and rhythm provide only modest information about the adequacy of alveolar ventilation. These deficiencies have particular significance in neurosurgery because of the frequent application of special techniques, the common occurrence of alterations in cardiac rate and rhythm, and the continuous necessity to provide adequate alveolar ventilation.

Although the authors recommend electrocardiographic monitoring in all neurosurgical procedures, it is particularly useful for the immediate recognition of cardiac arrhythmias secondary to intracranial manipulation. This occurs most commonly and with greatest significance in operations in the posterior fossa, because of pressure, distortion, or traction on the brain stem and cranial nerves. Other procedures or complications frequently associated with cardiac arrhythmias include orbital decompression, carotid ligation, sudden intracranial decompression, trigeminal nerve operations, tonsillar herniation, and air embolism. Stimu-

lation of the trigeminal nerve is a common cause of ventricular arrhythmias and is always associated with hypertension, perhaps a response to painful stimulation under light anesthesia rather than true reflex arrhythmia. Monitoring the electrocardiogram is also invaluable during induced hypothermia (for the recognition of both arrhythmias and shivering), induced hypotension, procedures associated with massive transfusion, and the localization of right atrial catheters or ventriculoatrial shunts.

The importance of adequate and proper ventilation in neurosurgery has been emphasized. The use of a mechanical ventilator provides an indirect but useful means of monitoring certain aspects of ventilation, including pressures, volume, and rate. A simple accurate means for continuous monitoring of Pa_{CO_2} would provide the ideal monitor. Detection of end-expired carbon dioxide with an infrared analyzer is useful for this purpose and may also aid in the recognition of venous air embolism (which causes an abrupt decrease in expired carbon dioxide). Direct measurement of Pa_{CO_2} is not always practical but is the most reliable method for evaluating adequacy of ventilation.

Direct, continuous monitoring of arterial pressure is indicated primarily in procedures requiring induced hypothermia or hypotension. This need not require elaborate equipment, and, as experience is gained, the indications may be expanded to include procedures in the posterior fossa and those associated with significant loss of blood. As in other operative procedures, knowledge of central venous pressure is of value in determining proper fluid and blood replacement. For this purpose, right atrial catheterization offers the additional option of monitoring central venous oxygen levels and, in the event of air embolism, will permit the aspiration of intracardiac air. Additional useful monitoring devices include the esophageal stethoscope and esophageal or rectal thermistors; the monitoring of temperature is particularly valuable in children and, of course, during induced hypothermia. Interest in the electroencephalogram as a clinical monitoring device has waxed and waned.[60] It is particularly useful in evaluating adequacy of cerebral circulation during carotid endarterectomy.

Interest has faded in monitoring the oxygen levels of jugular bulb blood as an index of cerebral blood flow. The validity of the method is based upon a number of assumptions, the most important of which are that the cerebral metabolic rate is steady, that there is no significant contamination by extracerebral blood, and that the sample is representative of "mixed" cerebral venous blood. The last of these is known to be false and may cause erroneous interpretations. Normally, two thirds of the blood collected by an internal jugular vein is from the ipsilateral hemisphere, hence complete mixing does not occur, and a single jugular sample may fail to reflect significant changes in flow occurring in the contralateral hemisphere. Of greater concern is the failure of oxygen levels of the jugular blood to reflect absence or diminution of flow to a part of the brain; in this event, if total flow remains unchanged, venous oxygen levels may actually increase because of a reduction in the amount of brain tissue that consumes oxygen. These sources of misinterpretation have been emphasized by Larson and co-workers; in their patients undergoing carotid endarterectomy, the measurement of oxygen levels of the jugular bulb was of little or no value.[22] Similarly, the detection of localized changes in cerebral blood flow during intracranial operations could not be accomplished by the monitoring of oxygen levels of jugular blood.

POSITION

Patients undergoing neurosurgical operations frequently must be placed in positions that may interfere with circulation and respiration. Respiratory mechanics may be altered by changes in the pulmonary blood volume, by interference with the movements of the thoracic wall and diaphragm, or by changes in lung volume. The distribution of pulmonary blood and of inspired gases may change with the posture of the anesthetized and ventilated patient; however, most of these changes can probably be adequately compensated for by judicious use of artificial ventilation. Usually, the normal anesthetized patient can compensate for the effects on the systemic circulation. Individuals with low cardiac reserve or inadequate nervous control of the peripheral circulation frequently cannot make appropriate adjustments. Immediate and sometimes dramatic effects, such as severe arterial hypotension, can result if the compensatory mechanisms fail, particularly during the positioning of the anesthetized patient. Adequate blood volume, occasional administration of vasopressors, and gradual rather than abrupt changes of body position allow the use, in most instances, of the position optimal for the operative procedure.

Improper positioning may result in injury to peripheral nerves (brachial plexus, common peroneal nerve, saphenous nerve, and so forth). Ocular complications such as retinal artery thrombosis may result from pressure over the eyeballs, particularly in conjunction with arterial hypotension. Closure of the eyelids after application of eye ointment usually will prevent corneal abrasions. Patients with systemic arteriosclerosis must be positioned with particular care to avoid arterial occlusion from pressure on diseased vessels.

For craniotomies done with the patient supine, a 10- to 15-degree elevation of the head will facilitate cerebral venous drainage. Venous pooling in the lower extremities can be minimized by correct wrapping of the legs with elastic bandages, applied while the patient is in the supine or slightly head-down position, before induction of anesthesia. No untoward alterations in circulatory or pulmonary function have been associated with the supine position.

The lateral position is likewise fairly benign as regards cardiopulmonary function. Hemodynamic studies in anesthetized (halothane) man in the right lateral position have shown a decrease in mean arterial pressure and systemic resistance, but an unchanged cardiac index.[13] Support of the pelvis and shoulder is necessary with this position and can be accomplished by means of sandbags and pillows. Excessive flexion of the head should be avoided so that cerebral venous drainage is not obstructed. The patient's head should be slightly elevated.

The prone position may compromise normal cardiopulmonary function. The flat prone position interferes with respiratory mechanics and possibly predisposes to atelectasis. It is particularly dangerous for the spontaneously breathing emphysematous patient who is primarily a diaphragmatic breather. Posner and co-workers found a decrease in total compliance of the chest in patients who were anesthetized, paralyzed, ventilated with a constant volume, and then turned from the supine to the prone position.[35] Abdominal compression may occur and result in obstruction of the inferior vena cava, which can cause arterial hypotension and excessive epidural bleeding. Various pads and devices have been described for support of the iliac crest and chest. Proper support of the iliac crest and the chest lessens the embarrassment to circulatory and respiratory function. Only the markedly obese patient presents an added risk.

The sitting position is preferred by many neurosurgeons for operations in the posterior fossa, middle fossa, and cervical spine because of improved venous drainage and better exposure. A variety of methods are available to hold the anesthetized patient in the sitting position. The legs should be wrapped with elastic bandages and placed at the level of the heart to facilitate venous return from the lower extremities. The patient should be put into the sitting position slowly, and the blood pressure measured frequently. With this precaution, arterial hypotension is rarely a problem. With the sitting position, however, even short periods of hypotension may result in cerebral hypoxia. The effect of the sitting position on internal carotid artery flow and pressure was recently determined in nine anesthetized and hyperventilated (Pa_{CO_2}, 22.5 mm of mercury) subjects.[52] Anesthesia (nitrous oxide and halothane) and hyperventilation alone resulted in an average decrease of 34 per cent in the internal carotid blood flow. The sitting position resulted in an additional reduction of 18 per cent. In healthy, unmedicated subjects, the change from the supine to the sitting position resulted in a decrease of 21 per cent in stroke volume and 10 per cent in cardiac index. An increase of 18 per cent in heart rate partially compensated for the decreased stroke volume.

Perhaps the greatest hazard associated with the sitting position is the potential for venous air embolism. This occurs most frequently in posterior fossa operations because of the greater likelihood of opening a noncollapsible venous channel (diploic veins and dural sinuses), which, in the presence of a negative venous pressure, may aspirate air. Prior to the introduction of ultrasonic (Doppler) devices for monitoring air embolism, the incidence of this complication in 751 posterior fossa explorations was reported to be 4.1 per cent, whereas in over 1200 cervical laminectomies and middle fossa explorations, only one episode of air embolism was recognized.[28] As recorded with a Doppler monitor, the true incidence of air embolism in all procedures performed in the sitting position approximates 25 per cent.[29] Obviously, the majority of these episodes are of no clinical significance.

Morbidity and death due to venous air embolism can be minimized by appropriate prophylactic measures, early diagnosis, and vigorous treatment. Useful prophylactic measures include proper positioning of the patient, wrapping of the legs with elastic bandages or the application of a "G" suit, maintenance of adequate blood volume, positive-pressure ventilation, intermittent compression of the internal jugular veins, frequent flushing of the operative wound with saline, and liberal application of bone wax. When, despite these measures, air embolism occurs, the presence of a right atrial catheter is useful both for early confirmation of the diagnosis and for treatment. The diagnosis should be first suspected when any sudden changes occur in the normal Doppler heart sounds. Later clinical signs include the development of a cardiac murmur; small volumes of air impart a tympanitic quality to the heart sounds, and with increasing volumes a coarse systolic murmur becomes evident. The classic "mill-wheel" murmur is not a consistent diagnostic sign and, when present, usually indicates a large volume of intracardiac air. Less consistent diagnostic signs associated with air embolism include arrhythmias (usually ventricular), hypotension, increased central venous pressure, cyanosis, and tachypnea. With a right atrial catheter, immediate and certain confirmation of a suspected diagnosis of venous air embolism can be achieved by aspirating air from the right atrium.

Treatment of air embolism should be directed at preventing further entry of air and dispersing or removing the intracardiac air. Prevention may be accomplished by a variety of measures designed to increase venous pressure in the operative wound, thus permitting identification and occlusion of the open venous channel. These measures include compression of the internal jugular veins, continuous positive-pressure ventilation, and lowering the patient's head. If a right atrial catheter is present, continuous aspiration will remove a portion of the intracardiac air; the remainder must ultimately be ejected into the pulmonary circulation. The administration of a vasopressor that has a positive inotropic action will aid the heart in ejecting the air as well as improve the perfusion pressure. If these measures are effectively implemented, the catastrophic events usually associated with air embolism can be avoided.

ANESTHETICS, CEREBRAL METABOLISM, AND BLOOD FLOW

There is no invariable response of either cerebral blood flow or metabolism to anesthesia; rather, a different response is associated with each agent and, in the frequent clinical circumstance of multiple anesthetic agents, the end-result may be unknown. Cerebral metabolism may be unchanged, depressed, or stimulated by anesthetic drugs. The most common response is metabolic depression and the most potent depressant drugs known are the barbiturates. Thiopental, in man, may reduce cerebral oxygen consumption as much as 55 per cent; however, the degree of metabolic (as well as functional) depression may be significantly reduced by the method of drug administration, because of the phenomenon of acute tolerance.[33] The volatile anesthetic agents such as halothane and ether have generally been reported to reduce cerebral oxygen consumption 10 to 20 per cent. When concentrations of these agents increase, further metabolic depression is slight, and in the case of ether and cyclopropane, a return to normal oxygen consumption has been observed at high concentrations. Nitrous oxide is an exceptional agent and has been found to increase cerebral oxygen consumption.[51] Other researchers have found either no change or minimal depression. Anesthetic agents other than the barbiturates cannot provide significant protection of the brain against hypoxic stress. Numerous animal studies have consistently shown that large doses of barbiturates do provide a degree of protection in models of both focal and global ischemia.[30,44] Clinical application of this possibly beneficial effect is controversial. Its potential applications include head trauma, acute stroke, and operative procedures during which a transient reduction in cerebral blood flow occurs (e.g., carotid endarterectomy).

The effect of anesthetic agents on cerebral circulation has not been as well documented as the metabolic effects, owing to the concomitant effects on cerebral vascular resistance produced by changes in perfusion pressure, arterial blood carbon dioxide tension, and metabolic rate. The barbiturates tend to reduce cerebral blood flow in relation to the reduced cerebral metabolic rate. The volatile agents in general decrease cerebral vascular resistance. Halothane, because of this, has been condemned by some for use in intracranial procedures. This objection is valid in the presence of spontaneous ventilation and a normal or elevated Pa_{CO_2}. Since anesthesia does not significantly alter the normal cerebral vascular response to carbon dioxide, the effects of halothane (and other agents) are countered by a moderate degree of hyperventilation.

Portions of this chapter are reproduced with permission from Anesthesiology, Vol. 30.

REFERENCES

1. Adams, R. W., Gronert, G. A., Sundt, T. M., Jr., and Michenfelder, J. D.: Halothane, hypocapnia, and cerebrospinal fluid pressure in neurosurgery. Anesthesiology 37:510–517, 1972.
2. Alexander, S. C., Cohen, P. J., Wollman, H., Smith, T. C., Reivich, M., and Vander Molen, R. A.: Cerebral carbohydrate metabolism during hypocarbia in man: Studies during nitrous oxide anesthesia. Anesthesiology, 26:624–632, 1965.
3. Allen, G. D., and Morris, L. E.: Central nervous system effects of hyperventilation during anaesthesia. Brit. J. Anaesth., 34:296–304, 1962.
4. Baker, G. S.: Physiologic abnormalities encountered after removal of brain tumors from the floor of the fourth ventricle. J. Neurosurg., 23:338–343, 1965.
5. Barach, A. L., Fenn, W. O., Ferris, E. B., and Schmidt, C. F.: The physiology of pressure breathing: A brief review of its present status. J. Aviat. Med., 18:73–87, 1947.
6. Bozza Marrubini, M.: General anaesthesia for in-

tracranial surgery. Brit. J. Anaesth., *37*:268–287, 1965.

7. Brown, A. S., and Horton, J. M.: Elective hypotension with intracardiac pacemaking in the operative management of ruptured intracranial aneurysms. Acta Anaesth. Scand., suppl. 23, pp. 665–670, 1966.

8. Clutton-Brock, J.: The cerebral effects of overventilation (preliminary communication). Brit. J. Anaesth., *29*:111–113, 1957.

9. Cohen, P. J., Wollman, H., Alexander, S. C., Chase, P. E., and Behar, M. G.: Cerebral carbohydrate metabolism in man during halothane anesthesia: Effects of Pa_{CO_2} on some aspects of carbohydrate utilization. Anesthesiology, *25*:185–191, 1964.

10. Dawson, B., Michenfelder, J. D., and Theye, R. A.: Effects of ketamine on canine cerebral blood flow and metabolism: Modification by prior administration of thiopental. Anesth. Analg., *50*:443–447, 1971.

11. Drew, C. E., and Anderson, I. M.: Profound hypothermia in cardiac surgery: Report of three cases. Lancet, *1*:748–750, 1959.

12. Eckenhoff, J. E., Enderby, G. E. H., Larson, A., Davies, R., and Judevine, D. E.: Human cerebral circulation during deliberate hypotension and head-up tilt. J. Appl. Physiol., *18*:1130–1138, 1963.

13. Eggers, G. W. N., Jr., deGroot, W. J., Tanner, C. R., and Leonard, J. J.: Hemodynamic changes associated with various surgical positions. J.A.M.A., *185*:1–5, 1963.

14. Elwyn, R. A.: Personal communication to the authors.

15. Enderby, G. E. H.: Safety in hypotensive anaesthesia. *In* Proceedings World Congress of Anaesthesiologists, 1955. Minneapolis, Minn., Burgess Pub. Co., 1956, pp. 227–230.

16. Galloon, S.: Controlled respiration in neurosurgical anaesthesia. Anaesthesia, *14*:223–230, 1959.

17. Gilbert, R. G. B., Brindle, G. F., and Galindo, A.: Anesthesia for Neurosurgery. Boston, Little Brown and Co., 1966.

18. Hayes, G. J., and Slocum, H. C.: The achievement of optimal brain relaxation by hyperventilation technics of anesthesia. J. Neurosurg., *19*:65–69, 1962.

19. Henriksen, H. T., and Jorgenson, P. B.: The effect of nitrous oxide on intracranial pressure in patients with intracranial disorders. Brit. J. Anaesth., *45*:486–492, 1973.

20. Kristiansen, K., Krog, J., and Lund, I.: Experiences with selective cooling of the brain. Acta Chir. Scand., Suppl. 253, pp. 151–161, 1960.

21. Larson, A. G.: Deliberate hypotension. Anesthesiology, *25*:682–706, 1964.

22. Larson, C. P., Jr., Ehrenfeld, W. K., Wade, J. G., and Wylie, E. J.: Jugular venous oxygen saturation as an index of adequacy of cerebral oxygenation. Surgery, *62*:31–38, 1967.

23. Lougheed, W. M., Sweet, W. H., White, J. C., and Brewster, W. R.: The use of hypothermia in surgical treatment of cerebral vascular lesions: A preliminary report. J. Neurosurg., *12*:240–255, 1955.

24. Lundberg, N., Kjällquist, Å., and Bien, C.: Reduction of increased intracranial pressure by hyperventilation: A therapeutic aid in neurological surgery. Acta Psychiat. Scand., *34*: suppl. 139: 1–64, 1959.

25. Mazze, R. I., Trudell, J. R., and Cousins, M. J.: Methoxyflurane metabolism and renal dysfunction. Clinical correlation in man. Anesthesiology, *35*:247–252, 1971.

26. Michenfelder, J. D., Gronert, G. A., and Rehder, K.: Neuroanesthesia. Anesthesiology, *30*:65–100, 1969.

27. Michenfelder, J. D., Kirklin, J. W., Uihlein, A., Svien, H. J., and MacCarty, C. S.: Clinical experience with a closed-chest method of producing profound hypothermia and total circulatory arrest in neurosurgery. Ann. Surg., *159*:125–131, 1964.

28. Michenfelder, J. D., Martin, J. T., Altenburg, B. M., and Rehder, K.: Air embolism during neurosurgery: An evaluation of right-atrial catheters for diagnosis and treatment. J.A.M.A., *208*:1353–1358, 1969.

29. Michenfelder, J. D., Miller, R. H., and Gronert, G. A.: Evaluation of an ultrasonic device (Doppler) for the diagnosis of venous air embolism. Anesthesiology, *36*:164–167, 1972.

30. Michenfelder, J. D., Milde, H. J., and Sundt, T. M., Jr.: Cerebral protection by barbiturate anesthesia. Arch. Neurol., *33*:345–350, 1976.

31. National Research Council: Summary of the National Halothane Study: Possible association between halothane anesthesia and postoperative hepatic necrosis. J.A.M.A., *197*:775–788, 1966.

32. Patterson, R. H., Jr., and Ray, B. S.: Profound hypothermia for intracranial surgery: Laboratory and clincal experiences with extracorporeal circulation by peripheral cannulation. Ann. Surg., *156*:377–391, 1962.

33. Pierce, E. C., Jr., Lambertsen, C. J., Deutsch, S., Chase, P. E., Linde, H. W., Dripps, R. D., and Price, H. L.: Cerebral circulation and metabolism during thiopental anesthesia and hyperventilation in man. J. Clin. Invest., *41*:1664–1671, 1962.

34. Plum, F., and Posner, J. B.: Blood and cerebrospinal fluid lactate during hyperventilation. Amer. J. Physiol., *212*:864–870, 1967.

35. Posner, A., Brody, D., and Ravin, M.: Effect of prone position with constant volume ventilation on paO_2 in man. Anesth. Analg. (Cleveland), *44*:435–439, 1965.

36. Rahn, H.: Body temperature and acid-base regulation. Pneumonologie, *151*:87–94, 1974.

37. Ritsema van Eck, C. R.: Neuroleptanalgesia. Int. Anesth. Clin., *3*:659–673, 1965.

38. Robinson, J. S., and Gray, T. C.: Observations on the cerebral effects of passive hyperventilation. Brit. J. Anaesth., *33*:62–68, 1961.

39. Rosomoff, H. L.: Distribution of intracranial contents with controlled hyperventilation: Implications for neuroanesthesia. Anesthesiology, *24*:640–645, 1963.

40. Rosomoff, H. L.: Adjuncts to neurosurgical anaesthesia. Brit. J. Anaesth., *37*:246–261, 1965.

41. Saidman, L. J., and Eger, E. I., II.: Change in cerebrospinal fluid pressure during pneumoencephalography under nitrous oxide anesthesia. Anesthesiology, *26*:67–72, 1965.

42. Shapiro, H. M.: Intracranial hypertension: Therapeutic and anesthetic considerations. Anesthesiology, *43*:445–471, 1975.

43. Small, J. M., and Stephenson, S. C. F.: Circulatory arrest in neurosurgery. Lancet, *1*:569–570, 1966.

44. Smith, A. L., Hoff, J. T., Nielsen, S. L., and Larson, C. P.: Barbiturate protection in acute focal cerebral ischemia. Stroke, *5*:1–7, 1974.

45. Smith, L. W., and Fay, T.: Observations on human beings with cancer, maintained at reduced temperatures of 75°-90° Fahrenheit. Amer. J. Clin. Path., *10*:1–11, 1940.

46. Sugioka, K., and Davis, D. A.: Hyperventilation with oxygen: A possible cause of cerebral hypoxia. Anesthesiology, *21*:135–143, 1960.

47. Sullivan, S. F., Patterson, R. W., and Papper, E. M.: Posthyperventilation hypoxia. J. Appl. Physiol., *22*:431–435, 1967.

48. Sundt, T. M., Jr., Sharbrough, F. W., Anderson, R. E., and Michenfelder, J. D.: Cerebral blood flow measurements and electroencephalograms during carotid endarterectomy. J. Neurosurg., *41*:310–320, 1974.

49. Symbas, P. N., Abbott, O. A., and Leonard, J.: The effects of artificial ventilation on cerebrospinal fluid pressure. J. Thorac. Cardiov. Surg., *54*:126–131, 1967.

50. Terry, H. R., Jr., Daw, E. F., Michenfelder, J. D., Baker, H. L., Jr., and Holman, C. B.: The evolution of anesthesia for neuroradiologic procedures. Surg. Clin. N. Amer., *45*:907–918, 1965.

51. Theye, R. A., and Michenfelder, J. D.: The effect of nitrous oxide on canine cerebral metabolism. Anesthesiology, *29*:1119–1124, 1968.

52. Tindall, G. T., Craddock, A., and Greenfield, J. C., Jr.: Effects of the sitting position on blood flow in the internal carotid artery of man during general anesthesia. J. Neurosurg., *26*:383–389, 1967.

53. Tinker, J. H., and Michenfelder, J. D.: Sodium nitroprusside: Pharmacology, toxicology, and therapeutics. Anesthesiology, *45*:340–354, 1976.

54. Ueyama, H., and Loehning, R. W.: Effect of hyperventilation on cerebrospinal fluid pressure and brain volume. Anesth. Analg. (Cleveland), *42*:581–587, 1963.

55. Uihlein, A., Owen, C. A., Jr., Cooper, T., and Thompson, J. H., Jr.: Bleeding tendencies associated with profound-hypothermia technics in neurologic surgery. Ann. N.Y. Acad. Sci., *115*:337–340, 1964.

56. Vandam, L. D., and Burnap, T. K.: Hypothermia. New Eng. J. Med., *261*:546–553, 595–603, 1959.

57. Werkö, L.: The influence of positive pressure breathing on the circulation in man. Acta Med. Scand., suppl. 193, pp. 1–125, 1947.

58. Whitwam, J. G., Boettner, R. B., Gilger, A. P., and Littell, A. S.: Hyperventilation, brain damage and flicker. Brit. J. Anaesth., *38*:846–852, 1966.

59. Wollman, H., Alexander, S. C., Cohen, P. J., Chase, P. E., Melman, E., and Behar, M. G.: Cerebral circulation of man during halothane anesthesia: Effects of hypocarbia and of d-tubocurarine. Anesthesiology, *25*:180–184, 1964.

60. Wyke, B.: Neurological principles in anaesthesia. *In* Evans, F. T., and Gray, T. C., eds.: General Anaesthesia, 2nd Ed. Washington, D.C., Butterworth & Co., Ltd., 1965, vol. 1, pp. 157–299.

31

GENERAL
OPERATIVE TECHNIQUE

A wide variety of neurosurgical operations have been performed during the centuries since prehistoric man first began trephination.[1-9] As a result of this broad experience, many safe and reliable techniques have been developed. The following is a discussion of basic neurosurgical procedures as practiced today.

CRANIAL OPERATIONS

Preoperative Preparation, Positioning, and Draping

After an appropriate diagnostic work-up, the neurosurgical patient is prepared for his operation. As with any other type of operation, the patient must give informed consent, but if he is unconscious or mentally incompetent, it must be obtained from the relative or institution that is legally responsible for him. His blood is typed and cross-matched, and, if possible, his oral intake is stopped at least eight hours before the operation. The pertinent x-ray films and brain scans are taken to the operating room.

In addition to the usual premedications for local or general anesthesia, it may be necessary to give special medications before certain operations. For example, cortisone acetate is usually given to patients scheduled for pituitary procedures (e.g., for an adult, 100 to 200 mg IM, 48, 24, and 2 hours before operation), and a steroid preparation may be given to patients with cerebral edema one or two days before operation (e.g., for an adult, dexamethasone sodium phosphate, up to 4 mg IM, every six hours, or methylprednisolone sodium succinate, up to 40 mg intramuscularly every six hours).

Immediately prior to operation, the appropriate areas, which have previously been clipped and washed, are carefully shaved. It may be desirable in some cases to clip and shave only one area of the scalp. For example, if only the posterior half is shaved, a woman undergoing suboccipital craniectomy can comb her remaining hair back after her bandage has been removed, with a better initial cosmetic result than if all her hair had been removed. The eyebrows should not be shaved, even when a supraorbital incision is to be made, because of the poor cosmetic result.

The lower extremities are wrapped with elastic bandages to prevent the pooling of blood in these limbs. Two sites for intravenous fluid administration should be prepared if unusual blood loss is anticipated. An intra-arterial catheter is inserted for monitoring the blood pressure and for obtaining samples for blood gas, serum osmolality, electrolyte determinations, and other biochemical studies if needed. If the operative site is to be elevated above the level of the right atrium, where air embolism might occur, a central venous catheter is inserted preoperatively. The position of the tip of the catheter within the right atrium is verified radiographically, and a Doppler monitor is attached to the anterior chest wall.[20]

After anesthesia has been induced, the eyes should be protected from accidental injury by a bland ophthalmic ointment and a cover over the closed eyelids. An indwelling catheter is placed in the urinary bladder if hypertonic solutions may be given intravenously during the operation, if excessive fluid loss and replacement are anticipated, if the operation will require more than four or five hours, or if the physical status of the patient requires close evaluation of fluid

---

R. H. WILKINS AND G. L. ODOM

balance. In order to assure adequate muscle relaxation or to be able to determine neuromuscular reversal if necessary, a nerve stimulator is used to monitor the motor response to ulnar nerve stimulation.

In many cerebral operations, the drainage of cerebrospinal fluid will greatly facilitate exposure and prevent cerebral herniation through the opening in the dura mater. In these cases, a lumbar puncture needle is introduced preoperatively and is connected by sterile plastic tubing to a stopcock so that lumbar drainage can be started and stopped at will during the operation. If the patient is to be on his side, folded sheets are used to protect the lumbar needle from the weight of the drapes. If he is to be supine, a split mattress may be used. As an alternative, a malleable spinal needle or a plastic spinal catheter can be employed instead of a regular spinal needle.

Correct positioning of the patient is essential to achieve maximum operative exposure and to avoid confusing distortions of normal anatomical relationships. If the patient is placed in the supine or lateral position, his head may be stabilized to some extent by placing it on a head ring. A pillow is placed between the patient's lower extremities if he is in the lateral position, and the area where the common peroneal nerve crosses the neck of the fibula is protected from the pressure of restraining straps. In the prone position, the patient's head may be supported by a pin-type head holder or a cerebellar frame, allowing the anesthetist access to the patient's face. Undue pressure on the patient's eyes by the cerebellar frame should be avoided. His shoulders, thorax, and iliac crests should be supported laterally, allowing the center of the thorax and abdomen room for respiratory excursions. Forward flexion of the head on the neck and caudal traction of the shoulders with wide adhesive tape increase the exposure in suboccipital and cervical operations, but pressure on the jugular veins should be avoided since this will increase intracranial venous pressure. In this position a footboard is usually advantageous to prevent the patient from sliding toward the foot of the operating table, especially if the head of the table is elevated during the operation.

The sitting or lounging position offers the advantage of decreased cranial venous pressure, with decreased operative blood loss. But it also has the distinct disadvantages of decreased cerebral arterial blood flow and possible venous air embolism or rapid ventricular decompression with subdural hematoma formation. For this position, a pin head holder (e.g., Gardner skull clamp) may be used to stabilize the patient's head. As in the prone position, flexion of the head on the neck will increase the suboccipital and cervical operative exposure.

The surgeon should look at the patient and examine his chart, x-ray films, and brain scans carefully just prior to operation to verify the side and location of the lesion. He should also remember two pertinent facts about craniocerebral topography (Fig. 31–1).[4] The fissure of Sylvius lies roughly along a line between the external angular process of the frontal bone and a point along the sagittal midline 75 per cent of the

Figure 31–1 Craniocerebral topography showing approximate locations of the sylvian and rolandic fissures (the former along a line between the external angular process of the frontal bone and a point on the sagittal midline 75 per cent of the distance from the nasion to the inion, the latter along the superior portion of a line between the sagittal midline about 2 cm posterior to the midpoint of the nasioiniac line and the middle of the zygomatic arch).

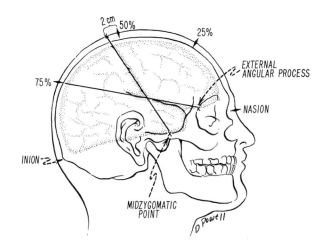

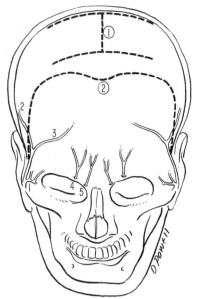

Figure 31–2 Basic incisions: (1), biparietal and (2), coronal. Arteries: 1, Superficial temporal; 2, parietal branch; 3, frontal branch; 4, supraorbital; 5, frontal.

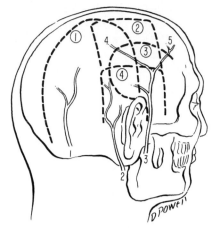

Figure 31–4 Basic incisions: (1), occipital; (2), parietal; (3) and (4), temporal. Arteries: 1, occipital; 2, posterior auricular; 3, superficial temporal; 4, parietal branch; 5, frontal branch.

total nasioiniac distance posterior to the nasion. The fissure of Rolando lies along the superior portion of a line beginning along the sagittal midline about 2 cm posterior to the midpoint of the nasioiniac line and extending laterally to cross the middle of the zygomatic arch. With these facts in mind, the surgeon should be able to plan a flap that will satisfactorily expose the pathological lesion without unnecessary exposure of the adjacent brain (Figs. 31–2 to 31–5).

The skin in the primary operative and appropriate donor areas (e.g., lateral thigh if a fascia lata graft to the dura is anticipated) is cleansed several times with antiseptic solutions. Care must be taken to keep these solutions out of the eyes. Tincture of iodine

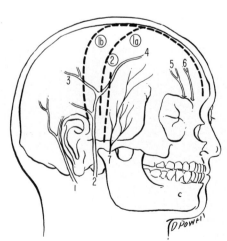

Figure 31–3 Basic incisions: (1a), standard frontal; (1b), large frontal; (2), temporal. Arteries: 1, posterior auricular; 2, superficial temporal; 3, parietal branch; 4, frontal branch; 5, supraorbital; 6, frontal. Nerves: 7, temporal branches of facial nerve.

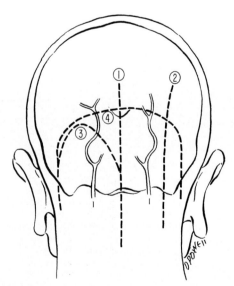

Figure 31–5 Basic incisions: (1), midline linear; (2), unilateral linear; (3), unilateral flap; and (4), bilateral flap. Arteries: 1, occipital.

may cause blistering of the skin and should be avoided in infants. A colorless antiseptic solution may be used on the face to avoid staining it (e.g., benzalkonium chloride in aqueous solution).

The proposed incision and appropriate landmarks, such as the sagittal midline, should be marked with a sterile dye. Cross marks should be made along the incision line every few centimeters to insure correct approximation of the edges of the scalp at the end of the operation. A sterile adhesive plastic film may be used to cover the cleansed areas after they have dried.

Appropriate sterile towels and drapes are then applied to isolate the operative field. These drapes are supported by an ether screen, poles, or angled bars to create a tent under which the anesthetist can reach the patient without entering the sterile operative field. The sterile portions of the suction and cautery lines are attached to their unsterile counterparts away from the operative field. Two suction lines should be set up if brisk hemorrhage might be encountered during operation, as from a ruptured intracranial aneurysm.

Illumination of the operative field is initially achieved by overhead lights, but as the operation proceeds, other methods, such as a head light or illuminated retractors, may be required. Magnification is also frequently advantageous during certain portions of a neurosurgical operation. Spectacles of various types are available for low-power magnification, and the operative microscope can be used to supply greater magnification as well as illumination of the operative field.[28,42,53]

The bactericidal effects of irradiation from ultraviolet lights in the operating room can be used during the operation, but the eyes and skin of all persons in the operating room must be protected against accidental burns.[32,52]

Exposure and Resection of the Brain

Each layer between the scalp and the brain presents a barrier against infection, and if an infection is localized to one plane, the underlying barrier should not be breached unless there is good evidence that infection is also present beneath it. For example, the arachnoid should be kept intact during the evacuation of a subdural empyema. If no such precautions are necessary, however, the brain can be exposed by the systematic opening of all the overlying tissue layers.

Whether or not general anesthesia is used, a local anesthetic agent may be injected along the proposed scalp incision for hemostasis as well as anesthesia. Such an injection will, however, limit the use of scalp clips because of the resulting local increase in the thickness of the scalp, so this technique is not used often.

In general, scalp incisions are either straight or are curved to outline a scalp flap that is based on a broad vascular pedicle (Figs. 31–2 to 31–5). Two incisions that meet or cross each other, such as Cushing's original crossbow incision, are now usually avoided because of poor healing at the angular tips of the scalp flaps. Excision of abnormal areas of the scalp (e.g., devitalized from trauma or distorted by an underlying neoplasm or encephalocele) should be as limited as feasible because of the difficulty encountered in closing even small scalp defects over the convex calvarium. In these situations, extensive undermining of the scalp, a relaxing incision elsewhere in the scalp, or a large scalp flap may be required for adequate closure. If it is possible, scalp incisions should be made so they will be hidden by the patient's hair when it grows back postoperatively.

As the scalp is incised, digital compression through sterile gauze pads or the plastic drape is maintained by assistants to control bleeding until the galea aponeurotica can be undermined a short distance on each side and hemostats or scalp clips can be applied (Fig. 31–6). These scalp clips should be used with care since they can lead to ischemic necrosis of the scalp edge if they are too tight. Exposed areas of the scalp should be covered with sterile skin towels. Large arteries supplying the scalp, such as the superficial temporal artery, should not be cut as the scalp is incised, if it is possible to avoid them. When they do cross the path of the incision they should be securely ligated or cauterized before they are divided.

The temporal and nuchal muscles should be incised in such a way that adequate

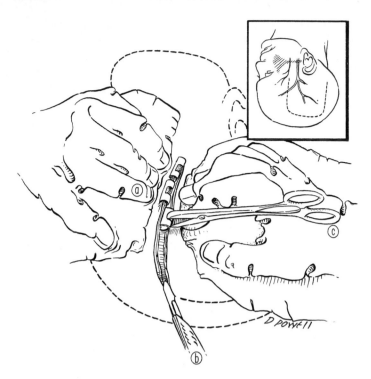

Figure 31–6 Standard craniotomy: (a), digital compression; (b), scalp incision; (c), application of scalp clips.

muscular and fascial cuffs are retained for closure of the wound. This applies in particular to incisions adjacent to the inferior temporal line and the superior nuchal line. The scalp, musculature, and periosteum can be reflected together, allowing the bone to be removed piecemeal or as a free bone flap. More commonly, the scalp is reflected first, and the bone flap is then hinged on the temporalis musculature and periosteum in order to preserve some of its blood supply and maintain its viability (Fig. 31–7). In this situation, the exposed surfaces of the galea aponeurotica, the periosteum, and the temporalis fascia will ooze blood and serum, and careful hemostasis with cautery and the temporary application of strips of oxidized cellulose is necessary to prevent operative blood loss as well as postoperative accumulation of fluid under the scalp flap. Occasionally the bone flap is elevated and reflected together with all the overlying soft tissues. Whenever the bone flap is hinged on the adjacent periosteum and musculature, it retains its vascularity and should be waxed to prevent continuous oozing of blood from its exposed surfaces.

Trephine openings are frequently made with the perforator and burr, as shown in Figure 31–8, or the combined D'Errico bit. Electrical and air drills are also used, but more attention is required to avoid dural laceration with these powerful instruments. After an adequate number of trephine openings have been made, the dura mater is carefully separated from the inner table of the skull along the lines of the proposed bony opening by using a suitable dissector. This maneuver, done to

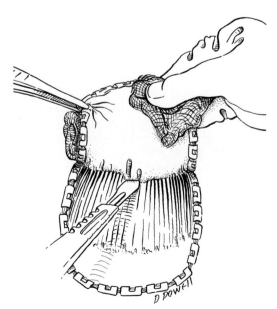

Figure 31–7 Standard craniotomy: reflection of the scalp flap (over rolled gauze to prevent ischemia due to angulation of the base of the flap).

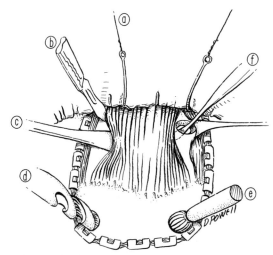

Figure 31–8 Standard craniotomy: (a), retraction of the scalp flap, which is wrapped in moist gauze and covered with a towel, by barbless fish hooks on rubber bands; (b), incision of the temporalis muscle; (c), separation of some of the muscle fibers from the bone with a periosteal elevator; (d) and (e), trephination with perforator and burr; (f), separation of the dura mater from the skull.

prevent accidental dural laceration when the overlying bone is sawed, is especially important at cranial suture lines, over the dural venous sinuses, and in areas where the dural is unusually thin (e.g., the frontal area in elderly individuals).

The bone is removed with rongeurs, or a bone flap is formed with a Gigli saw or an air-driven craniotome (Fig. 31–9). Saw cuts are made between the outermost edges of the burr holes to permit as large an exposure as possible. If only a small cranial opening is required, a crown trephine may be used to remove a circular button of bone, which may be replaced at the end of the operation.

If the edge is beveled as a bone flap is sawed, the flap will sit more securely when it is replaced. In general, areas of the skull over the dural venous sinuses or middle meningeal arteries are sawed last so that, if profuse bleeding occurs, the bone flap can be removed quickly and hemostasis achieved. When a bone flap is to be hinged laterally on the temporalis muscle, it can be divided along the other three sides and then broken across the thin squamous portion of the temporal bone by prying up its medial edge with periosteal elevators as the dura is gently stripped from the inner table of the bone flap with a suitable dissector (Fig. 31–10).

After the bone flap has been elevated, the margins of the bony openings are waxed to prevent diploic bleeding (Figs. 31–11 and 31–12). If the surgeon applies the wax with his finger, he should put a gauze sponge between his glove and the wax to prevent sharp bone spicules from tearing the glove. He may also apply the wax with a short segment of dental roll or a cotton pledget held with forceps.

If the bone flap is to be replaced at the end of the operation, a few small drill holes

Figure 31–9 Standard craniotomy: (a), linear subtemporal craniectomy with rongeurs; (b) and (c), beveled division of bone with a Gigli saw or a craniotome.

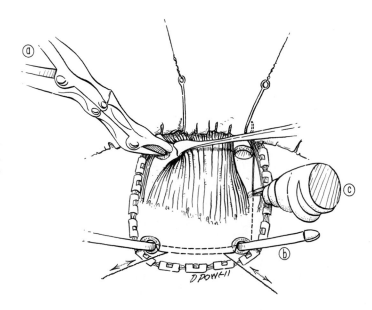

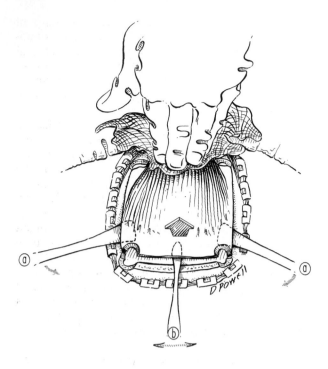

Figure 31–10 Standard craniotomy: (a), elevation of the bone flap; (b), separation of the dura mater from the flap.

are made in the skull around the periphery of the opening, avoiding contaminated areas such as the frontal sinus and mastoid air cells. The dura mater and brain are protected from injury, as each hole is drilled, by the temporary insertion of a metal ribbon or similar instrument immediately beneath the bone in the area being drilled. A

steel wire placed through each of these holes is bent double and is held out of the way with a hemostat. A small gauze pad beneath each wire protects it from contact with the potentially contaminated skin edge. Matching holes are drilled in the bone flap, and additional holes are made centrally so the dura mater can be sutured to

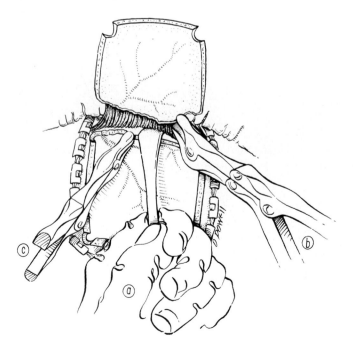

Figure 31–11 Standard craniotomy: (a), further separation of temporalis muscle from bone; (b) and (c), subtemporal craniectomy for postoperative decompression.

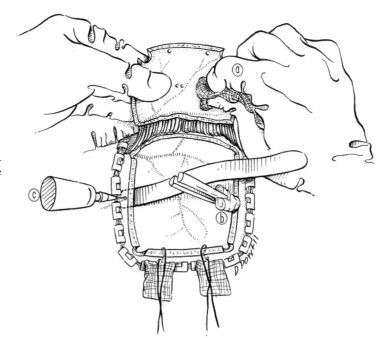

Figure 31–12 Standard craniotomy: (a) and (b), waxing of the bone; (c), drilling of wire holes.

the center of the bone flap when it is replaced at the end of the operation. A hinged bone flap is then wrapped in moist gauze and a surgical towel, and is retracted away from the operative field with barbless fishhooks or small towel clips on heavy rubber bands. A free bone flap is similarly wrapped and is placed on the instrument table.

In cases of cranial trauma, the opening of the skull may require a few additional maneuvers. Linear skull fractures may overlie dural lacerations, especially if the edges of the bone are separated by more than 1 or 2 mm. The surgeon should be careful in these areas not to insert a rongeur, Gigli saw, or craniotome through the dura as he is opening the bone. In the case of comminuted or depressed fractures, the trephine openings should be made and connected in normal bone adjacent to the traumatized area before removal of the fractured bone is begun. This will permit the surgeon to recognize the anatomical planes more easily and will give him adequate room to control bleeding or cerebral herniation if either occurs when the fractured bone fragments are removed. Irregular extensions of the craniectomy may also be required in order to follow underlying dural lacerations to their limits.

Bone involved by tumor or infection should be discarded after specimens have been taken for pathological or bacteriological examination. If possible, the line of bony resection should pass through normal bone adjacent to the involved area. A saw or craniotome should be used rather than rongeurs, which might squeeze the tumor cells or bacteria into the adjacent healthy bone during the removal of the diseased bone.

If an intravenous hyperosmotic agent is to be used to combat increased intracranial pressure during the operation, it is given slowly as the scalp and bone flaps are being turned so that its maximum effect is exerted as the cerebral cortex is exposed. For this purpose, 40 gm of urea can be given as a 30 per cent solution in a solvent containing 10 per cent dextrose or invert sugar. Mannitol, glycerol, or certain diuretics can also be used as dehydrating agents. Such an agent must, however, drip through an adequate intravenous line. Infiltration into the perivenous tissues may result in extensive sloughing.

Lumbar drainage is not begun until the surgeon is ready to open the dura mater, and it is done slowly in order to avoid possible uncal or tonsillar herniation. This drainage should be performed cautiously for other reasons as well. Rapid shrinkage of the brain may precipitate annoying extradural or subdural venous bleeding, and, in

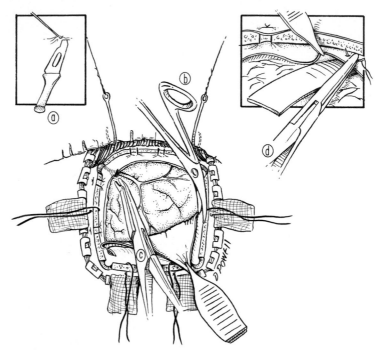

Figure 31–13 Standard craniotomy: (a) and (b), incision and division of the dura mater; (c), clip ligation of dural vessels; (d), suturing of the dura mater to the pericranium.

cases of intracranial aneurysm, may cause a perianeurysmal clot to be pulled away from the ruptured dome of the aneurysm, resulting in renewed arterial hemorrhage.

The dura mater is then picked up with a sharp hook and incised with a scalpel with a No. 15 blade (Fig. 31–13). In most supratentorial craniotomies, the dura is cut with scissors 1 to 2 cm within the entire circumference of the bony defect, except for a small pedicle on which it is reflected away from the exposed brain. Vessels in the dural margins are coagulated or occluded with tantalum clips. Large vessels are easily seen, but bleeding from small dural vessels may be identified more clearly as the dural edge is gently irrigated with clear fluid. Bleeding points on the dural surface should not be cauterized unless the underlying cerebral cortex can be protected from simultaneous thermal injury. In simple trephinations and suboccipital craniectomies, the dura mater may be opened in cruciate fashion instead of as a flap.

Veins bridging from the brain to the dural venous sinuses should be left intact if possible. The dural opening may therefore have to be contoured around these areas and around pacchionian granulations. If the bridging veins must be divided, they should be clipped or coagulated and cut a few millimeters from the venous sinus to avoid a rent in the sinus wall.

Bleeding from the pacchionian granulations or the dural sinuses usually can be controlled by strips of absorbable gelatin sponge and gentle compression. In addition, the head of the operating table may be elevated to reduce intracranial venous pressure, though this maneuver increases the risk of air embolization. When simpler methods fail, a tear in a dural sinus may be closed with sutures, with or without an interposed stamp of autogenous muscle. As a last resort, it may even be necessary to ligate the sinus. The superior sagittal sinus usually may be ligated without complication in its anterior third, but acute ligation at a more posterior point may lead to a severe neurological deficit due to venous stasis in both cerebral hemispheres.

After the dura mater has been opened, it is tacked up to the pericranium around the circumference of the bony opening with interrupted silk sutures to minimize operative and postoperative extradural bleeding. The dural flap is reflected away from the brain, and is covered with moist cotton strips to minimize shrinkage. In addition, the peripheral dural edges may be held back with temporary sutures if further exposure is necessary. Moist cotton strips may then be placed over the full thickness of the cutaneous, muscular, and bony edges of the cranial defect down to the brain, both to isolate the operative field and to prevent blood, pus, and other fluids from entering the subdural space or contaminating adjacent tissues.

The exposed brain should be constantly moistened by irrigation or by the application of moist cotton strips to prevent cortical injury due to drying. The irrigation fluid should be at a temperature of 105° to 115° F to be effective as a hemostatic agent, but fluid warmer than 120° F should not be used since this will damage neurons in the most superficial cortical layers.[47] With practice, the surgeon can judge the approximate temperature of the irrigation fluid by squirting a small amount on his gloved hand.

Frequently, extradural lesions can be exposed by simple retraction of the brain without cerebral resection. Strips of moist cotton, rubber, or a similar material should be placed between each retractor and the brain to prevent accidental cerebral laceration by the retractor. Lumbar drainage of cerebrospinal fluid and the intravenous administration of mannitol or urea markedly facilitate this cerebral retraction. If these techniques do not provide adequate exposure of the lesion, additional cerebrospinal fluid may be released by puncturing the adjacent subarachnoid cisterns or a cerebral ventricle.

Before any cortical incision is made, the exposed cerebral gyri should be identified anatomically for the surgeon's orientation, using landmarks such as the fissure of Sylvius, vein of Trolard, and vein of Labbé (Fig. 31–14). Electrical stimulation may also be used to identify the motor cortex.

The neurosurgeon's next task is to find the patient's lesion, which often does not present on the cortical surface. Widening or discoloration of the gyri in one area, however, usually indicates that a mass lies beneath them. If the cortical surface appears normal, palpation with the moistened gloved finger or the use of ultrasonic encephalography may disclose the underlying lesion. In patients undergoing cerebral ablations for the control of epileptic seizures, electrocorticography is a very sensitive guide to the abnormal areas. If no other method is sufficient, a blunt ventricular needle may be passed into the brain in several different directions. When it encounters the lesion, the cerebral dissection may be made along its course. A subcortical mass should be approached by the most direct route except when this is through a vital region such as a motor or speech area. In these cases, the cortical incision should be made in a less important area and the

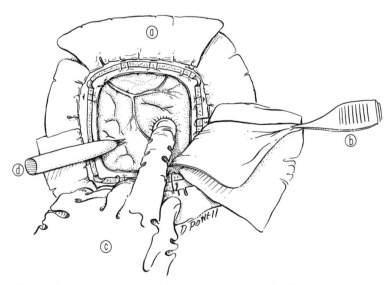

Figure 31–14 Standard craniotomy: (a), moist cotton strips; (b), reflection of the dural flap; (c) and (d), palpation and electrical stimulation of the brain.

dissection performed obliquely down to the lesion.

The cortex adjacent to the proposed cerebral incision or resection should be protected with moist cotton strips (Fig. 31–15). Then the cortical surface along the line of the proposed incision may be cauterized superficially to coagulate the small pial vessels. In general, as many of the larger cortical vessels as possible should be saved; the line of the incision should pass along the plateau of the gyri, avoiding the vessels hidden in the sulci. The larger blood vessels usually cannot be coagulated by simple surface cauterization. The pia mater must be opened and a small amount of adjacent gray matter removed by suction so that each of these vessels may be grasped with forceps and coagulated. Even this technique may not be sufficient for major arteries and veins, which must be clipped before they are cauterized and divided. In the case of vascular lesions or large cerebral resections, the major arteries should be divided before the veins to avoid vascular engorgement of the portion being removed. The pia mater and gray matter are usually incised with a scalpel. Normally the white matter is relatively avascular and soft, and it can be easily divided by any firm instrument such as a Penfield dissector or a metal suction tip. As the white matter along the

line of resection is removed by suction, the deep vessels tend to remain as a fragile network. It saves unnecessary and annoying bleeding if these vessels can be drawn against the sucker, cauterized, and divided before they are accidentally torn.

Moist cotton balls and patties are employed routinely during cerebral resections. They usually are used in combination with irrigation and suction to keep the field clear of blood and tissue debris. They are also used to tamponade individual bleeding vessels, or are placed into one area of a resection to restrict capillary oozing while another area is being dissected. If bleeding is pronounced, several cotton balls may be placed into the area to tamponade the vessels, and then, as these are removed one by one, hemostasis is achieved in each small sector uncovered. It is wise to use cotton balls and patties with attached sutures that are brought out through the cranial opening as a reminder to remove them before closure.

Irrigation may also be quite helpful during cerebral resections. This fluid can be used to rinse the operative field, and it can be pooled in a resected area so that residual bleeding from individual vessels can be identified as the blood streams out into the clear fluid. In addition, irrigation fluid at a temperature of 105° to 115° F has intrinsic

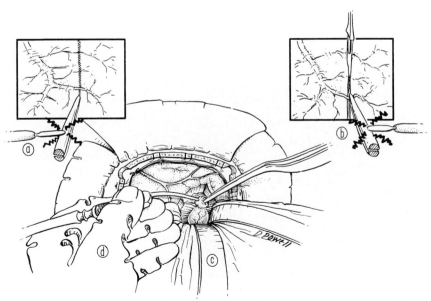

Figure 31–15 Standard craniotomy: (a), linear cauterization of the arachnoid, pia mater, and cortex; (b), cortical incision and cauterization of cortical vessels; (c), retraction of the brain; (d), suction in the depths of the wound.

hemostatic properties since it induces vascular constriction and hastens blood coagulation.[47]

Retractors are customarily used to separate the incised cerebral surfaces so that deeper areas may be seen. This should be done gently, using strips of cotton or rubber beneath the retractors to protect the brain from accidental laceration. The greatest degree of traction should be directed toward the lesion in order to spare relatively normal cerebral areas from undue compression. In particular, traction against the motor cortex should be avoided, since this may produce postoperative hemiparesis ("traction palsy"). During the resection of a brain tumor, the center of the neoplasm may be gutted or a neoplastic cyst aspirated to provide more room for dissection and reduce the amount of retraction required. If mechanically held retractors are used, they should be kept in place as short a time as possible. Excessive retraction reduces underlying local cerebral perfusion, especially when induced arterial hypotension is employed simultaneously.[21]

If a ventricle is entered, an attempt should be made to prevent blood and tissue debris from entering it by temporarily occluding the opening with a large cotton ball or some similar material. This maneuver will reduce the severity of the resulting postoperative sterile ventriculitis.

In cases complicated by incisural herniation of the uncus and hippocampal gyrus, these swollen structures must be disimpacted under direct vision to prevent progressive mesencephalic compression and death. Simple removal of the overlying lesion (e.g., epidural hematoma) is usually not adequate for this purpose.

When the cerebral resection has been completed, all residual bleeding should be controlled. Irrigation fluid placed into the surgical defect must remain clear before efforts at hemostasis are ended. Also, any blood that has entered the subdural space during the operation should be washed out. A final check should be made to be certain that all cotton balls and strips have been removed.

Closure of the Operative Defect

Frequently the flap of dura mater that was turned at the beginning of the operation

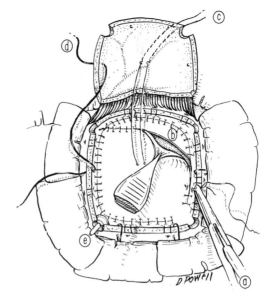

Figure 31–16 Standard craniotomy: (a), suturing of the dura mater; (b), dural graft; (c), central tack-up suture; (d), bone wires; (e), bottom of silicone rubber button.

is inadequate to fill the dural defect at the end (Fig. 31–16). The tack-up sutures cause retraction of the dural margins, and some shrinkage of the dural flap occurs despite its coverage with moist cotton strips during the operation. In this situation and when dural decompression is necessary, a dural graft can be inserted, using temporalis fascia, periosteum, fascia lata, or an artificial dural substitute. The dural flap and graft are usually sewn into position so that the suture line is watertight. In supratentorial operations, this dural closure prevents outward cerebral herniation and minimizes the formation of a cortical cicatrix. These considerations are not as important in the suboccipital area. The dura mater is sometimes left open after operations in the posterior fossa, and if an adequate closure of the nuchal muscles is achieved, no adverse effects can be detected. The dura mater is also usually left open beneath simple trephine openings and following subtemporal craniectomy for subdural hematoma.

The bone flap is wired back into place, and the dural flap is simultaneously sutured up to its central drill holes (Figs. 31–16 and 31–17). Silicone rubber or tantalum buttons, methylmethacrylate, or autogenous bone chips can be used to fill in the trephine openings and other bony defects for a better cosmetic result. Frequently, a portion of

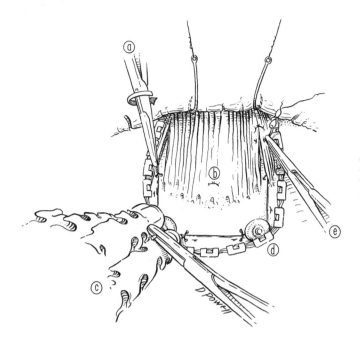

Figure 31–17 Standard craniotomy: (a), twisting the bone wires; (b), central tack-up suture; (c) and (d); application of button tops; (e), suturing of the temporalis muscle and fascia.

the bone under the temporalis muscle will be removed at some stage of the operation before the bone flap is closed, to provide a subtemporal decompression. This type of decompression has limited value, however, unless it is combined with dural grafting. In general, it is best to replace at least part of the bone flap after operations for malignant brain tumors in order to prevent a long terminal period with a large bulging scalp flap.

If there is marked cerebral swelling, the bone flap should be removed. It can be wrapped in sterile towels and a sterile plastic bag, stored in a freezer, and replaced at a later time.[41] As an alternative, this bone flap can be used as a model for the postoperative construction of a methylmethacrylate cranioplasty plate.[45]

Silk is frequently used for dural tack-up sutures and for closure of the dura, musculature, and scalp. In contaminated or infected cases, a less reactive type of suture material should be used, such as nylon or stainless steel wire. Interrupted inverted galeal sutures are an important part of the scalp closure in clean cases, but these buried sutures should not be used in the presence of gross contamination or infection, since they may form a nidus for subcutaneous or subgaleal abscesses. Even in clean cases, however, the use of an absorbable galeal suture (e.g., chromic catgut or

polyglycolic acid) rather than silk may reduce the incidence of postoperative wound infections.

If there has been gross bacterial contamination or infection, devitalized bone should not be replaced unless it is important for cosmetic reasons (e.g., portions of the supraorbital ridge). Similarly, plastics and other foreign materials should be avoided. Copious irrigation of the operative field with sterile Ringer's solution or isotonic saline at the various anatomical levels of the operation is advisable, and irrigation with a relatively nonepileptogenic antibiotic (e.g., bacitracin, 50,000 units in about 10 ml of sterile Ringer's solution or isotonic saline) may also be helpful. Iodoform gauze packing may be placed in the epidural space before the scalp is closed, with one end brought out through a dependent limb of the incision or a separate stab wound. It may then be withdrawn gradually over several days and perhaps replaced with fresh iodoform gauze. Cranioplasty should be delayed for at least 6 to 12 months in these cases to avoid the risk of a second infection around the cranioplasty plate.

As the scalp is closed, the skin clips or hemostats should be removed systematically in small groups to avoid continuous bleeding from the rest of the incision while one area is being sutured (Fig. 31–18). Ex-

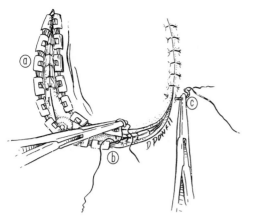

Figure 31–18 Standard craniotomy: (a), sutures in the temporalis fascia; (b), suturing of the galea aponeurotica; (c), suturing of the skin.

tensive cauterization of the bleeding scalp vessels is not advisable, since it may delay healing and result in sloughing along the scalp edges.

After the scalp has been sutured, sterile gauze pads, a loosely knit gauze wrap, and strips of adhesive tape are then applied. For the patient's comfort, his ears should be padded with cotton as the dressing is applied. An extra layer of fine-mesh gauze may also be wrapped over the dressing to hold it more firmly in place. This turban should come below the ears to keep the dressing from sliding off, but it should not be so tight that it is uncomfortable for the patient. As an aid to scalp hemostasis, if the bone flap has been replaced, an elastic bandage can be applied over the head dressing for a few hours postoperatively. Small scalp incisions can be covered by simple collodion or gauze and tape dressings. Intraoral incisions are usually closed with catgut sutures and require no dressing.

Ordinarily the gauze dressings are not taken off until it is time to remove the skin sutures. This is usually on the fifth day after operation for silk sutures in uncomplicated cases, or at a later time for nylon or wire sutures, especially if delayed wound healing is expected. The suture line should be painted with an antiseptic solution and the sutures removed, using sterile technique. Even a small stitch abscess, which would be only a nuisance elsewhere in the body, may lead to osteomyelitis of the bone flap and necessitate its removal.

When drains are used, they may be brought out through a dependent portion of the scalp incision or through a separate stab wound in a dependent area of the scalp. Drains in clean cases (e.g., from the subdural space after evacuation of a subdural hematoma) should be removed within 24 to 36 hours because of the danger of retrograde infection along the drain. Loose scalp sutures that are placed in each drain incision at the time of the operation should be tied as soon as the drain is removed to seal the incision. While the drains are in place, a bulky head dressing should be employed, and this should be changed whenever the drainage penetrates to the outer layers of gauze. Alternatively, a drain may be attached to a sterile collection device.

General Remarks about Specific Operative Approaches

Frontal Approach

A curved scalp incision is frequently used for a unilateral frontal approach (Fig. 31–3).[40] It arches posteriorly and then inferolaterally from a point on the forehead to end just anterior and superior to the ipsilateral ear. The vertical limb in the exposed portion of the forehead is least conspicuous if it is in the midline, and it will not result in denervation of any part of the frontalis muscle as will a more lateral incision. A coronal scalp incision, running from one anterior temporal area to the other at about the level of the coronal suture line, may be used for either unilateral or bilateral frontal operations (Fig. 31–2). This incision is entirely hidden behind the normal hairline, but is curved forward at the sagittal midline to allow easier anterior reflection of the frontal scalp.

With either type of incision, accidental injury to the anterior temporal branches of the facial nerve should be avoided by keeping the incision superior to the zygomatic process and no further than about 1.5 cm anterior to the ear. If these branches are damaged, noticeable postoperative paralysis of the ipsilateral frontalis muscle will result.

A supraorbital saw cut through the frontal bone should not enter the frontal sinus unless low exposure is necessary in a patient with large frontal sinuses (e.g., frontal craniotomy in an acromegalic patient). If the frontal sinus is entered, this contaminated area should be isolated from the sterile intracranial contents. The mucosa of the exposed portion of the sinus can be simply stripped away from the bone and collapsed if it has not been opened. If it has been opened, however, the mucosa in the sinus and any mucosal strips still adhering to the bone flap should be exenterated. In either case, the sinus can then be packed with autogenous muscle or gelatin sponge, or, if the mucosa has been opened, the sinus may be drained through the frontonasal duct into the nose, with or without the use of a small catheter. In sealing off a surgical opening into the sinus, a flap of frontal periosteum or temporalis fascia may be placed across the defect and sutured to the periosteum superiorly and the dura mater inferiorly.

If bifrontal bone flaps are made, the medial bony incision is made 1 to 2 cm lateral to the sagittal midline. This cut should be beveled so the two flaps can be wired tightly together at the end of the operation. The smaller bone flap is turned first, and then the superior sagittal sinus and dura mater are carefully separated from the sagittal sulcus and frontal crest of the remaining bone flap before it is similarly reflected laterally on its attached temporalis muscle fibers.

Parietal and Occipital Approaches

An inverted U-shaped parietal scalp incision is usually used (Fig. 31–4).[40] The base should not be narrower than the apex to insure against ischemia of the edges of the scalp flap. Since there is no parietal musculature on which to hinge a bone flap, a free flap of parietal bone is generally employed. Parasagittal lesions may be approached occasionally through a biparietal H-shaped flap or a unilateral flap that has been extended across the midline (Fig. 31–2).

The usual occipital scalp incision begins just above and lateral to the inion, and extends parallel to the midline into the posterior parietal region, where it curves temporally (Fig. 31–4). The bone flap is reflected laterally on the attached posterior fibers of the temporalis muscle.

In parietal and occipital operations, the superior sagittal and transverse sinuses should be carefully spared from injury because of the grave consequences of obstructing these venous channels.

Temporal Approach

Depending on the nature of the operation and the extent of exposure necessary, the temporal scalp incision can be linear, U-shaped, or in the configuration of a question mark (Figs. 31–3 and 31–4).[40] All three begin anterior to the superior portion of the pinna, and care must be taken to avoid injury to the temporal branches of the facial nerve. The linear incision extends directly toward the sagittal midline; the U-shaped incision arches superomedially, posteriorly, and then inferolaterally to end behind the ear; and the question mark incision curves posteriorly just above the ear and then turns superiorly, medially, and anteriorly to end in the anterolateral frontal area.

Since the squamous portion of the temporal bone is thin and the heavy temporalis muscle will provide postoperative protection of the underlying brain, craniectomy is frequently used in the temporal area rather than craniotomy. When subtemporal craniectomy is performed for retrogasserian neurotomy, bone should be removed down to the floor of the middle fossa to provide adequate exposure.

No matter which method of bony opening is used, the contaminated mastoid air cells should not be intentionally entered, and injury to the transverse sinus should be avoided. If the mastoid air cells are opened, they should be sealed off with bone wax.

Suboccipital Approach

In many suboccipital operations, supratentorial ventricular drainage is required to reduce increased intracranial pressure, especially if a ventriculogram has been performed preoperatively. At the beginning of the operation, an indwelling ventricular needle or catheter is inserted into the right lateral ventricle by way of a right occipital trephine opening so that the supratentorial ventricular pressure can be reduced at any time.

Several different types of incisions are used for suboccipital operations (Fig. 31–5).[22] Bilateral exposure is possible through a relatively avascular midline linear incision or a U-shaped incision arched across the inion and based inferolaterally at the mastoid tips. Unilateral exposure can be achieved through a unilateral linear or hockey-stick incision, or a narrow U-shaped flap that has its lateral limb in the mastoid region and its medial limb along the nuchal midline.

By any approach, the emissary veins in the mastoid, suboccipital, and condylar areas may be encountered. These must be controlled with cautery and bone wax to prevent significant venous bleeding. A cuff of nuchal musculature (the trapezius and semispinalis capitis medially; the sterno-cleidomastoid and splenius capitis laterally) should be left as the muscle is incised to insure adequate closure of the wound.

The bone in the suboccipital area is removed piecemeal with rongeurs after multiple trephine openings have been made. The posterior arch of the atlas may also be removed to provide adequate exposure and decompression. Injury to the vertebral artery must be avoided when this arch is uncovered and removed. Any mastoid air cells exposed during a suboccipital craniectomy should be plugged with bone wax. Besides creating a route of entry into the posterior cranial fossa for bacteria and air, an opening into these air cells can provide an avenue for the persistent leakage of cerebrospinal fluid into the middle ear, eustachian tube, and pharynx.

The dura mater is opened over one or both cerebellar hemispheres and tonsils. The dural leaves are turned back and sutured to the adjacent periosteum, fascia, or muscles. As the dural incision is carried inferiorly, the circular dural venous channels at the level of the foramen magnum should be clipped. Likewise, the occipital sinus should be ligated and divided if bilateral exposure is required. Transfixion sutures are useful for occluding the occipital sinus since they are less likely to slip off than is a tantalum clip. The posterior arachnoidal wall of the cisterna magna is opened to provide additional decompression and exposure of the posterior fossa.

The dura mater may be closed completely or may be left open at the completion of the suboccipital operation. If it is closed only partially, there is an increased tendency for cerebrospinal fluid to become trapped under the musculocutaneous flap. It is important that the nuchal muscles and scalp be closed well to prevent a cerebrospinal fluid fistula. If a ventriculocisternal shunt has been performed in association

with the procedure in the posterior fossa, the nuchal muscles must be closed snugly about the shunt tube to keep cerebrospinal fluid from dissecting superiorly along its course. If the cuff of fibromuscular tissue is inadequate for a firm closure, a row of drill holes may be made along the superior and lateral bony margins of the craniectomy defect so the nuchal muscles can be sutured to these margins instead.

After the cranial dressing has been applied, a "checkrein" of adhesive tape can be attached to this dressing and to the posterior cervical skin to prevent undue tension on a transverse suboccipital incision.

A few combined supratentorial-infratentorial approaches have been devised for exposure of lesions extending through the tentorial incisura, but these are seldom necessary. They are somewhat difficult technically and may be associated with injury to the transverse sinus. Also, if an incision is made to outline two adjacent scalp flaps (one supratentorial and one infratentorial), wound healing may not be optimal.

Basal Approach

Several types of operation may be performed through the base of the skull anterior to the foramen magnum.[27,47,48] The reader is referred to the references at the end of this chapter and to the other chapters in this book for the details of these procedures.

Postoperative Considerations

The very important subject of postoperative management is discussed elsewhere in this book. It does, however, seem appropriate to mention a few points about the postoperative care of the surgical flap or incision.[26,34,50]

If fluid collects in the subgaleal space beneath the patient's scalp flap, it should not be aspirated unless the incision is in danger of separation. This fluid will be gradually reabsorbed spontaneously, and the insertion of a needle through the potentially contaminated scalp is rarely justified because of the possible introduction of infection.

The postoperative leakage of cerebrospinal fluid through the scalp incision frequently indicates an inadequate closure of the dura mater, and perhaps of other layers of the wound as well. This complication usually can be controlled by placing additional sutures along the scalp incision. Occasionally the entire wound must be reopened for careful closure of each of its layers. Since persistently elevated cerebrospinal fluid pressure may also be a contributing factor, periodic lumbar punctures or continuous lumbar drainage may be used in reducing cerebrospinal fluid pressure to decrease its force against the healing wound. Antibiotics should be given until satisfactory healing has occurred.

If the leakage of cerebrospinal fluid is due to a wound infection, a more serious situation exists. The wound must be reopened, culture specimens must be taken, and the wound must then be thoroughly cleansed. A tight dural closure must be achieved, using relatively nonreactive suture material. The more superficial sutures and other foreign material should be removed. The scalp may then be closed with a single layer of interrupted wire sutures, with or without drains or packs. Antibiotic therapy should also be used under these circumstances.

Postoperative radiotherapy for intracranial tumors should be delayed until the operative incision is well healed in order to prevent wound dehiscence.

Reoperation may become necessary in the immediate postoperative period because of intracranial hemorrhage or edema of the brain. Subsequently, it may be required because of postoperative persistence or recurrence of the patient's original lesion, or because of complications such as infection or hydrocephalus. In general, portions of the patient's original operative incision are reopened, and it is a definite advantage to the surgeon if he has a detailed report of the original operation to review before the second procedure. If the bone flap has been removed previously, accidental dural laceration should be avoided as the scalp is reflected. In reoperations performed several months or years after the initial procedure, the dura mater may be quite adherent to the underlying cerebral cortex or neoplasm, necessitating careful dissection to separate the two. This dissection should be as limited as possible to prevent unnecessary cortical damage.

In closing a second operation done for acute postoperative hemorrhage or edema, it may be desirable to graft the dura mater and leave out part or all of the bone flap. When infection is present, all devitalized and foreign material should be removed except for the necessary dural and scalp sutures, which should be of a relatively nonreactive material. The infected wound should be treated as outlined previously.

SPINAL OPERATIONS

Preoperative Preparation, Positioning, and Draping

As for cranial operations, informed consent for a spinal operation is required. The patient's blood should be typed and cross-matched, his stomach should be empty, he should be given appropriate premedications, and his pertinent x-ray films should be taken to the operating room. Unless his lesion is close to the upper or lower end of the spinal column, where the surgeon can recognize the vertebral level exactly by counting up from the sacrum or down from the occiput, the patient's skin should be marked preoperatively at the level of the lesion, using radiographic identification. Just before the operation, the surgeon should consult the patient, his chart, and his x-rays to verify the side and level of his lesion.

General anesthesia is usually induced with the patient supine, and spinal anesthesia is achieved with the patient in the prone jackknifed or the lateral position. Patients with cervical fracture-dislocations are commonly intubated with a nasotracheal tube while they are still awake. Topical anesthesia is used, and a fiberoptic bronchoscope or laryngoscope may be employed to advantage. By this maneuver, the use of direct laryngoscopy with dangerous extension of the neck is avoided, and accidental aspiration of vomitus by the patient is minimized. As a last resort in this type of patient, a tracheostomy may be performed. A patient with a meningomyelocele may be intubated in the semilateral position to prevent unnecessary pressure on the spinal sac.

The patient's lower extremities are wrapped with elastic bandages to prevent pooling of blood in these limbs. As for other operations, the eyes of the anesthetized patient should be protected from accidental injury. For operations involving the spinal cord, it may be quite helpful, and even crucial to the success of the procedure, to monitor somatosensory evoked potentials during the operation. If so, the appropriate leads should be attached at this point.

Patients with spinal fractures or dislocations must be moved into position for operation with great care to avoid further injury to the spinal cord. Several strong persons, working simultaneously, should move the patient without unnecessary flexion, extension, or rotation of the spinal column. Cervical traction should also be maintained as the patient with cervical injuries is moved onto the operating table. The arterial blood pressure, central venous pressure, and electrocardiogram should be monitored carefully in quadriplegic or paraplegic patients, especially those exhibiting spinal shock.

Spinal operations are generally performed with the patient in a prone or sitting position, but anterior spinal discectomy and stereotaxic cervical cordotomy are done with the patient supine. Posterior spinal operations are accomplished by some surgeons with the patient in the lateral position.

If the prone position is used, the patient's trunk should be supported laterally on pads or folded sheets that allow space between them for free thoracic and abdominal respiratory excursions, avoiding compression of the inferior vena cava with its resulting distention of the intraspinal venous plexus. A footboard can be used to prevent the patient from sliding down the operating table if the head of the table is raised. Such elevation of the head can be used advantageously to reduce venous distention in the cervical area and to fill out the entire spinal subarachnoid space with cerebrospinal fluid to tamponade the extradural veins.

For most thoracic and lumbar operations done with the patient prone, the patient's head can be turned to the side and his arms extended to rest beside his head. Care must be taken to prevent overextension of the shoulder with pressure on or stretching of the vascular and nervous elements of the axilla. To avoid spinal rotation and distortion, upper thoracic and cervical operations should be performed with the patient's head flexed forward in the pin head holder

or on the cerebellar frame and with his arms by his sides. By the appropriate use of folded sheets and pads, an infant can be placed in a similar position on the operating table without the cerebellar frame. If the cerebellar frame is used, pressure on the patient's eyes should be avoided. Compression of the jugular veins by the mattress or pads should likewise be prevented in order to eliminate unnecessary cervical venous distention that might cause increased bleeding during the operation. Moderate caudal traction of the shoulders with wide adhesive tape can be used to increase the operative exposure in the cervical area, but the tape should not restrict respiratory movements of the posterior thorax and should not cover the iliac crests if an iliac bone graft is anticipated.

If cranial tongs for skeletal traction were inserted prior to operation, this traction can be maintained during the procedure by suspending the weight over a pulley attached to an extension beyond the cerebellar frame. The amount and direction of cervical traction can be altered to suit the surgeon during the operation.

During practically any spinal operation with the patient prone, the table may be flexed or extended, and the cerebellar frame or traction pulley may be lowered or elevated to separate or approximate the laminal arches. The surgeon can use these changes in position to gain a mechanical advantage. With the spine flexed and the laminal arches separated, the intervertebral disc is more easily exposed and dislocated facets can be more easily reduced. With the spine moderately extended, reduced facets can be locked in position and the laminal arches can be more easily wired or fused together.

The lateral position for spinal operations avoids a number of the problems encountered in the prone position. There is less jugular and caval venous obstruction, better control over the patient's airway, and natural drainage of blood and cerebrospinal fluid out of the wound. Subarachnoid-peritoneal shunts are performed in this position since it permits simultaneous exposure of the back and the abdomen. However, adequate bilateral exposure of the spine and spinal cord is usually more difficult by this approach.

The sitting position can also be used for

cervical spinal operations. As opposed to the prone position, there is less venous bleeding and little pooling of blood and cerebrospinal fluid in the wound. Yet there is a greater danger of cerebral ischemia, venous air embolism, and rapid loss of cerebrospinal fluid leading to an intracranial subdural hematoma.

After the patient has been positioned for operation, the primary and donor (e.g., iliac crests if a bone graft is anticipated) operative areas should be shaved and cleansed with antiseptic solutions. The anal area must be carefully excluded from the operative field with skin towels. Next, the important anatomical landmarks and the proposed incision line should be marked with a sterile dye. After the operative area is draped, the suction and cautery lines are attached, and the field is illuminated. As with cranial operations, ultraviolet lights may be used during spinal procedures for their bactericidal effects.

General Remarks About Specific Operative Approaches

Posterior Approach

The skin and subcutaneous tissues are usually divided in the longitudinal midline, although this incision may be deviated in an elliptical fashion around each side of a midline dermal sinus. One exception to this approach is the incision generally used for a meningomyelocele. A generous transverse incision is made for this, and its ends may be curved in opposite directions to create skin flaps adequate to cover the central defect left after the sac has been resected.

Superficial subcutaneous bleeding is controlled with hemostatic clamps. These are then laid back over sterile towels that are brought up to the edges of the wound on each side to cover all the previously exposed skin. The edges of the incision are retracted, and bleeding vessels in the deeper layers of the subcutaneous tissue are cauterized.

The next layer encountered is the fascial layer overlying the paravertebral muscles (lumbodorsal or nuchal fascia). This is divided in the midline in preparation for a bilateral laminectomy. If a hemilaminectomy is planned, however, the fascia is divided a few millimeters lateral to the midline, leaving a cuff to aid in suturing this fascia during closure of the wound. In the cervical area, dissection is then carried through the relatively avascular ligamentum nuchae down to the spinous processes.

The paravertebral muscles are stripped away from the spines and laminae. This step is usually performed with a periosteal elevator and gauze packs to bluntly dissect away the muscle fibers, and a scalpel or scissors to divide their tendinous insertions. If the posterior arches are open, however, as with a spina bifida, or are unstable, as with a spinal fracture, only sharp dissection under direct vision should be used. The paravertebral muscles should be stripped from the spinous processes in the acute angle between their insertions and the bone. If the scalpel or periosteal elevator is used in the opposite direction, it will tend to follow the direction of the fibers away from the vertebral spines out into the vascular muscle mass. Bleeding from the detached muscles is controlled by cautery and by temporarily packing the paravertebral gutters with gauze pads. These muscles are then retracted laterally and the laminae are cleaned of overlying connective tissue and fat out to and including the intervertebral facets. The transverse processes must also be exposed when a fusion of these elements is to be performed.

The exact vertebral level may be established by counting up or down from a recognizable landmark such as the occiput, the spine of C2, the spine of C7, or the sacrum. The level of a cervical operation may also be verified by examining preoperative anteroposterior and lateral roentgenograms to identify individual characteristics of the various cervical spines (i.e., long or short, single or bifid). In the thoracic area, the exact level is more difficult to establish; reference can be made to marks placed on the skin preoperatively. If there is any doubt about the exact vertebral level, however, roentgenograms should be made in the operating room, using a metal object to mark one of the spines or laminae.

If a wide opening between or through the spinal arches does not already exist, portions of them must be removed with rongeurs or drills to create an entrance into the spinal canal. As a general rule, as little bone as possible is removed to provide adequate exposure, especially if an ensuing posterior spinal fusion is planned. To uncover a posterolateral herniation of an intervertebral disc, it is generally necessary to excise only the edges of one or two laminae and perhaps a portion of the adjacent intervertebral facet. For unilateral cordotomy or rhizotomy, adequate exposure can be achieved by removing one or more laminae on just one side, but any larger procedure usually requires removal of the laminae, spines, and the attached ligaments of several vertebrae bilaterally.

The excision of the spinous processes is facilitated by the preliminary division of the supraspinous and interspinous ligaments. Similarly, removal of the laminal arches is made easier if a plane is first established between one of the laminae and its underlying ligamentum flavum. Since the ligamenta flava attach like shingles to the anterior surfaces of the superior laminae and the posterior surfaces of the inferior laminae, the inferior laminal edges are the more easily separated from these ligaments by the posterior approach. Thus, the removal of each lamina should begin along its caudal edge. Care must be taken to avoid compression of the spinal cord or nerve roots as the spines and laminae are removed. Typically, there is an emissary vein that perforates each lamina laterally. Bleeding from these veins and from the edges of the divided bones can be controlled with bone wax.

After the bony opening has been created, portions of one or more of the ligamenta flava should be removed. If two adjacent ligaments are exposed, a gap between them can usually be found, and, starting at that point, they can be peeled away from the underlying epidural veins. This is especially true in the cervical region where the ligamenta flava are not as well developed as in other areas of the spine. If only a single ligamentum flavum has been exposed, it should be elevated with a sharp hook or forceps and incised carefully to avoid accidental laceration of the underlying dura mater. This ligament should be cut in a plane perpendicular to its surface; if not, it may fray into laminations and prolong the time required for its removal.

No matter how the ligamenta flava are excised, care should be taken not to lacerate the underlying epidural veins. Bleeding from these vessels will obscure the operative field and will increase the risk of

paraplegia or quadriplegia due to the formation of a postoperative epidural hematoma.

If such a vein is accidentally opened, the bleeding usually can be controlled by compression. Direct pressure may be applied with a cotton patty; simultaneous compression of the spinal cord or its nerve roots must be avoided. As an alternative, the dura mater may be sutured laterally against the neighboring wall of the spinal canal after the dura has been opened. Pieces of gelatin sponge or oxidized cellulose may also be placed over the bleeding vein immediately before either of these maneuvers is performed. Frequently, individual epidural veins can be isolated and identified easily enough to permit clip ligation or cauterization of these structures. Before being cauterized, however, they should be held away from the adjacent dura mater to prevent thermal injury to the underlying nervous tissue. After the venous bleeding has been controlled, cotton strips are placed over the epidural space and intervertebral facets along each side of the exposed dura.

When the dura mater is to be opened, it may be picked up with a sharp hook, incised with a scalpel with a No. 15 blade, and divided with scissors or a blunt hook. It is frequently advantageous to leave the arachnoid membrane intact while the dura is being opened. By this maneuver, the hydrostatic pressure compressing the epidural veins is maintained and blood is kept out of the subarachnoid space. The cut edges of the dura mater are elevated and held apart with traction sutures. This provides exposure of the spinal cord and forms a small barrier to prevent the blood that collects in the depths of the incision from flowing over the surface of the cord. Usually, the dura is then tacked up to the adjacent periosteum and paravertebral muscles in several places along each side of the bony opening in order to minimize epidural venous bleeding.

If possible, the arachnoid should not be incised immediately beneath the dural opening. This will allow an intact strip of arachnoid to seal off the inner surface of the dural incision after the dura has been sutured shut. When the patient is in the sitting position, only a small arachnoidal opening should be made at first, to prevent the sudden loss of cerebrospinal fluid and the possible development of an intracranial subdural hematoma. If a spinal tumor is present, the initial arachnoidal opening should be made cephalad to it to avoid the occasional increase in neurological deficit associated with the release of cerebrospinal fluid below a spinal block.

The same techniques are applied in operating upon the spinal cord as upon the brain, but on a much smaller and more exact scale. The spinal cord is extremely sensitive to compression and other forms of injury, and the destruction of only a small amount of white or gray matter in the spinal cord may result in a significant neurological deficit. For this reason, great care must be taken to avoid injury to the normal nervous elements as pathological tissue is manipulated or removed from the spinal canal. Even minor retraction of the spinal cord may interfere with its function.

Adequate illumination is essential for this type of operation, and magnification can be of great value in avoiding unnecessary injury to normal structures. The cord should be kept moist with warm irrigation solution during the operation to minimize desiccation. Suction should be performed through a cotton patty to prevent accidental aspiration of normal nervous tissue. Cauterization should be as limited as possible and should be done with bipolar current and forceps with fine points. In order to avoid unnecessary hemorrhage, myelotomy should be performed in relatively avascular areas, and catheters should not be randomly passed into the epidural, subdural, or subarachnoid spaces away from the exposed areas of the spinal canal.

The dura mater may be left open at the end of the operation, but usually it is sutured shut to prevent blood and fibrous tissue from entering the subarachnoid space and cerebrospinal fluid from leaving it. If it appears that compression of the spinal cord might occur if the dura is sutured primarily, a graft of paravertebral fascia or an artificial dural substitute may be sutured into the dural defect. Whether or not a graft is used, a few of these dural sutures can also be tacked up to the overlying muscles as they are closed to aid in preventing postoperative epidural hemorrhage. Tantalum clips may be attached to the dura mater or paravertebral tissues to serve as postoperative radiographic markers.

If a posterior spinal fusion is planned, it can be done at this point. Next, the wound is carefully checked to make certain that all cotton strips and gauze sponges have been removed. The muscles, fascia, subcutaneous tissue, and skin are then sutured in anatomical layers. If a gap exists, as in the case of a meningomyelocele, additional maneuvers may be necessary to close it. Flaps of lumbodorsal or nuchal fascia can be elevated and sutured across such a defect. Also, the skin can be extensively undermined and cutaneous flaps can be created to obtain adequate coverage. Wire or another strong inert suture material should be used to close the laminectomy wound in debilitated patients and in those who will be given postoperative radiotherapy.

It is not advisable to place devitalized bone or foreign material into contaminated or infected laminectomy incisions. In these cases, the wound should be thoroughly irrigated with sterile Ringer's solution or isotonic saline before closure. An antibiotic solution, such as 50,000 units of bacitracin in 10 ml of fluid, may also be instilled into the wound. Because of the length of time required for a deep posterior spinal incision to fill with granulation tissue, an effort should be made to achieve some type of primary closure in minimally contaminated cases, using a relatively nonreactive suture material such as wire. If the wound is left open, it may be packed with iodoform gauze to reduce the numbers of bacteria present and to stimulate the formation of granulation tissue.[51]

In clean cases, the sterile gauze dressing placed on the skin incision is not disturbed until it is time for the skin sutures to be removed. For silk sutures in uncomplicated cases, this is usually on the sixth day after operation.

The postoperative management of patients with posterior spinal operations varies, depending on the nature of the pathological process and the location and extent of the operation. As soon as the effects of anesthesia have abated, the patient's neurological status should be tested. Frequent examinations should then be performed periodically over the ensuing hours and days to spot any neurological deterioration that may be a sign of a postoperative extradural hematoma.

Narcotics are usually necessary for postoperative analgesia, but because of possible respiratory depression from these drugs, they should not be given following a cervical laminectomy until the patient is awake and it is obvious that he is having no difficulty breathing. As after other types of operation, various measures should be taken to prevent postoperative pulmonary atelectasis and thrombophlebitis in the lower extremities. The paraplegic or quardiplegic patient will also require additional care, as discussed elsewhere in this book.

If the dura mater has not been opened and the bony resection has been minor, the patient can stand and walk with assistance within a day after the operation. Following extensive laminectomies, however, the patient is usually kept at bed rest for several days to allow the paravertebral muscles time to begin healing together before being subjected to their normal stresses and strains. A back or neck brace may also be of considerable value for mechanical support after some types of spinal procedures.

The postoperative leakage of cerebrospinal fluid through a laminectomy incision should be managed in the same way as when it occurs following a cranial operation.

If reoperation in the same area and by the same approach becomes necessary, the patient's previous incision may be reopened. As with cranial reoperations, a detailed report of the original operation is of value to the surgeon planning a second procedure. Dense fibrous connective tissue may be encountered against the dura mater where the laminae and ligamenta flava have been removed; such tissue may distort normal anatomical relationships. Therefore it is wise to begin a second exploration in relatively normal tissue adjacent to the scarred area and to extend the dissection gradually from normal anatomical planes into the scar. This maneuver will usually prevent accidental laceration of the dura mater and its contents.

Anterior Approach

The anterior approaches to the lower lumbar and lower cervical spine are considered in detail elsewhere in this book. Additional information may be found in the pertinent references at the end of this chapter.[25,30,43]

An anterior approach to the first two cervical vertebrae may be made through the oropharynx. This has been used primarily for the drainage of tuberculous and other types of abscesses, though a few surgeons have used this approach to resect tumors or to perform anterior spinal fusions. The procedure is not exceptionally difficult, but it is rarely necessary. Also, this approach is made through a contaminated area, with an appreciable chance of an operative infection.

Lateral Approach

The *direct lateral* approach to the spinal cord is made in some types of percutaneous stereotaxic cervical cordotomy. This, of course, does not involve an open operative exposure.

For some conditions, such as spinal tuberculosis or ruptured thoracic intervertebral disc, however, a *posterolateral* exposure of the spinal canal may be optimal. The details of these operations may be found in the appropriate references at the end of this chapter.[24,33,35]

More *extensive posterolateral and anterolateral* approaches have also been devised for the treatment of spinal tuberculosis and other spinal deformities, but these operations are primarily of interest to the orthopedic surgeon and are not discussed here.

SUMMARY

This chapter briefly outlines some of the techniques used in cranial and spinal operations. Specific operations are dealt with in subsequent chapters. Discussion of current techniques has been in general terms. These methods are under constant refinement and revision by practicing neurosurgeons and must be individualized according to the nature and location of the disease process, the physiological and psychological status of the patient, the skill and experience of the operating team, and the availability of various neurosurgical instruments and equipment.

It must also be stressed that skillful preoperative and postoperative management are necessary to achieve the best results from any type of neurosurgical operation, no matter how well the operative techniques have been performed.

The illustrations used in this chapter have been patterned primarily after those of Gurdjian and Thomas,[13] Cushing,[4] and Asenjo.[11]

REFERENCES

Historical

1. Bancroft, F. W., and Pilcher, C.: Surgical Treatment of the Nervous System. Philadelphia, J. B. Lippincott Co., 1946.
2. Bennett, G.: History. *In* Howorth, M. B., and Petrie, J. G., eds.: Injuries of the Spine. Baltimore, Williams & Wilkins Co., 1964, pp. 1–59.
3. Bick, E. M.: Source Book of Orthopaedics. 2nd Ed. Baltimore, Williams & Wilkins Co., 1948.
4. Cushing, H.: Surgery of the head. *In* Keen, W. W., ed.: Surgery, Its Principles and Practice. Philadelphia, W. B. Saunders Co., 1908, *3*:17–276.
5. Dandy, W. E.: Surgery of the brain. *In* Lewis' Practice of Surgery. Hagerstown, Md., W. F. Prior Co., Inc., 1932, *12*:1–682.
6. Elsberg, C. A.: Diagnosis and Treatment of Surgical Diseases of the Spinal Cord and Its Membranes. Philadelphia, W. B. Saunders Co., 1916.
7. Naffziger, H. C.: Brain surgery. Surg. Gynec. Obstet., *46*:241–248, 1928.
8. Walker, A. E.: A History of Neurological Surgery. Baltimore, Williams & Wilkins Co., 1951.
9. Wilkins, R. H.: Neurosurgical Classics. New York, Johnson Reprint Corp., 1965.

Review

10. Alexander, E., Jr.: Neurosurgical techniques, J. Neurosurg., *24*:818–819, 1966.
11. Asenjo, A.: Neurosurgical Techniques. Springfield, Ill., Charles C Thomas, 1963.
12. Crenshaw, A. H.: Campbell's Operative Orthopaedics. 5th Ed. St. Louis, C. V. Mosby Co., 1971.
13. Gurdjian, E. S., and Thomas, L. M.: Operative Neurosurgery. 3rd Ed. Baltimore, Williams & Wilkins Co., 1970.
14. Irsigler, F. J.: Allgemeine Operationslehre. *In* Olivecrona, H., and Tönnis, W., eds.: Handbuch der Neurochirurgie. Berlin, Springer-Verlag, 1960, Vol. IV, Part I, pp. 1–121.
15. Kempe, L. G.: Operative Neurosurgery. New York, Springer-Verlag, 1968–1970.
16. Krayenbühl, H.: Advances and Technical Standards in Neurosurgery. New York, Springer-Verlag. Vol. 1, 1974; Vol. 2, 1975.
17. Logue, V.: Operative Surgery, 14. Neurosurgery. 2nd Ed. Philadelphia, J. B. Lippincott Co., 1971.
18. Matson, D. D.: Neurosurgery of Infancy and Childhood. 2nd Ed. Springfield, Ill., Charles C Thomas, 1969.
19. Poppen, J. L.: An Atlas of Neurosurgical Techniques. Philadelphia, W. B. Saunders Co., 1960.

General

20. Albin, M. S., Babinski, M., Maroon, J. C., and Jannetta, P. J.: Anesthetic management of posterior fossa surgery in the sitting position. Acta Anesthes. Scand., *20*:117–128, 1976.
21. Albin, M. S., Bunegin, L., Dujovny, M., Bennett, M. H., Jannetta, P. J., and Wisotzky, H. M.: Brain retraction pressure during intracranial procedures. Surg. Forum, *26*:499–500, 1975.
22. Bucy, P. C.: Exposure of the posterior or cerebellar fossa. J. Neurosurg., *24*:820–832, 1966.
23. Burton, C. V., and McFadden, J. T.: Neurosurgical materials and devices. Report on regulatory agencies and advisory groups. J. Neurosurg., *45*:251–258, 1976.
24. Capener, N.: The evolution of lateral rachotomy. J. Bone Joint Surg., *36-B*:173–179, 1954.
25. Cloward, R. B.: The anterior approach for removal of ruptured cervical disks. J. Neurosurg., *15*:602–614, 1958.
26. Davidoff, L. M.: The brain and spinal cord. *In* Rothenberg, R. E., ed.: Reoperative Surgery. New York, Blakiston Div., McGraw-Hill Book Co., 1964, pp. 40–70.
27. Decker, R. E., and Malis, L. I.: Surgical approaches to midline lesions at the base of the skull: A review. Mt. Sinai J. Med., *37*:84–102, 1970.
28. Donaghy, R. M. P., and Yasargil, M. G.: Microvascular Surgery. Report of First Conference, October 1–7, 1966. Mary Fletcher Hospital, Burlington, Vermont. St. Louis, C. V. Mosby Co., 1967.
29. Ducker, T. B.: Tissue adhesives in neurosurgery. *In* Matsumoto, T., ed.: Tissue Adhesives in Surgery. Flushing, N.Y., Medical Examination Publishing Co., 1972, pp. 281–289.
30. Goldner, J. L., McCollum, D. E., and Urbaniak, J. R.: Anterior intervertebral discectomy and arthrodesis for treatment of low back pain with or without radiculopathy. Clin. Neurosurg., *15*:352–381, 1968.
31. Handa, H., Ohta, T., and Kamijyo, Y.: Encasement of intracranial aneurysms with plastic compounds. Prog. Neurol. Surg., *3*:149–192, 1969.
32. Hart, D., and Nicks, J.: Ultraviolet radiation in the operating room. Intensities used and bactericidal effects. Arch. Surg., *82*:449–465, 1961.
33. Hodgson, A. R., Stock, F. E., Fang, H. S. Y., and Ong, G. B.: Anterior spinal fusion. The operative approach and pathological findings in 412 patients with Pott's disease of the spine. Brit. J. Surg., *48*:172–178, 1960.
34. Horwitz, N. H., and Rizzoli, H. V.: Postoperative Complications in Neurosurgical Practice. Recognition, Prevention and Management. Baltimore, Williams & Wilkins Co., 1967.
35. Hulme, A.: The surgical approach to thoracic intervertebral disc protrusions. J. Neurol. Neurosurg. Psychiat., *23*:133–137, 1960.
36. Keener, E. B.: Regeneration of dural defects: A review. J. Neurosurg., *16*:415–423, 1959.
37. Light, R. U.: Hemostasis in neurosurgery. J. Neurosurg., *2*:414–434, 1945.
38. McFadden, J. T.: Metallurgical principles in neurosurgery. J. Neurosurg., *31*:373–385, 1969.
39. McFadden, J. T.: Tissue reactions to standard neurosurgical metallic implants. J. Neurosurg., *36*:598–603, 1972.
40. Odom, G. L., and Woodhall, B.: Supratentorial skull flaps. J. Neurosurg., *25*:492–501, 1966.
41. Odom, G. L., Woodhall, B., and Wrenn, F. R., Jr.: The use of refrigerated autogenous bone

flaps for cranioplasty. J. Neurosurg., *9*:606–610, 1952.

42. Rand, R. W.: Microneurosurgery. St. Louis, C. V. Mosby Co., 1969.

43. Robinson, R. A., and Southwick, W. O.: Surgical approaches to the cervical spine. Instr. Course Lect., *17*:299–330, 1960.

44. Rowe, S. N.: Types and positions of bone flaps for cranial surgery. Clin. Neurosurg., *13*:63–73, 1966.

45. Schupper, N.: Cranioplasty prostheses for replacement of cranial bone. J. Prosth. Dent., *19*:594–597, 1968.

46. Spiegel, E. A.: Development of stereoencephalotomy for extrapyramidal diseases. J. Neurosurg., *24*:suppl., 433–439, 1966.

47. Stevenson, G. C., Stoney, R. J., Perkins, R. K., and Adams, J. E.: A transcervical transclival approach to the ventral surface of the brain stem for removal of a clivus chordoma. J. Neurosurg., *24*:544–551, 1966.

48. Van Buren, J. M., Ommaya, A. K., and Ketcham, A. S.: Ten years' experience with radical combined craniofacial resection of malignant tumors of the paranasal sinuses. J. Neurosurg., *28*:341–350, 1968.

49. Vieth, R. G., Tindall, G. T., and Odom, G. L.: The use of tantalum dust as an adjunct in the postoperative management of subdural hematomas. J. Neurosurg., *24*:514–519, 1966.

50. Wright, R. L.: Postoperative Craniotomy Infections. Springfield, Ill., Charles C Thomas, 1966.

51. Wright, R. L.: Septic Complications of Neurosurgical Spinal Procedures. Springfield, Ill., Charles C Thomas, 1970.

52. Wright, R. L., and Burke, J. F.: Effect of ultraviolet radiation on postoperative neurosurgical sepsis. J. Neurosurg., *31*:533–537, 1969.

53. Yasargil, M. G.: Microsurgery, Applied to Neurosurgery. Stuttgart, Georg Thieme Verlag, 1969.

32

MICRO-OPERATIVE TECHNIQUE

A recent study of surgical services by the American College of Surgeons and the American Surgical Association ranked the application of microsurgical techniques to the treatment of vascular and neoplastic disorders of the nervous system among the first-order research advances in surgery in recent decades.[1] Microsurgery is defined as surgery done with the aid of the 3 to 40 times magnification provided by the operating microscope. Micro-operative techniques, the methods of accomplishing microsurgical procedures, require careful selection of the means of using magnification and the accurate use of microinstruments to obtain optimal results.

The advantages of micro-operative techniques in neurosurgery were first demonstrated during removal of acoustic neuromas.[20] The benefits of the magnified stereoscopic vision and the intense illumination provided by the microscope were quickly realized in other neurosurgical procedures. Microsurgery has not only improved the technical performance of many standard neurosurgical procedures; e.g., brain tumor removal, aneurysm obliteration, neurorrhaphy, and even lumbar and cervical discectomy, but in addition it has opened new dimensions previously unattainable to the neurosurgeon. With it, anastomosis of extracranial to intracranial arteries, transsphenoidal extirpation of sellar tumors with preservation of the pituitary gland, obliteration of previously inaccessible aneurysms, preservation of the facial and cochlear nerves in acoustic neuroma removal, and numerous other successful interventions in the areas of the brain and spinal cord are possible. It has improved operative results by permitting neural and vascular structures to be delineated with greater visual accuracy, deep areas to be reached with less brain retraction and smaller cortical incisions, bleeding points to be coagulated with less damage to adjacent neural structures, nerves distorted by tumor to be preserved with greater frequency, and anastomosis and suture of small vessels and nerves not previously possible. Its use has resulted in smaller wounds, less postoperative neural and vascular damage, better hemostasis, more accurate nerve and vascular repairs, and operations for some previously inoperable lesions. It has introduced a new era in surgical education by permitting the observation and recording, for later study and discussion, of minute operative detail not visible to the naked eye.

The use of micro-operative techniques has disadvantages. Training in the use of the microscope, microinstruments, and microsuture is required, as is a shift away from tactile-manual technique using fingers to one relying on vision-oriented instruments. The equipment is moderately expensive and requires added space in the operating room, and its care places an added burden on the nursing staff. The surgeon must keep head, eye, and shoulders in a constant position for long periods, which is fatiguing, and must maintain profound concentration. Distractions are poorly tolerated in operations under the microscope. It has been speculated that by prolonging some procedures, micro-operative techniques may increase the risks of anesthesia and infection. By allowing operations to be done through smaller openings, however, and by permitting increasing accuracy of dissection, they may reduce the duration of the procedure. Furthermore, any lengthening of the procedure by the use of microtechnique is progressively reduced as one gains experience.

A. L. RHOTON, JR.

Performing operations with loupes (magnifying lenses attached to eyeglasses) is a form of microsurgery.[11,23] Loupes are an improvement over the naked eye, but even when combined with a headlight, they lack many of the advantages of the microscope. Most surgeons are unable to use loupes that provide more than two to three times magnification, the lower limit of resolution provided by the operating microscope. For craniotomy many surgeons use loupes during the initial part of the operation and bring the microscope into the operative field just before or after opening the dura mater.

By no means has the final stage been reached on a subject as rapidly developing as microneurosurgery. It may be expected that the increasing applications of micro-operative technique will open further new avenues for neurosurgery. Texts on microneurosurgery are available for those desiring more information.*

TRAINING

Only when the surgeon has acquired proficiency in the use of the microscope should he undertake operations on patients. Clinical microtechnique should be applied first to procedures with which the surgeon is entirely familiar, such as excision of ruptured discs and the like, before expanding its use to new and technically more difficult procedures. Early in one's experience with the microscope, one tends to use it in less demanding situations and to discontinue its use when one encounters hemorrhage or problems of unusual complexity. Increasing experience, however, makes it apparent that bleeding is more accurately and quickly stopped under magnification and that the hemorrhage that occurs in operations performed under the microscope tends to be of lesser magnitude than that in operations done without magnification.

Neurosurgery demands of the surgeon such versatility with the microscope that special training in its use is needed. For operations on the eye and ear, the microscope is fixed in one position that varies only slightly from operation to operation. In neurosurgery, not only may the location of the operative site vary from procedure to

procedure, from the head to the spine or even to the distal parts of an extremity, but the depth of the operative field may vary from a few millimeters to several inches. The patient may be horizontal, so placed that the surgeon looks down on the operative site, or in the sitting position with the operative site directly in front of the surgeon. Because of the variety of operative sites in neurosurgery and the demands thus placed on the microscope, more training in its use is required for the neurosurgeon than for other specialists using it.

The surgeon should be knowledgeable about: (1) the basic optical and mechanical principles of the operating microscope; (2) the common types of mechanical and electrical failure that affect it and how to correct them; (3) the procedure of dismantling it into its component parts and supporting couplings and then rebuilding it (see Figs. 32–1 and 32–5); (4) the technique of removing the microscope from its stand and modifying it for use with the patient in either the horizontal or sitting position; (5) the selection of lenses, eyepieces, binocular tubes, light sources, stands, and accessories for different operations (see Figs. 32–2 to 32–4 and 32–6 to 32–8); and (6) the use of bipolar coagulators (see Fig. 32–9), air and electric drills, aneurysm clips and their appliers, self-retaining brain retractors (see Fig. 32–10), and other microsurgical instruments.

The laboratory provides a setting in which the mental and physical adjustments required for doing microsurgery can be mastered. For example, with the commonly used inclined binocular tube, the image is not in the surgeon's direct line of sight. Mental adjustment is required likewise to adapt to the expansion of the 6- to 60-mm field to become one's full horizon, with apparent speed of movement and physiological tremor being magnified proportionately.[6] Coordination must be increased and the speed of movement slowed in proportion to the magnification.

Training in the laboratory is essential before one undertakes microanastomotic procedures on patients (e.g., superficial temporal to middle cerebral artery anastomosis). These techniques cannot be learned by watching others do them; they must be perfected on animals. Furthermore, one should return to the laboratory for practice in order to maintain micro-operative dexterity and to test new instru-

---

* See references 10,13,17,19,28,36.

ments and suture material. Acquiring proficiency in the suture of small vessels may take a few days to several months of daily drill. Buncke, Chater, and Szabo suggest the ideal learning time for a motivated person working in a well-equipped laboratory as at least one month, and Yaşargil recommends several months of practice to master the technique of using an operating microscope.[6,37] Brief experience in a well-equipped laboratory is useful if it provides a plan for future learning.

The initial step in learning microsuture technique is to learn to tie knots with forceps under the microscope. Practice in tying knots can be initiated with 5-0 suture passed through a towel. Progressively smaller suture can then be used. After this has been mastered, 8-0 or 9-0 suture can be used to approximate the ends of small Silastic tubes. Eventually the surgeon should acquire experience with 7-0 through 11-0 suture and needles of various sizes.

The next step is to work with specimens of cerebral blood vessels taken from the middle cerebral distribution at autopsy. The ends can be anchored to a towel, the vessel transected, and the divided ends reapproximated under the microscope with 10-0 suture. The final step in learning microsuture technique is to perform an end-to-end and an end-to-side anastomosis on vessels approximately 1 mm in diameter, e.g., the carotid or femoral artery of the rat, with 10-0 suture and a suitable needle. All the cadaver and animal anastomoses should be opened longitudinally under the microscope to check for the accuracy of suture placement, thrombosis, and adventitial displacement internally.

Many useful exercises for the surgeon can be done with the rat, cat, rabbit, and dog.* Detailed descriptions of these laboratory procedures for small-vessel reconstruction are available. They include repair of a longitudinal incision, end-to-end and end-to-side anastomosis, patch grafting of an arterial defect, segmental arterial replacement with an artery or vein, by-pass procedures, duplication of an artery, preparation of a false aneurysm, reimplantation of limbs, and anastomosis between extracranial and intracranial arteries.

---

* See references 4–7,9,14,16,18,38,39.

After one is able to achieve a patent anastomosis on the carotid artery of the rat consistently, a superficial temporal to middle cerebral artery anastomosis can be done on a brain removed at autopsy; the middle cerebral branch is dissected free, and another arterial specimen the size of a superficial temporal artery is used to complete the procedure.

An operating exercise, which in many ways is similar to that required for the preparation of a cerebral aneurysm prior to ligation, is separation of the aorta and vena cava of the rat.[38] The remarkably thin wall of the rodent's vena cava, which is adherent to the adventitia of the aorta, provides an exceptional opportunity for the neurosurgeon to perfect his microtechnique. The goal is to isolate a length of aorta and vena cava without damage to the wall of either and without the use of electrocautery.

Dissection under the microscope of tissues taken from cadavers or at autopsy may increase one's skill. Performance of temporal bone dissection in the laboratory is an accepted component of the microsurgical training for otological operations, and such exercises are of value to the neurosurgeon.[24] One may gain skill in procedures in the cerebellopontine angle by dissecting temporal bone specimens and in transsphenoidal operations by dissecting sphenoid and sellar blocks.[30–33] A detailed microscopic exploration of the perforating branches of the circle of Willis and other common sites of aneurysm occurrence may improve one's technique with aneurysms.[26,34] As the need arises, other selected specimens may also be used to increase acquaintance with other operative sites; e.g., jugular foramen, cavernous sinus, pineal region, or ventricles.

NURSING

The surgical nurse plays an especially important role in microneurosurgery.[2,3] During an operation in which microtechnique is used, the surgeon is required to maintain head and body in a relatively fixed position over prolonged periods because indirect viewing of the operative field necessitates continuous observation of the operative field in order to coordinate hands and eyes. Hence, the nurse should make a constant effort to reduce the number of times the surgeon looks away from the microscope and to limit any distraction. The scrub nurse may need to guide the surgeon's hands to the operative field. Communication between them can be facilitated by a closed television system that allows the nurse to view the operative field displayed on a nearby monitor and thus to place the proper instrument in the surgeon's hands without obliging him to take his eyes away from the microscope (see Fig. 32–6C). She should know how to drape the microscope quickly, select and place aneurysm clips in the appropriate applier, pass instruments into the surgeon's hands ready for use without further manipulation, clean the tips of the bipolar forceps rapidly after each coagulation, place bits in the different microsurgical drills, clean microsurgical suction tips rapidly, pass cottonoids into the surgeon's forceps without requiring him to look away from the microscope, and unpack and place microsuture in the appropriate needle holder. A nurse can increase her knowledge and understanding of microtechnique by learning such techniques as suturing under the microscope in the animal laboratory.

The nurse should understand how each piece of equipment is to be used. She should be skilled in the operation and maintenance of the microscope, able to prepare it for the particular operation—including selecting the appropriate lenses—and able to ready it for use with the patient in the supine or sitting position. She should also be able to deal with commonly encountered mechanical and electronic malfunctions of the microscope, the bipolar coagulator, surgical drills, special suction and cautery devices, retractors, headholders, and other special instruments.

The circulating nurse or technician should be knowledgeable about all electrical and suction outlets in the room. She must be immediately available to adjust the bipolar coagulator and suction, rapidly change the microscope bulb or other light source, replace clouded or dirty objective lenses or eyepieces, adjust all foot pedals for the microscope or other microsurgical equipment, and locate additional equipment. The nurse should record the surgeon's eyepiece settings so that all replacement eyepieces are properly adjusted for use.

THE MICROSCOPE

Before a microscope for microneurosurgery is selected, other surgeons who are expert in the field should be consulted and the needs of the institution should be reviewed with various microscope distributors. The most important considerations in this selection are summarized by Urban. He writes,

A surgical microscope deemed suitable for microneurosurgery should be capable of providing the following:
1. A clear stereoscopic view of the operating field without discomfort to the surgeon;
2. Ample illumination at the surgical field without damage to tissue;
3. Homogeneous illumination of the field;
4. An objective lens that is interchangeable to permit changes in working distance from surgical microscope objective to the operating field;
5. Variable magnification either by a turret drum type or zoom type. Magnifications of approximately 3.5 to 25 × are ample;
6. A microscope that is well balanced and free in all axial motions; it should require a minimum amount of effort to position and should be capable of removal from the surgical field without delay;
7. A coaxial lamp assembly that is readily accessible in case of lamp failure, even though the surgical microscope is draped for sterility; and
8. A microscope assembly with provision to accept accessories including both film and electronic image formation, and an observation tube for direct view by an observer or assistant surgeon.[25]

The operating microscope consists of a series of lenses, aligned to give a stereoscopic image, and a built-in illumination system. It is a low-power microscope capable of being adjusted to give stepwise increases in magnification between 3 and 40 times.

The basic microscope, starting at the surgeon's eyes and moving toward the operative field, consists of: a set of eyepieces that can be adjusted to correct for myopia or hyperopia in either one or both of the surgeon's eyes, a binocular tube or head assembly into which the eyepieces fit and that can be adjusted to accommodate the surgeon's interpupillary distance, a magnification changer of either a zoom or turret assembly type, and an objective lens that determines the working distances between

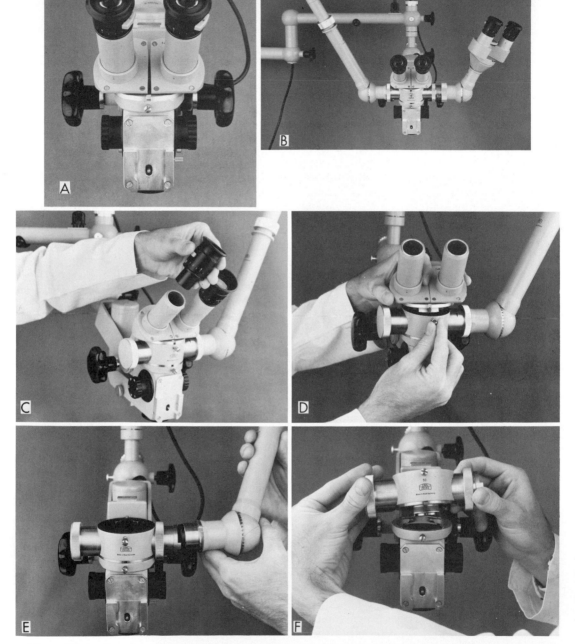

Figure 32–1 Steps in assembling operating microscope. *A*. Microscope viewed from surgeon's working position. Binocular tube above, microscope body below. Adjustable locks are on lower right of hand wheels on eyepieces. The hand wheels are rotated to bring image into focus. Large black knobs to each side of microscope are rotated to alter vertical height of microscope. Small black knobs to each side are rotated to change magnification. *B*. Beam splitter inserted between binocular tube and microscope body. Monocular observer tube on left and binocular observer tube on right of beam divider. *C*. High point eyepiece removed by gently withdrawing it from binocular tube. *D*. Binocular tube removed by loosening finger screw. *E*. Observer tube removed from beam splitter by loosening ring nut on beam splitter. *F*. Zeiss beam splitter removed after finger screw on front of microscope has been loosened.

Illustration continued on opposite page

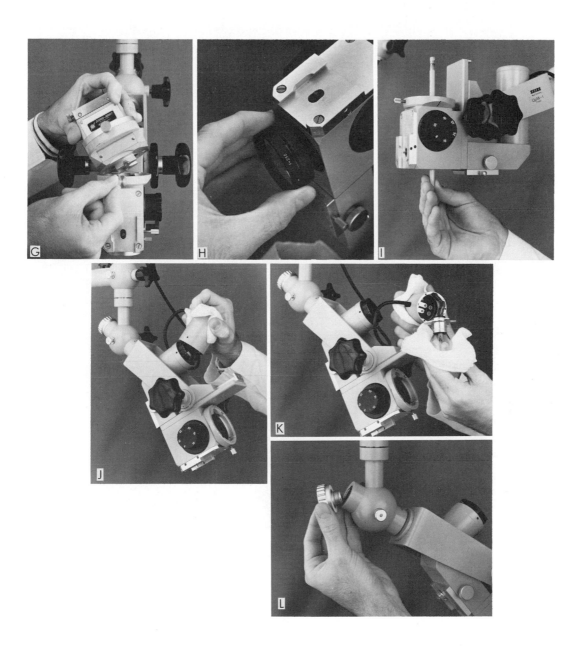

Figure 32–1 (*continued*) G. Urban beam splitter being removed. H. Objective lens rotated out of its socket in microscope housing. Focal length in millimeters is inscribed on side of objective lens. I. Pencil passed through lens changer at 16–16 position to illustrate that magnification at this setting determined by only eyepieces and objective lens. The 6–40 × and the 10–25 × positions contain telescopic lenses that increase or decrease the magnification, depending on which is rotated toward the binocular tube. J. Microscope bulb housing removed by rotating it clockwise. K. Light bulb removed from bulb housing by rotating it clockwise. Dry cloth is used to manipulate bulb because grease from hand shortens bulb life. L. First of two steps to remove microscope from stand by loosening retention bolt.

Illustration continued on following page

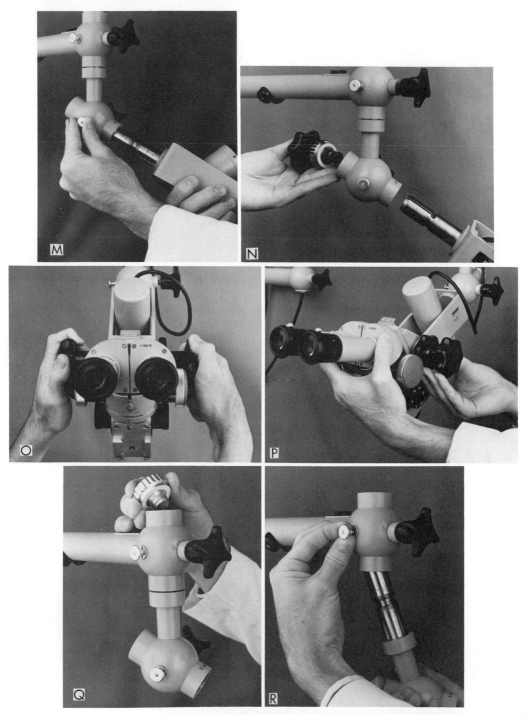

Figure 32–1 (*continued*)   *M*. Final step in removing microscope involves loosening black friction knob and pulling spring lock outward to free the microscope from its coupling. *N*. Spreader bolt used to attach microscope yoke to stand. Tightening bolt adjusts ease with which microscope yoke rotates in coupling. Adjusting this bolt allows the microscope to hold its position with accessories of different weights on each side and yet to rotate in its yoke under gentle pressure without loosening the friction locks. *O*. Hands on vertical control knobs. Rotating one knob or both knobs in same direction will alter the vertical position of the microscope. Rotating one knob while the other is fixed alters the ease of adjusting the vertical position of the microscope. *P*. Tightening the inner black knob on right side alters the ease with which microscope body rotates within its yoke. *Q*. First of two steps in unlocking coupling arms holding microscope involves removing hand bolt. *R*. Final step in removing coupling involves loosening black friction knob and opening spring lock.

the operative field and the microscope (Fig. 32–1).

The microscope most commonly used for neurosurgery, the Zeiss 1 (Carl Zeiss, Inc., New York, N.Y.), has magnification control settings of 6, 10, 16, 25, and 40, but these do not indicate the true magnification. The actual magnification is dependent upon the focal length of the objective lens, the eyepieces, and the magnification changer setting (Table 32–1). The eyepieces and objective lens usually selected for neurosurgery yield about half the magnification listed on the magnification control knob. Enlargement of the image is acquired at the expense of depth and breadth of field. Experience increases one's ability to work at the higher ranges of magnification with smaller, shallower fields.

Eyepieces and Microscope Focus

Eyepieces that magnify between 5 and 20 times are available (Fig. 32–1C). Those with a wide aperture, first developed for persons wearing eyeglasses, are now used routinely for all microscopes. Each eyepiece has a small hand wheel that is rotated to bring the image into focus. It is important that the eyepieces be properly set for each surgeon. These settings remain constant for each person and should be noted by the nursing staff so that eyepieces can be set correctly for the individual surgeon at the beginning of the procedure.

To determine the proper setting of the eyepieces, make a dot on a white piece of paper to use as a focus target and place the paper on a flat surface under the objective lens of the microscope. Set both eyepieces on 0 and the lens changer to 40 ×. Place the left eye over the left eyepiece and focus the microscope up and down to bring the dot into focus. Now, without moving the focus or the vertical adjustment of the microscope, rotate the changer to 6 × and adjust the hand wheel on the left eyepiece to obtain a sharp image of the dot. This setting will coincide with the sharp focus of the reticle if the eyepiece has one. Repeat checks should fall within ¼ diopter difference. Follow the same procedure with the right eye and eyepiece. Record the diopter ring settings for future use.

For a surgeon with normal vision the eyepiece diopter corrective scale on both lenses could be set at 0. This scale can be used to correct for simple myopia and hyperopia; however, most surgeons with these visual corrections prefer to wear their eyeglasses during the procedures because they can then visualize instruments and the operative field when looking away from the microscope. The surgeon with significant astigmatism should wear his glasses because the eyepieces do not provide any adjustment for it.

Binocular or Head Assembly

The binocular tubes into which the two adjustable eyepieces fit consist of two objective lenses and shclf-prism assemblies (the latter for proper orientation of the image) coupled with a means of adjusting the interpupillary distance to suit the operator (Figs. 32–1D, and 32–2A and B). There are two types of binocular tubes: the inclined and the straight. The binocular tube assembly is detachable, and depending on the nature of the operation, either straight or angled tubes can be utilized. The inclined binocular is usually used when the patient is in the horizontal position during operation. The inclined oculars are angled 45 degrees out of the plane in relation to the objective lens and light source. The straight binocular is used when a greater range of tilt of the microscope is required; it is routinely used if the patient is in the sitting position. The straight tube has the advantage that the image is oriented in the direct axis of the surgeon's vision, thus bringing his hand maneuvers into a plane congruous with the image he visualizes. It can be used for all operative fields, whereas the angled tube is awkward and impractical for use in procedures in the posterior fossa or with the patient sitting, although adaptation to the angled image from the inclined binoculars is not difficult for an experienced surgeon. For the beginner, it poses a problem that can be overcome by practice in the laboratory.

Both the inclined and straight binocular tubes are available in 125- and 160-mm focal length. The tube with the shorter focal length is more compact and provides less magnification and a larger field of view.

TABLE 32–1   TOTAL MAGNIFICATIONS AND OBJECT FIELDS OBTAINED*

OBJECTIVE $f_1 =$	EYEPIECES	APPROX. DIAM. OF ILLUM. FIELD	125 MM BODY TUBE — Magnification Changer Set to (Total Magnification / Approximate Diameter of Object Field)					160 MM BODY TUBE — Magnification Changer Set to (Total Magnification / Approximate Diameter of Object Field)				
			6	10	16	25	40	6	10	16	25	40
50mm	10×	8	10 / 20	15.5 / 13	25 / 8.0	40 / 5.0	64 / 3.1	12.5 / 16	20 / 10	32 / 6.2	52 / 3.8	82 / 2.4
	12.5×		12.5 / 16	20 / 10.5	32 / 6.4	52 / 4.0	82 / 2.5	16 / 13	25 / 8.0	40 / 5.0	66 / 3.1	105 / 2.0
	16×		15.5 / 12.5	25 / 8.0	40 / 5.0	64 / 3.1	100 / 2.4	20 / 10	32 / 6.2	52 / 3.8	82 / 2.4	130 / 1.5
	20×		20 / 9.5	31 / 6.2	50 / 3.8	82 / 2.4	130 / 1.5	25 / 7.6	40 / 4.8	64 / 3.0	105 / 1.9	165 / 1.15
100mm	10×	16	5.0 / 40	8.0 / 26	12.5 / 16	20 / 10	32 / 6.2	6.2 / 32	10 / 20	16 / 12.5	26 / 7.8	40 / 5.0
	12.5×		6.2 / 33	10 / 21	16 / 13	25 / 8.0	40 / 5.0	7.8 / 26	12.5 / 16	20 / 10	32 / 6.2	52 / 4.0
	16×		8.0 / 25	12.5 / 16	20 / 10	32 / 6.2	50 / 4.0	10 / 20	16 / 12.5	25 / 7.8	40 / 5.0	64 / 3.1
	20×		10 / 19	15.5 / 12.5	25 / 7.6	40 / 4.8	64 / 3.0	12.5 / 15.5	20 / 9.5	32 / 6.0	52 / 3.8	82 / 2.4
125mm	10×	20	4.0 / 52	6.2 / 32	10 / 20	16 / 12.5	25 / 7.8	5.0 / 40	8.0 / 25	12.5 / 15.5	20 / 10	32 / 6.2
	12.5×		5.0 / 42	7.8 / 26	12.5 / 16	20 / 10	32 / 6.4	6.2 / 32	10 / 20	16 / 12.5	26 / 7.8	40 / 5.0
	16×		6.2 / 32	10 / 20	16 / 12.5	25 / 7.8	40 / 5.0	8.0 / 25	12.5 / 16	20 / 10	32 / 6.2	52 / 3.8
	20×		7.8 / 24	12.5 / 15.5	20 / 9.5	32 / 6.0	50 / 3.8	10 / 19	16 / 12	25 / 7.6	40 / 4.6	64 / 2.9
150mm	10×	24	3.2 / 60	5.2 / 38	8.5 / 24	13.5 / 15	21 / 9.5	4.2 / 48	6.6 / 30	10.5 / 19	17 / 11.5	27 / 7.4
	12.5×		4.2 / 50	6.6 / 32	10.5 / 19	17 / 12	27 / 7.6	5.2 / 38	8.2 / 24	13.5 / 15	22 / 9.5	34 / 6.0
	16×		5.2 / 38	8.2 / 24	13.5 / 15	21 / 9.5	34 / 5.8	6.6 / 30	10.5 / 19	17 / 12	27 / 7.4	44 / 4.6
	20×		6.6 / 29	10.5 / 18	16.5 / 12	27 / 7.2	42 / 4.4	8.2 / 23	13 / 14.5	21 / 9.5	34 / 5.6	54 / 3.6
175mm	10×	28	2.8 / 72	4.4 / 46	7.2 / 28	11.5 / 17	18 / 11	3.6 / 56	5.6 / 36	9.0 / 22	14.5 / 13.5	23 / 8.5
	12.5×		3.6 / 58	5.6 / 36	9.0 / 23	14.5 / 14	23 / 9.0	4.4 / 46	7.2 / 28	11.5 / 18	18 / 11	29 / 7.0
	16×		4.4 / 44	7.0 / 28	11.5 / 18	18 / 11	29 / 6.8	5.6 / 36	9.0 / 22	14.5 / 13.5	23 / 8.5	36 / 5.4
	20×		5.6 / 34	9.0 / 22	14.5 / 13.5	23 / 8.5	36 / 5.2	7.2 / 27	11.5 / 17	18 / 10.5	29 / 6.6	46 / 4.2
200mm	10×	32	2.4 / 82	3.8 / 52	6.2 / 32	10 / 20	16 / 12.5	3.1 / 64	5.0 / 40	8.0 / 25	12.5 / 15.5	20 / 10
	12.5×		3.1 / 66	4.8 / 42	7.8 / 26	12.5 / 16	20 / 10	4.0 / 52	6.2 / 33	10 / 20	16 / 12.5	25 / 8.0
	16×		3.8 / 52	6.2 / 32	10 / 20	16 / 12.5	25 / 7.8	5.0 / 40	7.8 / 25	12.5 / 16	20 / 10	32 / 62
	20×		4.8 / 40	7.8 / 25	12.5 / 15.5	20 / 9.5	32 / 6.0	6.2 / 31	10 / 19	16 / 12	25 / 7.6	40 / 4.8
225mm	10×	36	2.2 / 90	3.4 / 58	5.6 / 36	9.0 / 22	14 / 14	2.8 / 72	4.4 / 46	7.0 / 28	11.5 / 17	18 / 11
	12.5×		2.8 / 74	4.4 / 46	7.0 / 29	11.5 / 18	18 / 11.5	3.6 / 58	5.6 / 36	9.0 / 23	14.5 / 14	23 / 9.0
	16×		3.4 / 58	5.6 / 36	9.0 / 22	14.5 / 14	23 / 9.0	4.4 / 44	7.0 / 28	11.5 / 18	18 / 11	29 / 6.8
	20×		4.4 / 44	7.0 / 28	11 / 17	18 / 10.5	28 / 6.8	5.6 / 34	9.0 / 22	14 / 13.5	23 / 8.5	36 / 5.2
250mm	10×	40	1.9 / 100	3.1 / 64	5.0 / 40	8.0 / 25	13 / 15.5	2.5 / 80	4.0 / 50	6.4 / 31	10 / 19	16.5 / 12.5
	12.5×		2.5 / 82	4.0 / 52	6.4 / 32	10 / 20	16 / 12.5	3.2 / 64	5.0 / 40	8.0 / 25	13 / 15.5	21 / 10
	16×		3.1 / 64	5.0 / 40	8.0 / 25	13 / 15.5	20 / 10	4.0 / 50	6.4 / 32	10 / 20	16.5 / 12	26 / 7.6
	20×		4.0 / 48	6.2 / 31	10 / 19	16 / 12	25 / 7.6	5.0 / 38	8.0 / 24	13 / 15	21 / 9.5	33 / 5.8
400mm	10×	64	1.2 / 165	2.0 / 105	3.1 / 64	5.0 / 40	8.0 / 25	1.55 / 130	2.5 / 80	4.0 / 50	6.4 / 31	10 / 20
	12.5×		1.55 / 130	2.5 / 82	4.0 / 52	6.4 / 32	10 / 20	2.0 / 105	3.1 / 66	5.0 / 40	8.0 / 25	13 / 16
	16×		2.0 / 100	3.1 / 64	5.0 / 40	8.0 / 25	13 / 15.5	2.5 / 80	4.0 / 50	6.4 / 31	10 / 20	16 / 12.5
	20×		2.5 / 78	3.8 / 50	6.2 / 31	10 / 19	16 / 12	3.1 / 62	5.0 / 38	8.0 / 24	13 / 15	20 / 9.5

* Courtesy of Carl Zeiss, Inc., New York, N.Y.

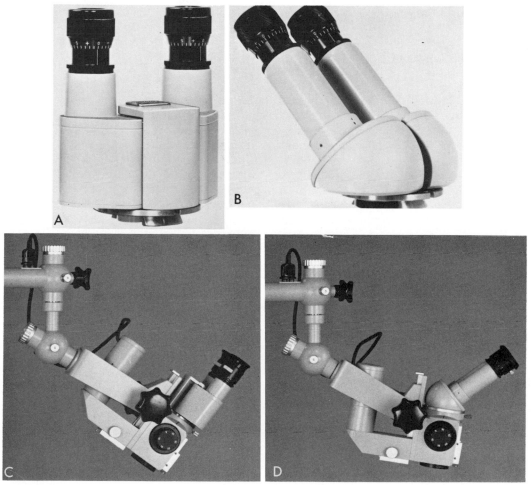

Figure 32–2 Binocular tubes with eyepieces inserted. Rotating hand wheel on eyepieces can be used to correct for hyperopia or myopia. *A*. Straight binocular tube. *B*. Inclined binocular tube. *C*. Microscope with straight binocular tube. *D*. Microscope with inclined binocular tube.

Objective Lens

The focal length of the objective lens determines the working distance between the lens and the operative field (Fig. 32–1*H*). Objective lenses ranging from 50 to 500 mm are available, but lenses of 200-, 250-, or 300-mm focal length are most suitable for neurosurgery. The focal length is stamped on the lens ring and corresponds to the distance between the operative site in focus and the lens. For a superficial operation such as a superficial temporal to middle cerebral artery anastomosis, a 200-mm objective can be used. A 250-mm objective lens is preferred for most other procedures except transsphenoidal operations, which require a 300-mm lens. An objective lens should be selected that not only allows easy passage of instruments between the microscope and the site of dissection without jarring the microscope but also provides for proper focusing at variable wound depths. The surgeon's arm length also affects the choice of focal length used.

Magnification Changer

The Zeiss I operating microscope, the instrument used by most neurosurgeons, is equipped with a turret drum type of magnification changer that is rotated by hand (Fig. 32–1I). The drum holds three optical assemblies (or telescopes) for each eye. Two of the three assemblies are capable of providing two different magnifications each, one high and one low, depending upon which direction the telescope is rotated end-to-end. The third assembly is an open tube and not a telescope. Thus, five different magnifications are made available by rotating the magnification drum to each of the six positions (6–10–16–40–25–16 ×) inscribed on the magnification drum. The reason that the six positions yield only five stages of magnification is that both 16 × positions provide clear passage through the drum, not utilizing any optics and therefore yielding only the magnification determined by the eyepieces, binocular tube, and objective lens. The other lens combinations in the drum increase or decrease this basic magnification. The six numbers listed on the changer represent true magnification only with the 200-mm objective lens and

20 × eyepieces; however, most neurosurgeons use 250- or 300-mm objectives and 10 × or 12.5 × eyepieces. These combinations yield approximately half the magnification inscribed on the changer knob. True magnifications are listed in Table 32–1. Enlargement of the image is always gained at the expense of depth of focus and breadth of field.

Zoom Microscopes

Zoom microscopes provide an alternative to the manual magnification changer (Fig. 32–3). The focusing adjustment, the magnification control knob (zoom), and the height of the microscope are automatically controlled by foot pedals. The microscope housing is necessarily much heavier, and because of this, the stand must be much heavier and more solidly built. The added weight and the heavier stand make the complicated diagonal movements needed in operations at the base of the brain more difficult to perform, and the difficulties are even greater if one needs to move back and forth rapidly between the surface and deep areas of the brain. Many neurosurgeons have found the foot controls difficult to use. These limitations have impeded wide acceptance of the zoom microscope in neurosurgery, although its use has been advocated by Pia.[27]

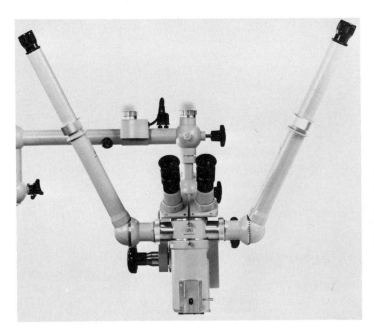

Figure 32–3 Zoom microscope with long monocular observer tubes attached on each side of beam splitter. The microscope body, between beam splitter and objective lens, is much larger and places surgeon's eyes farther from the operative site than model with turret lens changer if equal objective lenses are used. Zoom is adjusted with foot pedal.

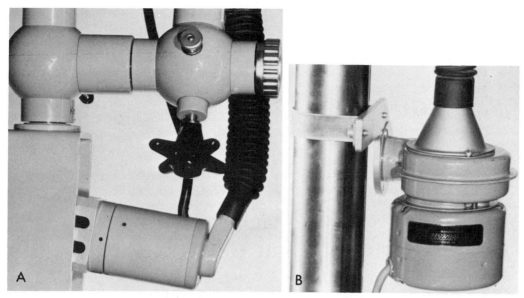

Figure 32-4   Suction system to cool light housing and prolong bulb life. *A*. Flexible black tube and connector cap attached to bulb housing. *B*. Suction tube connected to small motorized blower attached to microscope mounting pole.

Light System

The operating microscope should be equipped with coaxial lighting that provides an illuminated field that is concentric with the field of view. This is especially important in neurosurgery because, with minimal brain retraction, one can obtain excellent stereoscopic vision in deep, narrow exposures. The standard microscope is usually fitted with a simple transformer needed to illuminate a 30-watt bulb, which is adequate for operating in shallow fields at lower magnification without photography (Fig. 32–1*J* and *K*). For neurosurgery, however, a 50-watt bulb with power boosters is desirable. These lamps generate much heat, which accumulates under the microscope drapes; the heat should be dissipated to prolong bulb life. A suction cooling system containing a blower assembly mounted on the microscope column and attached to the lamp housing reduces the heat by sucking air through the lamp housing and out from under the microscope drape (Fig. 32–4).[35] A less expensive alternative is provided by leading a small latex tube from one of the holes of the light bulb housing into an operating room suction outlet. The heat can also be reduced by using a fiberoptic light designed to fit in the microscope light housing; however, this type of light is of lower intensity than can be obtained with the 50-watt 6-volt bulb needed for photography. A recent trend has been to attach an accessory fiberoptic light to the microscope body directly adjacent to the objective lens. This increases the illumination but has the disadvantage that the added light is not coaxial. Halogen light sources, said to be brighter than the 50-watt bulb, will soon be available.

Sterilization

To prevent contamination of the surgeon's hands and instruments by contact with the microscope demands great skill of the surgical nurse. Most surgeons prefer to drape the microscope with a neatly tailored sterile cloth or plastic covering that is carefully fitted to all its protrusions. A cotton drape made of stockinette has the advantage of having some ventilation, which reduces heat build-up under the drapes. Excessive heat can lead to drift and poor function of television cameras and reduce the length of life of light bulbs. Cloth drapes have the disadvantage of being porous, so if the fibers or the material is twisted the field becomes contaminated. Plastic drapes have the advantage of not allowing as frequent contamination of the operative field as porous drapes. If an unusual combination of accessories prevents use of a prefitted drape, one can use large garbage bags, which are slipped over the microscope and snugged up to it with a series of rubber bands. The author prefers clear plastic rather than an opaque drape because it permits easy manipulation of the friction locks and sidearms under direct vision. An easier method, but one that carries a greater risk of contamination, is to place molded sterilizable plastic or rubber caps over all the microscope control knobs that are touched during the operation. To prevent instruments from becoming contaminated against the objective lens, it should be covered with a sterilizable objective shell that covers the lens.

Manufacturers of the microscope have long recommended that instruments not be autoclaved, vapor sterilized, or gas sterilized; for over five years, however, one medical center has been using two ampules of ethylene oxide gas for 12 to 18 hours inside two plastic bags appropriately secured for this purpose. No heat or vapor is involved in this method, which obviates the necessity for draping if the microscope is used only once daily.[17]

Microscope Mount

An important decision is whether to place the microscope on a mobile floor stand or a fixed ceiling mount (Fig. 32–5C). The movable floor stand is essential if the microscope must be used in more than one operating room or shared with another surgical service. If the microscope is to be used for operations with the patient in the upright or sitting position, the mobile floor stand should be 200 centimeters or more in length if the surgeon's height requires it.

A ceiling mount may be superior to a floor mount if one always operates in the same room and the microscope need not be moved elsewhere. The ceiling mount simplifies introduction of the instrument into the operative field and provides increased maneuverability and stability. The expense and technical difficulties associated with its installation, however, may be prohibitive. The ceiling mount is three to five times as expensive as the floor stand; the variable cost depending on the construction needed to mount the microscope in the operating room ceiling. In selecting the position for a ceiling mount one needs to consider all aspects of the operating room utilization—including the overhead light system; the accessibility to suction, compressed air, electrical outlets, anesthetic gases, and leads to monitoring equipment; the table height customarily desired with the patient either sitting or lying down; and the positioning of the surgeon, anesthesiologist, and nurses during each type of operation. One should make sure that engineers can certify that ceiling vibrations will not be a problem.

The viewing portion of the microscope should have mobility through 120 degrees in the horizontal and 90 degrees in the vertical plane. It should lock instantly into a stable position from which it can be easily maneuvered and yet not be shifted by the surgeon looking into the eyepieces.

The friction locks on the microscope should be adjusted to give both mobility and stability. Mobility is needed so that the microscope can be easily maneuvered by hand without having to loosen or tighten the locks with each change of microscope position, and stability so that slight pressure on the surgeon's or assistant's eyepieces does not shift the position (Fig. 32–1L, M, N, and R).

Each time the position of the conventional microscope is readjusted, the surgeon has to lay down his instruments in order to free his hands. An average of 40 per cent of the operating time may be spent positioning the microscope. Because of this, Yaşargil developed a motorized microscope stand (see Fig. 32–5C).[40] A hand or mouth switch on the microscope unlocks the electromagnetic couplings to make it freely movable. The mouth switch is adjusted so that it fits comfortably into the surgeon's mouth as he views the operative field and is coupled to the microscope so that the bite of the teeth against it is sufficient to produce not only vertical but also complex diagonal movements. The microscope is balanced so precisely that unlocking the couplings does not produce movement but the gentlest pressure on the mouthpiece is sufficient to guide it. The motorized microscope stand can be adapted to floor stands or the ceiling mount. The disadvantages of such a unit are its large size, high cost, and sensitive balance mech-

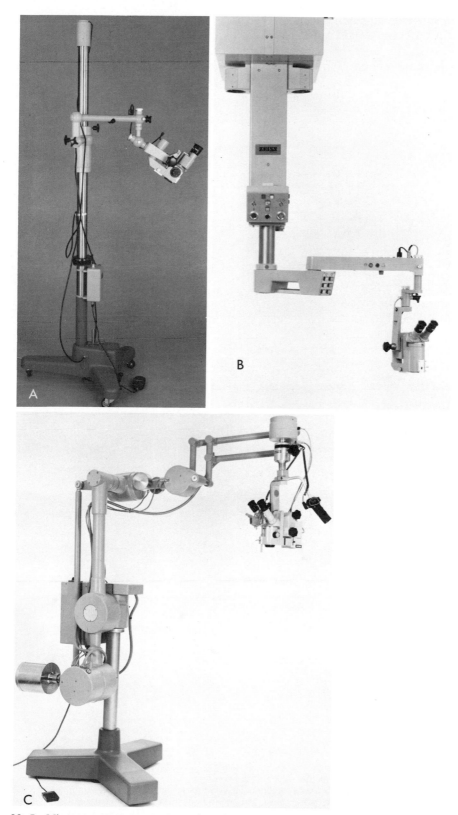

Figure 32–5 Microscope mounts. *A*. Operating microscope on floor stand. Straight-type binocular tube. *B*. Operating microscope on ceiling mount. Microscope of zoom type. *C*. Mobile microscope holder mounted on floor stand. Designed by Yaşargil.

anism that must be adjusted each time accessories of different weight are used.

Care of the Microscope

Urban has made the following suggestions for proper care of the operating microscope.

1. Keep all openings of the microscope covered at all times.

2. Examine objective lens for spots after each use and clean with water moistened cotton gauze.

3. When draping the microscope, allow ventilation of lamp housing to prevent overheating.

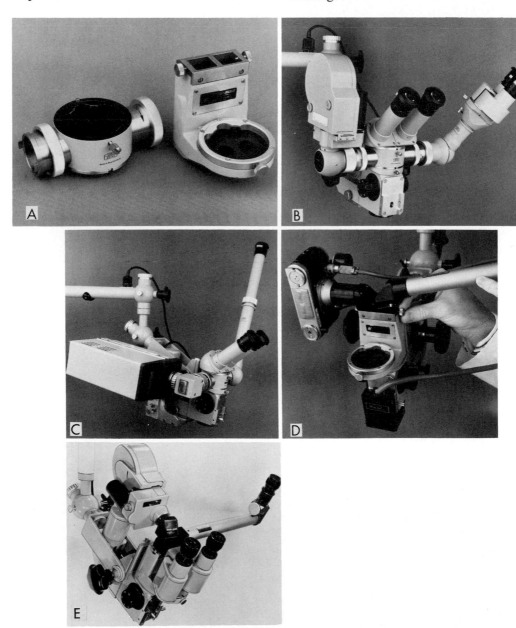

Figure 32–6 Beam splitters and accessories. *A*. Zeiss (*left*) and Urban (*right*) beam splitters. *B*. Movie camera on left side of Zeiss beam splitter; binocular observer tube on right. Cine adaptor between movie camera and beam splitter. *C*. Television camera on left and monocular observer tube on right side of beam splitter. Cine adaptor between camera and beam splitter. *D*. Still camera, 35 mm, and observer tube being attached to Urban beam splitter. Strobe light for photography is attached to microscope body. The binocular tube has been removed. *E*. Movie camera and Urban observer tube attached to Urban beam splitter.

Illustration continued on opposite page

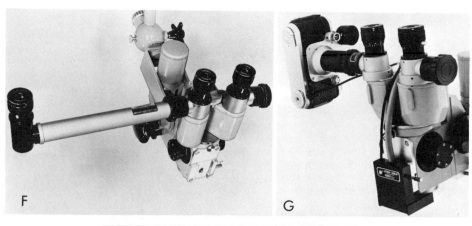

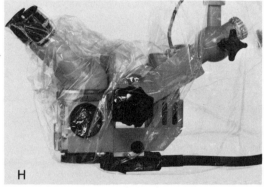

Figure 32–6 (*continued*)   *F*. Beam dividers have been placed in the two sides of the binocular tube. The right beam divider is capped and an Urban observer tube is attached on left. *G*. Thirty-five millimeter still camera attached to beam divider on left side of binocular tube. Beam divider on right side is capped. *H*. Rhoton fiberoptic accessory light attached to dovetail guide adjacent to objective lens. Microscope is draped with sterile clear plastic drape.

4. Do not leave the microscope uncovered when not in use.

5. Do not autoclave or gas vapor sterilize the microscope or accessories.

6. Do not use alcohol, ether, or acetone to clean the painted surfaces of the microscope.

7. Do not overtighten screws, friction locks, or hand wheels.[35]

Microscope Accessories

Accessories have been developed that allow the surgeon's assistants, the nurses, and others to observe the magnified image of the operation while it is in progress (Fig. 32–6). The surgeon can make a variety of permanent visual records of the procedure on film and magnetic tape by using a beam splitter, or divider, which consists of a semitranslucent mirror placed in the path of the incident light beam, a portion of which is thereby reflected into an accessory side tube. The beam divider is placed between the head of the microscope and the binocular tube (Figs. 32–1*B*, *F*, and *G*; 32–3; and 32–6*A* to *F*). Several types of beam dividers are available. The Urban type transmits the image away from the operator, and the accessories are attached to the beam splitter on the side of the microscope opposite the surgeon.* The Zeiss beam splitter directs the accessory images to the right and left sides of the microscope.† The most commonly used variety (50–50) directs half the light into an accessory side tube. A 70–30 beam splitter (30 per cent to the surgeon) allows more light for television, movie, or still cameras. The optical image seen by the surgeon is unaffected by the beam division

---

* Urban Engineering Co., Inc., Burbank, California.

† Carl Zeiss, Inc., New York, New York.

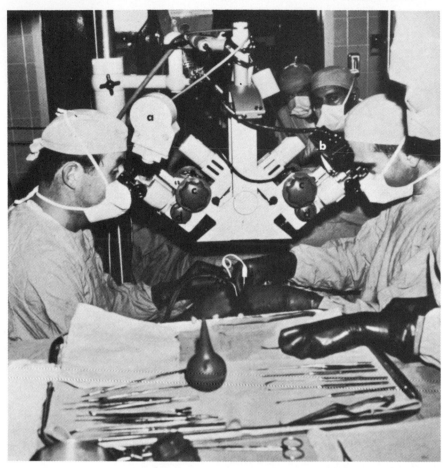

Figure 32–7   The Zeiss binocular diploscope being employed for the first time in October, 1967, during the removal of a spinal cord vascular anomaly by Drs. R. Rand and G. Yaşargil. Note the Urban motion picture camera, a, attached to the left eyepiece assembly and the Urban television camera, b, attached to the right side for closed-circuit television transmission. Sterile caps have been placed over the focusing knobs, c, and the magnifying turret knobs, d. (From Rand, R. W.: Experiences with microneurosurgery in spinal cord tumors and vascular malformation. *In* Rand, R. W., ed.: Microneurosurgery. St. Louis, C. V. Mosby Co., 1969, pp 210–219. Reprinted by permission.)

because it occurs in parallel between the microscope body and tube. The only effect observed by the operator is diminution of brightness. Utilization of the beam dividers does require a better light source, and it is for this purpose that the 50-watt 6-volt bulb and power pack have been developed by Urban.[35] The most common accessory attached to the beam splitter is an observer tube for the surgeon's assistant. Monocular and binocular observer tubes are available (Figs. 32–1E, 32–3, and 32–6B to F).

An interesting alternative to the observer tube is the binocular diploscope built in 1961 by Litton out of two operating microscopes coupled rigidly in an axis of 180 degrees (Fig. 32–7).[21] The two microscopes function independently, but the device is a helpful teaching aid in that the assistant obtains the same stereoscopic view of the operation as the surgeon. It is suitable only for those operations in which the surgeon and his assistant stand directly opposite one another. It has not gained wide use for neurosurgical procedures because microscope mobility is limited to less than desirable for many intracranial procedures and because diagonal movements are difficult to execute. Its greatest usefulness has been for spinal procedures in which the surgeon and the assistant stand facing each other on opposite sides of the patient. Lougheed has, however, used the diploscope for intracranial operative procedures on aneurysms.[21]

The other commonly used accessories are a 35-mm still camera, 16-mm and super 8 movie cameras, and black and white or color television cameras (Fig. 32–6*B, C, D, E,* and *G*). A photoadapter with a light intensity control (the f-stop shutter) must be placed between the Zeiss beam splitter and these accessories (but not between the Urban beam splitter and the accessories) (Fig. 32–6*B* and *C*). The surgeon can change the accessories depending on his interest and the needs of his assistants.

Instantaneous viewing of the procedure can best be facilitated by displaying the output of a television camera on a monitor in the operating room and, if desired, at a remote site. The output of the television camera also can be fed through a magnetic tape recorder and the operation recorded for review and study later (see Fig. 32–6*C*). Having a television screen in the operating room for immediate viewing by assistants, nurses, and anesthesiologists is an innovation that has increased knowledge of and interest in the operative procedures.

The number of commercial manufacturers producing television cameras adapted to the microscope is increasing. Prior to purchasing a camera, compare the various models by placing different types of camera on the two sides of the beam splitter and evaluating the images on comparable television monitors.

Two accessories, one on each side of the beam splitter, are commonly used; one may, however, desire three or more accessories such as a combination of a still 35-mm camera, a television camera, and an observer tube, or another consisting of a movie camera, a still camera, and an observer tube. This can be achieved by one of two means. An optical switch, built to accommodate two accessories, may be attached to either of the two ports of the Zeiss beam splitter. Adjusting the switch directs the image to either but not both of the accessories (Fig. 32–8). Another alternative permitting the use of three or four accessories is to place a beam divider in one or both sides of the binocular tube; thus two accessories may be attached to the conventional beam splitter between the binocular tube and the microscope body and another may be attached to each side of the binocular tube (see Fig. 32–6*F, G,* and *H*). Theoretically, four accessories could be used if beam switches were placed on each side of a conventional beam splitter or a beam divider was placed in each side of the binocular tube.

The attachment of multiple accessories has placed great demands on the lighting system and has reduced the light reaching the surgeon's eye. Initially, microscopes were equipped with 30-watt bulbs; however, 50-watt bulbs powered by transformers yielding greater voltage were introduced by Urban and are now built into most units. The increased light from the more powerful bulb has proved satisfactory for

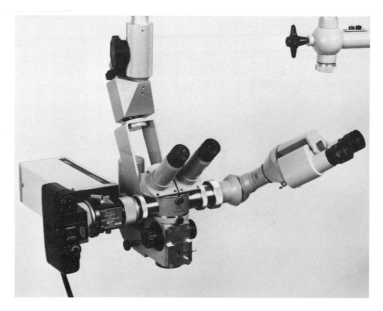

Figure 32–8 Photoadapter with optical switch attached to left side of beam divider; television and 35-mm camera are attached to the photoadaptor. Binocular observer tube is on right.

most applications. Still more light can be obtained by leaving the 50-watt light in the light housing and attaching a fiberoptic light to the microscope adjacent to the objective lens (Fig. 32–6*H*). Dual fiberoptic cables have also been developed; one may be inserted into the light housing and the other attached near the objective lens, or both may be attached near the objective lens. Having lights near the objective lens makes draping more difficult, and they also may limit the passage of instruments between the microscope and the operative field because they project downward from the microscope.

Because of inadequate light, reception from color television cameras is often good during surface operations but not deep procedures. Fox has summarized the methods for improving lighting for operating a microscope television camera as follows:

1. Use 50- instead of 30-watt bulbs.

2. Keep bulbs and optical system clean.

3. Discard bulbs with blue or dark spots in light image.

4. Use shorter focal length objective lens.

5. Use eyepieces with greater magnification. They require less magnification (and hence lose less light) inside microscope unit.

6. Avoid zoom lens system, which absorbs more light.

7. Use 30–70 beam splitter (70 per cent to side arms) instead of 50–50 beam splitter.

8. Open diaphragm of camera (but lose sharpness and depth of focus).

9. Properly adjust camera power supply and television monitor.

10. Turn off bright lights in operating room (better contrast; surgeon's pupils dilate, requiring less light).

11. Select efficient television camera that can operate with less light.

12. Make use of reflections in operative wound.

13. Remove black paint border around glass light deflector behind objective lens (some Zeiss microscopes).

14. Use add-on fiberoptic light sources.[17]

MICRO-OPERATIVE INSTRUMENTS

The role of the microscope has been stressed, but specific details of instrument

selection for microsurgery have received less attention. Achieving optimal results with micro-operative technique requires that the accurate use of appropriate microinstruments be combined with magnification. Originally, neurosurgery borrowed instruments from ophthalmological and otological surgeons and from jewelers. For new ideas, neurosurgeons should continue to scrutinize instrument developments by jewelers and the other surgical specialties. When new and unfamiliar instruments are selected, they should be tested in the laboratory prior to being used in the operating room. The surgeon should acquire a limited number of instruments for use while learning the basic micro-operative skills in the laboratory. The number and variety of instruments can then be expanded as needs and operative skill develop.

The neurosurgeon will need microscissors, microneedle holders, straight and bayonetted forceps with tips ranging from 0.3 to 2.0 mm, small suction tubes of 3, 5, and 7 French size (3 units on the French scale equals 1 mm outer diameter, i.e., 15 French equals 5 mm, and so forth), microdissectors and microforceps such as jeweler's forceps. Additional instruments include regular and microvascular clips, clip appliers, microsuture, self-retaining brain retractors, bipolar coagulators, continuous suction and irrigation units, nerve stimulators, microdrills, and dependable fixed head rests.

Conventional macro-operative instruments are designed with working tips as small as 2 to 3 mm. Most microinstruments are modifications of well-known macroinstruments, e.g., bayonet forceps and dissectors with miniature tips. One should try to obtain microinstruments with handles and designs similar to those one uses for operation without magnification. The instruments should have a dull finish because the brilliant light from highly polished instruments reflected back through the microscope can interfere with the surgeon's vision and detract from the quality of photographs taken through the microscope. Sharpness and sterilization are not affected by the dull finish.

The separation between the instrument tips should be only enough to allow them to straddle the tissue, the needle, or the thread in order to cut or grasp it accurately. Excessive opening and closing movements required by wide tip separation reduce the functional accuracy of the instrument during delicate manipulation under high magnification. The finger pressure required to bring widely separated tips together against firm spring tension often initiates a fine tremor and inaccurate movement. Micro-operative tissue forceps should have a tip separation of no more than 8 mm, needle holder tips should open no more than 3 mm, and scissor tips should open no less than 2 mm and no more than 5 mm depending on the length of the blade and their use.

The length of the instruments should be adequate for the particular task that is being contemplated. Standard jewelers forceps (11 cm in length) are barely long enough for use on the cerebral surfaces. Straight forceps, needle holders, and scissors approximately 18 cm in length are more satisfactory for use on the scalp and near, but not below, the surface of the brain. Bayonetted instruments (forceps, needle holders, and scissors) having 8-cm shafts (the length between the handles and tips) may be used near or just below the cortical surface, but a 10-cm length is needed for the cerebello-pontine angle, the sellar region, or near the circle of Willis. Bayonet instruments with shorter shafts (6 cm) are available; however, they are not commonly used nor do they have a significant advantage over straight instruments 18 cm in length. For trans-sphenoidal operations, instruments having shafts 9.5 to 12 cm long are needed.

Care of Microinstruments

Micro-operative techniques require new rigorous criteria of cleanliness, approximation, smoothness, and general excellence in performance of surgical instruments, which in turn demands correspondingly meticulous care of them. Special attention devoted to delicate microinstruments pays off in long and dependable service. The following are helpful points for their handling.[15,25,29]

1. A single person should be responsible for the care of the microinstruments. He or she must know the function of each and the types of soaps and oils that the manufacturer recommends for its care.

2. This person should insure that the instruments are carefully cleaned by hand or in an ultrasonic washer and thoroughly dried. Drying is especially important so that rust will not develop in small or concealed moving parts. Each instrument with removable parts should be disassembled before washing. Some require precleaning by hand with a soft, child-size toothbrush.

3. Microinstruments should have their own special washing baskets that separate them from each other. The instruments should never be stacked, dropped, or left loose to move around freely, thereby crushing or scratching each other.

4. Appropriately sized stylets must be used to clean open tubular instruments such as suction tips. Air pressure is also helpful in primary cleaning of inaccessible spots.

5. Instruments with moving parts should be carefully oiled with a special lubricant after each washing to insure that these parts move smoothly during the next operation.

6. A microinstrument should be used only for the purpose for which it was designed. A microneedle holder for 8-0 suture should never hold a 4-0 silk suture needle.

7. The special tray of microinstruments should be placed within the range of the surgeon only when the microscope is being used. On the tray the instruments should be carefully separated from each other. All sharp instruments should be positioned so their points are protected.

8. Between operations, each instrument should be inspected under the microscope for surface flaws (scratches, chips, indentations) and functional flaws (nonapproximation of forceps points, jerky movement of scissors or a noncutting area on their blades).

9. When not in use, clean, dry instruments should be stored in individual foam-lined boxes or compartments.

Bipolar Coagulator

The bipolar electrocoagulator is fundamental to the performance of micro-operative procedures because it allows accurate, fine coagulation of small vessels, minimizing dangerous spread of current that burns and damages surrounding tissues. Greenwood introduced its use to neurosurgery in 1940 and proved it to be safer in critical areas than "unipolar" coagulation.[12] Malis further refined the instrument by developing a unit providing better coagulation at the lowest voltage with the least muscle stimulation while restricting the current to

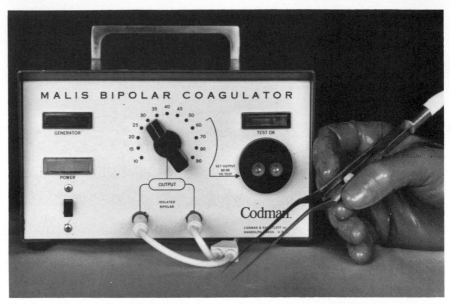

Figure 32–9   Malis bipolar coagulation unit with bayonet coagulation forceps attached.

the shortest path between the tips of the two blades of the forceps with no current of consequence flowing from tip to ground or from tip to patient (Fig. 32–9).[22]

The bipolar unit allows coagulation in areas where unipolar coagulation would be hazardous, such as near cranial nerves, within the ventricles, and around the brain stem. It is important to remember that when the electrode tips touch each other, the current is short-circuited and no coagulation occurs.

Surgeons with experience in conventional coagulation are conditioned to acquire maximal dryness at the surface of application, but with bipolar coagulation some moistness is preferable. Coagulation will take place even if the tips are immersed in saline, and indeed, keeping the tissue moist with local cerebrospinal fluid or saline irrigation during coagulation will reduce heating and minimize drying and sticking of tissue to the forceps. To avoid sticking after coagulation, the points of the forceps should be cleaned after each application to the tissue. If charred blood coats the tips, it should be removed with a damp cloth rather than by scraping with a scalpel blade because the blade may scratch the tips and make them more adherent to tissue during coagulation. The tips of the forceps

should be polished if they become pitted and rough after long use.

Bipolar coagulation may be more effective if it is applied in short bursts of less than one second each. Long bursts may be less effective, possibly because the short bursts allow for better dissipation of heat from the forceps and tissue. Because it is cumbersome to operate the coagulator foot switch in short bursts, Delong and Fox have developed a bipolar coagulation unit that automatically dispenses the current in short regular cycles.[8]

A special property of the coagulator enables the surgeon to coagulate the base of an aneurysm to form a "neck" without causing transmission of heat to the parent vessel and surrounding tissue.[41] This type of operation on aneurysms should be performed only after the surgeon has learned to use the technique in the laboratory and has observed its use clinically.

A series of bipolar forceps with blades ranging in length from 8 to 10 cm and having tips of 0.3 to 2.0 mm will allow coagulation of almost any size vessel encountered in a neurosurgical procedure. The forceps may be straight for surface work and of a bayonet shape for deeper operations. There should be enough tension in the handle of the forceps to allow the surgeon to control the distance between the tips, because no coagulation occurs if the tips touch or are too far apart. Some forceps, so attractive for their delicacv, compress with so little pressure that even with a delicate grasp one cannot avoid closing them during coagulation. The cable connecting the bipolar unit and the coagulation forceps should not be excessively long because longer cables can cause an irregular supply of current.[2] Both cables and forceps should be sterilized.

Brain Retractors

Self-retaining brain retractors have become indispensible to microneurosurgery because they allow the surgeon to work in a relatively confined space unhindered by an assistant's hand, and also because they are more dependable in maintaining constant, gentle retraction of the brain than the surgeon's or assistant's hand. Micro-operative procedures commonly require several hours of retraction, which can lead to severe edema and the need for brain resection. When self-retaining retractors are used, normal appearing brain is often found after removal of a retractor that has been in position for hours. The surgeon should learn to manipulate the retractor while looking through the microscope. The retractor should not be applied so firmly that it blanches the cortical vessels and causes infarction of the underlying brain. Infarction occurs infrequently if blood pressure is normal; however, if hypotension is used, as in aneurysm operations, inadequate perfusion under the retractor may cause infarction and subsequent hemorrhage after the retractor is removed. The self-retaining retractors are of two basic types. One employs a series of straight shafts attached by small clamps to give the correct arm length and configuration for holding the brain spatula in place (Fig. 32–10C). The other consists of a series of ball-and-socket units resembling a chain of pearls with an internal cable that, when tightened, will hold in the desired position. The most frequently used self-retaining brain retractor, the Leyla retractor designed by Yasargil, is of the ball-and-socket type (Fig. 32–10A and B). For some procedures the retractor may be attached directly to the craniectomy margin, but the small craniotomy openings often used for micro-operative procedures make this impractical. The author prefers to attach the retractor arm to a bar fixed to the operating table rather than to the craniectomy margin.

Head Fixation Devices

Under the operating microscope the slightest movement of the patient's head is magnified considerably. Microsurgery demands a precisely maintained position of the firmly fixed cranium whether one operates with the patient in the sitting, the supine, or the prone position. Fixation is best achieved by a pinion headholder in which the essential element is a clamp made to accommodate three relatively sharp pins (Fig. 32–11). The pins penetrate the scalp and are then firmly fixed to the outer table of the skull. When applied properly they allow wide access to any portion of the skull. When the pins are placed, care should be taken to avoid a spinal fluid shunt, surface vessels, thin bones such as the frontal and mastoid sinuses, and the thick temporalis muscle where the pin, however tightly the clamp is applied, tends to remain unstable. The pin should be applied well away from the eye or where it would be a hindrance to making the incision. Special shorter pediatric pins are available for thin skulls. The pins should not be placed over the thin skulls of some patients with a long history of hydrocephalus. After the clamp is secured on the head, it is loosely attached to a headholder fixed to the operating table and the final positioning is done.

This type of immobilization allows rapid intraoperative repositioning of the head. The clamp avoids the skin damage that may occur if the face rests against a padded head support for several hours. The skull clamps do not obscure the face during the operation as do padded headrests, thus permitting easy observation of facial movements when stimulating the facial nerve during an operation in the cerebellopontine angle. For transsphenoidal operations, the clamp should be placed so that it does not obscure the sella on intraoperative fluoroscopy.

Needles, Suture, and Needle Holders

The operating room should have readily available microsuture ranging from 6-0 to

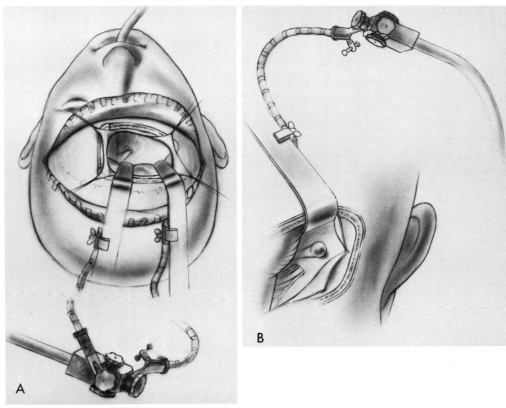

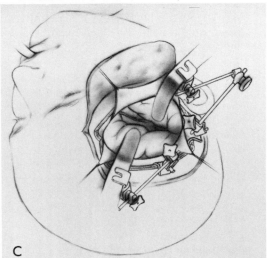

Figure 32–10 Self-retaining brain retractors. *A* and *B*. Leyla self-retaining brain retractor designed by Yasargil (Aesculap, Tuttlingen, Germany). The retractor arm shown here is locked to bar, which attaches to the operating table rather than directly to the bone margin. Attachments are available for locking the arm of the retractor to the craniotomy margin. *A*. Retractor as used for transfrontal operative appraoch to sella. *B*. Retractor placement for approach to cerebellopontine angle. *C*. Retractor made up of series of shafts and clamps as used for frontotemporal craniotomy. Retractors are clamped to craniotomy margin.

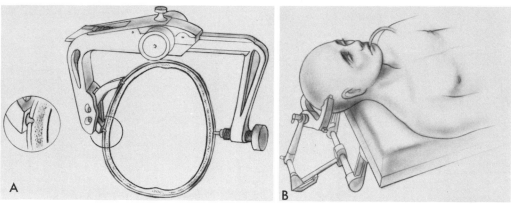

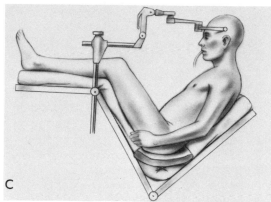

Figure 32–11 Pinion headholder used to immobilize head during micro-operative procedures. *A*. Pins penetrate scalp and are firmly fixed to the outer table of the skull. *B*. Pinion headholder as used for craniotomy in supine position or for transsphenoidal operations. For the latter, the headholder should be placed high enough on the head so that it does not obscure the sellar region on intraoperative fluoroscopy. *C*. Headholder as used for craniotomy in the sitting position.

10-0 on a variety of needles ranging in diameters from 50 to 130 μ. For the most delicate of suturing, as in a superficial temporal to middle cerebral artery anastomosis, nylon or Prolene suture of 22 μ diameter (10-0) on needles approximately 50 to 75 μ in diameter is used.

Table 32–2 gives recommended suture size in relation to the size of vessel.

The question arises whether to use a needle holder or a jewelers' forceps for grasping the microneedle. Buncke and co-workers note that jewelers' forceps afford less chance of damaging the vessel wall because they exert a gentler grasp on the needle, which will slip out of the needle holder if it is thrust in an incorrect direction.[4] The strong grip of a needle holder allows the needle to be forced through the wall in any direction and thus to damage the tissue. Most surgeons, however, have learned to use a microneedle holder very gently for microsuture. The needle holder handles should be round rather than flat or rectangular so that rotating them between the fingers yields a smooth movement that drives the needle easily (Fig. 32–12). There should

be no lock or holding catch on the microneedle. When such a lock is engaged or released, no matter how delicately it is made, the tip will jump, possibly causing misdirection of the needle or tissue damage.

TABLE 32–2 RECOMMENDED SUTURE SIZE IN RELATION TO VESSEL SIZE*

SUTURE SIZE	DIAMETER OF VESSEL (MM)	EXAMPLE OF BLOOD VESSEL SIZE
6-0	5.0–6.0	Common carotid artery
7-0	4.0 5.0	Internal carotid or vertebral artery
8-0	3.0–4.0	Basilar and middle cerebral artery
9-0	2.0–3.0	Anterior and posterior cerebral arteries
10-0	0.8–1.5	Sylvian and cortical arteries

MICROSURGERY SUTURE DIAMETERS	
Size	*Microns*
11-0	18
10-0	22
9-0	35
8-0	45

* From Yasargil, M. G.: Suturing techniques. *In* Microsurgery Applied to Neurosurgery. New York, Academic Press, 1969, pp. 87–124. Reprinted by permission.

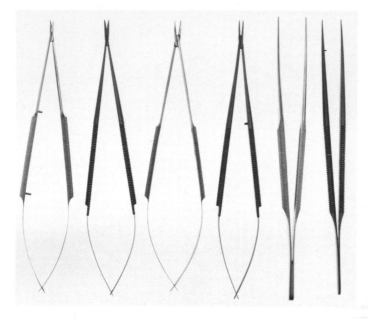

Figure 32–12 Straight round-handle scissors (two instruments on left), needle holders (middle two instruments), and forceps (two instruments on right) for microvascular operations. The instrument on the left of each pair is made of stainless steel; the one on the right weighs less, being made of titanium.

Jewelers' forceps or straight needle holders are suitable for handling microneedles near the cortical surface. For deeper applications bayonet needle holders with fine tips may be used (Fig. 32–13). For tying microsuture, microneedle holders, jewelers' forceps, or tying forceps may be used. Tying forceps have a platform in the tip to facilitate grasping the suture; however, most surgeons prefer to tie suture with jewelers' forceps or fine needle holders.

Bayonet Forceps

Standard and bipolar bayonet forceps with 8- and 10-cm blades in a variety of tip sizes ranging from 0.3 to 2.0 cm are needed.

Three-tenths millimeter tips are like those found on jewelers' forceps and are suitable for the finest work. The bayonet forceps should be properly balanced so that, when its handle rests across the radial side of the middle finger and the web between the thumb and index finger, it remains there without falling forward when the grasp of the index finger and thumb is released. Poor balance prevents the delicate grasp needed for micro-operative procedures. Some surgeons prefer the recently introduced round-handle bayonet forceps because they allow finer movement; it is possible to rotate these instruments between the thumb and forefinger rather than having to rotate the entire wrist (Fig. 32–13).

It is preferable to test forceps for tension and tactile qualities by holding them in the

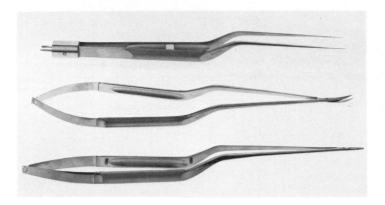

Figure 32–13 Bayonet bipolar coagulation forceps (*top*), scissors (*middle*), and needle holder (*bottom*) with round handles. The working distance from handle to tip is 8 cm, suitable for most neurosurgical operations. For deeper work similar instruments with 10-cm shafts are used. For surface work straight, not bayonetted, instruments such as those shown in Figure 32–12 are used.

gloved rather than the naked hand. Forceps resistance to closure that is perceived as adequate in the naked hand may become almost imperceptible in the gloved hand. The forceps may be used to develop tissue planes by inserting the partially closed forceps between the structures to be separated and releasing the tension so that the blades open and separate the structures. This form of dissection requires greater tension in the handles than is found in some delicate forceps.

Suction and Suction Irrigation Equipment

The most commonly used suction tubes, the 9 and 10 French sizes of the Frazier and Adson types, are too large for many micro-operative procedures. Stretched nerve fascicles or small vessels can easily become entrapped in such large tubes. Suction tubes of 3, 5, and 7 French size of the type one customarily uses are needed for operations under the microscope. The French designation applies to the outer diameter of the instrument; 3 French is equivalent to 1 mm outer diameter, 15 French has an outer diameter of 5 mm, and so forth. A No. 3 French tube is preferred when using suction near cranial nerves or an anastomosis to the middle cerebral artery.

A suction system with a mechanism to control the negative pressures to very low levels is needed. The suction should be finely adjusted to eliminate the hazard of fine neural and vascular structures being entrapped and damaged. Many neurosurgical suction tubes are constructed to allow regulation of suction strength by adjustment of the degree to which the thumb occludes an air hole. If one relies on this technique, the hole should be large enough for removal of one's thumb to reduce suction to near zero. In place of wall suction some surgeons prefer an electric suction pump easily regulated by adjusting the dials on the pump.[2,41]

A continuous stream of irrigating fluid can be helpful during part of the procedure; it discourages the formation of small blood clots and their adherence to the dissected surfaces; it also increases the effectiveness of the bipolar coagulation forceps and reduces the adhesiveness of the tips to tissue.

Constant bathing by cerebrospinal fluid will have the same effect.

Irrigation with physiological saline is also helpful in cooling the drill, which may transmit heat to nearby neural structures, and in washing bone dust from the incision (Fig. 32–14D). The irrigation should be regulated so that the solution does not enter the operative field unless the surgeon removes his finger from the suction release hole. Some drills have a built-in irrigation system that directs the fluid toward the burr under pressure to insure optimal cleaning of the burr while irrigating the operative field.

Cutting Instruments

A fresh No. 11 or 15 blade on a suitable handle is adequate for most micro-operative procedures requiring a knife (Fig. 32–15A and C). For more delicate cutting, a razor blade fragment or diamond knife is recommended. Razor knife holders are designed both to crack off a blade fragment of the proper size and shape and to hold the fragment for making the incision. The length and width of the blade fragment is determined by how the blade is held when it is cracked. With practice a wider or narrower, shorter or longer blade fragment can be prepared. To crack accurately, a razor blade must be hardened and brittle with a higher carbon content than the average stainless steel shaving blade. Blades that crack cleanly without bending are being manufactured especially for use in preparing razor knives, and some manufacturers offer precut razor blade fragments. The fragment should be examined carefully under magnification before its use.

Diamond knives have the sharpest cutting edges; however, their use is limited by the cost. Diamond knives are usually prepared by the manufacturer in a holder with a protective cover. The protective cover should be removed and replaced by only the surgeon, and the instrument should be trusted to only the most reliable operating room personnel.

Scissors with fine blades on straight and bayonetted handles are frequently used in micro-operative procedures. Cutting should be done by the distal half of the blade (Figs. 32–12, 32–13, and 32–15H). If the scissors open too widely, both cutting abil-

Text continued on page 1190

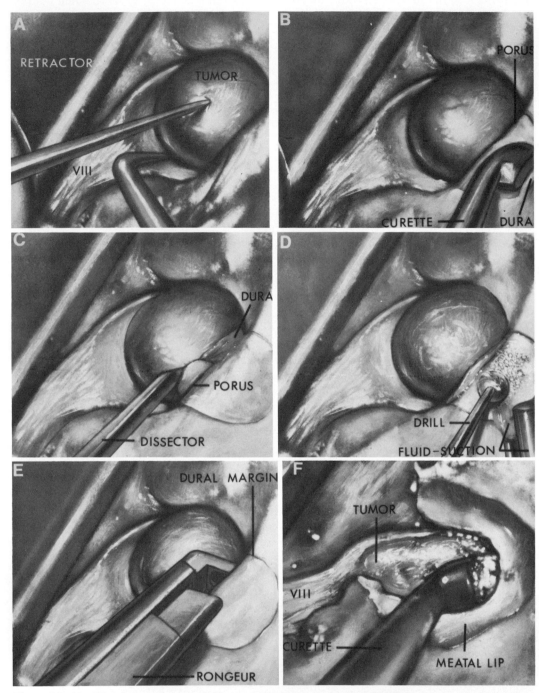

Figure 32–14 Microinstruments as used in cerebellopontine angle. Photographs were retouched from 16-mm movie frames taken at the time of removal of acoustic neuroma in right cerebellopontine angle. This operation resulted in preservation of the facial, acoustic, and vestibular nerves. Orientation is as shown in Figure 32–10*B*. *A*. Small pointed instruments called needles separating tumor from eighth nerve (VIII). Straight needle retracts the tumor, and a 45-degree-angled needle develops a cleavage plane between the tumor and the nerves. *B*. Microcuret with a 1.5-mm cup strips dura mater from posterior meatal margin. *C*. Round dissector 1 mm in diameter separates dura mater from bone at the porus and within the meatus. *D*. Drilling away the posterior margin of the meatus. Suction irrigation cools and removes bone dust. *E*. Alternative method of removal of posterior lip by using a Kerrison rongeur with a 1-mm side bite. *F*. Microcuret with 1.5-mm cup removes the last bit of bone from the posterior meatal wall.   *Illustration continued on opposite page*

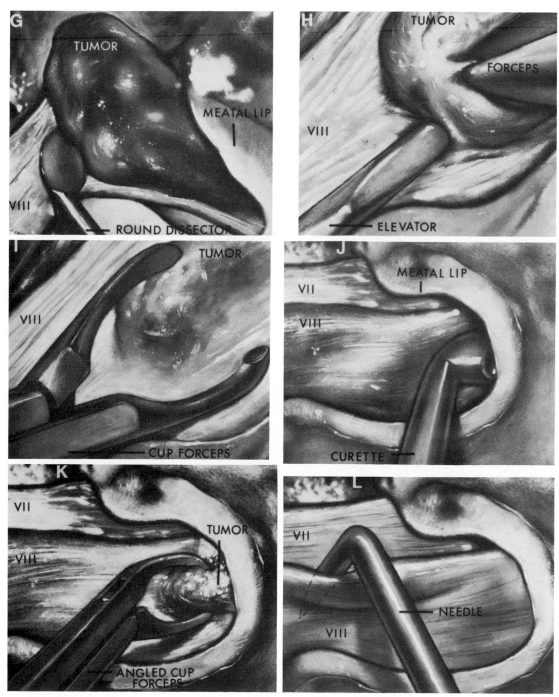

Figure 32–14 (*continued*) *G*. One-millimeter round dissector separates eighth nerve (VIII) and tumor. *H*. Elevator with a 1-mm-wide tip separating tumor and eighth nerve. *I*. Microcup forceps with 0.5-mm cup removing nodule of tumor from nerve. *J*. Microcuret reaches into meatus behind the eighth nerve to bring nodule of tumor into view. Facial nerve (VII) is anterior and superior to vestibulocochlear nerve (VIII). *K*. Microcup forceps angled to right removes last remaining tumor from the lateral part of the meatus. *L*. Angled needle examines the area between facial (VII) and vestibulocochlear (VIII) nerves for residual tumor. (From Rhoton, A. L.: Microsurgical removal of acoustic neuromas. Surg. Neurol., 6:211–219, 1976. Reprinted by permission.)

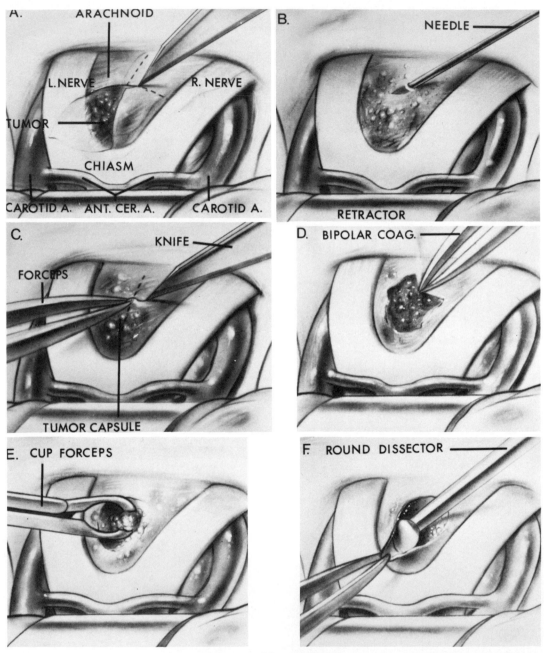

Figure 32–15   Microoperative instruments as used for transfrontal approach to a suprasellar tumor. Orientation and exposure as shown in Figure 32–10A. A. Arachnoid incised with No. 11 knife blade so that it is not removed but is left over the optic nerves as a protective layer. B. Tumor aspirated as cyst prior to starting removal. C. Tumor capsule incised with No. 11 blade. D. Bipolar coagulation used on bleeding points on capsule. E. Micro-cup forceps used to remove tumor within capsule. F. Small round dissector used to push tumor inferiorly for removal.
Illustration continued on opposite page

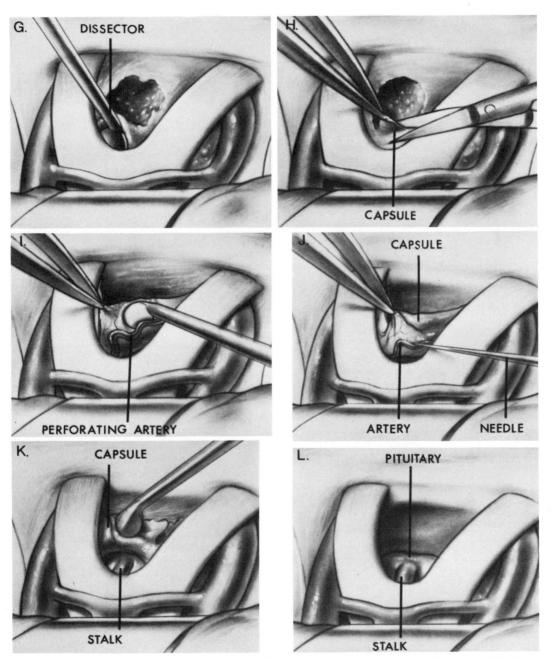

Figure 32–15 (*continued*) *G.* Capsule pushed inferiorly away from chiasm with round dissector. *H.* Portion of capsule being excised with bayonet microscissors. *I.* Perforating artery being dissected away from tumor capsule with a round dissector. *J.* Perforating vessel being removed from capsule with a needle dissector. *K.* Capsule depressed inferiorly with round dissector and pituitary stalk exposed. *L.* Removal complete. (From Rhoton, A. L., and Maniscalco, J. E.: Microsurgery of the sellar region. *In* Glaser, J., ed.: Neuro-Ophthalmology. Vol. IX. St. Louis, C. V. Mosby Co., 1977. Reprinted by permission.)

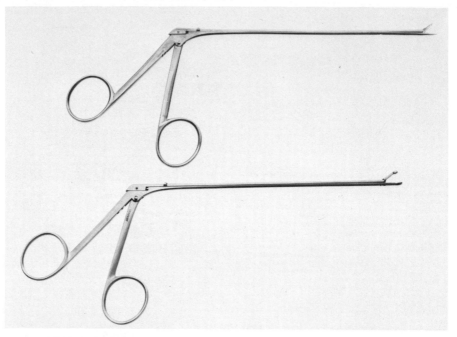

Figure 32–16   Alligator-type scissors (*top*) and cup forceps (*bottom*) suitable for cutting or grasping in deep narrow openings. Cup forceps with cups 1 to 3 mm in diameter are needed for transsphenoidal operations.

ity and accuracy suffer. Delicate cutting near the surface such as opening the middle cerebral artery for anastomosis or embolectomy should be done with straight, not bayonetted, scissors with fine blades approximately 5 mm long that open approximately 3 mm (see Fig. 32–12). Only delicate suture and tissue should be cut with such small blades. For deep areas such as the cerebellopontine angle or sellar region use bayonet scissors with curved and straight blades (see Fig. 32–13). The blade should measure 14 mm in length and should open approximately 4 mm. Scissors on an alligator-type shank with a long shaft may be needed for cutting in deep and narrow openings, as in transsphenoidal operations (Fig. 32–16).

Drills

A drill frequently is used during micro-operative procedures for removing the sphenoid ridge, the clinoid process, the wall of the internal acoustic meatus, or other protrusions of the cranial base (see Fig. 32–14D). After a drill has reduced the thickness of an area like the posterior lip of the internal acoustic meatus, a Kerrison microrongeur with a 1-mm lip or a microcuret may be used to remove the remaining thin layer of bone (Fig. 32–14E and F).

A drill that will reverse its direction is preferred to one that cuts in only one direction. Most electric but only a few air drills are reversible, and for that reason electric drills have been best suited to micro-operative procedures. The operation should be so planned that the burr rotates away from critical structures so that if skidding occurs it will be away from them. Diamond burrs are used near important structures. One should become acquainted with and skilled in the application of the drill in the laboratory prior to using it in a neurosurgical operation.

Drills are available that function at speeds from 6000 to nearly 100,000 rpm. At speeds greater than 25,000 rpm the bone melts away so easily that the drill poorly transmits the tactile details of bony structure to the surgeon's hand. Speeds less than 25,000 rpm should be used for delicate procedures in which tactile control of the drill is important. A diamond bit used at speeds below 8000 rpm is preferable for the most delicate bone removal.

Hold the drill like a pen and cut with the side rather than the end of the burr. Use a large burr when possible. The greatest accuracy and control of the drill is obtained at higher speeds if a light brush action is used to remove the bone. Dangerous skidding may ensue at lower speeds because greater pressure is needed to cut the bone. Avoid running the burr across bone by using light, intermittent pressure rather than constant pressure of the burr on one spot. Overheating near nerves may damage them. Constant suction irrigation with physiological saline reduces heat transmission to nearby neural structures. Keep the teeth of the burr clean of bone dust. A coarse burr that clogs less easily is harder to control and runs across bone more easily, but this is reduced with irrigation. Do not use a burr blindly to make a long deep hole, but keep the field beveled and as wide open as possible. Use a small curet to follow a small track rather than pursuing it with a drill. Clean away bone dust because of its potent osteogenic properties.

Curets

Small curets are sometimes used for removing the last shell of bone between the drill surface and the optic canal or internal acoustic meatus or for removing a clinoid process (Figs. 32–14B, F, and J, and 32–17). A straight curet is satisfactory for this although 45-degree angled curets may be needed for special purposes such as curetting a tumor from the sphenoid ridge, the lateral margin of the acoustic meatus, or other areas on the cranial base. Curets with tips as small as 1.5 mm are available (Fig. 32–17). Hold the curet so the cutting edge is in full view and try to cut with the side rather than the tip. Apply pressure parallel to or away from important structures rather than perpendicularly toward them. Properly sharpened curets cut with less pressure and are safer than dull ones. Try to use the largest curet that will do the job.

Dissectors

The most widely used neurosurgical dissectors are of the Penfield or Freier type; however, the size and weight of these instruments makes them unsuitable for microdissection around small tumors and aneurysms (Fig. 32–17). The smallest Penfield dissector, the No. 4, has a width of 3 mm. For microdissection one needs dissectors with tips 1 and 2 mm wide. Spatula dissectors similar to, but smaller than, the No. 4 Penfield dissector are needed for defining the neck of an aneurysm and separating it from adjacent perforating arteries. Round-tipped dissectors resembling the Sheehy canal knives are used for separation of tumor from nerve (see Figs. 32–14C and G, and 32–15F, I, and K). An alternative method of fine dissection is to use the straight, pointed instruments that the author calls needles (see Figs. 32–14A and L, and 32–15J). It may be difficult to grasp the margin of the tumor with forceps; however, a small needle dissector introduced into its margin may be helpful in retracting the tumor in the desired direction (see Fig. 32–14A). This type of pointed instrument can also be used to develop a cleavage plane between tumor and arachnoid membrane, nerves, and brain.

Any vessel that stands above the surface of the capsule should be dealt with initially as if it were a brain vessel that runs over the tumor surface and can be preserved with accurate dissection. One should try to displace the vessel and adjacent tissue off the tumor capsule toward the adjacent neural tissues by using a small dissector after the tumor has been removed from within the capsule. Vessels, which initially appeared to be adherent to the capsule, often, when dissected free of the capsule, prove to be neural vessels on the pial surface.

If the pia-arachnoid membrane is adherent to tumor capsule or if there is a mass of tumor within the capsule preventing collapse of the capsule away from nerves, chiasm, or other structures, there is a tendency to apply traction to both layers and to tear neural vessels running on the pial surface. Prior to separating the pia-arachnoid from the capsule, it is important that all of the tumor be removed so that the capsule is so thin that it is almost transparent. If one is uncertain about the margin between the capsule and the pia-arachnoid membrane, several sweeps of a small dissector through the area will help clarify the appropriate plane for dissection.

Cup Forceps

A cup forceps such as that used for intervertebral disc removal is commonly used

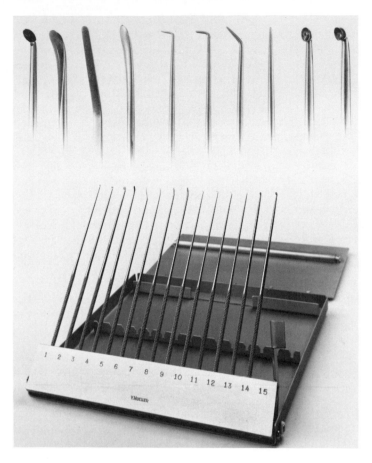

Figure 32–17 Microdissectors for neurosurgery. Beginning on left (*top*) are four types of dissectors: round, spatula, flat, and micro-Penfield in that order. The next two instruments are sharp and blunt microhooks, and the next two are angled and straight needle dissectors. The two instruments on right are straight and angled microcurets. Storage case of type shown (*bottom*) permits easy access to instruments and yet protects the delicate tips when not in use.

for removal of tumors (see Figs. 32–14*I*, 32–15*E*, and 32–16). The most frequently used cup forceps have a tip 3 mm wide, which is suitable for the intracapsular removal of large tumors. For removal of small tumors or small fragments of tumor in critical locations such as on cranial nerves, in the acoustic meatus, or within the ventricles, cup forceps having a diameter of 1.0 to 2.0 mm are used. For grasping small bits of tumor directly on or within cranial nerves the 1.0-mm cup forceps is used. The 2-mm tip is suitable for the intracapsular removal of some small tumors. Angled microcup forceps enable one to reach around a corner to grasp tissue or remove tumor. A cup forceps angled to the right is used to reach laterally to the right, e.g., to reach posterior to the facial and acoustic nerves in the right acoustic meatus, and the cup forceps angled to the left is used on the left side (see Fig. 32–14*K*). The angled cup forceps can also be used to reach to either side of a small capsular opening for intracapsular re-

moval or for reaching laterally into an intervertebral foramen for disc removal.

REFERENCES

1. American College of Surgeons and the American Surgical Association. Surgery in the United States. A Summary Report of Surgical Services in the United States. 1975.
2. Bader, D. C. H.: Microtechnical nursing in neurosurgery. J. Neurosurg. Nurs., 7:22–24, 1975.
3. Bader, D. C. H.: Microsurgical treatment of intracranial aneurysms. J. Neurosurg. Nurs., 7:25–27, 1975.
4. Buncke H. J., and Murray, D. E.: Small vessel reconstruction. *In* Rand, R. W. ed.: Microneurosurgery. St. Louis, C. V. Mosby Co., 1969, pp. 183–192.
5. Buncke, H. J., and Schulz, W. P.: The suture repair of one millimeter vessels. *In* Donaghy, R. M. P., and Yasargil, M. G., eds.: Micro-Vascular Surgery. St. Louis, C. V. Mosby Co., 1967, pp. 24–35.
6. Buncke, H. J., Chater, N. L., and Szabo, Z.: The complete teaching manual of microvascular surgery. Microvascular Research Laboratory, R.

K. Davies Medical Center, San Francisco, California, October 1974 (unpublished data).

7. Buncke, H. J., Cobbett, J. R., Smith, J. W., et al.: Techniques of microsurgery. Pamphlet published by Ethicon, Inc., Somerville, N.J., 1968.

8. DeLong, W. B., and Fox, J. L.: Automatic cycling bipolar coagulation. Surg. Neurol., 8:15–16, 1977.

9. Donaghy, R. M. P.: Patch and by-pass in microangional surgery In Donaghy, R. M. P., and Yasargil, M. G., eds.: Micro-Vascular Surgery. St. Louis, C. V. Mosby Co., 1967, pp. 75–86.

10. Donaghy, R. M. P., and Yasargil, M. G., eds.: Micro-Vascular Surgery. St. Louis, C. V. Mosby Co., 1967.

11. Drake, C. G.: Surgical treatment of acoustic neuroma with preservation or reconstitution of the facial nerve. J. Neurosurg., 26:459–464, 1967.

12. Greenwood, J.: Two point coagulation. A new principle and instrument for applying coagulation current in neurosurgery. Amer. J. Surg., 50:267, 1940.

13. Handa, H., ed.: Microneurosurgery. Baltimore, University Park Press, 1973.

14. Hardy, J.: Preparation of aneurysm in the rat. Lecture delivered as guest instructor, Theodore Gildred Microsurgical Education Center, University of Florida, Gainesville, Florida, November 1975.

15. Hodges, G.: The TLC of instruments for eye surgery. Point of View, Vol 4, No 6. Somerville, N.J., Ethicon, Inc., 1968.

16. Jacobson, J. H.: The development of microsurgical technique. In Donaghy, R. M. P., and Yasargil, M. G., eds.: Micro-Vascular Surgery. St. Louis, C. V. Mosby Co., 1967, pp. 4–14.

17. Joint Committee for Stroke Resources: Guidelines for treatment of neurovascular disease (Part I). Stroke, 1977.

18. Kohdadad, G.: Microvascular surgery. In Rand, R. W., ed.: Microneurosurgery. St. Louis, C. V. Mosby Co., 1969, pp. 170–182.

19. Koos, W. T., Böck, F. W., and Spetzler, R. F., eds.: Clinical Microneurosurgery. Stuttgart, Georg Thieme Verlag, 1976.

20. Kurze, T.: Microtechnique in neurological surgery. Clin. Neurosurg., 11:128, 1963.

21. Lougheed, W. M., and Marshall, B. M.: Management of aneurysms of the anterior circulation by intracranial procedures. In Youmans, J. R., ed.: Neurological Surgery. Vol. II. Philadelphia, W. B. Saunders Co., 1973, pp. 731–767.

22. Malis, L. I.: Bipolar coagulation in microsurgery. In Yasargil, M. G., ed.: Microsurgery Applied to Neurosurgery. New York, Academic Press, 1969, pp. 41–45.

23. Ojemann, R. G., Montgomery, W. W., and Weiss, A. D.: Evaluation and surgical treatment of acoustic neuroma. N. Eng. J. Med., 287:895–899, 1972.

24. Pait, T. G., and Rhoton, A. L.: Microsurgical anatomy and dissection of the temporal bone. Surg. Neurol., 8:363–391, 1977.

25. Perkins, J. J.: Principles and Methods of Sterilization in Health Sciences. Springfield, Ill., Charles C Thomas, 1969, Chapter 10.

26. Perlmutter, D., and Rhoton, A. L.: Microsurgical anatomy of the anterior cerebral-anterior communicating-recurrent artery complex. J. Neurosurg., 45:259–272, 1976.

27. Pia, H. W.: The microscope in neurosurgery. In Handa, H., ed.: Microneurosurgery. Baltimore, University Park Press, 1973, pp. 3–7.

28. Rand, R. W., ed.: Microneurosurgery. St. Louis, C. V. Mosby Co., 1969.

29. Rand, R. W.: Microneurosurgery instrumentation. In Rand, R. W., ed.: Microneurosurgery. St. Louis, C. V. Mosby Co., 1969, pp. 21–37.

30. Rhoton, A. L.: Microsurgery of the internal acoustic meatus. Surg. Neurol., 2:311–318, 1974.

31. Rhoton, A. L.: Microsurgical removal of acoustic neuromas. Surg. Neurol., 6:211–219, 1976.

32. Rhoton, A. L., and Maniscalco, J. E.: Microsurgery of the sellar region. In Neuro-Ophthalmology. Vol. IX. St. Louis, C. V. Mosby Co., 1977.

33. Rhoton, A. L., Harris, F. S., and Renn, W. H.: Microsurgical anatomy of the sellar region and cavernous sinus. Clin. Neurosurg., 24:54–85, 1977.

34. Saeki, N., and Rhoton, A. L.: Microsurgical anatomy of the upper basilar artery and the posterior circle of Willis. J. Neurosurg., 46:563–578, 1977.

35. Urban, J. C.: The surgical microscope, its use and care. In Rand, R. W., ed.: Microneurosurgery. St. Louis, C. V. Mosby Co., 1969, pp. 9–20.

36. Yasargil, M. G., ed.: Microsurgery Applied to Neurosurgery. New York, Academic Press, 1969.

37. Yasargil, M. G.: Suturing techniques. In Yasargil, M. G., ed.: Microsurgery Applied to Neurosurgery. New York, Academic Press, 1969, pp. 87–124.

38. Yasargil, M. G.: Experimental microsurgical operations in animals. In Yasargil, M. G., ed.: Microsurgery Applied to Neurosurgery. New York, Academic Press, 1969, pp. 60–79.

39. Yasargil, M. G.: Experimental small vessel surgery in the dog including patching and grafting of cerebral vessels and the formation of functional extra-intracranial shunts. In Dohaghy, R. M. P., and Yasargil, M. G., eds.: Micro-Vascular Surgery. St. Louis, C. V. Mosby Co., 1967, pp. 87–124.

40. Yasargil, M. G.: Development of a motorized microscope stand. In Koos, W. T., Böck, F. W., and Spetzler, R. F., eds.: Clinical Microneurosurgery. Stuttgart, Georg Thieme Verlag, 1976, pp. 3–4.

41. Yasargil, M. G., Fox, J. L., and Ray, M. W.: The operative approach to aneurysms of the anterior communicating artery. In Krayenbuhl, H., ed.: Advances in Technical Standards in Neurosurgery. Vol. II. New York, Springer-Verlag, 1975.

33

INTERVENTIONAL NEURORADIOLOGY

An intravascular approach to a vascular lesion is not new. As early as 1929, fragments of muscle were released into the circulation to help obliterate a carotid-cavernous fistula. Interest remained restricted until Luessenhop published a series of articles in the 1960's detailing his techniques and results in the treatment of previously untreatable intracranial arteriovenous malformations by using intravascular embolization of Silastic spheres.[26,28–30] The results were excellent. During the past decade, his techniques have been enlarged upon and simplified, new embolization materials have been introduced, and magnetically guided catheters for intracranial navigation have appeared as well as catheters with balloons that can be detached. A small revolution in the management of complex vascular lesions affecting the central nervous system has occurred. This chapter outlines this new approach and provides guidelines for its use.

HISTORICAL PERSPECTIVE

Brooks, in 1931, reported embolizing muscle into a carotid-cavernous fistula.[4] Several other reports appearing during the following years have described this technique, and it is outlined in Chapter 15. Luessenhop and Spence reported a case of artificial embolization of a cerebral arteriovenous malformation with silicone pellets. The technique required general anesthesia, an operative exposure and catheterization of the external carotid artery, and courage on the part of the surgeon and the patient.[28]

Through the next decade, Luessenhop and his colleagues published extensively on their results, confirming without a doubt the validity of their approach.[26,29,30] In 1968, Doppman and his colleagues and Newton and Adams reported embolization of a spinal cord malformation.[12,33] Remarkably, in the later case, the lesion was primarily supplied by the anterior spinal artery. In 1970, Hilal and his colleagues reported on embolization of extracranial vascular anomalies and neoplasms.[23] Numerous reports have since appeared on modifications of the techniques and embolization materials.[9–11] Embolization is widely used for problems outside the nervous system.[2,15] Most recent efforts have been directed toward the development of a reliable detachable balloon catheter and better materials for embolization.[22,34,36,37]

TECHNICAL CONSIDERATIONS AND MATERIALS

Embolization, whether it is performed percutaneously or by an open operative procedure, requires close coordination of effort between the surgeon and the radiologist. Catheter selection, preparation, and placement are crucial to achieving success. Throughout the procedure, sterile techniques must be used. Superselective arteriography must be available prior to embolization and must be carefully studied. It is far too time-consuming and wearing on the patient and the clinician to perform angiography and embolization at one session. Embolization is almost always performed

W. J. MICHELSEN AND S. K. HILAL

through a catheter inserted into the femoral artery.[25] The authors usually use a No. 9 catheter inserted with a Mylar sheath. This catheter is used for Silastic sphere embolization. If spheres larger than 2.5 mm are necessary a No. 10 or even a No. 12 can be used, but with a higher degree of risk to the femoral artery. Double-lumen balloon catheters varying in size from No. 2 to No. 6 French can also be used through this catheter. In all cases, a flushing solution with heparin is used.

There is a wide variety of materials available for embolization. The oldest material is muscle, which was used for carotid-cavernous fistulas.

The authors have tried to restrict their material to Silastic spheres and liquid Silastic.[13,24] Previously Gelfoam was used, but this material has many disadvantages. It is difficult to render radiopaque and is dangerous to use. Also, it is resorbed in four to six weeks and therefore is not a permanent solution for an arteriovenous malformation. It can be used to obliterate tumor blood supply if a subsequent operation is to be performed promptly. Its wide availability is an advantage.

Silastic spheres remain the material of choice for intracranial arteriovenous malformations. The spheres are radiopaque; they are manufactured in an excellent variety of sizes, are easily delivered, and are well tolerated. A disadvantage is that they are not thrombogenic.

Liquid Silastic is an almost ideal material for embolization of extracranial tumors, dural arteriovenous malformations, and spinal arteriovenous malformations. Its viscosity can be made quite low, the time course of polymerization can be varied almost infinitely, and when tantalum powder is added its visualization under fluoroscopy is excellent. A major disadvantage is discoloration of the skin if the material goes to vessels supplying such an area. Another disadvantage becomes apparent when the material is injected into a tumor. When polymerized, Silastic is a soft rubberlike substance, and the usual techniques for tumor removal do not work well. Ring forceps and sissors are more useful than a sucker or cutting cautery in removing the tumor that has been made tough by the Silastic.

New catheters are being studied for use intracranially. Catheters with magnetic tips are useful for navigating into the anterior cerebral artery and also the anterior spinal artery. Detachable balloon catheters have been extensively used in Europe and Russia, but several difficulties remain.[33] The ability to detach a balloon reliably remains a problem, as does keeping the balloon inflated. Magnetic and balloon techniques hold great promise for the future, however.[1,5,22,38]

APPLICATIONS OF EMBOLIZATION

Embolization is useful as a treatment alone or as an adjunct to operative therapy.[2,18,20] It is most often used in the latter situation. It has proved to be useful in treatment of a variety of lesions including intracranial and spinal arteriovenous malformations, dural arteriovenous malformations, arteriovenous malformations of the scalp and face and neck, extracranial tumors including meningiomas, carotid body and glomus jugulare tumors, and extraspinal lesions such aneurysmal bone cysts, giant cell tumors, hemangiomas of vertebral bodies, and other highly vascular lesions. As each type of lesion requires a different therapeutic approach, they are discussed individually in that fashion.

Embolization of intracranial arteriovenous malformations is still considered to be experimental, and a detailed informed consent form and a strict protocol should be used. It is also helpful to go through a lengthy educational process with the patient prior to hospitalization. Embolization is a treatment for intracranial arteriovenous malformations, but not a cure, and it does have complications, although few.[16,27]

The evening before embolization each patient receives 25 mg of diazepam (Valium) orally and 16 mg of dexamethasone. The morning of the procedure atropine and dexamethasone, 10 mg, are given intramuscularly, and in the x-ray suite droperidol, 5 mg intravenously, and fentanyl in an appropriate dose are given. Supplemental fentanyl is given as necessary. Dexamethasone, 4 mg every six hours, is given for two days after the procedure and then discontinued. The patients are usually hospitalized three to four days.

Intracranial Arteriovenous Malformations

Luessenhop and Presper have graphically illustrated the geometry of intracranial arteriovenous malformations that are amenable to embolization with Silastic spheres.[27] Lesions that are large and involve the middle cerebral artery beyond its trifurcation are easily embolized (Fig. 33–1). Certain radiographic considerations must be noted, however. A small number of patients have a severe stenosis of the middle cerebral artery and its bifurcation-trifurcation with the malformation distal. Embolization in such a situation will lead to a catastrophe. Prior to embolization of any malformation in the middle cerebral distribution, Caldwell views must be obtained. A second type of malformation that is hazardous to embolize in the middle cerebral distribution has one large feeding artery and several small feeding vessels. Obliteration of the large artery leads to increased flow through the smaller vessels and may result in a disastrous hemorrhage.

Embolization is discontinued when one sphere goes astray. This almost never causes neurological defect, an experience shared with several other groups.[25,27,29] If a considerable portion of the malformation remains at the time of stopping, the patient is discharged and readmitted to the hospital several weeks later for a second procedure. This approach gives the circulation time to adjust. If operative intervention is contemplated, a period of four to six weeks is allowed to elapse between embolization and operation.

When an arteriovenous malformation has a large contribution from the middle cerebral artery and the posterior cerebral artery, it is preferable to embolize the posterior cerebral artery first (Fig. 33–2). This can be done with excellent success, and less than 15 per cent of patients develop any visual field disturbance even with complete obliteration of the posterior cerebral circulation. Difficulty is rare because these patients have an excellent collateral supply to the calcarine area from both the middle and anterior cerebral arteries.

When the anterior cerebral artery is the major contributing vessel, embolization is not useful, as the geometry of the vessel is unfavorable for the pellets to negotiate. Small balloon catheters and magnetic catheters hold promise for the future in this situation.

Lesions in which the major contribution is from the lenticulostriate vessels and the thalamic perforating arteries are not suitable for embolization.

Great vein of Galen malformations in which the posterior cerebral circulation is a major factor are very suitable for embolization (Fig. 33–3B). By using both open and percutaneous techniques it is possible to reduce headaches, reverse heart failure, and improve cerebral perfusion. It is important to remember that these patients cannot tolerate a large fluid load, and therefore multiple procedures often are necessary.

Embolization as the only treatment has

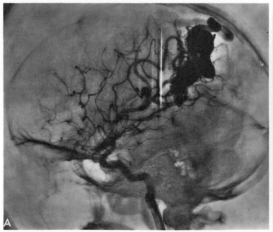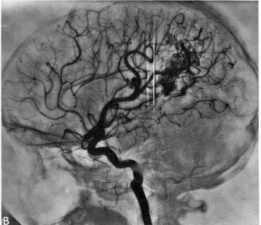

Figure 33–1   *A.* Large arteriovenous malformation supplied by anterior and middle cerebral arteries. *B.* After Silastic pellet embolization.

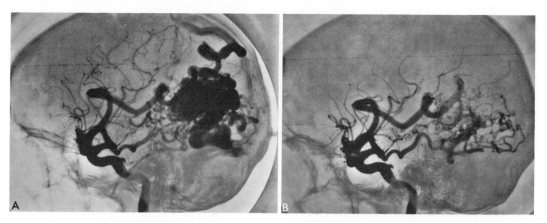

Figure 33–2 *A*. Large arteriovenous malformation involving middle and posterior cerebral arteries. *B*. After embolization; headache and seizures were relieved and no visual disturbance occurred.

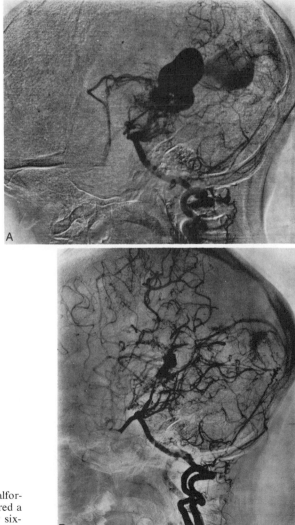

Figure 33–3 *A*. Vein of Galen arteriovenous malformation. *B*. After embolization. The patient suffered a hemorrhage at age 1. No further problems after six-year follow-up.

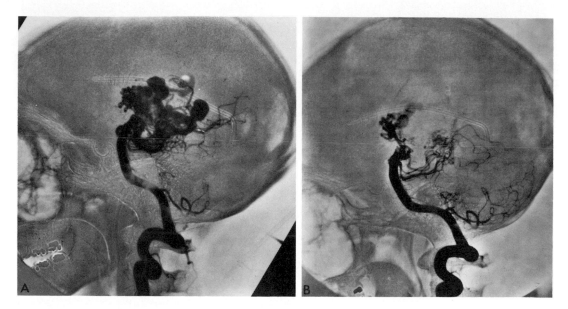

Figure 33–4 *A*. Deep basal ganglia arteriovenous malformation. *B*. After embolization. Improvement in hemiparesis after procedure.

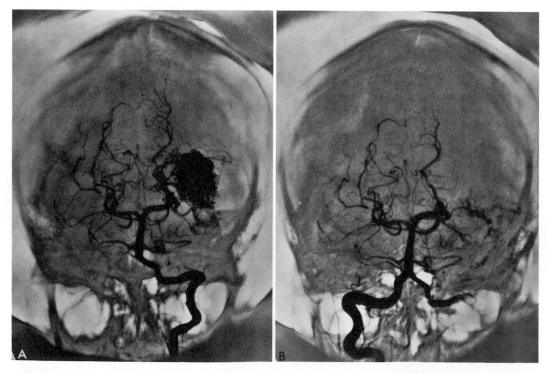

Figure 33–5 *A*. Dominant temporal lobe arteriovenous malformation in a 17-year-old girl with frequent seizures. *B*. After embolization, seizures have stopped.

been used primarily when a lesion was inoperable (Fig. 33–4). Approximately 50 per cent of lesions treated by the authors become operable after embolization. The rare patient with a progressive neurological deficit is often dramatically improved by embolization, and long-term follow-up has demonstrated that the improvement is maintained. Similarly, seizure reduction can be achieved with embolization alone and, as shown by long-term follow-up, is excellent (Fig. 33–5).

Spinal Arteriovenous Malformations

Spinal arteriovenous malformations are difficult operative problems.[6,7,11,12] Embolization techniques offer an excellent and often dramatic alternative. For embolization to be helpful and safe, careful spinal angiography must be performed. The precise anatomy of the anterior spinal artery must be noted. Lateral films must be obtained. Often, when the lateral film is difficult to obtain, an oblique projection is useful.

Spinal arteriovenous malformations occur most frequently in the thoracic cord, next most frequently in the thoracolumbar area, and least frequently in the cervical area. Those in the cervical area have blood supply from major vessels such as the vertebral artery, thyrocervical trunk, and costocervical trunk. Those in the thoracic and thoracolumbar area are fed by radicular arteries. Thoracic cord lesions are mostly supplied by dorsal arteries, whereas those in the thoracolumbar region (conus) are supplied by anterior and posterior spinal arteries. The venous drainage of these malformations is impressive but of little relevance to their treatment.

Embolization with Silastic liquid may result in dramatic reversal of long-standing neurological deficit and obliteration of

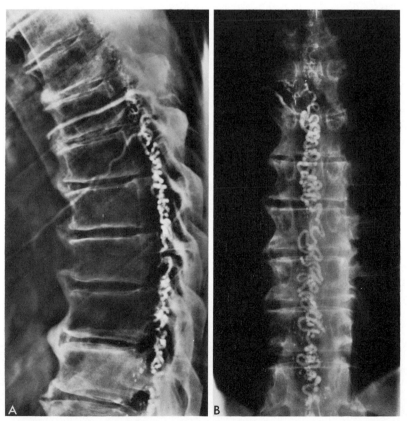

Figure 33–6 Large spinal arteriovenous malformation completely obliterated by Silastic liquid. Patient recovered from paraplegia to an ambulatory state.

these lesions.[12,13,24,33] This is particularly true in thoracic lesions (Fig. 33–6). The Silastic is placed within the malformation itself, and the lesion is obliterated. This procedure requires great skill on the part of the radiologist in wedging a catheter into the appropriate feeding vessel. It also requires precise timing of the hardening of the Silastic liquid.

Early attempts at embolization of spinal arteriovenous malformations were performed with Gelfoam.[8] Six weeks later the malformation recanalized. It is interesting that Djindjian reported that embolization of these lesions was a failure, as they all became symptomatic again after a few weeks. He had used Gelfoam.[6] It is therefore crucial that a permanent material be used for this application of embolization. It is the authors' belief that almost all spinal arteriovenous malformations can be managed with embolization.

Dural Arteriovenous Malformations

Dural arteriovenous malformations are not yet clearly defined in terms of their natural history and deleterious effects.[31,32] Most commonly they result in a bruit if the occipital artery is involved, or chemosis, exophthalmos, and glaucoma if the anterior meningeal circulation feeds into the cavernous sinus. Some of these lesions are obliter-

ated by angiography, others involute by themselves, and still others remain static. As a result, it is difficult to decide when to treat these patients.

When a lesion involves the cavernous sinus and results in a painful, unattractive eye, embolization is performed. If intraocular pressure threatens vision, treatment is undertaken. The lesions draining into the cavernous sinus are difficult to obliterate entirely, as often one or more branches of the cavernous carotid artery are involved. The authors have not been aggressive with these lesions because their potential for harm is unclear.

Dural arteriovenous malformations involving the occipital artery and the lateral sinus are easily managed with embolization alone (Fig. 33–7). Such patients are often "driven crazy" by the noise in the ear, and as the treatment is simple, they should be treated early. These patients must be forewarned that they will suffer from a painful scalp neuralgia in the distribution of the greater occipital nerve for several weeks after the procedure. Numbness often appears in the distribution of this nerve and probably is due to an infarction of the nerve itself.

Extracranial and Extraspinal Neoplasms

Vascular neoplasms such as basal meningiomas, glomus jugulare tumors, aneurys-

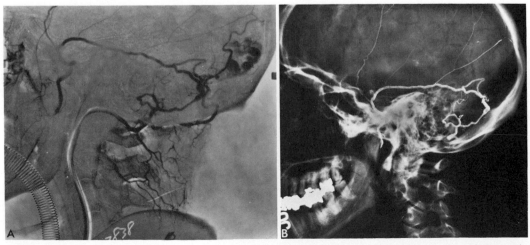

Figure 33–7   *A.* Dural arteriovenous malformation supplied by occipital artery. Patient had cerebellopontine angle syndrome. *B.* After embolization with Silastic liquid, complete recovery.

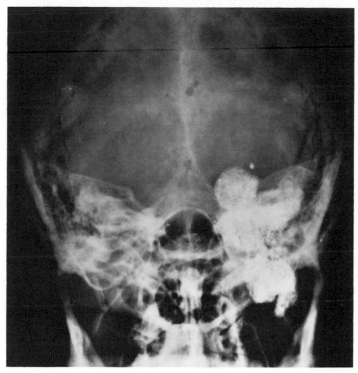

Figure 33–8 Large glomus tumor completely filled with Silastic liquid. Note large intracranial component.

mal bone cysts, and vertebral hemangiomas are difficult operative problems. For extracranial neoplasm, the external carotid artery has been ligated in the neck, a maneuver of dubious value. Embolization is quite helpful in the management of these lesions.[15,18,19,23,24] There are important qualifications to be noted, however, and the techniques vary according to the location of the lesion.

Meningiomas of the pterion are an example. The meningeal supply to these tumors can be embolized with ease. But, it is important that the embolic material remain mostly outside the lesion in the feeding vessels, virtually depriving the lesion of its blood supply. When this is done correctly, infarction of the lesion will follow, and its removal will be greatly eased. If the lesion is filled with the Silastic liquid, however, the tumor will be expanded and an emergency situation will be created.

Glomus jugulare tumors are difficult to manage.[11,23] Most of these lesions are within bone, but some expand into the posterior and middle fossae. Because this tumor consists virtually of sinusoids filled with blood and some of the supply can be intracranial, the authors attempt to fill the entire tumor with Silastic (Fig. 33–8). Even with this manuever, tumor tissue taken at operation has grown in tissue culture. When the lesion is filled with Silastic, operative removal is more troublesome because of the "rubbery" nature. This change in its consistency, however, is a small price to pay for improving an otherwise difficult situation. Another advantage is that this technique may also render these lesions more susceptible to the effects of irradiation.

When a glomus jugulare tumor is embolized with Silastic, pre-existing mild cranial nerve weakness often is accentuated. This is particularly true of the seventh and tenth nerves. Probably this worsening is due to tumor expansion and compression. Occasionally, filling of the stapedial artery with Silastic occurs when embolization of these tumors is performed. Filling of this artery also causes facial weakness that recovers in six weeks. If the glomus tumor is large and compressing the brain stem, the embolization is done to occlude the feeding vessels without allowing the material to enter the tumor. On more than one occasion, patients have been relieved of their symptoms with embolization alone, but long-term follow-up has demonstrated recurrence.

Glomus jugulare tumors are extremely difficult to manage even with both embolization and operation. This subject is discussed further in Chapter 107.

Aneurysmal bone cysts, hemangiomas of bone, and giant cell tumors often cause spinal cord compression and are hazardous to operate upon because of bleeding. Selective angiography will reveal a direct blood supply. Embolization will reduce the bleeding substantially. It is useful in these cases to obliterate as many feeding vessels as possible without further increasing the bulk of the tumor. As operative intervention is often mandatory and urgent, Gelfoam is an acceptable material to use. None the less, Silastic liquid is the preferred embolic agent. Symptoms of cord compression can be reversed with this technique.[18,20]

COMPLICATIONS OF EMBOLIZATION

Complications of embolization are rare but they may be catastrophic. The complications of angiography alone must be included.[15,20,27] Fatal cases of intracranial hemorrhage have occurred. Transient neurological deficits may be caused by stray emboli, but the authors have seen a virtual cessation of this complication with the routine medication used in their operations for intracranial arteriovenous malformations.

Embolization of extracranial lesions has resulted in one death and one serious neurological deficit in the authors' patients, whereas other groups have reported no complications. Gelfoam was used in both of the cases in which the outcome was adverse.

Skin discoloration and cranial nerve palsy have been observed when liquid Silastic was used. These complications have been eliminated by employing the techniques described earlier. No instances of vascular occlusive disease have occurred in the authors' patients from the use of large catheters, but this remains a distinct possibility. Infection, although a possibility, has not been observed.

SUMMARY

Embolization techniques are available for the management of vascular lesions of the nervous system and its surrounding structures. Close cooperation between the clinician and radiologist is imperative. A variety of embolic materials are available, but Silastic pellets and liquid Silastic are the preferred agents. Complications are few, but are important. These techniques may be curative or may be useful as an adjunct to operation.

REFERENCES

1. Alksne, J. F.: Magnetically controlled intravascular catheter. Surgery, 64:339, 1968.
2. Baum, S., and Nusbaum, M.: Control of gastrointestinal hemorrhage by selective mesenteric arterial infusion of vasopressin. Radiology, 98:497–505, 1971.
3. Boulos, R., Kricheff, I. I., and Chase, N. E.: Value of cerebral angiography in the embolization treatment of cerebral arteriovenous malformations. Radiology, 97:65, 1970.
4. Brooks, B.: Discussion of paper by L. Noland and A. S. Taylor. Trans. Southern Surg. Ass., 43:171, 1931.
5. Cares, H. I., Hale, J. R., Montgomery, D. B., et al.: Laboratory experience with a magnetically guided intravascular catheter system. J. Neurosurg., 38:145, 1973.
6. Debron, G.: Presented at the Symposium on Aneurysms, Arteriovenous Malformation and Carotid-Cavernous Fistula. University of Chicago, November 16–17, 1977.
7. DiChiro, G., and Wener, L.: Angiography of the spinal cord; a review of contemporary techniques and applications. J. Neurosurg., 39:1, 1973.
8. Djindjian, R.: Angiography of the Spinal Cord. Paris, Masson & Cie.; Baltimore, University Park Press, 1970.
9. Djindjian, R., Cophignon, J., Rey, A., et al.: Superselective arteriographic embolization by the femoral route in neuroradiology; study of 50 cases—II, embolization in vertebromedullary pathology. Neuroradiology, 6:132, 1973.
10. Djindjian, R., Cophignon, J., Rey, A., et al.: Superselective arteriographic embolization by the femoral route in neuroradiology; study of 50 cases—III, embolization in craniocerebral pathology. Neuroradiology, 6:143, 1973.
11. Djindjian, R., Cophignon, J., Theron, D., et al.: Embolization by superselective arteriography from the femoral route in neuroradiology; review of 60 cases—I, technique indications, complications. Neuroradiology, 6:20, 1973.
12. Doppman, J. L., DiChiro, G., and Ommaya, A.: Obliteration of spinal cord arteriovenous malformation by percutaneous embolization. Lancet, 1:477, 1968.
13. Doppman, J. L., DiChiro, G., and Ommaya, A.: Percutaneous embolization of spinal cord arteriovenous malformations. J. Neurosurg., 34:48, 1971.
14. Doppman, J. L., Zapol, W., and Pierce, J.: Transcatheter embolization with a silicone rubber

preparation; experimental observations. Invest. Radiol., 6:304, 1971.

15. Grace, D. M., Pitt, D. F., and Gold, R. E.: Vascular embolization and occlusion by angiographic techniques as an aid or alternative to operation. Surg. Gynec. Obstet., 143:469–482, 1976.

16. Heinz, E. R.: Neuroradiologic special procedures. In Meaney, T. F., Lalli, A. F., and Alfidi, R. J., eds.: Complications and Legal Implications of Radiologic Special Procedures. St. Louis, C. V. Mosby Co., 1973, p. 47.

17. Hekster, R. E. M., Lutendijk, W., and Matricall, B.: Transfemoral catheter embolization; a method of treatment of glomus jugulare tumors. Neuroradiology, 5:208, 1972.

18. Hekster, R. E. M., Lutendijk, W., and Tan, T. I.: Spinal cord compression caused by vertebral hemangioma relieved by percutaneous catheter embolization. Neuroradiology, 3:160, 1972.

19. Hekster, R. E. M., Matricali, B., and Lutendijk, W.: Presurgical transfemoral catheter embolization to reduce operative blood loss. Technical note. J. Neurosurg., 41:396, 1974.

20. Hilal, S. K., and Michelsen, W. J.: Therapeutic percutaneous embolization for extra-axial vascular lesions of the head, neck and spine. J. Neurosurg., 43:275–287, 1975.

21. Hilal, S. K., Michelsen, W. J., and Driller, J.: POD catheter; a means for small vessels exploration. J. Appl. Physiol., 40:1046, 1969.

22. Hilal, S. K., Michelsen, W. J., Driller, J., and Leonard, E.: Magnetically guided devices for vascular exploration and treatment. Radiology, 113:529–540, 1974.

23. Hilal, S. K., Michelsen, W. J., Mount, L., et al.: Therapeutic embolization of vascular malformations of the external carotid circulation; clinical and experimental results. Presented at the Eleventh Symposium Neuroradiologicum, Goteborg, Sweden, 1970.

24. Hilal, S. K., Sane, P., Michelsen, W. J., and Kosseim, A.: The embolization of vascular malformations of the spinal cord with low-viscosity silicone rubber. Neuroradiology, 16:430–433, 1978.

25. Kricheff, I. I., Madayag, M., and Braunstein, O.: Transfemoral catheter embolization of cerebral and posterior fossa arteriovenous malformations. Radiology, 103:107, 1972.

26. Luessenhop, A. J.: Artificial embolization for cerebral arteriovenous malformations. Progr. Neurol. Surg., 3:320, 1969.

27. Luessenhop, A. J., and Presper, J. J.: Surgical embolization of cerebral arteriovenous malformations through internal carotid and vertebral arteries; long term results. J. Neurosurg., 42:443, 1975.

28. Luessenhop, A. J., and Spence, W. T.: Artificial embolization of cerebral arteries; report of use in a case of arteriovenous malformation. J.A.M.A., 172:1153, 1960.

29. Luessenhop, A. J., Gibbs, M., and Velasquez, A. C.: Cerebrovascular response to emboli, Observations in patients with arteriovenous malformations. Arch. Neurol. (Chicago), 7:264–274, 1962.

30. Luessenhop, A. J., Kachmann, R., Shelvin, W., and Ferrero, A. A.: Clinical evaluation of artificial embolization in the management of large cerebral arteriovenous malformations. J. Neurosurg., 23:400, 1965.

31. Mahaley, M. S., and Boone, S. C.: External carotid-cavernous fistula treated by arterial embolization. J. Neurosurg., 40:110, 1974.

32. Michelsen, W. J., and Hilal, S. K.: Management of arteriovenous malformations of the orbit. In Jakobiec, F., and Jones, I., eds.: Ocular and Adnexal Tumors. New York, Aesculapius Publishing Co., 1978.

33. Newton, T. H., and Adams, J. E.: Angiographic demonstration and nonsurgical embolization of spinal cord angioma. Radiology, 91:873, 1968.

34. Serbinenko, F. A.: Balloon catheterization and occlusion of major cerebral vessels. J. Neurosurg., 41:125, 1974.

35. Sokoloff, J., Wickbom, I., McDonald, D., et al.: Therapeutic percutaneous embolization in intractable epistaxis. Radiology, 111:285–287, 1974.

36. Taren, J. A., and Gabrielsen, T. O.: Radio-frequency thrombosis of magnetic catheter. Science, 168:138, 1970.

37. Yodh, S. B., and Wright, R. L.: Experimental evaluation of synthetic adhesives by intra-arterial injection. Neurochirurgia, 13:118, 1970.

38. Yodh, S. B., Pierce, N. T., Weggel, R. J., et al.: A new magnetic system for "intravascular navigation." Med. Biol. Eng., 6:143, 1968.

Index

In this index page numbers set in *italics* indicate illustrations. Page numbers followed by (t) refer to tabular material. Drugs are indexed under their generic names when dosage or action or special use is given. The abbreviation vs. is used to indicate differential diagnosis.

INDEX